Microneurosurgery of Cerebellopontine Angle

José Manuel González-Darder

Microneurosurgery of Cerebellopontine Angle

Springer

José Manuel González-Darder
Department of Neurosurgery
Hospital Clínico Universitario de Valencia
Valencia, Spain

ISBN 978-3-032-03090-0 ISBN 978-3-032-03091-7 (eBook)
https://doi.org/10.1007/978-3-032-03091-7

This Springer imprint is published by the registered company Springer Nature Switzerland AG
The registered company address is: Gewerbestrasse 11, 6330 Cham, Switzerland

Prologue

Neurosurgery is a surgical specialty that is highly demanding for the neurosurgeon and high risk for the patients. The history of modern neurosurgery is short, about a hundred years, and during all this time neurosurgeons have fought to improve the technical quality of neurosurgical procedures and patient safety. One of the areas where this struggle has been most difficult is in the cerebellopontine angle.

The mortality rate of patients undergoing craniotomy was over 80% in the last years of the nineteenth century, being reduced to 40% in the first years of the twentieth century thanks, among others, to advances in asepsis, antisepsis, topographic localization of neural structures and intracranial lesions by craniometry. However, at that time, the mortality rate of patients undergoing posterior fossa surgery was still around 75%. This mortality rate was drastically reduced by the innovations of Harvey Cushing and Walter Dandy to less than 10%. Mortality has been subsequently reduced by new improvements, and nowadays it is anecdotal.

Numerous advancements have improved the results of individuals undergoing neurosurgical therapy for surgical diseases of the cerebellopontine angle. It is important to keep in mind that the surgical microscope was first used in neurosurgery in 1957 by William F. House and Theodore Kurze to treat vestibular nerve schwannomas. Today, all neurosurgery procedures are performed utilizing microsurgical techniques. The most advanced method for diagnosing cerebellopontine angle lesions is magnetic nuclear resonance, which has supplanted traditional neuroradiological, electrophysiological, and otological methods. The lateral suboccipital approach, with minor modifications since its proposal by Walter Dandy, is the approach of choice for lesions of the cerebellopontine angle and brainstem. Robotic-assisted surgery, neuronavigation, and endoscopy have all added subtleties to the strategy in this respect. In vestibular nerve schwannomas, however, one of its most common and effective indications is stereotactic radiosurgery, which was developed by Lars Leksell. Lastly, a special class of diseases known as cranial rhizopathies are found in the cerebellopontine angle. These diseases have such a distinct pathophysiology that, following the suggestion of James Gardner and Peter Jannetta, microvascular decompression of the cranial nerve roots is thought to be a remarkable and successful treatment for them. The modern anatomical-surgical study of the region based on Albert Rhoton's postulates, however, has, in our judgment, had the biggest influence on neurosurgery of the cerebellopontine angle.

For several neurosurgeons, the cerebellopontine angle is the primary area of attention, and these findings support this claim. In the past 15 years, the author has operated on every patient and case in this book at the University Clinical Hospital of Valencia in Spain. The implementation of all hospital departments' human and material resources—especially those related to neurosurgery, neurology, otology, diagnostic imaging, anesthesiology, postoperative critical care, rehabilitation, and radiosurgery—leads to the successful completion of complex cases involving neurosurgery. The chief neurosurgery residents and the young neurosurgeons throughout the first several years have been crucial to the surgical approach, assistance, wound closure, and postoperative care of the patients. In all of them, the author of the majority of the anatomical dissections gathered in the book, Dr. Pau Capilla-Guasch, must be commended for his outstanding work as an assistant and collaborator in recent years.

The book is organized in chapters according to the pathology, preferably including those processes that can be resolved with a standard retrosigmoid approach and the far-lateral approach. The chapters have a similar internal structure, with an emphasis on providing a thorough explanation of each step of the surgical process. This is bolstered by numerous pictures, and the last chapter is devoted to providing illustrative examples.

Everything points to microneurosurgery of cerebellopontine angle lesions as the key component of treatment for these lesions in the upcoming decades. This, along with radiosurgery and a successful patient selection process that only requires image observation, enables the safe and effective management of all patients.

Department of Neurosurgery
Hospital Clínico Universitario de Valencia
Valencia, Spain

José Manuel González-Darder

Contents

1 Microsurgical Anatomy of the Cerebellopontine Angle

1.1 Introduction

The cerebellopontine angle, a component of the posterior fossa, has complex anatomy that every neurosurgeon must comprehend. This is where several prevalent neurosurgical disorders can be found, such as vestibular schwannomas, the main pathology of the cerebellopontine angle, meningiomas, pontine cavernomas, aneurysms, cranial nerve rhizopathies, and epidermoid cysts. Therefore, a complete understanding of the microsurgical anatomy around the cerebellopontine angle is necessary in order to create a rigorous surgical plan.

Since the inception of microneurosurgery, neuroanatomy has been examined from a microsurgical perspective. This led to the emergence of major schools of neuroanatomy, most notably the one led by Albert Rhoton (1932–2016) [5]. Because of his extensive dissections and guided study, neuroanatomy has been meticulously systematized for microsurgical applications. All neurosurgeons receive their education and training primarily in the cerebellopontine angle using this method, which blends laboratory, microsurgery, and neuroanatomy. On the one hand, becoming proficient in microsurgical methods will allow for safe passage through the neurovascular components of the cerebellopontine angle, sometimes in confined areas distant from the surgical approach's surface. Conversely, the neurosurgeon who has the best three-dimensional understanding of anatomical structures will be able to understand the architecture that has been warped by the pathology they are treating and use that information to reason and determine the safest course of action.

This chapter presents the anatomy of the cerebellopontine angle from a microneurosurgical perspective, using a few anatomical pictures to provide the reader a clear and distinct grasp of the three-dimensional intricacy of the cerebellopontine angle. Following Rhoton's idea helps us comprehend the need to identify anatomical areas for several reasons. When doing microneurosurgery, neurosurgeons use craniotomies, which are cranial openings in the skull that only reveal a part of the cerebral region. Neurosurgeons must find anatomical reference points in this narrow surgical field so that they can mentally map the complete microneuroanatomy while performing the surgery. Additionally, the surgical microscope has gradually reduced the size of the apparent surgical windows, making it possible to view only a small portion of the anatomy. Additionally, rather than always approaching disease from the same surgical approach, neurosurgeons may change the patient's perspective throughout the same surgical approach due to the mobility of modern surgical instruments. A neurosurgeon can also select different entrance sites and different routes to attain the same deep aim in order to view the same anatomy from multiple perspectives. For all of these reasons, neurosurgeons can

J. M. González-Darder, *Microneurosurgery of Cerebellopontine Angle*,
https://doi.org/10.1007/978-3-032-03091-7_1

gain a better understanding of three dimensions by using familiar anatomical features to describe anatomical spaces. Another reason is that a significant amount of the pathology modifies the natural morphology and anatomy of the cerebellopontine angle. Therefore, having anatomical reference points to assist in characterizing these locations is essential to treating these lesions successfully. After the lesion is removed, the problem has been resolved, and the anatomy needs to return to its normal state [2, 5, 6].

1.2 Boundaries of the Cerebellopontine Angle

The cerebellopontine angle is compared with a dihedral angle (Fig. 1.1). The posterior wall, also known as the squama of the occipital bone, is relatively wide and is used for surgical access. However, the cerebellopontine angle steadily narrows until it reaches the deepest point at the petroclival fissure, where it is quite constricted. In general, and from a neurosurgical standpoint, the cerebellopontine angle is the section of the infratentorial space or posterior fossa located between the lateral side of the cerebellum and brainstem and the medial surface of the petrosal portion of the temporal bone or petrosal bone. The floor communicates to the spinal space via the foramen magnum and is composed of the inner surface of the occipital bone's squama. The roof is formed by the caudal surface of the cerebellar tentorium, which is connected to the supratentorial area via the tentorial foramen. The cerebellopontine angle's medial surface represents the brainstem's anterolateral aspect. The cerebellum's lateral or petrosal aspect is the surface that also corresponds with the medial limit of the cerebellopontine angle. The medial face of the petrosal bone and the occipital bone form the lateral wall of the cerebellopontine angle. This area is coated in dura mater and has multiple orifices that allow cranial nerves to leave the cerebellopontine angle. The inferior surface of the tentorium corresponds to the roof of the cerebellopontine angle. The remainder of the roof of the cerebellopontine angle is open and corresponds to the tentorial foramen, also known as Pacchioni's foramen. The foramen has three cisterns: interpeduncular, ambiens, and quadrigeminal. The petroclival fis-

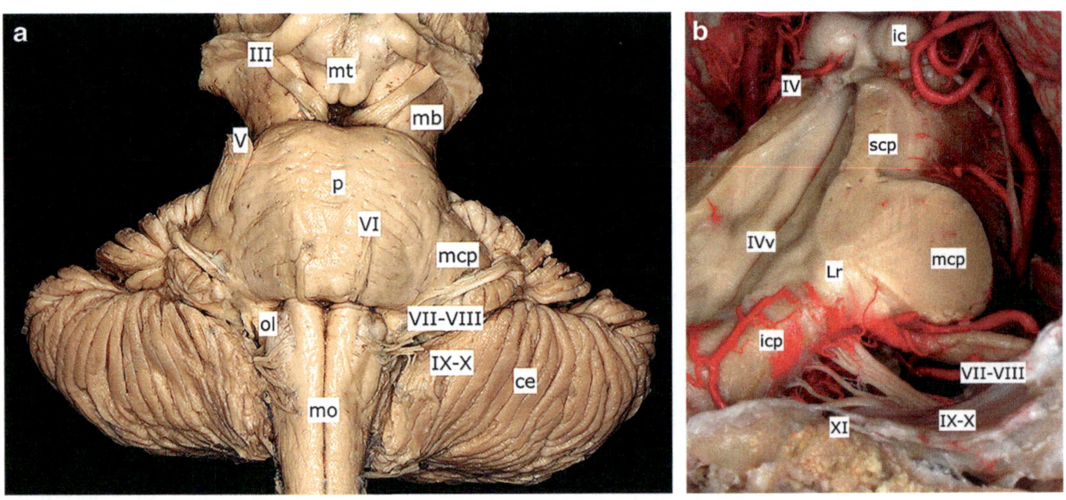

Fig. 1.1 Anatomy. (**a**) Anterior view of the brainstem and cerebellum. (**b**) Overview of the right cerebellopontine angle after removal of the cerebellum (III oculomotor nerve; IV trochlear nerve; V trigeminal nerve; VII–VIII facial-vestibulocochlear complex; IX–X glossopharyngeal and vagal nerves; XI accessory nerve; IVv fourth ventricle; ce cerebellum; mb midbrain; ic inferior colliculus; icp inferior cerebellar peduncle; Lr Luschka recess; mcp middle cerebellar peduncle; mo medulla oblongata; mt mammillary tubercles; ol olive; p pons; scp superior cerebellar peduncle)

sure is a cleft that separates the petrous bone and the clivus. It extends from the jugular foramen below to the apex of the petrous bone above, forming the narrowest and deepest portion of the cerebellopontine angle.

1.2.1 Lateral Wall: Posterior Face of the Petrous Bone

The lateral aspect of the dura mater-covered petrosal and mastoid parts of the temporal bone, where the jugular and internal auditory foramina are prominent, is the lateral surface of the cerebellopontine angle. The internal auditory meatus and canal, via which the facial and vestibulocochlear nerves enter, are the most crucial neurosurgical components of this lateral wall. A transverse crest splits the fundus of the canal into an upper and a lower part, and one vertical crest, also known as Bell's bar, further divides the upper half of the internal auditory canal fundus into two halves. The anterosuperior quadrant receives the facial nerve, the anteroinferior quadrant receives the cochlear nerve, the posterosuperior quadrant receives the superior vestibular nerve, and the posteroinferior quadrant receives the inferior vestibular nerve. The internal auditory meatus is an important anatomical site because it gives anatomical access to the contents of the internal auditory canal. The posterior semicircular canal is situated lateral to this posterior ridge of the canal, which may include pneumatized mastoid cells. The endolymphatic duct is situated inferolaterally to the meatus, while the subarcuate eminence is situated just above it. Lastly, the jugular bulb may approach the posterior border of the meatus quite closely if it is excessively high. There is a prolongation of the arachnoid that extends like a glove finger inside the internal auditory canal, and the entire inner surface of the canal is coated with dura mater.

A gap between the temporal and occipital bones at the base of the skull is known as the jugular foramen or posterior lacerated foramen. The sigmoid sinus, jugular bulb, inferior petrosal sinus, and lower cranial nerves, including the glossopharyngeal, vagal, and spinal nerves, as well as other less important anatomical features like Arnold's or Jacobson's nerves, the cochlear aqueduct, and a few minor arterial branches, all pass through the jugular foramen. However, only the entry of the cranial nerves is visible when the jugular foramen is approached from the cerebellopontine angle because the majority of it is concealed by dura mater. All of the remaining anatomical components of the lateral aspect of the cerebellopontine angle are also covered by the dura mater. To reach the jugular foramen, the sigmoid sinus passes through a bone groove. The endolymphatic sac, situated between the layers of the dura mater, occupies the space inferolateral to the internal auditory meatus and extends toward the sigmoid sinus. Via the endolymphatic duct, the endolymphatic sac exchanges fluids with the inner ear vestibule. Lastly, the tiny subarcuate artery enters through the subarcuate fossa, which is lateral to the meatus.

1.2.2 Medial Wall: Cerebellum and Brainstem

1.2.2.1 Cerebellum

The cerebellum occupies a great part of the posterior cranial fossa and relates to the cerebellopontine angle. The most complex of the three surfaces of the cerebellum is the suboccipital, which confronts the inner side of the occipital bone and is situated posterior to the sigmoid sinus and caudal to the transverse sinus. The falx cerebelli lies in the posterior cerebellar notch, a vertical depression along the midline. Deep indentations known as the vermis-hemispheric fissures divide the cerebellar hemispheres from the vermis. At the notch, the vermian surface appears to be diamond-shaped. The bottom part, which protrudes inferiorly between the cerebellar tonsils, is referred to as the uvula, and the top part is called the pyramid. The nodule is hidden beneath the uvula and is the most caudal part of the vermis. The vallecula, a subarachnoid area, is between the tonsils and is connected to the fourth ventricle via the foramen of Magendie.

The inferior semilunar lobule and portions of the tonsils, superior, and biventral lobules make up the hemisphere. The folium, tuber, pyramid, and uvula (from cranial to caudal) make up the vermian portion. The suboccipital fissure is the main fissure that separates the anterior and posterior portions of the suboccipital surface of the cerebellum. This fissure splits the tuber and pyramid at the vermian level and the inferior semilunar and biventral lobes at the hemisphere level. The most noticeable features are the cerebellar tonsils, a hemisphere component that blocks access to the fourth ventricle's caudal area. The amygdaline peduncle, a bundle of white matter fibers, connects each tonsil, an ovoid structure situated in the inferomedial portion of the suboccipital surface, to the cerebellum via its superolateral border.

The petrosal aspect of the cerebellum forms part of the lateral boundaries of the cerebellopontine angle. This area is split by a usually conspicuous grove, the petrosal sulcus. This sulcus has the shape of a V, with the angle superficial. Therefore, the sulcus opens as it goes deep, until it reaches the middle cerebellar peduncle and the trigeminal nerve on its way to Meckel's cave. The petrosal fissure divides the cerebellar petrosal surface into the superior and inferior sections. This fissure is divided into two branches: a lower branch that divides the cerebellum from the middle cerebellar peduncle and the pons, and an upper branch that separates the cerebellum from the pons. The choroid plexuses protrude into the angle under the flocculus, and the inferior branch of the petrosal fissure enters the lateral recess of the fourth ventricle and links with the cerebellopontine angle via the Luschka foramen. Choroid plexus exits through the Luschka's recesses of the fourth ventricle since the plexus arises in the tela coroidea that forms part of the roof of the fourth ventricle.

1.2.2.2 Brainstem

The brainstem is divided into three main structural parts: the midbrain, the protuberance (or pons of Varioli), and the medulla oblongata, which are separated by grooves or sulci. Between the pons and the cerebral peduncle lies a depression known as the pontine-mesencephalic sulcus. The medullary-pontine sulcus then separates the pons from the medulla oblongata. The anatomical limit between the cerebellum and brainstem is marked by the apparent exit of the trigeminal nerve in the pons, which extends laterally with the middle cerebellar peduncle. The anterolateral side of the medulla oblongata and the pons comprise the deepest component of the medial wall of the cerebellopontine angle.

1.2.2.2.1 Sulci of the Brainstem

The pontine-mesencephalic sulcus is where the oculomotor nerves emerge from the interpeduncular fossa. This is an interesting location since it is the place of the posterior perforating area, where multiple perforators originating from the basilar artery enter; the basilar artery divides into both posterior cerebral arteries, and the superior cerebellar artery emerges.

The medullary-pontine sulcus appears to be the anatomical origin of the abducens, facial, and vestibulocochlear cranial nerves. The abducens nerve is positioned along the midline, while the facial and vestibulocochlear nerves are located farther laterally, in the supra-olivary fossa.

1.2.2.2.2 Pons

The medulla oblongata and the midbrain are separated by the pons, the central section of the brainstem. The medullary-pontine sulcus limits the anterior surface caudally, whereas the pontine-mesencephalic sulcus limits the anterior surface cranially. The rostral cranial and caudal surface bounds are defined by an imaginary line caudally to the superior colliculi and another caudally at the level of the lateral angles of the fourth ventricle. The clivus supports the anterior face of the pons, which is convex in the transverse plane. The pyramidal tract is located on either side of the basilar sulcus, which runs down the center along the pons. The cerebellar peduncle is where the lateral surface of the pons extends laterally. The anatomical lateral boundary of the pons is arbitrarily defined as the apparent exit of the trigeminal root.

1.2.2.2.3 Medulla Oblongata

The medulla oblongata is shaped like a cone. It is bounded superiorly by the pontine-medullary sulcus and inferiorly by a conventional horizontal plane that passes over the first cervical spinal nerve, right below the decussation of the pyramids, where it continues with the cervical spinal cord. The transition between the spinal cord and the medulla oblongata corresponds to an imaginary bony plane traveling between the superior edge of the posterior tubercle of the atlas and the central portion of the anterior arch of the atlas.

The anterolateral surface of the medulla oblongata has a complex anatomical arrangement and comprises the following structures from the midline: anterior median sulcus; anterior pyramid; anteromedial or pre-olivary sulcus, from which the fibers of the hypoglossal nerve emerge; inferior olive; posterolateral or retro-olivary sulcus, from which the fibers of the glossopharyngeal, vagal, and accessory nerves exit; and lastly, the cuneate fasciculus or Burdach's fasciculus. The inferior cerebellar foramen, also known as the foramen of Vicq-d'Azyr, is the cranial end of the median anterior sulcus, which is located in the midline and extends cranially to the medullary-pontine junction. The pyramids' decussation interrupts this sulcus caudally. On either side of this sulcus are the anterior pyramids. Near the pyramids, in the medullary-pontine-medullary sulcus, is where the abducens nerve exits. The anterolateral sulcus, sometimes referred to as the pre-olivary sulcus or hypoglossal sulcus, is situated laterally and divides the medullary olive from the pyramid. The posterolateral sulcus, also known as the retro-olivary sulcus, is located in the dorsal part of the medullary olive and is the origin of the glossopharyngeal, vagal, and accessory lower cranial nerves, adjacent to the spinocerebellar tract. The facial nerve and the intermediate nerve of Wrisberg originate in the supra-olivary fossa, a depression that separates the superior end, which does not reach the pons. The vestibulocochlear nerve arises from the lateral medullary fossa, a tiny, depression-like region posterior to the supra-olivary fossa.

The restiform body, also referred to as the inferior cerebellar peduncle, extends to the lateral recesses, where the fibers bend dorsally to enter the cerebellum from the lateral margins of the lower half of the fourth ventricle. It is made up of external arcuate fibers, posterior spinocerebellar tract fibers, and cerebello-olivary fibers.

From the superior portion of the olivary body, caudal to the facial nerve's origin, arises the glossopharyngeal nerve. The lower medulla, the upper cervical spinal cord segments, and the bottom two-thirds of the medullary olive are the origins of the accessory spinal nerve. Because they frequently form a single bundle of nerves, it can be challenging to distinguish the roots originating from the retro-olivary sulcus from the vagal nerve roots. The hypoglossal nucleus, situated at the level of the hypoglossal triangle on the floor of the fourth ventricle, is where the roots of the hypoglossal nerve begin. At the level of the caudal two-thirds of the olivary body, these roots emerge through the pre-olivary sulcus before entering the hypoglossal canal.

1.2.2.2.4 Internal Organization of the Brainstem

The brainstem contains a number of neurological structures, such as nuclei and intricately interlaced tracts of ascending, descending, and transverse fibers. Therefore, microneurosurgical access to intrinsic lesions of the brainstem can only be made via a limited number of safe paths based on anatomical references. Next, we describe the anatomical relationships of these secure routes to the brainstem [3, 4, 8].

The *lateral mesencephalic sulcus* is the safe route of entry into the anterolateral midbrain. The lateral mesencephalic sulcus separates the peduncular and tegmental portions of the midbrain from the medial geniculate body of the thalamus to the pontine-mesencephalic sulcus. It is tracked by the lateral mesencephalic vein and crossed by the posterior cerebral artery in its cranial portion and by the trochlear nerve and superior cerebellar artery in its caudal portion, thus having a supratentorial and an infratentorial portion. The sulcus measures about 10 mm, and the working channel is about 8 mm long. The trochlear and oculomotor nuclei are located about 9.5 mm deep from the lateral mesencephalic sulcus.

In the pons, the pyramidal tract divides into several fascicles, which reassemble in the anterior area of the medulla oblongata. A portion of the medullary-level fibers move posteromedially to generate the pyramidal decussation. The motor nuclei of the pons are where the corticopontine tract, which is composed of a second pair of descending fibers, ends. Transverse extensions then appear and proceed to the contralateral cerebellum via the middle cerebellar peduncle. The corticomedullary tracts for the medullary nuclei and the corticospinal tract can be projected onto the surface of the pons, situated between two hypothetical lines: a medial one that connects the most medial point of the pontine-mesencephalic sulcus to the point where the pyramid joins the medullary-pontine sulcus, and a lateral one that connects the pontine-mesencephalic sulcus and the lateral portion of the peduncle to the point where the pyramid joins the medullary-pontine sulcus. The safe entry zone in the pons is the *peritrigeminal area*, which is a triangle with a lower base that runs from the flocculus to the lateral edge of the pyramid and corresponds to the medullary-pontine sulcus. The external limit of the previously established pyramidal tract forms its medial side, while a line that runs through the internal border of the exit from the pons of the trigeminal nerve and the external edge of the pyramid forms its lateral side. The floor of the triangle is made up of the fibers of the middle cerebellar peduncle. Deep within the peritrigeminal area is the motor and sensory nucleus of the trigeminal nerve. The distance between the pyramidal tract and the inner border of the trigeminal nerve is 4–5.5 mm. Reaching the trigeminal nucleus only requires a depth of 4–9.5 mm caudally and 10–13 mm cranially.

The safe entrance zone in the medulla oblongata is the *retro-olivary sulcus and the olive* itself within the two outer thirds of its transverse dimension, since damage to the olive does not seem to result in neurological symptoms. Between the inferior olive and the corticospinal tract, at the level of the pre-olivary sulcus, the fibers of the hypoglossal nerve arise in the lower medulla between the pyramid and the olive. Behind the inferior olive, within the medulla oblongata, the spinothalamic tract ascends. The fibers and nuclei of the lower cranial nerves exit through the retro-olivary sulcus and are located in the medulla oblongata behind the spinothalamic tract. The olive measures approximately 13 mm in length, 7 mm in width, and 2.5 mm in thickness.

1.2.3 Roof: Tentorium and Tentorial Incisura

The caudal, or inferior, face of the tentorium is the larger portion of the roof of the cerebellopontine angle. The tentorium covers the tentorial surface of the cerebellar hemispheres and is attached to the petrosal bone edge, forming the superior petrosal sinus. Just in the apex of the petrosal bone, it leaves a hole to allow the trigeminal root access to the Meckel's cave. Medially, the tentorium leaves a broad opening, termed Pacchioni's oval foramen, which is the communication between the supratentorial and infratentorial cavities and facilitates the passage of the midbrain.

The remaining space between the midbrain and the tentorial edge is a very narrow anatomical region, named the tentorial notch or tentorial incisura. This tentorial incisura is divided into three sections: anterior, protected by the interpeduncular cistern; lateral, protected by the crural and ambiens cisterns; and posterior, tectal or pineal, protected by the quadrigeminal cistern.

The lateral incisura corresponds to the lateral zone of the midbrain and the mesial part of the temporal lobe and faces the cerebellopontine angle. The medial side of the region is formed by the lateral face of the midbrain and the superior face of the pons, separated by the pontine-mesencephalic sulcus, which is located at the level of the free edge of the tentorium. In the midbrain, two zones can be distinguished: an anterior one, formed by the cerebral peduncle, and a posterior or tegmental one, separated by a vertical depression or lateral mesencephalic sulcus, usually traversed by the lateral mesencephalic vein. The roof of the lateral fissure is formed by the optic tract and the lower portion of the thalamus with the lateral and medial geniculate nuclei.

This lateral incisure, in its supratentorial portion, is related to the mesial face of the temporal lobe formed by the uncus and the parahippocampal gyrus. In its most anterior portion, the uncus protrudes through the tentorial notch, and the free edge of the tentorium marks a groove on it in a high percentage of cases. Behind the uncus, the mesial surface of the temporal lobe is actually formed by three longitudinal strips arranged one above the other. The lowest and closest to the tentorial edge is formed by the parahippocampal gyrus; the middle one is formed by the dentate gyrus, and finally, the upper strip is formed by the fimbria of the fornix.

In its infratentorial portion, the lateral aspect of the lateral incisure forms the cerebellomesencephalic fissure, which separates the anterosuperior portion of the cerebellum from the lateral aspect of the mesencephalic tegmen. The trochlear nerve runs through the region, separating the posterior cerebral and superior cerebellar arteries, until it enters through the lower border of the tentorium to reach the cavernous sinus. In the most anterior portion of the region, the anterior choroidal artery runs, a direct branch of the internal carotid artery, reaching the inferior choroidal point. Further back, the posterior cerebral artery enters the lateral incisure in its P2 segment, which runs around the midbrain, from where cortical branches, the medial and lateral posterior choroidal arteries, and the thalamogeniculate artery emerge. The trigeminal nerve runs through the infratentorial portion of the region toward Meckel's cave, and also in the infratentorial portion of the region, the superior cerebellar artery is found before its bifurcation into its two terminal branches, superior and inferior. The main vein of the lateral tentorial incisure is the Rosenthal basal vein, which runs along the roof of the region over the posterior cerebral artery until it drains into the Galen vein. The lateral tentorial incisure is occupied by the crural and ambient cisterns. The crural cistern is anterior and is located between the uncus and the cerebral peduncle. Behind, the ambiens cistern occupies the region up to the quadrigeminal cistern. The ambient cistern extends above and below the free edge of the tentorium.

1.2.4 Floor: Foramen Magnum

The dura mater covers the occipital bone, which encircles the foramen magnum and forms the floor of the cerebellopontine angle. The clivus is the most anterior portion, and the jugular tubercle, a bony protuberance that extends laterally with the squamous portion of the occipital bone, is next in line. The jugular tubercle is situated between the hypoglossal canal below and the jugular foramen above.

1.3 Contents of the Cerebellopontine Angle

Contents of the cerebellopontine angle are cranial nerves, arteries, veins, and cisterns (Fig. 1.1).

1.3.1 Cranial Nerves

This section will go into great detail about the relationships and courses of each of the cranial nerves. Knowing the anatomy of the cranial nerves is crucial because it makes it easier to locate these structures when normal anatomy is moved or deformed by pathology, and nerves are especially safe anatomical references due to their low variability (Fig. 1.2).

1.3.1.1 Trochlear Nerve or Fourth Cranial Nerve

The trochlear nerve is probably the one that is furthest distant from the majority of lesions that impact the cerebellopontine angle. It is situated in the upper neurovascular compartment, and when viewed from the infratentorial compartment, its trajectory is related to the superior cerebellar artery and the tentorium edge.

Origin: The trochlear nerve begins in the quadrigeminal cistern, in the inferolateral portion of the inferior colliculus.

Course: The nerve originates at the medial border of the tentorium and goes through the ambiens and crural cisterns. It is closely related to the posterior cerebral artery, choroidal arteries,

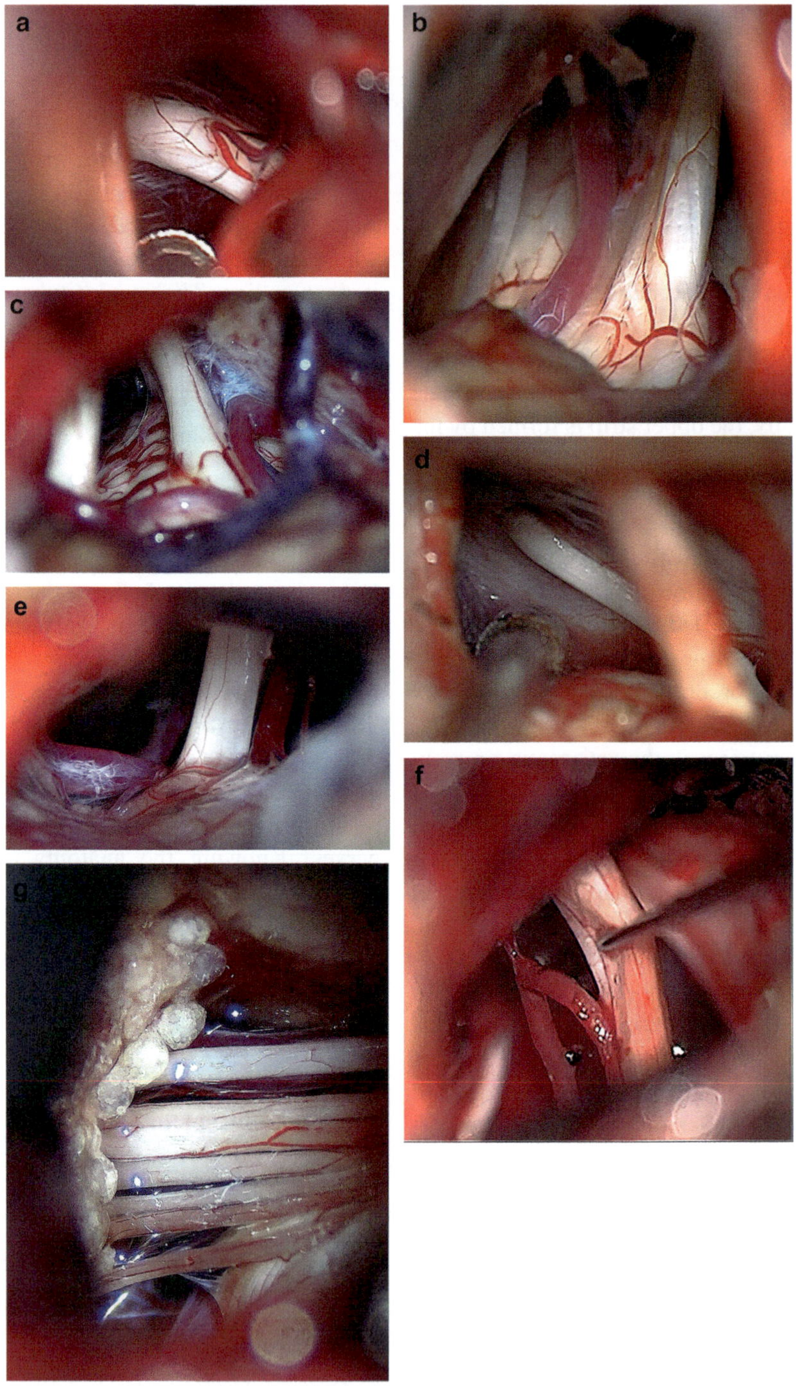

Fig. 1.2 Operative pictures displaying the cranial nerves in their cisternal trajectory via a retrosigmoid route. (**a**) Oculomotor nerve. (**b**) Trochlear nerve. (**c**) Trigeminal nerve. (**d**) Abducens nerve. (**e**) Vestibulocochlear nerve. (**f**) Facial nerve. (**g**) Rootlets of the glossopharyngeal and vagal nerves, along with the choroid plexus. (**h**) Glossopharyngeal, vagal, and accessory nerves. (**i**) Accessory and hypoglossal nerves. (**j**) Hypoglossal nerve

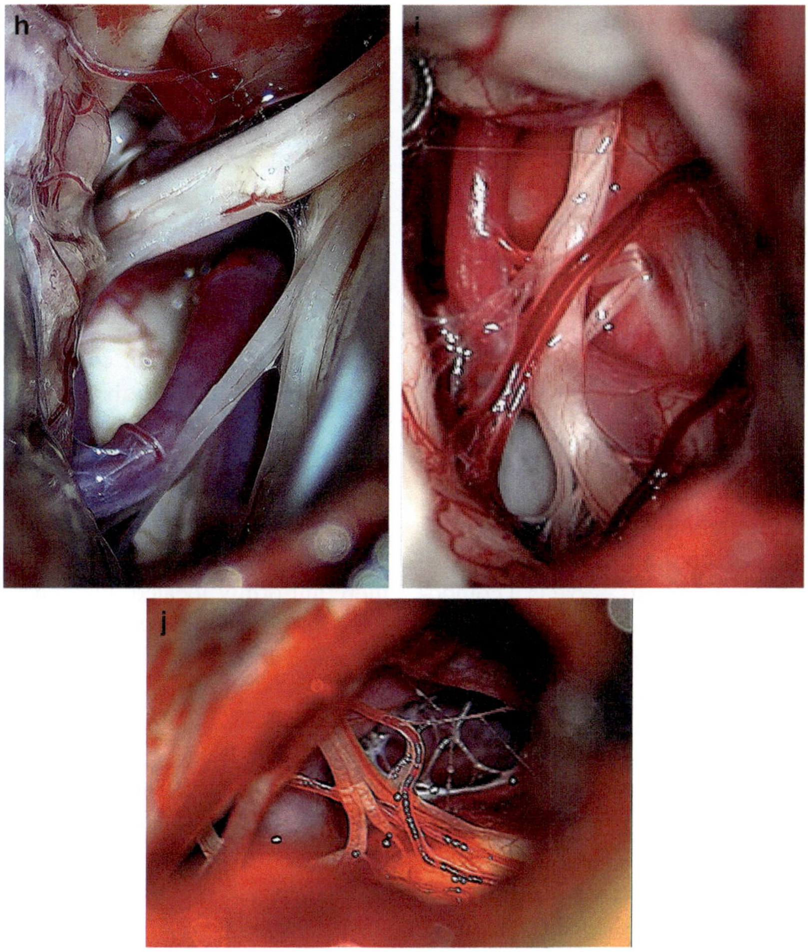

Fig. 1.2 (continued)

superior petrosal vein, and superior cerebellar artery.

Pathology. The trochlear nerve may be cranially dislocated by large and giant vestibular schwannomas or meningiomas of the cerebellopontine angle. Given the placement of the fourth cranial nerve and its small diameter, extreme caution must be used when operating on the cranial pole of these tumors. Because of its delicate nature, even minor touching or inadvertent aspiration might cause traction damage to the nerve.

1.3.1.2 Trigeminal Nerve or Fifth Cranial Nerve

With a small motor root, the trigeminal nerve is mainly sensory. The trigeminal nerve is a component of the upper neurovascular complex, and the superior cerebellar artery and the superior petrosal vein complex are frequently related to its root entry zone near the pons.

Origin: It begins at the middle cerebellar peduncle, anterior to the quadrilateral lobe of the cerebellar hemisphere.

Course: The trigeminal nerve projects anteriorly until it reaches Meckel's cave, following a superolateral trajectory along its cisternal route around the pons. It travels from the posterior fossa to the middle fossa via the porus trigemini, toward the Meckel's trigeminal cave near the apex of the petrosal bone. Here, the nerve gives rise to the three branches of the gasserian ganglion: the ophthalmic (V1), maxillary (V2), and mandibular (V3).

Pathology: Vascular compression of the trigeminal nerve root is a frequent occurrence in this area. It is brought on by the caudal loop of the superior cerebellar artery, which can make extremely tight contact between the artery and the nerve. Trigeminal neuralgia may result from arterial compression in certain situations. Neuralgia brought on by venous compression can also be produced by the superior petrosal vein complex, which can form a complicated venous network that engulfs and surrounds the nerve root.

1.3.1.3 Abducent Nerve or Sixth Cranial Nerve

The lateral rectus muscle is innervated by the abducens nerve, also known as the external ocular motor nerve. The abducens nerve is a component of the middle neurovascular complex in the cerebellopontine angle region.

Origin: It has the most medial placement within the posterior fossa of all the cranial nerves, and it exits almost midline of the medullary-pontine sulcus.

Course: The nerve travels in a caudocranial direction from its origin to the Dorello's canal via the prepontine cistern. Dorello's canal is the name given to a narrow, arch-shaped osteofibrous ridge near the apex of the petrosal bone, through which the abducens nerve travels just before entering the cavernous sinus.

1.3.1.4 Facial and Vestibulocochlear Nerves, Seventh and Eighth Cranial Nerves, or Facial–Vestibulocochlear Complex

These nerves belong to the intermediate neurovascular complex described by Rhoton, along with the anteroinferior cerebellar artery, and are the target of most microneurosurgical approaches to the cerebellopontine angle.

Origin: More laterally than the abducens nerve, at the medullary-pontine sulcus, directly above the supra-olivary fossa, are the exits of the facial and vestibulocochlear nerves. The origin of the facial nerve is situated inferiorly and somewhat anteriorly to the vestibulocochlear nerve exit.

Course: One to two millimeters before the vestibulocochlear nerve emerges from the brainstem, the facial nerve begins its journey from the brainstem close to the lateral end of the medullary-pontine sulcus. The facial and vestibulocochlear nerves are farther apart at the medullary-pontine sulcus, but they get closer as they run to the internal acoustic meatus. A variable number of rootlets with adhesions to each of the two nerves that lie between them make up the intermediate nerve of Wrisberg. The facial, cochlear, superior vestibular, and inferior vestibular nerves are located inside the internal acoustic canal after they enter through the meatus. The fundus of the canal, which is separated into upper and lower halves by a horizontal bony lamina called the falciform crest or transverse crest, is where these nerves are more uniformly located, just when they enter in the bone. The upper part contains the facial and superior vestibular nerves. The vertical crest, also known as Bell's bar, is a vertical bony lamina that separates the facial nerve from the superior vestibular nerve. The cochlear and inferior vestibular nerves are situated anterior to the inferior vestibular nerve and caudally to the transverse crest, respectively.

Pathology: The vestibular nerve is the origin of the vestibular schwannoma, the most prevalent tumor in the cerebellopontine angle.

1.3.1.5 Glossopharyngeal, Vagal, and Accessory Nerves, or Ninth, Tenth, and Eleventh Cranial Nerves, or Lower Cranial Nerves

The inferior neurovascular complex includes these three cranial nerves, which are closely associated with the posterior inferior cerebellar artery.

Origin: The retro-olivary sulcus is the common origin of the so-called lower cranial nerves, which include the glossopharyngeal nerve, vagal nerve, and accessory nerve. The glossopharyngeal nerve normally arises from the superior portion of the olivary body, caudal to the origin of the facial nerve, as a single root, though it can sometimes emerge as two. As the glossopharyngeal nerve travels to the jugular foramen, it passes ventral to the choroid plexus.

On its journey to the jugular foramen, the vagal nerve passes anterior to the choroid plexus after emerging from the upper part of the olive as a bundle of roots caudal to the glossopharyngeal nerve. The lower two-thirds of the olivary body in the medulla oblongata and the upper segments of the cervical spinal cord are the origin of the medullary rootlets of the accessory nerve.

1.3.1.6 Hypoglossal Nerve, or Twelfth Cranial Nerve

The hypoglossal cranial nerve is the most caudal cranial nerve and is the cranial nerve with the shortest cisternal path until the bone.

Origin: The hypoglossal nerve exits via the pre-olivary sulcus at the caudal two-thirds of the olivary body.

Course: Before arriving at the hypoglossal canal, hypoglossal nerve rootlets cross behind the vertebral artery. The nerve roots may not be in contact with the vertebral artery when it is short and straight; if the artery is convoluted, the roots may be displaced posteriorly. The roots usually form two bundles before entering the hypoglossal canal.

1.3.2 Arteries

The vertebrobasilar system includes the arteries located at the level of the cerebellopontine angle. It is crucial to comprehend their position and pathways to enhance methods for microneurosurgical dissection at this level for a safe surgery (Fig. 1.3).

1.3.2.1 Vertebral Artery

Originating from the big thoracic vessels, the two vertebral arteries (VAs) ascend through the transverse foramina of the first six cervical vertebrae and then pass through the dura mater between the superior border of the posterior arch of the atlas and the occipital condyle. The extradural vertebral artery splits into three sections in its trajectory. From its starting point in the large cervicothoracic trunks, segment V1 climbs to the transverse foramen of C6. On occasion, though, it may pass via the fifth, fourth, or seventh cervical vertebrae's transverse foramen. Despite its frequent structural variants, it typically arises from the posterosuperior portion of the subclavian artery. The artery is situated between the longus colli and anterior scalene muscles, as well as between the internal jugular vein and the vertebral veins. The transverse foramina of the first six cervical vertebrae are typically where segment V2 starts until the transverse foramen of the atlas. The area pertaining to the craniovertebral junction is known as segment V3. It stretches from the transverse foramen of C1 to the dural entrance. Deep within the suboccipital muscular triangle, it extends medially between the occipito-atlantal joint and the lateral mass of the atlas, arriving at the superior boundary of the posterior arch of the atlas. A rich venous plexus encircling the artery anastomoses with the deep cervical and epidural veins. The posterior meningeal and also branches to the deep cervical musculature originate from the last extradural segment, and, on occasion, the posterior spinal and posterior inferior cerebellar arteries arise at this level [1].

The final section, segment V4, is intradural and runs anterior to the dentate ligament and the spinal segment of the accessory nerve. This segment is a component of the inferior neurovascular complex of Rhoton. In relation to the medulla oblongata, it is further separated into two segments: anterior and lateral.

- The lateral medullary segment begins at the dural entrance and extends laterally and cranially along the lateral medullary surface, reaching the pre-olivary sulcus, which is situated between the medullary pyramid and the medullary olive.
- The most distal part of the vertebral artery is the anterior medullary segment, which begins at the level of the pre-olivary sulcus and extends anteriorly between the hypoglossal nerve's roots. It then crosses the medullary pyramid and joins the contralateral vertebral artery at the level of the medullary-pontine sulcus.

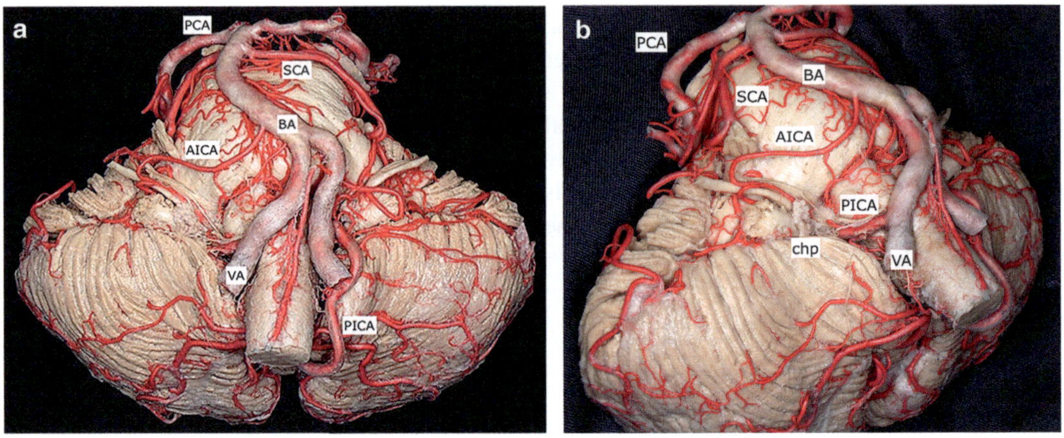

Fig. 1.3 Arteries of the brainstem and cerebellum injected with red silicone. (**a**) Anterior view. (**b**) Anterolateral view (AICA anteroinferior cerebellar artery; BA basilar artery; PCA posterior cerebral artery; PICA posteroinferior cerebellar artery; SCA superior cerebellar artery; VA vertebral artery; chp choroid plexus)

1.3.2.2 Posteroinferior Cerebellar Artery

Among the cerebellar arteries, the posteroinferior cerebellar artery (PICA) has the most intricate and diverse course. It is also a component of the inferior neurovascular complex.

Origin. The posteroinferior cerebellar artery often comes from the vertebral artery in the intradural space close to the caudal part of the medullary olive, but it is relevant to remember that in 10–15% of cases, the artery may have an extradural origin.

Course and segments: The posteroinferior cerebellar artery splits into five segments along its lengthy course.

- The anterior surface of the medulla oblongata is encircled by the anterior medullary segment of the artery. It passes across the hypoglossal nerve's roots as it encompasses posteriorly. The posteroinferior cerebellar artery may occasionally arise posterior to the roots of the hypoglossal nerve rather than from the anterior area of the medulla, in which case the anterior medullary segment would not be present.
- The artery passes behind the roots of the lower cranial nerves and then continues laterally to the most conspicuous point of the medullary olive, marking the beginning of the lateral medullary segment.
- The amygdalo-medullary segment begins as soon as it passes behind the lower cranial nerve roots and continues all the way to the cerebellar tonsils.
- The most intricate posteroinferior cerebellar artery segment is the telo-velo-amygdalar segment. It begins in the caudal part of the cerebellar tonsil and extends along the roof of the fourth ventricle. It comes to an end when the artery leaves through the opening between the tonsil, vermis, and cerebellar hemisphere and reaches the suboccipital surface of the cerebellum.
- Lastly, the cortical segment includes the terminal cortical branches and starts where the posteroinferior cerebellar artery branches leave the fissure between the tonsil, vermis, and cerebellar hemisphere.

1.3.2.3 Basilar Artery

At the level of the medullary-pontine sulcus in the prepontine cistern, the two vertebral arteries unite to produce the basilar artery (BA). It travels cranially straight or slightly curved till it reaches the interpeduncular cistern. It should be noted that a large curvature may cause the basilar artery to be displaced to one side in older patients with extensive arteriosclerosis. Therefore, in order to establish a surgical strategy and prepare for an unexpected contact with the artery, it is essential to individualize the vascular anatomy in older patients.

The P1 segment of both posterior cerebral arteries (PCA) originates from the basilar artery, bifurcating at the level of the interpeduncular cistern. A number of branches, including circumferential and paramedian perforating arteries that supply the majority of the pons and midbrain, emerge from the basilar artery as it passes through the prepontine and interpeduncular cisterns. The anteroinferior cerebellar artery, the superior cerebellar artery, and occasionally the internal auditory artery are some of the major branches that emerge from the basilar artery.

1.3.2.4 Anteroinferior Cerebellar Artery

The anteroinferior cerebellar artery (AICA) is a component of the middle neurovascular complex.

Origin. According to a study by Yasargil, duplicated (20%) or even triplicated arteries (20%) can occur, whereas their absence (2%), on the other hand, is far less prevalent. Although it can occasionally emerge from the higher or even lower third of the basilar artery, the anteroinferior cerebellar artery typically begins in the middle third.

Course and segments. The artery splits into the rostral and caudal major trunks in the cisternal space at the level of the cerebellopontine angle. The facial and vestibulocochlear cranial nerves are closely related to the rostral trunk. The bottom portion of the petrosal surface of the cerebellum, which includes the choroid plexus and a section of the flocculus, is supplied by the caudal trunk. Following the point of bifurcation, the anteroinferior cerebellar artery splits into four separate segments:

- The clivus and the convex portion of the pons are separated by the anterior pontine segment. Usually, this segment comes into contact with the abducens nerve.
- Starting at the anterolateral edge of the pons, the lateral pontine segment passes above, below, or in between the vestibulocochlear and facial cranial nerves as it passes through the cerebellopontine angle. The choroid plexus that protrudes from the foramen of Luschka, the lateral recess, and the internal acoustic meatus are all strongly associated with this arterial segment. It can be divided into premeatal, meatal, and postmeatal sections based on where it is in relation to the internal acoustic meatus. The labyrinthine artery, which nourishes the facial nerve, vestibulocochlear nerve, and vestibulocochlear labyrinth; recurrent perforating arteries; and the subarcuate artery are some of the branches that emerge from this section. The premeatal portion of the lateral pontine segment is the most typical origin of the labyrinthine, or internal auditory, artery, which enters the internal auditory canal.
- To reach the middle cerebellar peduncle and the cerebello-pontine fissure, the artery passes either caudally or rostrally around the flocculus, in the flocculonodular segment.
- Lastly, the distal branches of the anteroinferior cerebellar artery, which supply the petrosal surface of the cerebellum, correlate to the cortical segment.

1.3.2.5 Superior Cerebellar Artery

Origin. The superior cerebellar artery (SCA) begins caudal to the bifurcation of the basilar artery. The P1 segment of the posterior cerebral artery may occasionally be the direct source of this artery.

Course and segments. The oculomotor, trochlear, and trigeminal cranial nerves are usually closely related to the superior cerebellar artery, and occasionally they are even in contact with the artery. Anatomically, it is associated with the superior cerebellar peduncle, the tentorial surface, the upper half of the fourth ventricle's roof, and the cerebello-mesencephalic fissure. The artery begins its journey caudally to the oculomotor nerve in the interpeduncular cistern, directly in front of the midbrain. Following its cranial origin, it passes cranially to the trigeminal nerve and caudally to the trochlear nerve before circling the brainstem close to the ponto-mesencephalic sulcus. Along its path, the artery splits into the caudal and rostral major trunks. The caudal trunk irrigates the upper portion of the suboccipital surface, whereas the rostral trunk nourishes the vermin and paravermal areas of the cerebellum. Additionally, it produces perforating branches that nourish the cerebellar peduncles and brainstem.

The superior cerebellar artery has these segments:

- The ponto-mesencephalic anterior section begins at the basilar artery, where the artery originates, and travels caudally to the oculomotor nerve before arriving at the anterolateral part of the brainstem.
- The pontine-mesencephalic lateral segment extends caudally to the lateral portion of the upper half of the pons from the anterolateral edge of the brainstem. This caudal loop of this segment projects and occasionally comes into close contact with the trigeminal nerve root.
- The cerebello-mesencephalic segment is parallel to the cranial course of the posterior cerebral artery and Rosenthal's basal vein. This segment runs distally along the upper part of the cerebello-mesencephalic fissure and deep within it before arriving at the anterior area of the caudal tentorial surface.
- The distal branches that supply the tentorial surface of the cerebellum are part of the cortical segment. Vermal and hemispheric are the two groups into which these cortical arteries split. Three hemisphere branches—lateral, intermediate, and medial—as well as two vermal arteries—medial and paramedial—are part of the most typical arterial distribution.

1.3.2.6 Perforating Arteries

The posterolateral portion of the medulla oblongata is supplied by a large number of perforating arteries from the vertebral artery and the posteroinferior cerebellar artery, with some from the anteroinferior cerebellar artery. The perforating arteries from the vertebral artery arise both proximally and distally from the exit of the posteroinferior cerebellar artery. The anterior spinal artery also gives off perforators to the medulla oblongata. The perforating arteries from the posteroinferior cerebellar artery arise mainly from the tonsillar-medullary segment, while they are less numerous in the anterior medullary and lateral medullary segments and absent distally. The distribution of the perforating arteries from the vertebral artery and the posteroinferior cerebellar artery is balanced, such that the more proximal the origin of the posteroinferior cerebellar artery, the more numerous the perforating arteries from the vertebral artery. The compensatory capacity for countercurrent retrograde filling from the distal posteroinferior cerebellar artery in case of proximal occlusion of the same is very limited, and the anastomoses between the perforating arteries are very inefficient, so they are considered terminal arteries.

The pontine arteries are direct branches of the basilar artery that run parallel to the pons, surrounding it and running above the pia mater, and are therefore called circumferential perforating arteries. The short circumferential perforating arteries run through the pia mater and supply the anterolateral part of the pons. The long circumferential perforating arteries are larger and reach further, to the lateral side of the pons. The most constant circumferential arteries are, in a craniocaudal direction, the posterolateral pontine artery, the lateral pontine artery, and, finally, the medullary-pontine artery.

The paramedian perforating arteries are small branches that originate from the basilar artery and enter directly into the brainstem, without having any route along the pial surface. They are classified into three groups according to their area of entry into the brainstem. The proximal perforators originate from the bifurcation of the basilar artery and enter the posterior perforated substance of the interpeduncular sulcus. The caudal group is formed by several branches that end in the foramen cecum of the medullary-pontine sulcus and the lower half of the pons at the level of the medial basilar sulcus. Finally, the central group is more numerous and powerful, entering through the upper half of the medial basilar sulcus of the pons.

The perforating arteries around the distal portion of the basilar artery are numerous, of very different origin and destination, and, more importantly, of great clinical relevance. The perforating arteries originating from the P1 segment of the posterior cerebral artery constitute the main group and can be grouped into the following: posterior thalamic perforating arteries, thalamogeniculate arteries, and peduncular perforating arteries. The posterior thalamic perforating arteries emerge from the proximal portion of the P1 segment and enter the midbrain through the posterior perforated substance, interpeduncular fossa, and medial surface of the cerebral peduncles. Occasionally, all the perforating arteries emerge grouped into a single trunk that arises from the P1 segment of one of the two posterior cerebral arteries, forming the so-called artery of Percheron. The thalamogeniculate perforating arteries have an ascending course and go directly to the lateral geniculate nucleus that is above the posterior cerebral artery. The circumferential perforating arteries have a horizontal course and, according to their length, are classified as short and long. Finally, the posterior cerebral artery gives rise in the P2A segment to the posteromedial choroid artery that accompanies the posterior cerebral artery surrounding the midbrain until reaching the pineal region, where it penetrates the choroid web of the roof of the third ventricle.

1.3.3 Veins

The veins of the posterior fossa are essential for safe microneurosurgery in the cerebellopontine angle. These veins are significant both anatomically and clinically because of their strong relationships with the nearby neurovascular elements. The superficial, deep, brainstem, and bridge veins are the four primary venous groups that make up this region's venous system. The venous sinus of Galen, petrosal sinuses, and tentorial sinuses are the three main venous drainage groups into which all of these veins eventually empty (Fig. 1.4).

1.3.3.1 Superficial Veins

The superficial veins group drains the cerebellar cortex. Superficial veins are divided into three groups according to their connections to the cortical areas of the cerebellum that they drain: the suboccipital, petrosal, and tentorial veins. The cerebellar tentorial surface is drained by the tentorial veins; the superior vermian vein and the superior hemisphere vein are the main veins in this group. The cerebellar suboccipital surface is drained by the suboccipital veins; the inferior vermian vein and the inferior hemisphere vein are the principal veins in this group. The cerebellar petrosal surface is drained by the petrosal veins; the anterior hemisphere veins are the main veins in this group.

1.3.3.2 Deep Veins

Between the brainstem and the cerebellum, there are three deep fissures harboring significant veins of the deep venous group: the cerebellomedullary, the cerebello-pontine, and the cerebello-mesencephalic fissures. A particular vein that is intimately associated with the surrounding areas is located within each of these fissures.

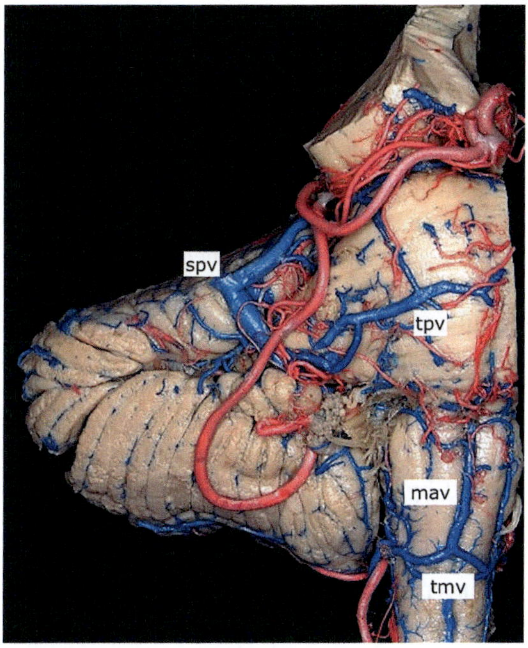

Fig. 1.4 Anterior view of the brainstem and cerebellum veins injected with blue silicone (mav medullary anteromedial vein; spv superior petrosal vein complex; tmv transverse medullary veins; tpv transverse pontine vein)

The cerebello-mesencephalic fissure vein, which is connected to the upper portion of the fourth ventricle's roof, emerges from the cerebello-mesencephalic fissure. The vein that runs along the cerebello-medullary fissure is located in close proximity to the lower portion of the fourth ventricle's roof. The lateral recess and the lateral walls of the fourth ventricle are associated with the cerebello-pontine fissure vein, which runs inside the fissure. Several proximal branches are received by each of these main veins on their way along the fissures. The cerebello-mesencephalic fissure contains the superior cerebellar peduncle vein. The cerebello-medullary fissure contains the inferior cerebellar peduncle vein. The cerebello-pontine fissure contains the middle cerebellar peduncle vein. Furthermore, this deep venous group also includes the amygdalar veins.

1.3.3.3 Brainstem Veins

The names of the veins that drain the brainstem are defined by three main features: the area of the brainstem that they drain (medulla oblongata, pons, or midbrain), the surface that they drain (lateral, anteromedial, or anterolateral), and, finally, if they project longitudinally or transversally.

The principal longitudinal veins of the brainstem are located in the anteromedial surface of the pons and midbrain, which are drained by the pontomesencephalic anteromedial vein. The anteromedial surface of the medulla oblongata is drained by the medullary anteromedial vein. The medullary anterolateral vein is also known as the retro-olivary vein because of its position behind the medullary olive.

The principal transversal veins of the brainstem are described. The cerebellar peduncles are drained by the peduncular veins. The posterior connecting vein of the brainstem is known as the posterior communicating vein. The pontine-mesencephalic sulcus is home to the sulcal pontine-mesencephalic vein. The lateral parts of the pons drain through the transverse pontine veins. The medullary-pontine sulcus is home to the sulcal medullary-pontine vein. The transverse medullary veins drain the lateral areas of the medulla oblongata.

1.3.3.4 Major Drainage Groups and Bridge Veins

The farthest branches of the previously mentioned venous groups terminate to produce the bridge veins draining to the dural venous sinuses and intradural venous lakes. The vein of Galen and the tentorial and superior, and inferior petrosal sinuses form the main drainage groups into which these veins will empty. The superficial veins of the tentorial surface and the deep veins of the cerebello-mesencephalic fissure are among the veins that make up the galenic group and converge into the vein of Galen. The posterior branches of the tentorial surface and the superficial veins of the suboccipital surface will be drained by the tentorial group. Every vein that empties into the superior and inferior petrosal sinuses is a member of the petrosal drainage group. The deep veins of the cerebello-pontine and cerebello-medullary fissures, the superficial veins of the lateral cerebellar area, and the majority of the drainage veins of the brainstem will drain here.

The superior petrosal venous complex, which empties into the superior petrosal sinus, is the most significant venous channel in the upper portion of the cerebellopontine angle. Typically, two or more veins that emerge from the surface of the brainstem or cerebellum unite to form a single drainage channel, also known as a Dandy vein. Occasionally, the superior petrosal sinus receives drainage from two or more separate trunks. The site of entry of the main vein or veins in the superior petrosal sinus is variable and can be medial, above, or lateral in relation to the internal acoustic meatus. There may also be a close connection between the trigeminal root and the pontine-trigeminal vein, which ends in the superior petrosal sinus complex.

1.3.4 Cisterns

The microneurosurgical treatment of disorders involving the cerebellopontine angle depends on an understanding of the anatomy of the posterior fossa cisterns. Between the arachnoid and the pia mater, the subarachnoid space extends from the base of the brain around the brainstem and the tentorial incisura to create cisterns, which are compartments that hold cerebrospinal fluid (CSF). The cisterns are traversed by the main intracranial arterial vessels and all cranial nerves. Lesions at the cerebellopontine angle can be more easily accessed when the cistern walls are opened to allow cerebrospinal fluid to be drained. Accessing certain cisterns for cerebrospinal fluid evacuation may occasionally be challenging. For instance, when using a retrosigmoid approach to approach a large acoustic schwannoma, a neurosurgeon must focus on the caudal portion of the approach. Then, with the help of a retractor, a microdissector, and an aspirator, it is possible to open the cerebello-medullary cistern to remove cerebrospinal fluid, which relieves pressure and keeps the cerebellopontine angle easier to mobilize and remove the tumor. Arterial and venous vessels and cranial nerves implicated in the various disorders are being exposed to travel through the cerebellopontine angle only after the microsurgical dissection and opening of the cisterns. To enhance operating conditions, the cisterns should be thought of as connected compartments that must be opened one after the other in order to remove cerebrospinal fluid and examine their contents.

Moreover, different tumors have a particular preference to occupy or displace specific cisterns. Because of this, Rhoton divides tumors into five categories according to how they relate to the cisterns: tumors that grow inside one cistern, tumors that grow inside one cistern but displace others, tumors that grow across multiple cisterns, tumors that grow in adjacent structures but penetrate the cisterns, and tumors that grow in adjacent structures but only displace the cisterns without penetrating them. For instance, when a tiny vestibular schwannoma expands, it may compress or spread to nearby peripheral cisterns. Initially, it grows inside the cerebellopontine cistern. The anterior pontine arachnoid membrane, the lateral medullary-pontine arachnoid membrane, and the lateral pontine-mesencephalic arachnoid membrane can all be compressed by vestibular schwannomas. Multiple cisterns are frequently the site of epidermoid cyst growth, which can also cause anatomical and arachnoid membrane distortion. Though they can spread into other cisterns, such as the premedullary, interpeduncular, ambiens, and quadrigeminal cisterns, these tumors are usually seen in the posterior fossa, specifically in connection to the cerebellopontine, cerebello-medullary, and prepontine cisterns. Conversely, meningiomas usually originate from nearby structures outside the cisterns, but when they grow, they have the potential to move into the cisterns. The cisterns are typically kept anatomically maintained in procedures involving unruptured aneurysms or microvascular decompression of cranial nerves.

The subarachnoid space of the posterior fossa is divided into compartments or cisterns. Membranes separate these cisterns. The chiasmatic cistern and the interpeduncular cistern are separated by the Liliequist membrane; the prepontine cistern and the cerebellopontine cistern are separated by the anterior pontine membrane; the ambiens cistern and the cerebellopontine cistern are separated by the lateral pontine-mesencephalic membrane; the premedullary and prepontine cisterns are separated by the medial medullary-pontine membrane; and the cerebellopontine cistern and the cerebello-medullary cistern are separated by the lateral medullary-pontine membrane.

1.3.5 Interpeduncular Cistern

The cisternal transition between the supratentorial and infratentorial areas is marked by the interpeduncular cistern, which is situated between the cerebral peduncles in the anterior tentorial incisura. Its superior border is located at the third ventricle's floor, on the posterior limit of the mammillary bodies. Its bottom border is located at the pontine-mesencephalic sulcus level. The interpeduncular cistern divides with the ambiens and crural cisterns, which encircle the midbrain and temporal lobe in the tentorial incisura. The oculomotor nerves act as anchors for the Liliequist membrane and run along the cistern's lateral walls. The mesencephalic membrane, which divides the interpeduncular cistern from the prepontine cistern, and the diencephalic membrane, which divides the interpeduncular cistern from the chiasmatic cistern, are the two discrete components of this membrane.

Neurovascular components of the upper complex, including the superior cerebellar artery and its perforating branches, are located in the interpeduncular cistern. The posterior thalamic-perforating arteries, the top of the basilar artery, the P1 segment of the posterior cerebral artery, the posteromedial choroidal artery, the peduncular veins, the posterior communicating artery, the anteromedial pontomesencephalic arteries, and the pontine-mesencephalic sulcus vein are additional structures.

1.3.6 Prepontine Cistern

The prepontine cistern is situated in front of the rostral aspect of the pons. The mesencephalic membrane of Liliequist separates it from the interpeduncular cistern cranially, while the medullary-pontine sulcus marks its caudal border. The cerebello-pontine cisterns, which are divided by the anterior pontine membranes, form the lateral borders of the cistern. The basilar artery, which gives rise to the anterior inferior cerebellar artery, passes through the cistern, which is devoid of cranial nerves.

1.3.7 Cerebellopontine Cistern

Because the structures contained by the cistern are most closely associated with diseases in this region, the cerebellopontine cistern is the most pertinent from a microneurosurgical standpoint at the level of the cerebellopontine angle. The lateral pontine-mesencephalic membrane divides the cistern from the ambiens cistern cranially, while the lateral mesencephalic-pontine membrane, which spans the subarachnoid space between the vestibulocochlear and glossopharyngeal nerves, divides it from the cerebello-medullary cistern caudally. The anterior pontine membrane divides the cistern from the prepontine cistern, which limits it medially. The cerebellopontine fissure is formed laterally by the cistern's extension between the cerebellum and the lateral side of the pons.

The trigeminal nerve passes along the superolateral portion of the cistern after emerging from the anterolateral surface of the pons at the middle level, roughly near the upper border of the middle cerebellar peduncle. Just lateral to the anterior pontine membrane, the abducens nerve ascends medially within the cistern after beginning at the medullary-pontine sulcus. Just cranial to the lateral medullary-pontine membrane in the lower part of the cistern are the origins of the facial and vestibulocochlear nerves. Additionally, the flocculus extends into the cistern behind the vestibulocochlear and facial nerve exit. In terms of vascular elements, the anterior inferior cerebellar artery and the superior cerebellar artery travel through this cistern. The veins that make up the superior petrosal vein complex also converge here, encircling the trigeminal nerve before emptying into the superior petrosal sinus.

1.3.8 Premedullary Cistern

The premedullary cistern is situated behind the caudal part of the clivus and in front of the medulla oblongata. The medial medullary-pontine membrane divides it from the prepontine cistern, and its cranial border is located at the level of the medullary-pontine sulcus. It shares a lateral border with the cerebello-medullary cisterns in the posteroinferior part of the olivary body, immediately in front of the glossopharyngeal, vagal, and accessory nerves that emerge from the retro-olivary sulcus. The premedullary cistern extends caudally into the anterior spinal cistern without being blocked by arachnoid membranes. The hypoglossal nerve travels laterally via this cistern between the medullary pyramids and the inferior part of the olivary body after its exit at the pre-olivary sulcus. As the vertebral artery ascends via the foramen magnum, it enters the cistern. The anterior spinal artery, which runs from the premedullary cistern to the anterior spinal cord, is formed by the union of the two spinal arteries, branches of the two vertebral arteries, in the lower part of the cistern.

1.3.9 Cerebello-Medullary Cistern

From the standpoint of the retrosigmoid approach, the cerebello-medullary cistern is very important since it enables the neurosurgeon to open it early on and release cerebrospinal fluid, which relaxes the posterior fossa. The cerebello-medullary cistern is situated caudal to the point where the medulla oblongata and pons meet. The lateral medullary-pontine membrane divides it from the cerebellopontine cistern. The foramen magnum is at the level of its caudal border. The olivary body borders the cistern in the middle, and it reaches the biventral lobe of the cerebellum on the side. This cistern is where the glossopharyngeal, vagal, and medullary portions of the accessory nerves travel before arriving at the jugular foramen. The spinal part of the accessory nerve enters the cerebello-medullary cistern after ascending via the spinal cisterns. At the lower edge of this cistern, the V3 segment of the vertebral artery penetrates the dura mater to reach the posterior fossa. It then quickly leaves it to enter the premedullary cistern. The posterior inferior cerebellar artery travels posteriorly around the medulla to reach the cisterna magna after entering the cistern between the roots of the lower cranial nerves that emerge from the retro-olivary sulcus.

1.3.10 Cisterna Magna

The vermis of the cerebellum and the medulla oblongata are situated behind the cisterna magna. The foramen magnum and its arachnoid membranes at this level are closely connected. One feature of this cistern is the arachnoid membranes' remarkable thickness, which defines the posterior border of the foramen of Magendie and adheres laterally to the medulla and cerebellar tonsils. This cistern connects to the cerebello-medullary fissure ventrally and extends into the posterior spinal cistern caudally. Near the point where the posterior inferior cerebellar artery splits into a medial branch that irrigates the vermis and a lateral branch that irrigates the cerebellar tonsil and a portion of the suboccipital surface of the cerebellum, the artery enters the cistern.

1.4 Neurovascular Groups

Albert Rhoton classified the neurovascular content of the cerebellopontine angle into three groups [5].

- The *superior neurovascular complex* consists of the superior cerebellar artery and its branches, the trochlear nerve, and the trigeminal nerve, as well as the superior petrosal vein complex.
- Together with the anterior inferior cerebellar artery, the *intermediate neurovascular* complex consists of the abducens nerve, the facial nerve, and the vestibulocochlear nerve. The cerebellopontine fissure vein, which is generated by the confluence of multiple smaller veins and runs cranially toward the superior petrosal venous complex, is the main conduit for the venous drainage of this middle level of the cerebellopontine angle. The vein of the middle cerebellar peduncle is another venous channel that runs cranially toward the superior petrosal complex after starting in the medullary-pontine sulcus.
- Finally, the posterior inferior cerebellar artery and the glossopharyngeal nerve, vagal nerve, spinal or auxiliary nerve of Willis nerve, and hypoglossal nerve comprise the *lower neurovascular complex*. Venous drainage of the inferior compartment of the cerebellopontine angle is done through small veins that converge into the inferior petrosal sinus.

1.5 Cerebellopontine Angle Compartments

A three-dimensional understanding of the connections between the brainstem, cerebellar surfaces, cranial nerves, and cerebellar arteries is necessary to optimize surgical approaches to the cerebellopontine angle. Thus, the neurovascular compartments were described by Rhoton in his attempt to systematize the study of microsurgical anatomy: a superior compartment associated with the superior cerebellar artery; a middle compartment associated with the anterior inferior cerebellar artery; and an inferior compartment associated with the posterior inferior cerebellar artery.

- The upper portion of the pons, trigeminal nerve, trochlear nerve, superior cerebellar artery, and superior petrosal vein complex are all parts of the *superior compartment*. At the intersection of the anterolateral surface of the pons and the upper border of the middle cerebellar peduncle, the posterior root of the trigeminal nerve emerges from the brainstem and ascends obliquely from the anterolateral part of the pons to the petrosal apex of the temporal bone and leaves the posterior fossa and enters the middle fossa before entering Meckel's cave. The trochlear nerve runs parallel to the tentorial edge. The brainstem is normally surrounded by the superior cerebellar artery. The superior cerebellar artery may occasionally come into close contact with the trigeminal nerve, usually over the superior or superomedial edge of the nerve, due to a pronounced loop projecting caudally. The petrosal vein, also known as the superior petrosal vein complex, is usually created by the intersection of several venous tributaries. The most common tributary veins are those from the middle cerebellar peduncle, the lateral portion of the cerebellar hemisphere, the pontine transverse veins, the pontine-trigeminal veins, and the veins of the cerebellopontine fissure.
- The anterolateral inferior surface of the pons, the anteroinferior cerebellar artery, the middle cerebellar peduncle, the cerebello-pontine fissure, the petrosal surface of the cerebellum, the abducens nerve, the facial nerve, and the vestibulocochlear nerve are all components of the *middle compartment*. The anteroinferior cerebellar artery emerges from the basilar artery at the level of the pons. It then proceeds along the middle cerebellar peduncle's surface and passes through the cerebellopontine fissure to irrigate the petrosal surface of the cerebellum. The anteroinferior cerebellar artery often travels around the brainstem and passes caudally to the facial and vestibulocochlear nerves. In some cases, though, it travels cranially to these nerves. When performing surgical approaches to the middle compartment, the petrosal surface of the cerebellum is the most important area to consider. It faces medially to the brainstem and the fourth ventricle and anteriorly to the posterior aspect of the petrosal bone. The amygdala, flocculus, quadrangular, simple, biventral, superior, and inferior semilunar lobes, as well as the wings of the central lobe, make up the petrosal surface of the cerebellar hemisphere. The petrosal fissure, which separates the upper and lower parts and is often referred to as the horizontal or cerebello-pontine fissure, is the biggest fissure on this surface. This split between the superior and inferior semilunar lobes. The vein of the medullary-pontine sulcus, the vein of the cerebello-medullary fissure, the vein of the middle cerebellar peduncle, and the vein of the cerebellopontine fissure are located at the level of the middle neurovascular complex, surrounding the pons. The facial and vestibulocochlear nerves, emerging from the medullary-pontine sulcus, are intimately associated with each of these veins.
- The upper anterolateral surface of the medulla oblongata, the inferior cerebellar peduncle, the cerebello-medullary fissure, the suboccipital surface of the cerebellum, the glossopharyngeal, vagal, accessory, and hypoglossal nerves, and the posterior inferior cerebellar artery are all components of the *inferior compartment*. The posteroinferior cerebellar artery is closely related to the cerebello-medullary fissure and has the most intricate and winding path among the cerebellar arteries. While an extradural origin from the vertebral artery has also been reported in as many as 10% of cases,

it often begins at the level of the lower part of the olivary body from the vertebral artery. Glossopharyngeal, vagal, and accessory nerves are grouped in their exit through the jugular foramen and referred to as low cranial nerves. This inferior compartment continues with the upper cervical spinal compartment.

1.6 Key Messages

- *The cerebellopontine angle is a small and highly intricate anatomical region.*
- *A safe microneurosurgery of lesions in this topography is contingent upon a three-dimensional understanding of the anatomy of the cerebellopontine angle.*
- *The cerebellopontine angle is typically divided into three zones or compartments, each of which contains representative neurovascular groups.*
- *The brainstem, cerebellum, and nerves have a very rigid anatomical organization, while the arteries are more variable. The veins are anarchic.*
- *The cisterns, which contain cerebrospinal fluid and neurovascular elements, are also anatomically relevant components.*

References

1. Arnautovic K, Al-Mefty O, Pait TG, Krisht AF, Husain HM. The suboccipital cavernous sinus. J Neurosurg. 1997;86:252–62.
2. González-Darder JM, Quilis-Quesada V, Capilla-Guasch P, de Oliveira E. Abordajes neuroquirúrgicos de la patología craneal y cerebral. Barcelona: Elsevier España; 2020.
3. Prats-Galino A, de Soria G, Notaris G, Puig J, Pedraza S. Functional anatomy of subcortical circuits issuing from or integrating at the human brainstem. Clin Neurophysiol. 2012;123:4–12.
4. Recalde RJ, Figueiredo EG, De Oliveira E. Microsurgical anatomy of the safe entry zones on the anterolateral brainstem related to surgical approaches to cavernous malformations. Neurosurgery. 2008;62(3 Suppl 1):9–15.
5. Rhoton AL Jr. The posterior fossa: microsurgical anatomy & surgical approaches. Neurosurgery. 2000;47(3 Suppl):S1–S279. https://doi.org/10.1097/00006123-200009001-00013.
6. Ribas G, Yasuda A, Peace D, Rhoton AL. Microsurgical anatomy of the cerebellopontine angle and its suboccipital retromastoid approaches. In: Bambakidis NC, Megerian CA, Spetzler RF, editors. Surgery of the cerebellopontine angle. Shelton: BC Decker Inc; 2009. p. 11–30.
7. Tanriover N, Abe H, Rhoton AL Jr, Kawashima M, Sanus GZ, Akar Z. Microsurgical anatomy of the superior petrosal venous complex: new classifications and implications for subtemporal transtentorial and retrosigmoid suprameatal approaches. J Neurosurg. 2007;106:1041–50.
8. Yagmurlu K, Rhoton AL, Tarinover N, Bennett JA. Three-dimensional microsurgical anatomy and the safe entry zones of the brainstem. Oper Neurosurg. 2014;10:602–20.

2 Retrosigmoid Approach

2.1 Introduction

One of the most traditional and practical cranial approaches is the lateral suboccipital approach, which is primarily utilized for the surgical management of disease involving the cerebellopontine angle. Because it is done medial to the sigmoid sinus in the dural phase and medial to the mastoid in the bony phase, this technique is often referred to as the retromastoid or retrosigmoid approach (Fig. 2.1).

Vestibular schwannomas, benign schwannomas that primarily arise in the superior vestibular nerve in the internal auditory canal but spread to the cerebellopontine angle as they grow, are the prototypical neurosurgical pathology of the pontocerebellar angle. Meningiomas, epidermoid cysts, schwannomas of various cranial nerves and metastases, and fourth ventricle tumors that infiltrate the cerebellopontine angle through the Luschka foramina are among the additional tumors discovered in this area. Rare arteriovenous malformations of the cerebellopontine angle and vertebral artery or posterior inferior cerebellar artery aneurysms are examples of vascular disease, which are uncommon. Nowadays, several lesions on the anteromedial surface of the medulla oblongata or the pons can be safely accessed through the cerebellopontine angle. The lateral suboccipital approach is also used to surgically treat cranial neuropathies caused by neurovascular compression, such as trigeminal neuralgia caused by compression of the trigeminal root, hemifacial spasm caused by compression of the facial nerve, intractable vertigo or tinnitus caused by compression of the eighth cranial nerve, neuralgia caused by compression of the glossopharyngeal nerve, or compression of the medulla that is associated with cases of essential hypertension. Lastly, the lateral suboccipital approach can be combined with more cranial approaches to create the family of petrous approaches and, finally, with more caudal approaches for the extreme lateral or far-lateral approach to the foramen magnum.

When modern neurosurgery first emerged in the 1920s, Harvey Cushing and Walter Dandy were the world leaders in treating vestibular schwannomas with neurosurgery. Cushing advocated a broad medial suboccipital approach with radical tumor removal, but Dandy carried out a unilateral suboccipital procedure with internal tumor decompression. The advent of microneurosurgical techniques utilized in otology by Rand and Kurze in the 1960s marked a significant improvement in the surgical technique, which in turn led to a greater degree of tumor resection and, more significantly, better clinical results. The incidence and severity of neurological sequelae have been reduced more recently with the use of imaging techniques like magnetic resonance imaging (MRI) and high-resolution computed tomography (CT) in the preoperative evaluation of patients and intraoperative

J. M. González-Darder, *Microneurosurgery of Cerebellopontine Angle*,
https://doi.org/10.1007/978-3-032-03091-7_2

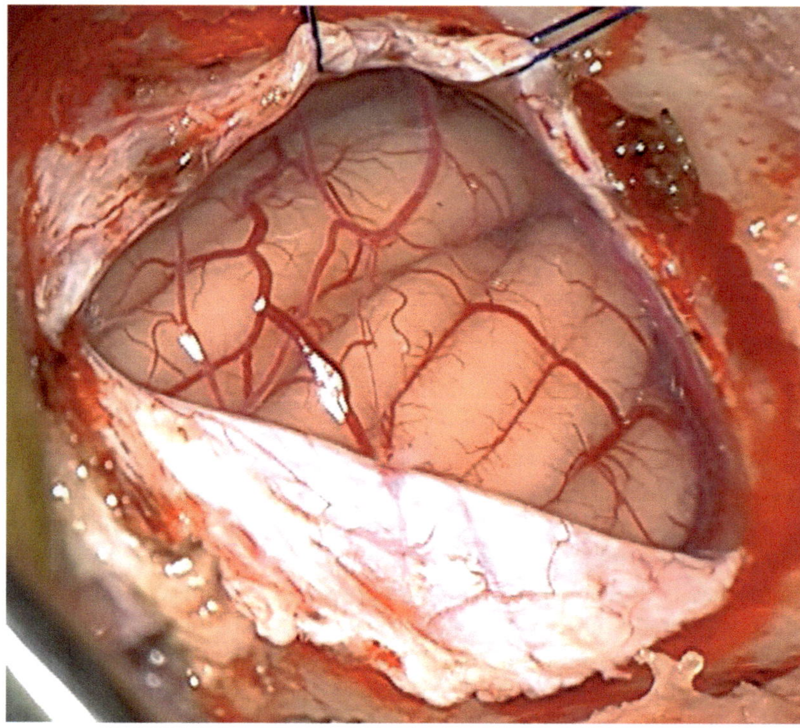

Fig. 2.1 Right side retrosigmoid craniotomy

neurophysiological monitoring for real-time control of cranial nerve function.

2.2 Anatomical Considerations

The ensuing chapters will explore the majority of the anatomical features of the retrosigmoid approach, with a focus on neurovascular interactions [3, 6]. Only the most pertinent anatomical aspects associated with the surgical technique of the approach will be discussed in this section [1, 3, 4, 7, 9].

2.2.1 Bone Relationships

A craniotomy that resects a portion of the occipital, parietal, and temporal bones around the angle created by the transverse and sigmoid sinuses is the core of the lateral suboccipital approach. The *asterion*, which is the cranial point where the parietomastoid, occipitomastoid, and lambdoid or parietooccipital sutures converge, is a bone point to this anatomical zone (Fig. 2.2). The transverse and sigmoid sinuses, as well as the location of the craniotomy for the lateral suboccipital approach, are anatomically related to the asterion. The lambdoid suture extends laterally from the midline's lambda point to the asterion, connecting the parietal bone to the occipital bone's squama. The occipitomastoid suture lies between the mastoid section of the temporal bone and the squama of the occipital bone, and it runs inferiorly from the asterion to the jugular foramen. Lastly, the mastoid part of the temporal bone and the mastoid border of the parietal bone are connected by the parietomastoid suture. The asterion is situated about 1 cm behind where the sigmoid and transverse sinuses converge.

The superior and inferior nuchal or occipital lines are the most significant bony features on the outside surface of the lateral part of the occipital bone's squama. The insertion of the sternocleidomastoid and trapezius muscles marks the superior nuchal line, which is an imaginary line that joins the asterion and the external occipital protuberance. The major and minor rectus muscles delineate the inferior nuchal line, while the sple-

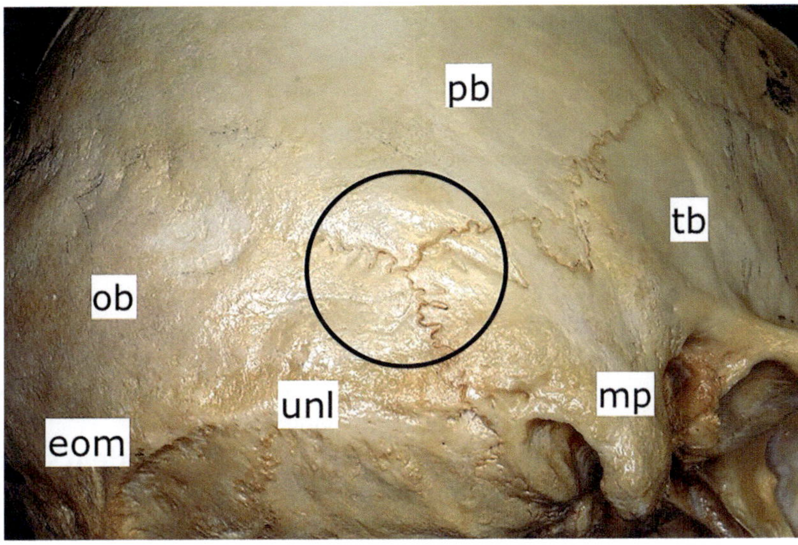

Fig. 2.2 Cranial view around asterion (circle) (external occipital protuberance; mp: mastoid process; ob: occipital bone; pb: parietal bone; tb: temporal bone; unl: upper nuchal line)

nius capitis and superior oblique muscles insert below the superior nuchal line and above the inferior one. The posterior belly of the digastric muscle is inserted into a notch or groove on the posteroinferior surface of the mastoid. The mastoid emissary vein of the sigmoid sinus typically corresponds to an aperture in the occipital bone. There are other interesting features on the inside of the occipital bone, particularly the horizontal canal or groove that contains the transverse sinus and, after passing through the occipitomastoid suture, curves inferiorly to contain the sigmoid sinus. The mastoid antrum is the largest and most stable of the many pneumatized mastoid cells that make up the mastoid. These cells vary greatly in size, number, and location.

2.2.2 The Dural Sinuses

The lateral sinus, which is made up of a horizontal portion known as the transverse sinus and a vertical section known as the sigmoid sinus, is the dural sinus associated with the lateral suboccipital approach. The Herophilus press, where the occipital, straight, and superior sagittal sinuses intersect, is where the transverse sinus starts. Along the insertion of the tentorium cerebelli, the transverse sinus extends laterally and horizontally in a channel or groove etched into the inner surface of the occipital bone. The mastoid emissary vein is received by the sigmoid sinus as it travels vertically in a groove or channel carved on the inner face of the mastoid section of the temporal bone, leading to the internal jugular vein bulb. An abrupt shift in the lateral sinus's direction is implied by the point of transition between its two sections. A number of pertinent anatomical peculiarities are present at this point: the dural sinus's direction shifts from horizontal (transverse sinus) to vertical (sigmoid sinus); the lateral sinus no longer has a relationship with the tentorium; the superior petrosal sinus drains at this level; and, lastly, this angle is near the cranial point asterion, a significant anatomical point of surgical importance. The Citelli sinodural angle is the name of this pertinent anatomical region, which has surgical implications. It is defined in anatomy as the angle formed by the middle fossa's dura mater and the transverse sinus, which indicates the end of the middle fossa when the superior petrosal sinus reaches it. It is the angle formed by the mastoid tegmen and the lateral sinus in mastoid surgery. The presigmoid approach is of interest in neurosurgery because it corresponds to the superior angle of Trautman's presigmoid triangle and indicates the arrival of the superior petrosal sinus to the lateral sinus, exactly where it changes direction from transverse to vertical.

2.2.3 Cranial Points

On the posterosuperior border of the external auditory meatus, the asterion—the confluence of the lambdoid, occipitomastoid, and parietomastoid sutures—is the most significant cranial point. It is situated approximately 6.5 cm from the inion or external occipital protuberance, 5 cm from the tip of the mastoid, and 4.5 cm from the suprameatal crest or Henle's spine. Above the point where the transverse and sigmoid sinuses converge is the asterion. Since the asterion is the traditional bone reference point for lateral suboccipital craniotomy, there are numerous ways to find it so that the first trepanation hole for the craniotomy can be placed. Regretfully, numerous anatomical investigations reveal frequent structural differences between the dural sinuses and asterion. Furthermore, during surgical procedures, it is frequently impossible to identify the asterion on the skull's surface. Nevertheless, several helpful cranial references can be outlined. The theoretical line that connects the asterion with the inion is the lower boundary of the transverse sinus. At a cranial position where the occipitomastoid suture intersects with a line drawn between the inion and the tip of the mastoid, the sigmoid sinus crosses the suture. Last but not least, the emissary mastoid vein's foramen, which is often situated at the middle of a line formed between the inion and the mastoid tip, is a significant but highly variable site. A dural fold and the underlying preoccipital notch, which loosely delineates the border between the temporal and occipital lobes, correspond to the asterion at the intracranial level. When placing lateral suboccipital craniotomy and trepanation holes, all of these bone references can be useful. The most anterior part of the tentorium's insertion on the inner surface of the calvarial bone, or the most posterior point of the petrous part with respect to the calvaria, can also be identified as the cranial point of external projection of the posterior border of the temporal bone's petrous portion. This point is situated 1 cm above the place where the parieto-mastoid and parieto-squamous sutures converge. The supramastoid crest, a component of the root of the zygomatic arch, marks the confluence of the aforementioned sutures, which is located in a palpable depression approximately 4 cm above the posterior section of the mastoid tip. The point specifically projects internally into the superior part of the inferior temporal gyrus, more medially with the parahippocampal gyrus and the fusiform gyrus at the level of the ventricular atrium [3, 8].

2.3 Retrosigmoid Approach

2.3.1 Patient's Position

There are various positions used for this approach: semi-sitting, prone, lateral, supine, and park bench have all been utilized. Selection is done considering factors pertaining to the anesthetics, type of pathology, and tumor size, but also related to the comfort of the patients and the surgeon's preferences. For the majority of patients, we employ the supine position with the head turned contralaterally. The patient is positioned with the neck stretched horizontally and the trunk raised by around 30°. The neck is then flexed once the head has been turned contralaterally. The surgeon may work comfortably in this position while sitting with their arms supported, and the patient's positioning is simple. The issues with this position include the possibility that patients who are obese or have cervical stiffness may not be able to rotate their necks excessively, which could kink their vertebral arteries or impair their ability to drain their jugular veins. By moving the operating table in the other way or using a pillow to elevate the contralateral shoulder, these limits can be overcome. Additionally, anesthetic issues may arise from the semi-sitting and prone postures because getting the patient into either one is difficult and painful for the surgeon. The prone position lacks arm support for the surgeon, and the semi-sitting position causes blood and washing saline to pool at the bottom of the surgical area. In patients who are obese or have short necks and prominent shoulders, the lateral decubitus position is extremely time-consuming and may cause discomfort for the surgeon.

2.3.2 Planning Before Surgery

In order to determine the measurement of distances of interest for surgery, a CT scan of the skull with a bone window is crucial for the preoperative assessment. The line connecting the sigmoid sinus with the apex of the petrous ridge marks the plane of the medial surface of the petrous section of the temporal bone, which is 32° from the midline. On average, the internal auditory canal's posterior wall is 11 mm in diameter, while the internal acoustic meatus's maximum diameter is 8 mm. A line drawn from the medial edge of the sigmoid sinus to the canal, passing through the posterior limit of the labyrinth, indicates the portion of the internal auditory canal's posterior wall that can be drilled without endangering auditory function. When the jugular bulb is positioned high, there is also a chance of damage. In 15% of cases, a jugular bulb can be seen at the level of the internal auditory canal, and in another 15%, it can be seen higher. CT provides a good assessment of the mastoid cells' expansion and pneumatization, and in 40% of instances, pneumatized cells are seen near the tip of the petrous bone above the internal auditory canal. Vascular MRI can also be used to determine the relative dominance of the sigmoid sinus, which is equal in 20% of instances and greater on the right in 40% of cases.

2.3.3 Skin Incision and Soft Tissue Dissection

Our standard retroauricular and retromastoid skin incision is done two fingerbreadths behind the ear, beginning just above the external auditory canal and ending at the tip of the mastoid, either straight or slightly curved. It is deepened cranially to the occipital bone periosteum, after which the insertions of the deeper and sternocleidomastoid muscles are sectioned and laterally separated following periosteal detachment. Our incision extends caudally to the occipital artery and its satellite veins, which pass beneath the digastric muscle and then cross the field superomedially.

2.3.4 Craniotomy

The dura mater of the posterior fossa is accessible at the lower margin of the angle produced by the transverse and sigmoid sinuses through a trephine hole positioned underneath the asterion. Using this hole as a guide, young individuals can have a craniotomy that is tailored to the posterior margin of the sigmoid sinus and the lower edges of the lateral sinus, using the asterion as a cranial anatomical landmark reference. However, since it can be challenging to identify the cranial sutures in the operating setting, the asterion's bony markers are typically useless. Using a high-speed motor and a burr with a diameter of 4–6 mm, we often make a large hole in the occipital squama, far from the hypothesized location of the dural sinuses, until we reach the dura mater. Then, using a finer burr, we expose a few millimeters of the transverse and sigmoid sinuses by moving superiorly and laterally. The size and topography of the pathology that needs to be treated determine the medial and caudal extensions. More distally, the condylar vein can be seen passing through the bone, and the caudal bone resection typically stops at the point where the occipital squama becomes horizontal.

Three issues may arise during the craniotomy. Entry into the mastoid cells, which are sealed by muscle and/or surgical wax, is the first and most frequent. Finding the mastoid emissary vein within the bone's thickness is the second step. If the vein is considerable in size, it must be skeletonized and coagulated before being retracted over the dural sinus. The size of an unintentional laceration of the dural sinuses determines how to manage this uncommon complication. Small cuts can be closed with a stitch or vascular miniclip, coated with hemostatic material, or coagulated with bipolar. Direct suturing should be used to treat large cuts following extensive bone drilling that exposes the sinus. In the event of a dominating asymmetric sinus, packing will be avoided since it can result in thrombosis and severe neurological symptoms.

2.3.5 The Dura Mater Opening

The dura mater opens up a few millimeters around the dural sinuses, with releasing incisions up to the dural sinuses. The dura mater flap is withdrawn medially, and traction sutures are placed on the dura mater that remains surrounding the sinuses.

2.3.6 Cisternal Navigation

The space available in the cerebellopontine angle after dural opening is variable and different from the anatomical studies (Fig. 2.3). It can be very narrow because cisterns are frequently occupied by the tumor pathology to be treated. Venous drainage is sometimes rendered ineffective by the lack of muscular relaxation enforced by neurophysiological monitoring in the cerebellopontine angle. The cerebellum is significantly displaced when large tumors are present and occupies the surgical field. Because of all of this, safe surgery depends on the cerebrospinal fluid draining from the cisterns. Only in anatomical studies, lesions of small size or approaches for microvascular decompression can the anatomy of the cerebellopontine angle be freely exposed (Fig. 2.3). The first maneuver is to release cerebrospinal fluid (CSF) from the cisterns, and to reach the cisterns, the cerebellum must be mobilized. Initially, the cerebellum is raised superomedially with a retractor to reach the lateral cerebello-medullary cistern and drain cerebrospinal fluid at this level. Tension is released, and the retractor can be repositioned to open the cerebellopontine angle and reveal its anatomical structures by sectioning the existing arachnoid bands between the tumor, cranial nerves, arteries, and the cerebellum. Lastly, a self-retaining retractor is used to hold the cerebellum in place after it has been moved to the proper position.

The cerebellum is displaced inferomedially when the spatula is positioned parallel to the superior petrosal sinus to reach the upper neurovascular complex region, such as for microvascular decompression of the trigeminal root (Fig. 2.4). The lateral side of the cerebellum, which is shifted laterally, is where the spatula is inserted when treating the middle neurovascular complex area, as is the case with vestibular schwannomas (Figs. 2.5 and 2.6). Lastly, the spatula is positioned inferolaterally, and the cerebellum is raised superomedially if the lower neurovascular complex area is addressed, as is required for the clipping of posterior inferior cer-

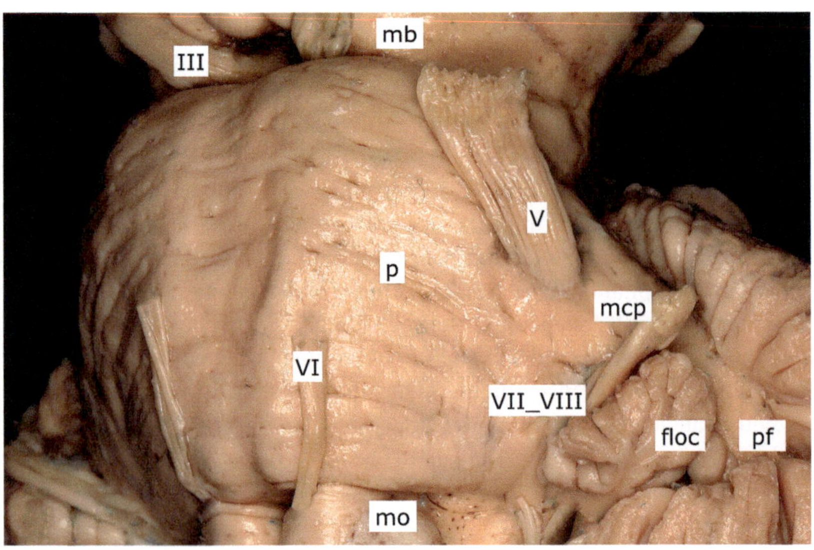

Fig. 2.3 Anatomical view of the left cerebellopontine angle (III: oculomotor nerve; V: trigeminal nerve; VI: abducens nerve; VII-VIII: facial-vestibulocochlear complex; floc: flocculus; mb: middle brain midbrain; mcp: middle cerebellar peduncle; mo: medulla oblongata; p:: pons; pf: petrosal fissure)

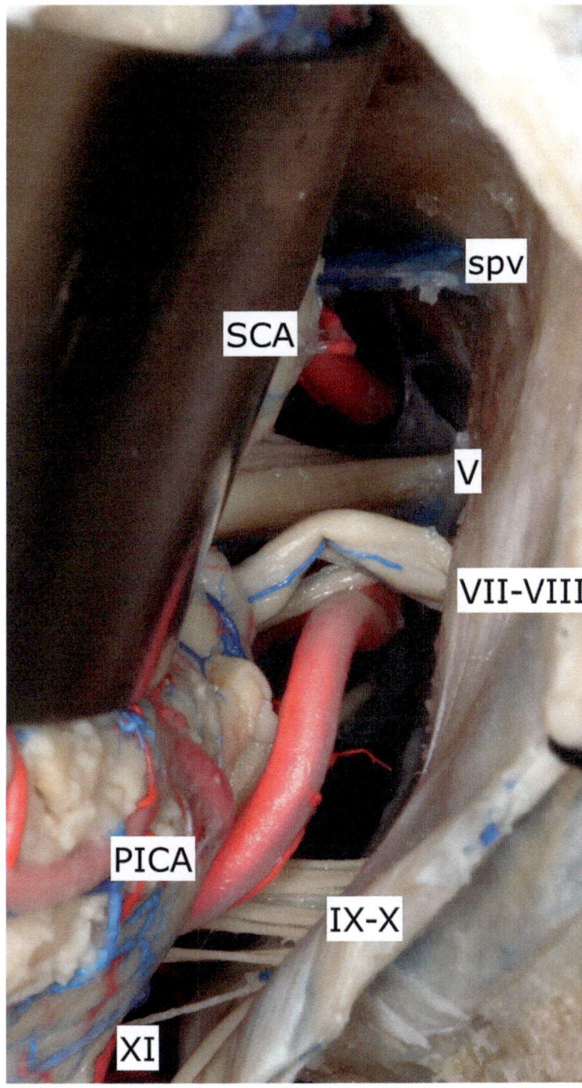

Fig. 2.4 Anatomical overview of the right cerebellopontine angle accessed by a retrosigmoid approach (V: trigeminal nerve; VII-VIII: facial-vestibulocochlear complex; IX-X: glossopharyngeal and vagal nerves; XI: accessory nerve; SCA: superior cerebellar artery; spv: superior petrosal vein; PICA: posteroinferior cerebellar artery)

ebellar artery or vertebral artery aneurysms (Fig. 2.7). During extended periods of surgery, relaxation, adjustment, and even elimination of retraction are recommended to avoid excessive cerebellar injury.

2.3.7 Intraoperative Neurophysiological Monitoring

Intraoperative neurophysiological monitoring makes surgery for cerebellopontine angle lesions safer for the patient. Intraoperative neurophysiological monitoring options include stimulation of the median and/or posterior tibial nerves to study long ascending pathways with somatosensory potentials (SSEP); transcranial cortical electrical stimulation and peripheral electromyographic recording in muscles dependent on cranial nerves (corticomedullary pathway) and/or spinal nerves (corticospinal pathway) (TcMMEP); brainstem auditory evoked potentials (BAEP) to study the auditory pathway; free-sweep electromyography of muscles dependent on cranial nerves; and, lastly, electromyographic recording of muscles through direct electrical stimulation of cranial nerves. The neurophysiological study's design is

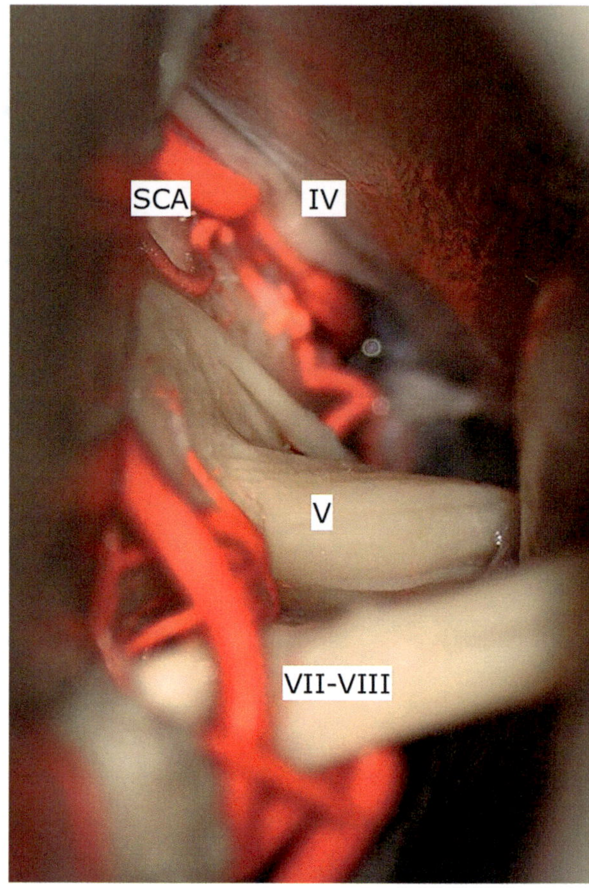

Fig. 2.5 Anatomical view of the upper compartment of right cerebellopontine angle accessed by a retrosigmoid approach (IV: trochlear nerve; V: trigeminal nerve; VII-VIII: facial-vestibulocochlear complex; SCA: superior cerebellar artery)

tailored, but it must always involve direct electrical stimulation of the facial and trigeminal nerves as well as free electromyographic scanning. Electromyographic electrodes can be positioned on the appropriate homolateral or contralateral muscles to monitor any other cranial nerve. Homolateral auditory potentials are evaluated when hearing preservation is needed, and the patient retains nerve auditory conduction with morphologically maintained potentials in preoperative studies. In addition to somatosensory and/or motor potentials, contralateral auditory potentials are captured for functional monitoring of the brainstem in the event of hearing loss or the absence of detectable potentials. Pathological activity resulting from tonic (or trains) or phasic (or bursts) nerve irritation can be identified in the sweep electromyographic study. Rapid trains or bursts of potentials are known as neurotonic discharges. There are single or repeated bursts that last less than 200 ms and have frequencies between 30 and 100 Hz. They can be brought on by rubbing, contact, traction, or any other mechanical stimulus applied to the nerve. Additionally, there are larger bursts, usually lasting 1–30 s, which could be a sign of increased nerve aggression. Furthermore, when the motor axon is mechanically stimulated, trains of waves with an entirely asynchronous beat may emerge. Although neurotonic discharges are useful, nerve injury is not always indicated by them, nor is it excluded by their absence. With a sensitivity and specificity of about 90%, type A neurotonic discharges—sinusoidal, symmetric sequences, high frequency [60–210 Hz], and low amplitude [100–200 μV]—have been linked to postoperative motor deficits and have been linked to nerve compression, traction, or intense ischemia that

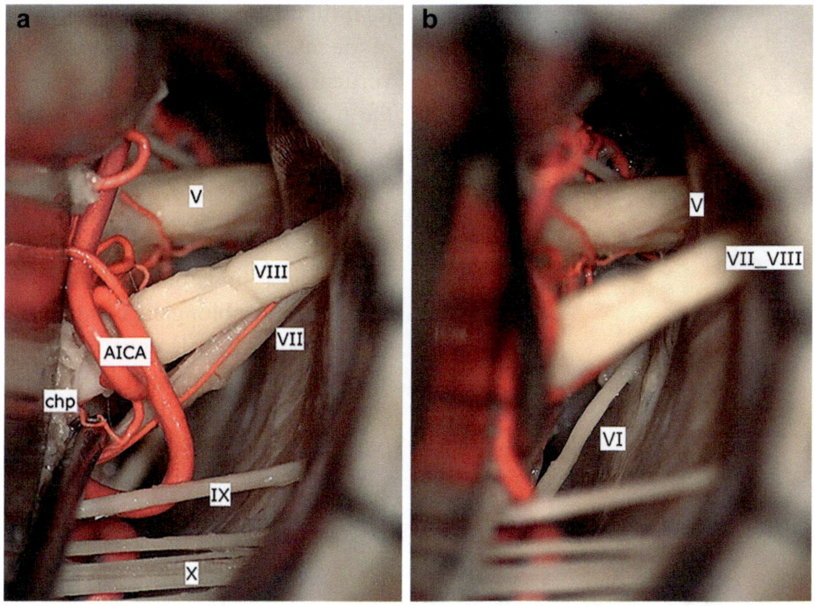

Fig. 2.6 Anatomical view of the middle compartment of the right cerebellopontine angle accessed by a retrosigmoid approach. (**a**) Superficial overview of the neurovascular elements. (V: trigeminal nerve; VII: facial nerve; VIII: vestibulocochlear nerve; IX: glossopharyngeal nerve; X: vagal nerve; AICA: anteroinferior cerebellar artery; chp: choroid plexus). (**b**) Deeper focus to show the abducens nerve (V: trigeminal nerve; VI: abducens nerve; VII_VIII: facial and vestibulocochlear nerves)

results in areas of persistent depolarization and metabolic changes. The bursts are variable-duration motor unit discharges that are triggered simultaneously by the stimulation of many nerve axons. Bone drilling, tumor evacuation, irrigation, retraction, or tumor dissection from the nerves may all result in a decline in electrical activity. Auditory potentials can be deteriorated by the spasm of tiny arterioles, particularly the internal auditory artery. Motor and somatosensory potentials are steadier.

2.3.8 Accesses

Although the retrosigmoid approach provides a broad view of the anatomy and diseases of the cerebellopontine angle, specific microsurgical techniques can be used to access a variety of specific restricted or hidden anatomical locations. The transmeatal, suprameatal, and anterolateral accesses to the brainstem are a few of these; they will be discussed in the relevant chapters.

The most useful access is the transmeatal access to the internal auditory canal to expose the intracanalicular portion of the vestibular schwannomas (Fig. 2.8). The access is based on the anatomical identification of the Tübingen line. This line facilitates the identification of the internal auditory canal on the posterior aspect of the petrosal bone during the retrosigmoid approach. This line serves as an anatomical landmark readily discernible in both cadaveric examinations and the microneurosurgical retrosigmoid approach. This observation is based on the identification of several vertical folds of the dura mater on the posterior wall of the petrosal bone, which converge cranially at a similar level, delineating a boundary above which the dura mater appears smooth due to its continuous adhesion to the bone. This line serves as a secure reference for accessing the internal auditory canal, as the removal of the dura mater above it facilitates bone drilling, granting access to the caudal limit of the internal auditory canal. The extent of bone drilling to reach the dura mater of the canal is

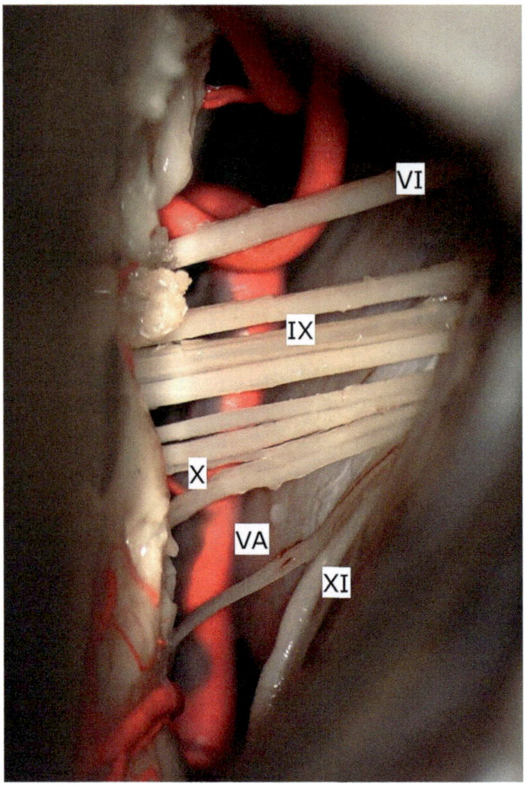

Fig. 2.7 Anatomical view of the lower compartment of the right cerebellopontine angle accessed by a retrosigmoid approach (VI: abducens nerve; IX: glossopharyngeal nerve; X: vagal nerve; XI: accessory nerve; VA: vertebral artery)

contingent upon the thickness of the posterior wall, which may consist only of solid bone or incorporate pneumatized cells.

The suprameatal access is useful to reach the upper petroclival region and the ostium of Meckel's cave, where the trigeminal root enters and, therefore, to resect some petroclival meningiomas. The suprameatal access is possible after the drilling of the suprameatal tubercle. This compact, highly variable bony protrusion obstructs access to the trigeminal nerve, prepontine cistern, and clivus, which are situated medially in the standard retrosigmoid approach. The tubercle is constrained cranially by the border of the petrosal bone, which is the location of the superior petrosal sinus. It is constrained caudally by the internal acoustic meatus, laterally by a vertical line that passes through the external border of the internal acoustic meatus, and medially by a vertical line that extends from the medial side of the trigeminal fissure, which is the medial limit of the trigeminal foramen through which the trigeminal root enters Meckel's cave.

Access to the anterolateral aspect of the brainstem allows a direct way to a great number of intra-axial lesions placed in the midbrain, pons, and medulla oblongata using the so-called safe entry zones. The safe entry to the brainstem using a retrosigmoid approach is the anterolateral sulcus in the midbrain; the peritrigeminal area in the pons and the olive in the medulla oblongata.

2.3.9 Closure

The closure of the craniotomy involves the meticulous sealing of all exposed mastoid cells. Even if there are no obvious exposed cells, surgical wax is used to close the bone. A free muscle or fascia graft is typically used to ensure that the dura mater closes airtight. A free bone flap is put back in place if one has been obtained. Surgical cement is used to fill the bone defect if the bone has been drilled to create the cranial opening. As an alternative, a titanium mesh can be affixed. All of these elements are affixed to the craniotomy's margins using tiny screws, and the dead space can be filled with bone dust and hemostatic substance. Soft tissues are closed by layers and skin with loose stitches.

2.4 Complications, Prevention, and Management

The retrosigmoid approach is a safe procedure, but there is some morbidity related to the procedure [2, 5, 10]. Cerebrospinal fluid fistula is the most common approach-related complication (refer to cases 3 and 9 in Chap. 21). Compressive dressings and postponing the removal of skin sutures can stop leaks through the incision, which are caused by the subarachnoid space communicating with the outside through the surgical

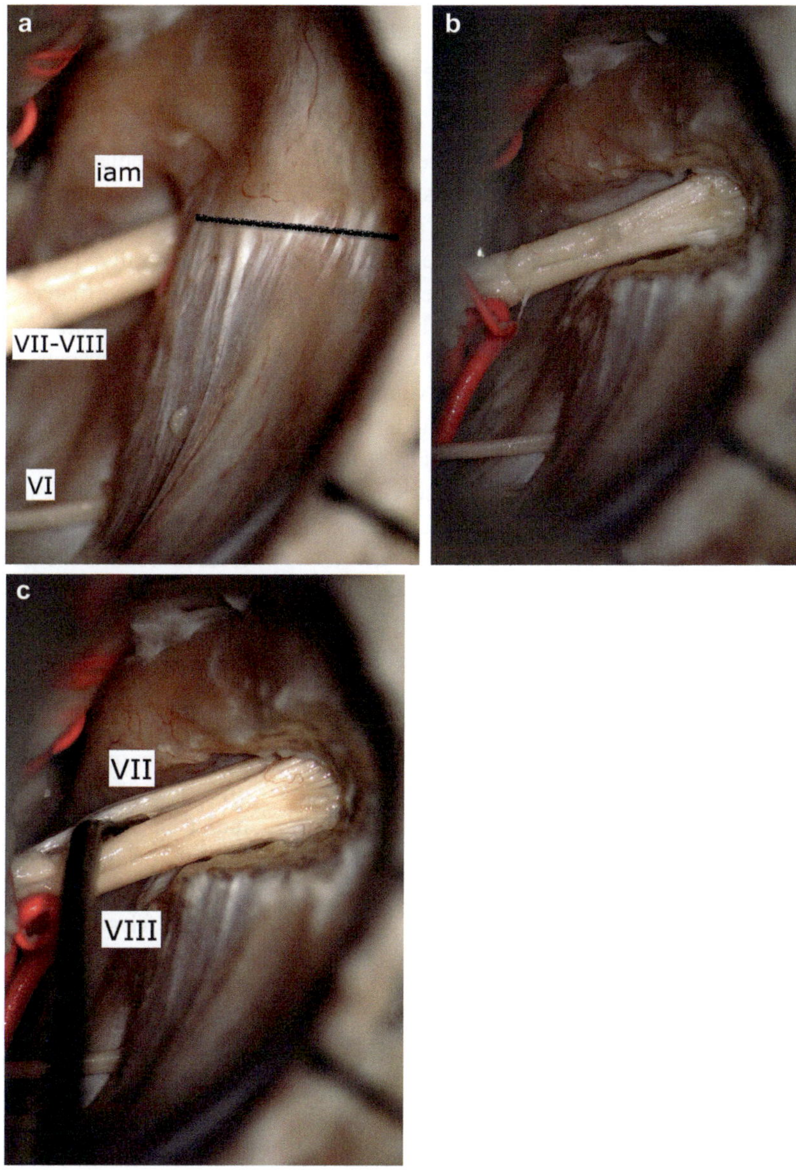

Fig. 2.8 Anatomical view of the transmeatal access in the right side. (**a**) Tübingen line; (**b**) Opening of the internal auditory canal: (**c**) Dissector separating the facial and vestibulocochlear nerves. (VI: abducens nerve; VII: facial nerve; VIII: vestibulocochlear nerve; VII-VIII: facial-vestibulocochlear complex; iam: internal auditory meatus)

wound. Rhinoliquorrhea is caused by the open cells in the middle ear communicating with the subarachnoid space. The Eustachian tube transports cerebrospinal fluid to the nasopharynx. A ruptured eardrum that permits cerebrospinal fluid to flow from the middle ear into the external ear is the cause of otoliquorrhea, which is an uncommon condition. Communication must be through the mastoid cells opened during craniotomy or through the petrosal cells opened during drilling of the petrosal bone. Because pneumatized mastoid cells vary greatly in size, location, and number, they often open during craniotomy. If the mastoid cells extend into the posterior edge of the internal auditory canal, a specific scenario is the opening of the cells during the milling of this region. Ten percent of cases result in a postoperative cerebrospinal fluid fistula. Cerebrospinal fluid fistula can be avoided by carefully closing the open cells with surgical wax or pieces of muscle or fat graft, hermetically sealing the dura mater, and performing a preoperative CT scan to evaluate the state of the cells. Treatment is based on bed rest, external lumbar drainage, and antibiotic prophylaxis.

Neurological impairments can occasionally result from obstruction of the superior petrosal venous complex. All of the veins and venous channels of the cerebellopontine angle should generally be respected to the greatest extent feasible. Certain meningiomas and the microvascular decompression of the trigeminal nerve may require the sacrifice of the superior venous complex. Due to the unpredictability of venous drainage, the clinical effects are unexpected. However, if symptoms do appear, they include headache, vomiting, and abnormalities of the cerebellum and auditory system. If a severe cerebellar infarction develops, the illness may be deadly.

Lastly, headaches are a rare but severely incapacitating side effect for individuals. Usually a unilateral suboccipital headache, it has been connected to the neck muscles' traction on the dura mater during closure. It is advised that the bone defect from the craniectomy be filled with acrylic cement or covered with titanium mesh to separate the soft tissues from the dura mater and the muscle-aponeurotic scar.

2.4.1 Other Approaches

2.4.1.1 The Presigmoid Approach

For big tumors, or to increase access to the posterior fossa, the presigmoid and retrosigmoid approaches are combined. Compared to the retrosigmoid approach, the incision made in the retroauricular skin is wider and more curved. The posterior boundary of the external auditory canal is seen when the bone is periosteally stripped, and the posterosuperior angle of Henle's spine is identified. Resecting the layer of cortical mastoid bone in a triangle that is designated below a horizontal line that crosses above the external auditory canal and behind a line that crosses behind the external auditory canal to the tip of the mastoid is known as a simple mastoidectomy. The mastoid's whole bone, which is often made up of thin septa that make up the mastoid cells, is then drilled all the way down to compact bone, which is particularly dense in the otic capsule and surrounding the semicircular canals. The facial nerve's tympanic section is located deep at the level of Henle's spine and emerges under the lateral semicircular canal. The largest and most stable mastoid cell, the mastoid antrum, is located more laterally. The fine cortical bone of the presigmoid dura mater of the posterior fossa, also known as Trautman's triangle, is drilled beneath it. The superior petrosal sinus above, the sigmoid sinus behind, the jugular bulb at the inferior angle, and the compact bone of the labyrinth in front form the boundaries of the Trautman triangle. A diamond bur is used to release the sigmoid sinus from the bone that surrounds it, which is located behind the Trautman triangle. As in the previously described lateral suboccipital craniotomy, the entire sinus is exposed, and the retrosigmoid dura mater is reached behind it. The transverse sinus is reached by the sinus's exposure in the proximal direction, whereas the jugular bulb is reached by the exposure in the distal direction. The presigmoid and retrosigmoid dura mater can be opened by either ligating and sectioning the sigmoid sinus or by leaving it intact.

2.4.1.2 The Paramedian Suboccipital Approach

This method is a limited variant that permits access to particular intrinsic or extrinsic lesions of the upper compartment of the cerebellopontine angle or the cerebellar hemispheres. The patient can be positioned either prone or semi-sitting, with the head slightly bent and turned 20° to the side of the lesion. By elevating the body and separating the shoulder, we can prevent the discomfort of these situations by using the supine position with the head tilted to the opposite side and slightly flexed. A vertical incision is made halfway between the midline and the retroauricular region. The muscles are retracted and separated from the bone plane. A trephine hole is formed 1–2 cm below the superior nuchal line, and the craniotomy is completed using a vertical saw, extending if required to the occipital foramen, midline, or retromastoid region. The dura mater is opened longitudinally a few millimeters below the transverse sinus, and the cisterna magna can be opened medially to drain the cerebrospinal fluid if necessary. A retractor is placed infratentorially over the cerebellar hemisphere directed paramedially toward the ispsilateral tectal region and posterolateral tentorial incisure. Bridging veins are coagulated and severed.

2.5 Key Messages

- *The lateral suboccipital approach, also known as the retromastoid or retrosigmoid approach, is the universal approach to the cerebellopontine angle.*
- *The approach is based on anatomical references.*
- *Complications include cerebrospinal fluid fistula, venous thrombosis, and headache.*

References

1. Bambakidis N, Megerian CA, Spetzler RF, editors. Surgery of the cerebellopontine angle. Springer Nature: Chaim; 2018.
2. Brennan JW, Rowed DW, Nedzelski JM, Chen JM. Cerebrospinal fluid leak after acoustic neuroma surgery: influence of tumor size and surgical approach on incidence and response to treatment. J Neurosurg. 2001;94:217–23. https://doi.org/10.3171/jns.2001.94.2.0217.
3. González-Darder JM, Quilis-Quesada V, Capilla-Guasch P, de Oliveira E. Abordajes neuroquirúrgicos de la patología craneal y cerebral. Barcelona: Elsevier España; 2020.
4. Koos WT, Pernezcky A. Suboccipital approach to acoustic neurinomas with emphasis on preservation of facial nerve and cochlear nerve function. In: Rand RW, editor. Microneurosurgery. St Louis: Mosby; 1985. p. 335–65.
5. Nonaka Y, Fukushima T, Watanabe K, Friedman AH, Sampson JH, Mcelveen JT Jr, et al. Contemporary surgical management of vestibular schwannomas: analysis of complications and lessons learned over the past decade. Neurosurgery. 2013;72(2 Suppl Operative):103–15; discussion ons115. https://doi.org/10.1227/NEU.0b013e3182752b05.
6. Rhoton AL Jr. The posterior fossa: microsurgical anatomy & surgical approaches. Neurosurgery. 2000;47(3 Suppl):S1–S279. https://doi.org/10.1097/00006123-200009001-00013.
7. Parkinson D. The posterior cranial fossa: microsurgical anatomy and surgical approaches. Neurosurgery. 2001;48:1196. https://doi.org/10.1097/00006123-200105000-00064.
8. Ribas G, Yasuda A, Peace D, Rhoton AL. Microsurgical anatomy of the cerebellopontine angle and its suboccipital retromastoid approaches. In: Bambakidis NC, Megerian CA, Spetzler RF, editors. Surgery of the cerebellopontine angle. Shelton: BC Decker Inc; 2009. p. 11–30.
9. Samii M, Gerganov V. Surgery of cerebellopontine angle lesions. Berlin/Heidelberg: Springer-Verlag; 2013.
10. Samii M, Matthies C. Management of 1000 vestibular schwannomas (acoustic neuromas): surgical management and results with an emphasis on complications and how to avoid them. Neurosurgery. 1997;40(1):11–21. https://doi.org/10.1097/00006123-199701000-00002.

Far-Lateral Approach

3

3.1 Introduction

The so-called far-lateral approach makes it easier to access the occipitocervical junction region and the lateral and anterior regions of the foramen magnum (Fig. 3.1). It is also known as *extreme lateral inferior transcondylar exposure* (ELITE) because it is essentially a lateral and inferior or cervical extension of the lateral suboccipital approach, anatomically centering the access on the occipital condyle, which is often partially resected. Before the intradural phase, a number of extradural extensions can be carried out from this point. The lateral advancement of approaches to the foramen magnum to provide a better angle of attack for lesions located in its anterior and anterolateral part is reflected in the far-lateral approach shown below. The approach's two main steps—the partial resection of the occipital condyle and the mobilization of the V3 segment of the vertebral artery—were first suggested by Wolfgang Seeger and Bernard Georges, respectively. Roberto Heros was the pioneer of this philosophy, arguing for an aggressive resection of the occipital bone.

Extradural and intradural lesions in the suboccipital area, foramen magnum, occipitocervical junction, and lower portion of the clivus can be treated with the far-lateral approach. The foramen magnum, especially the lower section of the clivus and the occipital condyles, can be affected by a variety of skull base lesions. Chordoma, chondrosarcoma, and metastases—which can spread to the jugular foramen or impact the odontoid or atlas—are the most prevalent tumor types. This approach is the only way to treat bone tumors that affect the distal part of the clivus and spread to one of the condyles. Meningiomas, schwannomas, or neurofibromas of the hypoglossal cranial nerve and first spinal roots, epidermoid cysts extend to the cervical region, or hemangioblastomas are the most frequent intradural tumors. Vascular diseases, such as complex dural arteriovenous fistulas at the junction of the medulla oblongata and spinal cord, arteriovenous malformations in the region, or aneurysms of the vertebral or posterior inferior cerebellar arteries, less commonly necessitate the far-lateral approach. Lastly, the far-lateral approach can be used to treat certain occipitocervical junction abnormalities that require decompression of the foramen magnum.

3.2 Anatomical Considerations

There are three stages to the surgical technique from an anatomical perspective. With a superficial, intermediate, and deep muscular plane (suboccipital muscle triangle) and close ties to the vertebral artery, the first phase is primarily muscular and finishes at the bony plane of the occipitocervical junction. The transcondylar, supracondylar, paracondylar, and infracondylar

J. M. González-Darder, *Microneurosurgery of Cerebellopontine Angle*,
https://doi.org/10.1007/978-3-032-03091-7_3

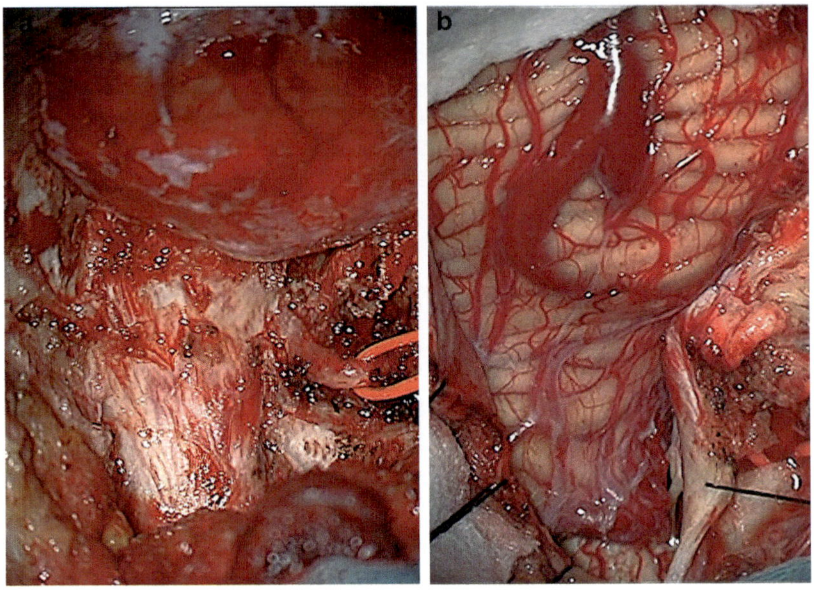

Fig. 3.1 Surgical right far lateral approach. (**a**) Picture displaying the surgical field after removal of the occipital bone and the posterior arch of the atlas. The vertebral artery has been isolated and secured with a rubber band. (**b**) Picture displaying the surgical field after opening of the dura mater, in a case of arteriovenous malformation

extensions are included in a second stage of extradural dissection. The relationships with the vascular and neurological structures are exposed during the third and last phase, which is intradural [1, 5, 8].

3.2.1 Soft Tissues and Muscle Relationships

Although most of the muscles in the area do not require individual muscle-by-muscle dissection during the surgical approach, a thorough understanding of them is useful. The flat muscles comprise the superficial layer, whereas the nuchal long muscles constitute the intermediate layer. The *trapezius muscle* medially and the *sternocleidomastoid muscle* laterally are the most superficial muscles. The external surface of the mastoid and the external segment of the superior nuchal line are where the sternocleidomastoid muscle inserts. The medial component of the superior nuchal line and the exterior occipital protuberance are where the trapezius muscle inserts. The superoexternal oblique fibers of the *splenius capitis muscle*, which stretch upward and outward from the midline, are visible between the anterior border of the trapezius muscle and the posterior border of the sternocleidomastoid muscle. Therefore, directly under the sternocleidomastoid, the splenius capitis muscle also inserts into the mastoid and superior nuchal line. Below this initial layer of flat superficial muscles, there is a group of intermediate long muscles that extend caudally to insert into the processes of the cervical and thoracic vertebrae. These muscles insert into the squama of the occipital bone between the superior and inferior nuchal lines (*major complex muscle or semispinalis capitis*) and into the mastoid process (*splenius cervicis muscle or splenius colli* and *minor complex muscle or longissimus capitis*). The posterior belly of the *digastric muscle* and the *elevator scapulae muscle* attach to the mastoid process more laterally. The occipital artery enters the field beneath the posterior belly of the digastric muscle, passing through the muscular insertions of the superior occipital line, travels above and cranially to the superior oblique muscle, and arrives at the occipital region. There is a thick layer of fibroadipose tissue that contains a rich venous plexus between the layer of the deep muscles and the layer of the intermediate muscles that have been described.

The *rectus capitis posterior major muscle* medially and above, the *obliquus capitis superior muscle* above and laterally, and the *inferior oblique muscle* below and laterally form the layer of deep muscles that make up the so-called suboccipital triangle (Fig. 3.2a). These muscles are all highly strong despite their short length and conical shape. The rectus capitis posterior major extends upward and outward to terminate behind the inferior occipital line, inserting at the apex of the axis's spinous process. From the tip of the atlas's transverse process, the *superior oblique muscle* extends to the occipital bone before terminating above and laterally at the larger posterior rectus muscle's insertions. Lastly, the *inferior oblique muscle* extends upward and outward to the posterior and inferior surfaces of the transverse process of the atlas from the lateral surface of the spinous process of the axis. Two additional short muscles of interest are located in this region. Inside the major rectus muscle's insertion, the *rectus capitis posterior minor muscle* stretches from the tubercle of the posterior arch of the atlas to the occipital bone. Lastly, the

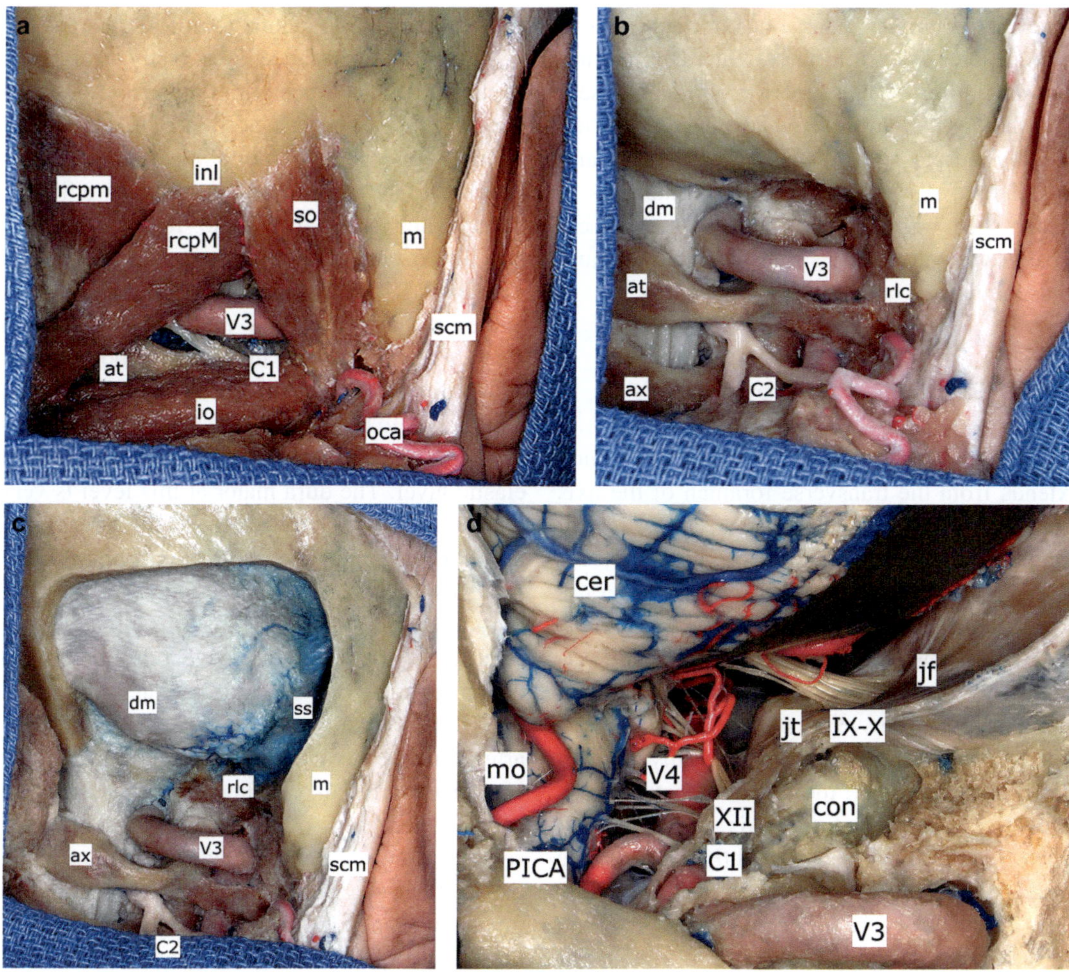

Fig. 3.2 Anatomical right far lateral approach. (**a**) Muscular triangle. (**b**) Extradural view. (**c**) Suboccipital craniotomy. (**d**) Intradural view. (IX-X: glossopharyngeal and vagal nerves; XI: accessory nerve; XII: hypoglossal nerve; C1: first spinal nerve; C2: second spinal nerve; PICA: posteroinferior cerebellar artery; V3: V3 segment of the vertebral artery; V4: V4 segment of the vertebral artery; at: posterior arch of the atlas; ax: lamina of the axis; cer: cerebellum; con: occipital condyle; dm: dura mater; inl: inferior nuchal line; io: inferior oblique muscle; jf: jugular foramen; jt: jugular tuberculum; m: mastoid process; mo: medulla oblongata; oca: occipital artery; rcpm: rectus capitis posterior minor muscle; rcpM: rectus capitis posterior major muscle; scm: sternocleidomastoid muscle; so: superior oblique muscle; ss: sigmoid sinus; rlc: rectus lateralis capitis muscle)

posterior border of the jugular foramen is related to the *rectus capitis lateralis muscle* insertion, which runs from the transverse process of the atlas to the jugular tubercle of the occipital bone. The vertebral artery and the first spinal nerve are located within the fibroadipose tissue that makes up the suboccipital triangle. This tissue also has a rich venous plexus. The muscles that make up the suboccipital triangle must be separated and retracted to reveal its contents and floor. The rectus capitis posterior minor muscle, which stays in the midline, is revealed when the rectus capitis posterior major muscle separates from the occipital bone and folds inferiorly. Lateral retraction and separation of the superior oblique muscle from the occipital muscle reveal the rectus capitis lateralis muscle, which stays in the deepest and most lateral region. The lamina of the axis is finally seen when the inferior oblique muscle separates from the atlas's transverse process and folds medially.

3.2.2 Extradural Vertebral Artery

The vertebral artery in its V3 segment—which extends from the transverse foramen of the axis until it crosses the dura mater—is the primary component of the suboccipital triangle (Fig. 3.2a, b). Here, the diameter of the vertebral artery is 4–5 mm, with the left side—referred to as dominant in this context—often being larger. The vertebral artery makes four turns over its course: the first is at the transverse foramen of the axis, where it moves vertically and laterally upward and slightly posterior; the second is between the transverse foramen of the axis and the atlas, where it goes upward and slightly anterior; the third is at the artery's exit from the atlas's transverse foramen, where it becomes horizontal and moves medially applied in the atlas's posterior arch groove; and the fourth and final turn takes place around the occipital condyle, leaving the vertebral artery at the point where it will perforate the dura mater. Over its whole length, the vertebral artery is encircled by a dense venous plexus and applied to a variety of bony and articular structures.

The vertebral artery passes lateral to the atlantoaxial joint and in front of the second spinal root in the area between the axis's transverse foramina and the atlas. Medial to the rectus capitis lateralis muscle, the vertebral artery and its venous plexus are surrounded by a genuine periosteal fibrous ring in the transverse foramen of the atlas. The artery travels through the transverse foramen of the atlas and then rests in an osteofibrous canal that is made up of the posterior occipitoatlantal ligament above and the posterior arch of the atlas groove below. The artery passes behind the occipitoatlantal joint and the atlas lateral mass in this instance. In as many as one-fifth of cases, the atlas's posterior arch groove is a real bone channel. The last portion of the vertebral artery before its entry into the dura mater is attached to the occipitocervical joint by a fibrous band called the retroglenoid ligament, which may also occasionally be found ossified. Through a dural ring that encircles it, the vertebral artery passes through the dura mater. The vertebral artery's adventitia and media layer both drastically thin out at a variable distance of around 5 mm prior to hitting the dura mater. The same is true for the media's elastic fibers and the external elastic layer. The dura mater at this level is very thick and contains between its layers the continuation of the venous plexus of the vertebral artery that surrounds it in its extracranial portion. The intradural vertebral artery has thus already separated from the surrounding venous plexus and possesses the wall structure of an intracranial artery. Additionally, there is an autonomic periarterial nerve plexus around the vertebral artery. Numerous arterial branches, both constant and variable, are released by the vertebral artery's V3 section. Between the two transverse foramina in the vertical segment of the vertebral artery, a muscular branch that is caudally associated with the second spinal nerve and a radiculomuscular branch that is cranially related to the same branch arise. Another muscle branch and the posterior meningeal artery arise in the horizontal portion of the vertebral artery. The extradural origin of the posterior spinal artery and the posterior inferior cerebellar artery can be found in addition to these constant branches.

3.2.3 First and Second Spinal Nerves

The nervous elements of the suboccipital triangle are the first and second cervical spinal nerves. The first nerve becomes extradural, accompanying the vertebral artery on its ventral side, exiting through the dural ring described above, and distributing to the deep muscles of the occipital triangle. The second nerve becomes extradural in the atlantoaxial space, with its ganglion visible behind the atlantoaxial joint. Immediately after, the nerve divides into an anterior branch and a posterior branch. The anterior branch is related to the vertical portion of the vertebral artery between the transverse foramina of the axis and the atlas and is distributed to the cervical musculature. The posterior branch runs beneath the inferior oblique muscle and then turns upward to divide into two branches, one lateral that distributes to the neck muscles and another medial, much thicker, which forms the greater occipital nerve, or Arnold's suboccipital nerve, taking an upward and medial direction, passing through the major complex muscle and the trapezius muscle to end by distributing to the skin of the occipital region. The entire suboccipital triangle is filled with fibroadipose tissue with abundant veins. At the bottom of the triangle is the occipitoatlantal membrane, which extends between the posterior surface of the foramen magnum and the posterior arch of the atlas. However, this membrane laterally leaves a wide opening through which the muscular arterial branches of the horizontal segment of V3 segment of the vertebral artery and the first cervical nerve exit.

3.2.4 Bone and Joint Relationships

The far-lateral approach has the occipito-atlantal joint (C0-C1) condyle as its bony reference target, formed between the occipital condyle and the glenoid cavity of the superior face of the lateral mass of the atlas. The occipital condyles are located in the anterolateral portion of the margin of the occipital foramen, have an oval shape and a size of about 24 mm, and are oriented forward and medially, forming an angle of 45° with respect to the sagittal plane. The occipital condyle is traversed by the anterior condylar canal or hypoglossal canal, which has a forward and outward direction forming an angle of about 45° with the sagittal plane. Above the occipital condyle, the bony margin of the occipital or foramen magnum is already present. The most anterior part of the foramen magnum corresponds to the clivus, and laterally, the jugular tubercle, a bony prominence that continues laterally with the squamous portion of the occipital bone, is located. The jugular tubercle is located between the jugular foramen above and the hypoglossal canal below. At the back of the condyle, there is a depression where the posterior condylar foramen is located, through which the emissary condylar vein passes, connecting the vertebral venous plexus with the sigmoid sinus.

The superior surface of the lateral mass of the atlas has a concave excavation that articulates with the occipital condyle. The surfaces of both occipitoatlantoid joints are contained within the surface of a theoretical sphere, which explains the wide range of motion of the occipitocervical junction. The inferior surface of the lateral mass of the atlas has a nearly flat or slightly concave articular surface oriented downward, medially, and slightly backward, which articulates with the atlas forming the atlantoaxial joint (C1-C2). The lateral masses of the atlas are connected by the posterior arch and the anterior arch. The posterior arch has a posterior tubercle where the rectus capitis posterior minor muscle is inserted, and on the side, it has a canal through which the vertebral artery runs medially from the transverse foramen. The atlantoaxial joint is complex, as in addition to the described atlantoaxial joint, the atlanto-odontoid joint must also be considered. Indeed, the odontoid process of the axis has two articular surfaces, one posterior, which is related to the transverse ligament that connects both lateral masses of the atlas, and another anterior, which is related to the inner surface of the anterior arch of the atlas. From the tip of the odontoid process extends the apical ligament, median occipito-odontoid, or suspensory ligament of the odontoid, which reaches the tip of the clivus. On both sides are the alar or lateral occipito-odontoid ligaments. On a more superficial plane, the atlas and axis are joined by powerful ligaments. The most important is the *cruciate ligament*, formed by a strong transverse part or transverse ligament, which emits ascending fibers to the inferior border of the clivus and other descending fibers that reach the posterior face of the axis. Above, the occipital and the axis are also united by the medial and lateral occipito-axoidal ligaments and, finally, by the posterior longitudinal vertebral ligament that extends from the posterior face of the body of the third cervical vertebra to the clivus, whose upper portion forms the so-called *tectorial membrane* covering the cruciform ligament. In front, the occipitocervical junction is also secured by a powerful anterior occipitocervical ligament between the clivus and the anterior arch of the atlas. Finally, the posterior occipitoatlantal ligament between the posterior margin of the foramen magnum and the posterior arch of the atlas should be considered, which is the equivalent of the yellow or interlaminar ligament of the rest of the lower vertebral segments. The joints between the condyle and the lateral mass of the atlas, between the lateral mass of the atlas and the axis, and those established between the odontoid process with the transverse ligament and the anterior arch of the atlas are of the amphiarthrodial type, with their articular cartilage, synovial membrane, and articular capsule [4, 6, 8, 9].

3.3 Far-Lateral Approach

The far-lateral approach is justified by the need to handle extradural or intradural disease in the area by gaining access to the anterior and anterolateral parts of the foramen magnum [2, 5, 8]. Prior to the dura mater opening, bone must be resected during the extradural phase in order to provide room. Hemilaminectomy of the atlas and lateral suboccipital craniotomy are included in the extent of bone excision in the cranio-caudal direction. The lateral expansion of the bone resection to reach extra- or intradurally the most anterolateral and anterior area of the foramen magnum is the unique feature of the far-lateral technique, which explains its name. This makes it easier to open the dura mater as laterally as feasible, usually medial to the vertebral artery entry, and permits wide access to the intradural pathology.

3.3.1 Patient's Position

The far-lateral approach can be performed by placing the patient in different positions, and the final choice of the operative position depends on various factors. The lateral position is laborious and must ensure good padding of the axilla and contralateral arm, or leave it below the level of the operating table. The supine position with the head turned or the table rotated about 45° is also laborious and can compromise respiratory function in obese patients. The semi-sitting position with the head turned, the semi-prone position (*park bench*), or the prone position with the table rotated about 45° are also alternatives. In any case, to facilitate access to the suboccipital and lateral cervical region, lateral flexion and contralateral flexion with contralateral rotation of the neck are necessary. However, excessive rotation of the neck can cause a large number of problems: compromise of venous drainage with cerebral edema; excessive stretching of the vertebral artery in its course between axis and atlas; and, finally, the displacement of the transverse process of the atlas that moves below the mastoid or that will hinder the exposure of the vertebral artery in the transverse foramen of the atlas. In general, prone positions favor venous bleeding from the distended venous plexuses of the muscular planes, around the vertebral artery, and through the emissary veins while protecting against gas embolism. On the contrary, the semi-sitting position favors venous return, and bleeding is less, but measures to prevent the risk of gas embolism must be increased. The surgeon positions himself laterally above the patient's shoulder, and the dissection is directed cranially, which facilitates access to the deeper regions. On the contrary, the surgeon's position at the vertex proposed by others, with caudal direction of the dissection complicates the work in the final phases of the approach.

3.3.2 Planning Before Surgery

Imaging studies allow for determining the location and extent of the lesion to preoperatively plan the approach and necessary extensions for its removal in an individualized manner. For the bone study, high-resolution computed tomography (CT) is important for three-dimensional reconstruction. The bone study allows for the identification of structural alterations that, added to those produced by the approach, will determine the need and type of postoperative stabilization. The course and bony relationships of the vertebral artery are studied with CT angiography and three-dimensional reconstruction. Preoperative digital subtraction angiography (DSA) is necessary in vascular lesions and jugular bulb tumors, and may be of interest in meningiomas or metastases to consider the indication for preoperative embolization of the arterial afferents. The external anatomical landmarks of interest are the mid-nuchal line marked by the external occipital protuberance and the spinous process of C7, the tip of the mastoid, and the prominence produced by the transverse process of the atlas on the lateral aspect of the cervical region below the mastoid. Finally, it is necessary to assess the pertinence of intraoperative neurophysiological monitoring of the long pathways and the lower cranial nerves, especially the accessory and hypoglossal nerves.

3.3.3 Skin Incision and Soft Tissue Dissection

There are several incisions recommended for this approach. We prefer the suboccipital horseshoe incision, which starts at the midline about 5 cm below the external occipital protuberance, follows the superior occipital line horizontally to the mastoid, and continues vertically about 5 cm below the tip of the mastoid towards the cervical region in front of the sternocleidomastoid muscle, reaching below and passing in front of the transverse process of the atlas, which can be easily palpated in the lateral cervical region. The skin flap is reflected downwards and medially to expose the superficial musculature with the trapezius and sternocleidomastoid muscles. The dissection of the superficial and intermediate muscle layers can be done muscle by muscle or, more comfortably, by detaching the sternocleidomastoid muscle from the mastoid and moving it forward, folding all the remaining muscles of the superficial and intermediate layers medially over the nuchal line in a block. It is advisable to leave a muscular border on the bony plane to facilitate closure. A variant is the hockey stick incision, which starts at the tip of the mastoid and ascends to follow the nuchal line to the external occipital protuberance, descending along the midline to the spinous process of C7. In this case, the skin flap and the superficial and intermediate muscles are retracted laterally alongside the sternocleidomastoid muscle, which can complicate deep access due to the interposition of the flap. In case the far-lateral approach is combined with a petrous approach, the incision can be in the shape of a C, starting in the retroauricular region and extending to the laterocervical region through the tip of the mastoid. Finally, the option of a vertical linear paramedial incision is simpler and quicker, but the thickness of the cervical musculature makes it advisable to avoid it again for working in the deep area.

Once the superficial and intermediate muscles have been retracted, the deep muscles and the suboccipital triangle are exposed. The muscles are detached and mobilized as previously described: the rectus capitis major muscle is detached from the occipital bone and folded inferiorly; the superior oblique muscle is detached from the occipital bone and folded laterally; finally, the inferior oblique muscle is detached from the transverse process of the atlas and folded medially. Removing the fibroadipose tissue that fills the suboccipital triangle reveals the vertebral artery surrounded by its venous plexus. This venous plexus and the muscular and dural branches of the vertebral artery must be completely or partially removed to mobilize the vertebral artery and identify the occipitocervical joint and thus the occipital condyle (Fig. 3.2c).

3.3.4 Vertebral Artery Mobilization

The objective of the mobilization of the vertebral artery is to identify its entry into the dura mater to remove the necessary bone to allow the opening of the dura mater immediately medial to the artery. The vertebral artery is mobilized by freeing it from the transverse foramen of the axis to the dura mater. The posterior edge of the atlas transverse foramen is milled or removed with a fine laminotome. The artery is freed from the osteofibrous canal of the posterior arch of the atlas by sectioning and removing the posterior occipitocervical ligament. The artery is followed medially to its entry into the dura mater. Finally, the artery is freed up to the transverse foramen of the axis, removing the abundant venous plexus in the area and dissecting and mobilizing the second spinal nerve. Now it is also possible to identify the lateral atlantoaxial joint. A rubber is passed under the vertebral artery, allowing it to be mobilized cranially or caudally. The mobilization of the artery is much broader if a total or partial resection of the ipsilateral half of the posterior arch or hemilaminectomy of the atlas is performed. It is necessary to recognize, and in this case respect, an extradural origin of the posterior inferior cerebellar artery.

3.3.5 Craniotomy

The exposure and resection of the occipital bone depend on the type of pathology and can be extended unilaterally from the midline to the edge of the transverse and sigmoid sinuses (Fig. 3.2c). An essential aspect is that the lateral suboccipital craniectomy always includes the radical drilling of the occipital foramen rim as far as possible, before any extradural extension, as these may be unnecessary after the radical removal of the margins of the foramen magnum. The lateral suboccipital craniotomy can also extend upwards to the transverse sinus, outwards to the sigmoid sinus, and medially to the midline. The retrosigmoid lateral suboccipital craniectomy can be extended with a presigmoid approach, associating a mastoidectomy that exposes the sigmoid sinus, the presigmoid dura mater, until skeletonizing the facial nerve canal or mobilizing it. The craniectomy is performed with a high-speed motorized vertical saw, entering and exiting through a couple of bone notches carved into the edge of the occipital foramen. Alternatively, it can be supported by a trephine hole.

The lateral retrosigmoid craniotomy is usually associated with an ipsilateral resection of the posterior arch of the atlas and, if necessary, the lamina of the axis. Laminectomy can be done in small pieces using the chisel, gouge, and laminotome. This technique is currently out of use, and laminoplasty is more frequently employed. The bone obtained during a laminectomy should be preserved for eventual use as a fusion element. Laminotomy involves the en bloc resection of the lamina and the spinous process. It is achieved with a high-speed motor equipped with a very small-diameter burr, which cuts the laminae at the level of their junction with the articular masses. This cut can also be made with a fine vertical cutting saw mounted on a pediatric craniotomy attachment. A notch is made on each side at the lower edge of the most lateral part of the plate, and it is cut in an upward direction. The lamina can also be cut gradually with a 1 mm laminotome. In this way, as many laminae as desired can be cut. Once the bone cut is completed, the interlaminar, interspinous, and supraspinous ligaments are cut proximally and distally, obtaining all the laminae in a single piece. Laminotomy is faster and safer than laminectomy, has less blood loss, and allows, if appropriate, the repositioning of the laminae at the end of the procedure to reconstruct the canal and protect its contents from cervical musculature and its scar.

3.3.6 Extradural Extensions

The pathology to be treated, whether it involves intradural or extradural lesions, determines whether other bony elements, such as the occipital condyle, jugular tubercle, joints, upper cervical laminae, and processes that are part of the atlas and axis, should be removed and to what extent. The occipital condyle can be exposed by medially and downward mobilization of the vertebral artery, and at this moment, the extradurally extended far-lateral approach described by Albert Rhoton can be performed before opening the dura mater. There are three extensions: *transcondylar*, resecting part of the occipital condyle towards the hypoglossal canal; *supracondylar*, resecting the jugular tubercle of the occipital bone towards the jugular foramen; *paracondylar*, laterally towards the jugular bulb; and finally, *infracondylar*, milling the lateral mass of the atlas towards the odontoid process.

Drilling the posterior part of the occipital condyle all the way down to the hypoglossal canal is the transcondylar extension. Once the cortical bone of the condyle is drilled, cancellous bone is found until reaching a second layer of cortical bone that corresponds to the hypoglossal canal. Given its trajectory, it is possible to remove the posteromedial third and the posterolateral two-thirds of the condyle to completely expose the posterior cortical bone of the hypoglossal canal. The resection of one-third of the condyle allows for the creation of additional space between the extradural vertebral artery and the lateral bony limit of the foramen magnum, facilitating the extradural exposure of the hypoglossal nerve, as well as increasing the intradural exposure after the opening of the dura mater. If the cortical bone of the hypoglossal canal is extensively resected, the venous plexus and the meningeal artery that run within the hypoglossal canal are exposed. These structures can be coagulated, exposing the hypoglossal nerve and ultimately enabling its mobilization to accomplish a total condylectomy, which would allow access to the inferior part of the clivus and the anterior part of the foramen magnum. Extradural and intraosseous excision are carried out as needed in cases of bone pathology affecting the clivus and foramen magnum.

Resecting the jugular tubercle, a bony prominence medial to the lateral portion of the jugular foramen and lateral to the clivus, which continues laterally with the squamous portion of the occipital bone, allows for a supracondylar extension. It is crucial to observe the relationships of the jugular tubercle with the lower cranial nerves, particularly the accessory nerve. Therefore, the nerves, although not visible as they are on the other side of the dura mater, must be protected from pressure, stretching, or the heat produced by milling. Similarly, it should be kept in mind that the jugular bulb is located in the jugular foramen, just lateral to the jugular tubercle. The extradural removal of the jugular tubercle substantially increases intradural exposure after the opening of the dura mater.

The jugular foramen can be exposed more widely thanks to the paracondylar extension. To do this, the rectus capitis lateralis muscle must be detached extradurally from the posterior border of the jugular foramen. Once the rectus capitis lateralis muscle is resected and the jugular foramen is opened medially, it is possible to identify the posterior portion of the transition between the jugular vein, jugular bulb, and sigmoid sinus, while the lower cranial nerves occupy a more anterior plane. This approach is facilitated by the prior mobilization of the vertebral artery, freeing it from the transverse foramen of the atlas, as otherwise, the surgical room is minimal.

Infracondylar extension is necessary when the lateral mass of the atlas is affected by the pathological process, when extradural access to the periodontoid region is desired, and when an intradural lesion extends to the upper cervical space. The drilling of the lateral mass of the atlas can be extended forward to the anterior arch, outward to the transverse foramen, and, if necessary, to remove the transverse process to mobilize the vertebral artery, and finally, caudally to the atlantoaxial joint. The way that provides access to the odontoid is thus opened, as the insertion of the transverse ligament in the lateral mass has been released.

3.3.7 The Dura Mater Opening

For the approach to intradural pathology, the dura mater is opened vertically, starting in the suboccipital region behind the sigmoid sinus and continuing to the cervical region just medial to the entry of the vertebral artery. If necessary, the dura mater can be opened circularly around the vertebral artery for additional mobilization. The dura mater of the posterior fossa is opened as described in the retrosigmoid approach, and both incisions are connected. Traction sutures are placed at the edges of the dura mater.

3.3.8 Cisternal Navigation

The vertebral artery immediately passes to the premedullary cistern when the dura mater is opened, granting access to the intradural space at the level of the lateral cerebello-medullary cistern. The arachnoid bands and layers are cut to expose the neurovascular anatomical structures as well as the lesion. The pathology-focused chapters include descriptions of the anatomical neurovascular relationships (Fig. 3.2d).

3.3.9 Closure

The closure of the dura mater must be watertight, and the bone from the craniotomy and laminoplasties is replaced using cranial miniplates. The dead space can be filled with free fat graft from the abdominal wall. The detached deep muscles are repositioned, and the intermediate and superficial layers are closed en bloc using the muscle rim left at the opening. It is advisable to leave a drain in the deep cervical epidural plane.

3.4 Complications, Prevention, and Management

The retrosigmoid approach is a safe procedure, but there is some morbidity related to the procedure. Complications are similar to those described for the retrosigmoid approach, particularly cerebrospinal fluid (CSF) fistula, wound complications, and neck pain. The most relevant complication is occipitocervical instability [4, 7, 9–11].

Decompression of the posterior fossa, especially the far-lateral approach, is one approach to the skull base that can result in abnormalities in the biomechanics of the occipitocervical junction. External orthoses, such as the Philadelphia collar or the Halo cranio-thoracic vest, can be used to correct the preoperative instability. Occipitocervical internal fixation is the recommended surgical treatment for postoperative instability. Biomechanical studies have measured the different levels of instability caused by the far-lateral approach's subsequent damage to the muscles, ligaments, and joint components. Resection of 50% of an occipital condyle increases flexion-extension (150%), lateral inclination (40%), and axial rotation (30%), and if more than 75% of the condyle is resected, it significantly increases atlantoaxial axial rotation. The unilateral section of an alar ligament produces a modest increase in axial rotation, but the bilateral section significantly increases all movements at the atlantoaxial level. The destruction of the atlas increases flexion-extension (50%) and lateral inclination (20%). While odontoidectomy does not enhance axial rotation, it does significantly increase translation in the sagittal axis (12.7 mm), lateral (6.7 mm), and rostro-caudal (2.0 mm). The biomechanical effect of transverse ligament resection is comparable to that of odontoidectomy. Muscle detachment and retraction, especially if intense and sustained, as often occurs in the far-lateral approach, produce ischemia and muscle devascularization, which are followed by a greater or lesser degree of muscle atrophy and fibrosis, resulting in muscle dysfunction. The muscles of the superficial, intermediate, and deep layers achieve neck extension when they act symmetrically and extension, lateral inclination, and contralateral rotation when they act unilaterally or asymmetrically. The degree of muscle damage, the extent of condyle resection, the occipitocervical and atlantoaxial joints, the odontoid, and ligament damage will all contribute to the potential instability, which will be determined by the structural destruction that is carried out. This will be in addition to any neuromuscular weakness or osteoarticular involvement that results from the pathology that is being treated surgically.

Occipitocervical stabilization with internal fixation can be done with transarticular screws or with bars attached to screws with different bony anchors (occipital squama and condyle; lateral mass of the atlas; pedicle, articular masses, or lamina of the axis, and more caudal vertebrae). In the design of the stabilization surgery, it must be considered that the far-lateral approach is unilateral, so stabilization is usually performed in a second surgical stage, keeping the patient protected until that moment with an external orthosis. Moreover, it must be taken into account that some of the bony anchorage points may have been destroyed by the pathology that necessitated the surgery or removed by the approach itself.

3.5 Other Approaches

The lateral-far approach is a versatile technique that must be specifically designed for each patient and can also be combined with other skull base approaches involving the jugular foramen, posterior fossa, retro or presigmoid of the pontocerebellar angle, petrous bone, and even subtemporal [3].

3.6 Key Messages

- *The far-lateral approach is the approach to the occipitocervical region, being useful for lesions around the foramen magnum and extending from the cerebellopontine angle to the spine.*
- *The approach is based on anatomical references.*
- *The most relevant complication is occipitocervical instability.*

References

1. Arnautović KI, al-Mefty O, Pait TG, et al. The suboccipital cavernous sinus. J Neurosurg. 1997;86:252–62. https://doi.org/10.3171/jns.1997.86.2.0252.
2. Babu RP, Sekhar LN, Wright DC. Extreme lateral transcondylar approach: technical improvements and lessons learned. J Neurosurg. 1994;81:49–59. https://doi.org/10.3171/jns.1994.81.1.0049.
3. Baldwin HZ, Spetzler RF, Wascher TM, et al. The far-lateral-combined supra- and infratentorial approach: clinical experience. Acta Neurochir. 1995;134:155–8. https://doi.org/10.1007/BF01417683.
4. Benke M, Yu WD, Peden SC, et al. Occipitocervical junction: imaging, pathology, instrumentation. Am J Orthop (Belle Mead NJ). 2011;40:E205–15.
5. González-Darder JM, Quilis-Quesada V, Capilla-Guasch P, de Oliveira E. Abordajes neuroquirúrgicos de la patología craneal y cerebral. 2nd ed. Barcelona: Elsevier España; 2020.
6. Joaquim AF, Ghizoni E, Rubino PA, et al. Lateral mass screw fixation of the atlas: surgical technique and anatomy. World Neurosurg. 2010;74:359–62. https://doi.org/10.1016/j.wneu.2010.05.010.
7. Lopez AJ, Scheer JK, Leibl KE, et al. Anatomy and biomechanics of the craniovertebral junction. Neurosurg Focus. 2015;38:E2. https://doi.org/10.3171/2015.1.FOCUS14807.
8. Rhoton AL Jr. The posterior fossa: microsurgical anatomy & surgical approaches. Neurosurgery. 2000;47(Suppl 3):S1–S279. https://doi.org/10.1097/00006123-200009001-00013.
9. Rocha R, Safavi-Abbasi S, Reis C, et al. Working area, safety zones, and angles of approach for posterior C-1 lateral mass screw placement: a quantitative anatomical and morphometric evaluation. J Neurosurg Spine. 2007;6:247–54. https://doi.org/10.3171/spi.2007.6.3.24.
10. Steinmetz MP, Mroz TE, Benzel EC. Craniovertebral junction: biomechanical considerations. Neurosurgery. 2010;66(Suppl 3):7–12. https://doi.org/10.1227/01.NEU.0000366109.85796.42.
11. Vender JR, Rekito AJ, Harrison SJ, et al. The evolution of posterior cervical and occipitocervical fusion and instrumentation. Neurosurg Focus. 2004;16:E9. https://doi.org/10.3171/foc.2004.16.1.10.

4 Cerebellopontine Angle, Vestibular Schwannoma, and Retrosigmoid Approach

The cerebellopontine angle is an anatomical area of the cranial posterior fossa where the vestibular nerve schwannoma grows and is microsurgically removed by the neurosurgeon through a retrosigmoid approach. This simple chained reasoning is true in most cases, but not all tumors of the cerebellopontine angle are vestibular schwannomas; not all schwannomas of the cerebellopontine angle arise from the vestibular nerve; and not all vestibular schwannomas are removed by a retrosigmoid approach, nor is the retrosigmoid approach used exclusively for the removal of vestibular schwannomas. However, it is true that from a historical point of view, these three elements—anatomy, pathology, and approach—have been intimately related.

4.1 Cerebellopontine Angle

The concept of the cerebellopontine angle, outlined as a well-defined anatomical area with its own pathology associated with a distinctive symptomatology and which posed a need for a specific neurosurgical approach for its resolution, was built over a few decades, from the beginning of the nineteenth century to the mid-twentieth century [2–7]. By the early twentieth century, it was established that tumors existed in the cerebellopontine angle, originating extracerebellarly and possibly associated with the acoustic nerve. During that period, the cerebellopontine angle anatomical region was referred to by a different designation. In 1903, Ziehen referred to this area with the term *angulus pontis*, *receptaculum pedunculorum,* or *acoustic region*. Hartmann, in 1902, named the tumors of those areas as *acoustic-cerebellar recess tumors* or simply *recess tumors*, and French authors referred to them as *tumeurs cerébello-protubérantiélles*. Nonetheless, it was Henneberg and Koch in 1902 who originally employed the word we presently utilize for tumors of the cerebellopontine angle, in German *Kleinhirnbrtickenwinkeltumor*. At this time, it was common to use the term *acoustic neuroma* for any tumor that grew in the cerebellopontine angle, assuming they originated in the acoustic nerve. The anatomical concept was poorly defined, with both the *angle* and *corner* used to describe the intersection of the cerebellar flocculus, the middle cerebellar peduncle, and the medulla oblongata olive, a description that became logically warped with the growth of a tumor in the region. In 1917, Harvey Cushing (1869–1939) distinctly articulated the conceptual characteristics of *cerebellopontine angle tumors* for the first time, emphasizing the necessity to differentiate intracerebellar tumors from extracerebellar tumors within the posterior fossa. Furthermore, he specified that cerebellopontine

J. M. González-Darder, *Microneurosurgery of Cerebellopontine Angle*,
https://doi.org/10.1007/978-3-032-03091-7_4

tumors should be considered separately, with those originating from the acoustic nerve being particularly notable [2].

4.2 Vestibular Schwannoma

There are numerous uncertainties around the timing of the initial description of a vestibular schwannoma. The deficiency in understanding arises from the necessity of reading ancient medical texts through the lens of contemporary knowledge of that era. A lesion is nowadays defined as a vestibular schwannoma when it fulfils specific histological, diagnostic, and clinical criteria; however, the definitive identification of these criteria in historical medical writings is challenging and subject to the reader's or researcher's biases and interests. In numerous instances, there exist peculiar clinical descriptions that may evoke the present clinical symptomatology of a substantial vestibular schwannoma; nevertheless, there is often an absence of histopathological analysis, and when such analysis is available, the diagnosis is characterized by ambiguous and outdated nomenclature. The descriptions of the limited cases that underwent surgery are equally ambiguous. Consequently, the numerous observations gathered possess solely speculative significance.

To evaluate this matter, we have examined the bibliographic data and references presented by Cushing in his 1917 monograph, *Tumors of the Acoustic Nerve and the Syndrome of the Cerebellopontile Angle*, taking into account the author's rigor and the closer chronological proximity of his historical review while seeking these original bibliographic sources, now in the public domain and available online, to verify the information provided [2]. The initial point is the identification of vestibular schwannoma as a distinct tumor lesion. The most valuable historiographical sources are several cases documented before Cushing, accompanied by illustrations or photographs of the patient's necropsy, clearly depicting the lesion situated at the cerebellopontine angle. Based on this criterion, the earliest definitive description of a cerebellopontine angle tumor potentially corresponding to a vestibular schwannoma can be attributed to Jean Cruveilier (1835–1842). In his work, *Anatomie Pathologique du Corps Humain*, which comprises 200 annotated plates illustrated by Antoine Chazal, he meticulously delineates the clinical progression and autopsy findings of a benign fibrous tumor arising from the posterior aspect of the petrosal bone, exerting pressure on the cerebellum and pons. He notes the loss of the facial and acoustic nerves at their entry into the petrosal bone, where the internal auditory canal is enlarged (Fig. 4.1) [1]. Subsequently, many British, German, and French authors also document such cases in autopsy examinations.

The understanding of the disease's natural history, coupled with an increase in pathological findings and the emergence of brain localization ideas at the close of the twentieth century, prompted several authors to advocate for the diagnosis of vestibular schwannoma in living patients based on clinical symptoms. In this regard, all evidence suggests that Oppenheim was the first to ascertain that a patient had a vestibular schwannoma, publishing his findings in 1890 alongside a diagram illustrating the tumor's location and an illustration of the necropsy specimen, which unequivocally confirms its correspondence to a vestibular schwannoma (Fig. 4.2) [9]. In 1900, von Monakow presented a novel instance of clinical description and anatomic–clinical association derived from necropsy, wherein he delineated and illustrated a lesion in the right cerebellopontine angle, which he termed an *acoustic neuroma* (Fig. 4.3) [11]. The histological diagnosis of vestibular schwannoma was established in 1900; nevertheless, for many years, there were uncertainties in differentiating it from meningioma, leading to the usage of various terminologies to describe this tumor from a histopathological perspective. In 1907, Murri published a patient's detailed medical history in a lengthy paper and asked, "But where is the tumor?" concluding that "As a consequence of these considerations we are fined to a diagnosis of a tumor situated in the left half of the cerebellum, comprising the left side of the pons and bulb." The patient underwent surgery days later,

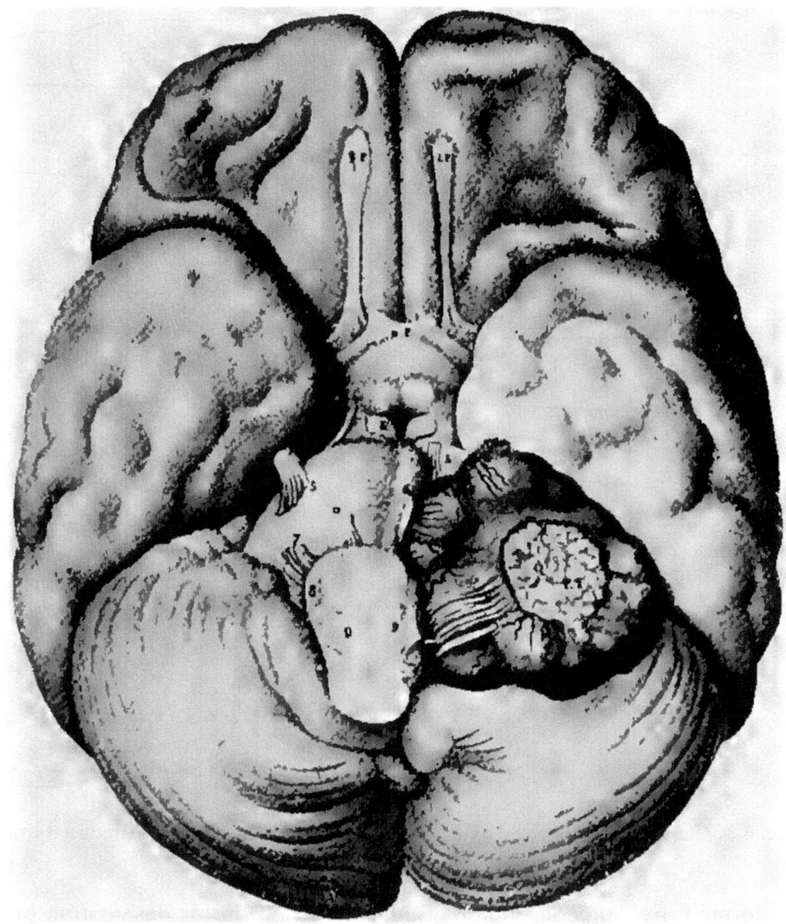

Fig. 4.1 Cerebellopontine angle tumor (left side, in place). (Reproduced from Cruveilhier [1])

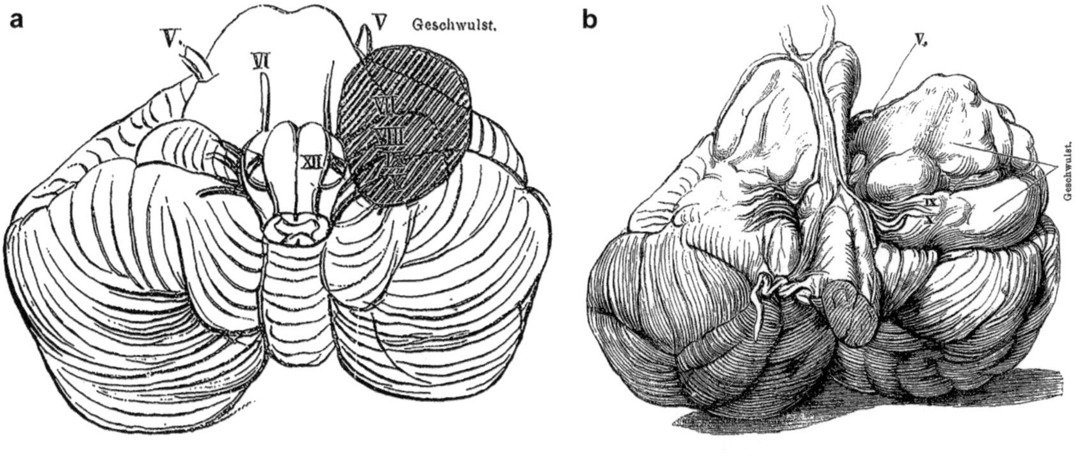

Fig. 4.2 Cerebellopontine angle tumor (left side), in place (**a**) and anatomic drawing (**b**). (Reproduced from Oppenheim [9])

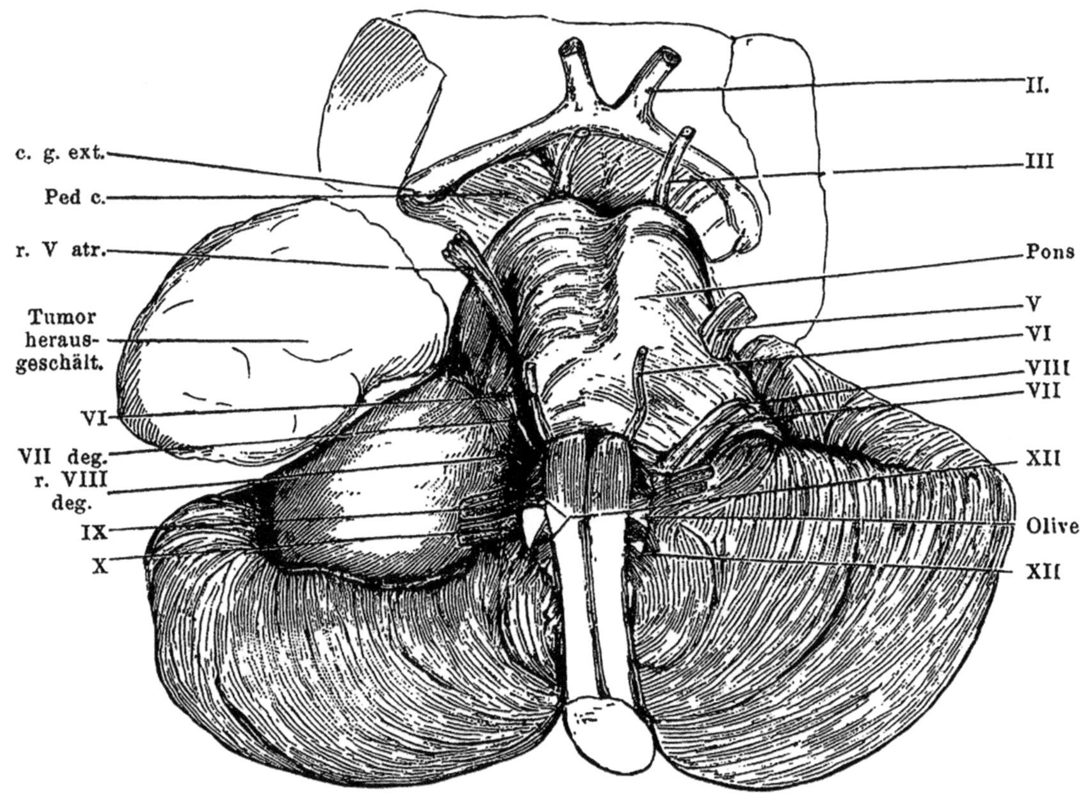

Fig. 4.3 Cerebellopontine angle tumor (right side), turned cranially. (Reproduced from Von Monakow [11])

performed by surgeon Guido Bendani, who excised a portion of a fibrosarcomatous tumor from the left cerebellum via craniotomy, as complete resection was unfeasible. One month post-surgery, the patient remained alive and in improved condition compared before the intervention [8].

The third milestone following the lesion's identification and diagnosis pertains to the initial documented effort at surgical resection. During that period, the suggestion for a potential surgical resection and the planning of the surgical intervention were formulated following the surgeons' examination of necropsies of deceased patients with the lesion remaining either wholly or partially intact. The tumor's association with the branches of the basilar artery, as demonstrated in these necropsy studies, prompted Cushing to liken the tumor's position at the cerebellopontine angle to a fence during the bloody Battle of Gettysburg in the American Civil War, resulting in his designation of the cerebellopontine angle as the "bloody angle," a term that has persisted for decades.

During the final decade of the nineteenth century, instances of surgical intervention for lesions clinically identified as vestibular schwannoma are documented; however, a series of perplexing circumstances arise: the tumor is absent during surgery, the patient succumbs during the procedure, the tumor appears to be embedded within the cerebellum, the pathological diagnosis is more consistent with meningioma (endothelioma), alongside other cases of partial resection yielding ambiguous outcomes, such as the patient being "better than worse" post-operation. In his 2013 review of the history of cerebellopontine angle surgery, Madjid Samii [10] examined the authorship of the inaugural definitive surgery for a vestibular schwannoma and concluded that Victor Horsley was the first surgeon to execute a complete resection of a vestibular schwannoma in 1905 at the National Hospital in London, despite the patient being significantly impaired due to an ischemic lesion likely resulting from injury to the anterior inferior cerebellar artery. Subsequent years saw an enhancement in expertise about the surgical management of vestibular schwannomas. Tumors were clinically detected and confirmed using standard skull X-rays, utilizing specific radiological projections and comparisons with the ostensibly healthy side to reveal the enlargement of the internal auditory meatus. During the International Congress of Medicine in London in 1913, the preeminent surgeons of the era showcased their surgical outcomes, which were marked by an intolerable mortality rate: Horsley from London reported 15 cases with a 67% mortality rate; Eiselberg from Vienna presented 17 cases with a 77% mortality rate; and Krause from Berlin documented 31 cases with an 84% mortality rate.

4.3 Surgical Approaches

4.3.1 Unilateral Retrosigmoid Approach

The tumor excision was performed by these pioneering surgeons using a unilateral suboccipital retrosigmoid approach. Nonetheless, other possibilities existed based on the surgeons' tastes and inventions. The intervention may be conducted in one or two parts; the initial stage involves craniotomy, followed by the second stage, which entails tumor resection a few days later. Anesthesia may be classified as local or general, with the available options at the time being ether or chloroform. The patient was often seated, with an assistant securely holding and positioning the patient's head for optimal visibility for the surgeon. The skin incision typically resembled a horseshoe or hockey stick form. Following the elevation of the nuchal muscles and their detachment from the occipital bone along the skin incision line, craniotomy was performed in two methods. The first method involves creating a burr hole or trephination, which is subsequently widened with bone gouge forceps until the dural sinuses are revealed. The second involves performing an osteoplastic craniotomy by creating burr holes connected with a Gigli saw or bone forceps until the base of the bone flap may be shattered. The occipital bone was bent caudally toward the soft tissues to which it was attached. Upon the incision of the dura mater, the tumor was excised by attempting to enucleate it en bloc with the finger. Each physician possessed distinct tastes and implemented enhancements in subsequent surgeries informed by cadaver studies or prior surgical experiences. Feodor Krause advocated for local anesthesia, osteoplastic craniotomy, and two-stage surgery. Nonetheless, there were numerous arguments both in favor of and against this strategy. A significant difficulty with the surgical techniques of the era was the hemorrhaging of soft tissues, bone, and brain, which, coupled with unreliable anesthesia, often resulted in acute intraoperative or postoperative shock, accounting for nearly all perioperative mortality. Soft tissue hemostasis was attained with the local injection of saline or cocaine solution or by the application of a hemostatic cuff, which was not particularly suitable for this surgical field. Hemostasis was ultimately attained by packing the wound with hemostatic gauze, which was left protruding from the depth of the wound. A common strategy to avert hemorrhage and ensuing hemodynamic shock was to increase the speed of the tumor excision, whereas some surgeons proposed a two-stage resection approach.

The unilateral approach facilitated a more expedited surgical procedure compared to the bilateral approach. The unilateral approach necessitated the exposure of the lower border of the transverse sinus and the medial border of the sigmoid sinus through an osteoclastic craniectomy using a gouge or an osteoplastic craniotomy with interconnected holes created by a saw or bone forceps, allowing for extension in the caudal and medial directions as required by the surgeon. Surgeons of that era noted the challenge of the lateral suboccipital approach due to the bone's thickness, leading to a propensity for medial craniotomy extension, which positioned the posterior aspect of the petrous bone at a distance, necessitating consistent digital access to the tumor via the cerebellum, usually partially removed. Anatomical and necropsy studies indicated that the rational method for reaching vestibular schwannoma was to explore, via digital palpation, the interval between the posterior surface of the petrosal bone and the cerebellum. This was only achievable when the approach was like the relatively regular cranial nerve neurectomies conducted at that time, particularly advantageous when the patient was seated; however, the presence of a tumor occupying the cerebellopontine angle obscured all visibility. Krause delineates and fabricates spatulas that facilitated the separation of the cerebellum in pursuit of the cranial nerves and advocates for medial separation of the cerebellum during the resection of cerebellopontine angle tumors, which were enucleated en-bloc using a broad curette when the tumor was firm, and the tumor was diminished with an innovative suction apparatus when the tumors were pliable [7]. Additional overarching issues that obscured the prognosis and were well recognized by contemporary surgeons included the constraints in topographic diagnosis, the characteristics of the lesion, and the patients' poor overall health, with many presenting at a low level of consciousness or following a prolonged period of functional and general decline. Fraenkel's 1904 paper candidly illustrates the challenges faced by surgeons of the era in addressing vestibular schwannomas. He concludes that the "clinical syndrome of cerebellar angle tumor is well defined and that the diagnosis can be made with virtually complete certainty, that since it is a benign non-infiltrating tumor it can be surgically enucleated, but that its deep and close-to-vital-centers location imposes serious difficulties for a safe removal." Ultimately, Fraenkel advocates for a unilateral approach using a finger inserted between the posterior aspect of the petrous bone and the cerebellum to reach the tumor, which can be removed "without compromising the vital centers" [6]. Krause detailed the excision of two cerebellopontine angle tumors by the same technique employed for vestibulocochlear nerve neurectomy, performed via a unilateral osteoplastic craniotomy, with the patient in a seated position and the head stabilized by an assistant who adjusted it as required. The method is thoroughly delineated in his book *Surgical Operations of the Head*, initially published in German in 1906 (Fig. 4.4) [7].

4.3.2 Trans-Labyrinthine Approach

As early as 1904, Panse advocated for the removal of tumors via the petrosal bone, notwithstanding the inevitable loss of hearing capacity in all patients. Facial nerve paralysis was likewise an obligatory consequence at that time. Nonetheless, the principal objections to this method included the limited depth and narrowness of the surgical field, the unavoidable postoperative cerebrospinal fluid fistula leading to meningitis in most patients, and the absence of any indirect cranial decompression for the patient. The petrosal approach was concurrently linked with the lateral suboccipital approach, necessitating the ligation and division of the sigmoid sinus.

4.3.3 Cushing's Bilateral Suboccipital Approach

Concurrent with the aforementioned techniques, certain surgeons employed a bilateral suboccipital approach, notably advocated and meticulously delineated by Cushing in his 1917 treatise on vestibular schwannomas [2]. The bilateral suboccipital approach may be performed via osteoplastic or osteoclastic craniotomy. The initial procedure involved a broad horseshoe incision, ligation of both occipital arteries, and the creation of three trephine openings—one medial and two lateral—above the torcula and transverse sinuses, which were connected using a Gigli saw or bone forceps and extended caudally with bone forceps toward the posterior margin of the foramen magnum. A substantial musculoskeletal and cutaneous flap was lifted in a caudal direction (Fig. 4.5). This was a significant method for that era, serving as the initial step before the incision of the dura mater and excision of the tumor. Conversely, osteoclastic craniotomy was executed via a

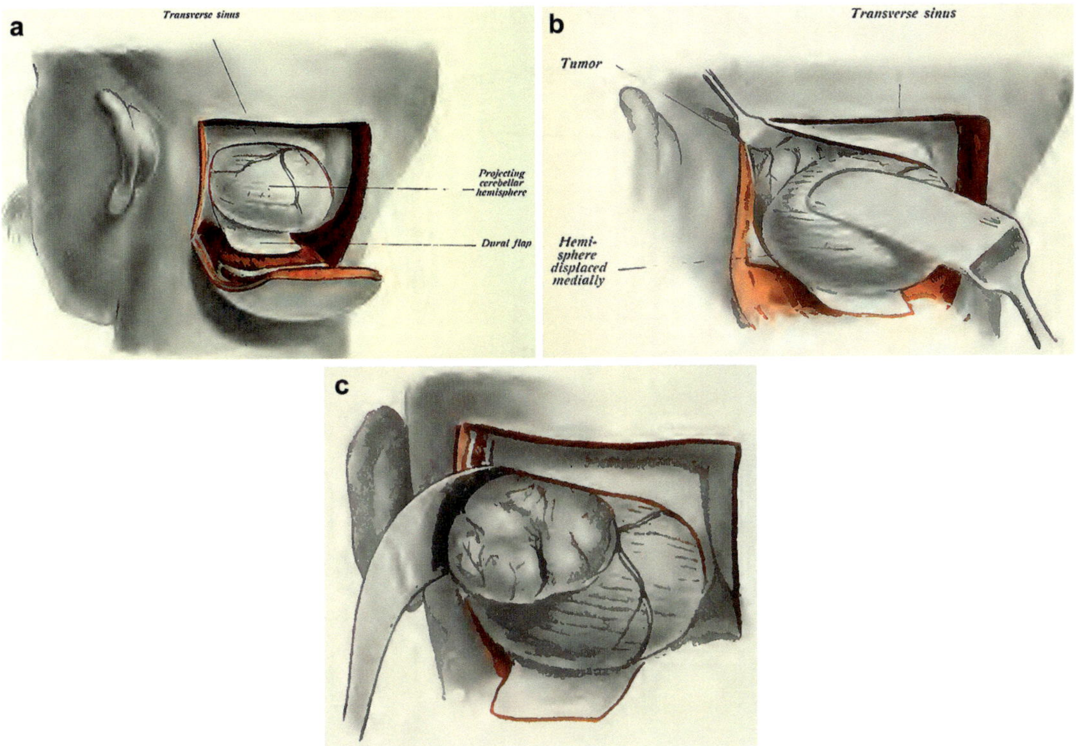

Fig. 4.4 Unilateral suboccipital osteoplastic approach. (**a**) Exposure of the left cerebellar hemisphere. (**b**) Exposure of the tumor. (**c**) Enucleation of the tumor with a large dull curette. (Reproduced from Krause and Heymann [7])

T-incision, meticulously debriding the occipital bone subperiosteally from the neck muscles, which were laterally retracted. The bone was excised using gouge forceps from two trephine apertures created in both occipital bones, extending in all directions for the requisite distance (Fig. 4.6). At that time, it was a challenging method, yet less sanguinary, more adaptable, and swifter than osteoplastic craniectomy.

Cushing asserted that the bilateral osteoclastic method possessed numerous advantages compared to the unilateral technique, which he detailed in his publication.

The bilateral method facilitates the simultaneous exploration of both cerebellar hemispheres, which is advantageous due to the unreliability of topographic diagnosis at that time. It also facilitates the contralateral displacement of the unaffected cerebellar hemisphere during the examination of the afflicted side. It facilitates the swift regulation of intracranial pressure through the excision of the bony margins of the foramen magnum and the posterior arch of the atlas, enabling the caudal opening of the dura mater significantly beyond the limitations of the osteoplastic approach, thereby promoting the decompression of the medulla oblongata. He contends that osteoclastic craniotomy is significantly less hemorrhagic and expedited compared to osteoplastic craniotomy, hence allowing tumor excision to be performed in a single surgical session. Ultimately, osteoplastic craniectomy provides the patient with significant and swift cranial decompression post-surgery, particularly in cases of incomplete excision or as a palliative intervention. At this juncture, Cushing proposed a ground-breaking approach that enhanced the safety of the procedure, as he highlighted the complications associated with complete resection (via digital or instrumental enucleation) of the tumor, asserting, “I doubt very much, unless some more perfected method is devised, whether

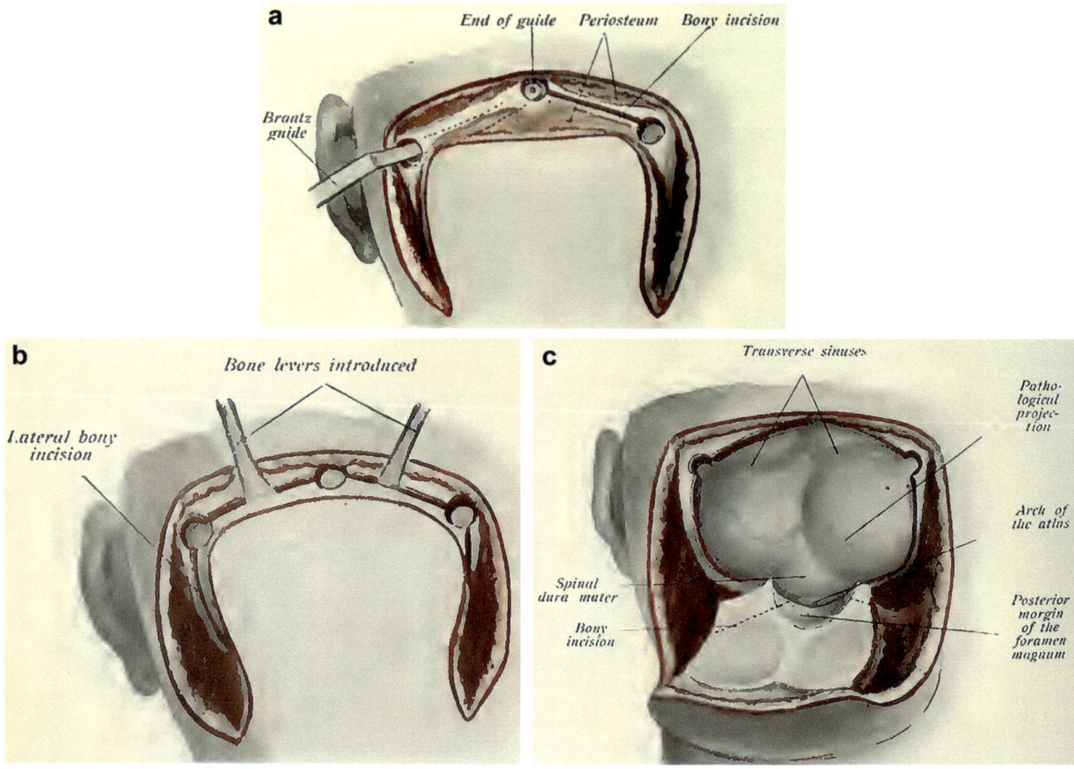

Fig. 4.5 Bilateral suboccipital osteoplastic approach. (**a**) Three drill holes were made; on the left, the dura is being separated, and on the right, the bony incision is completed. (**b**) Prying up the bone plate. (**c**) The cerebellar fossae of the occipital bone turned down. (Reproduced from Krause and Heymann [7])

one of these lesions can with safety be totally enucleated." Following a series of arguments against complete resection, he concluded, "Owing to these considerations, we have come in recent years to abandon the idea of an extirpation, and the usual custom is to bluntly incise or even to bisect the lesion after it has been as fully exposed as possible, and by an intracapsular procedure to enucleate as much of the contents as possible." For this internal decompression, he advocates for opening the capsule and intratumorally emptying it with a spoon while retaining the tumor capsule in situ. Upon completion of the decompression, the closure was executed in layers, with the dura mater remaining open, and a plaster bandage was applied encompassing the cranial, cervical, scapular, and upper thoracic regions. Through this method, he realized a significant reduction in operative mortality, which reached 15.4% in his cohort of 29 operated patients, largely attributing this outcome to the patients' poor health status at the time of surgery.

4.3.4 Dandy's Unilateral Suboccipital Approach

Confronted with this surgical treatment protocol centered on patient safety, as formulated by Cushing, and involving subtotal excision via a bilateral suboccipital approach, the complaint over the years was the nearly unavoidable recurrence of the tumor. Due to Walter Dandy's personality and the intricate dynamics of the relationship between Cushing and Dandy, it was Dandy who instituted and ultimately realized a paradigm shift in the surgical management of vestibular schwannoma through complete resection via a unilateral suboccipital approach. Dandy

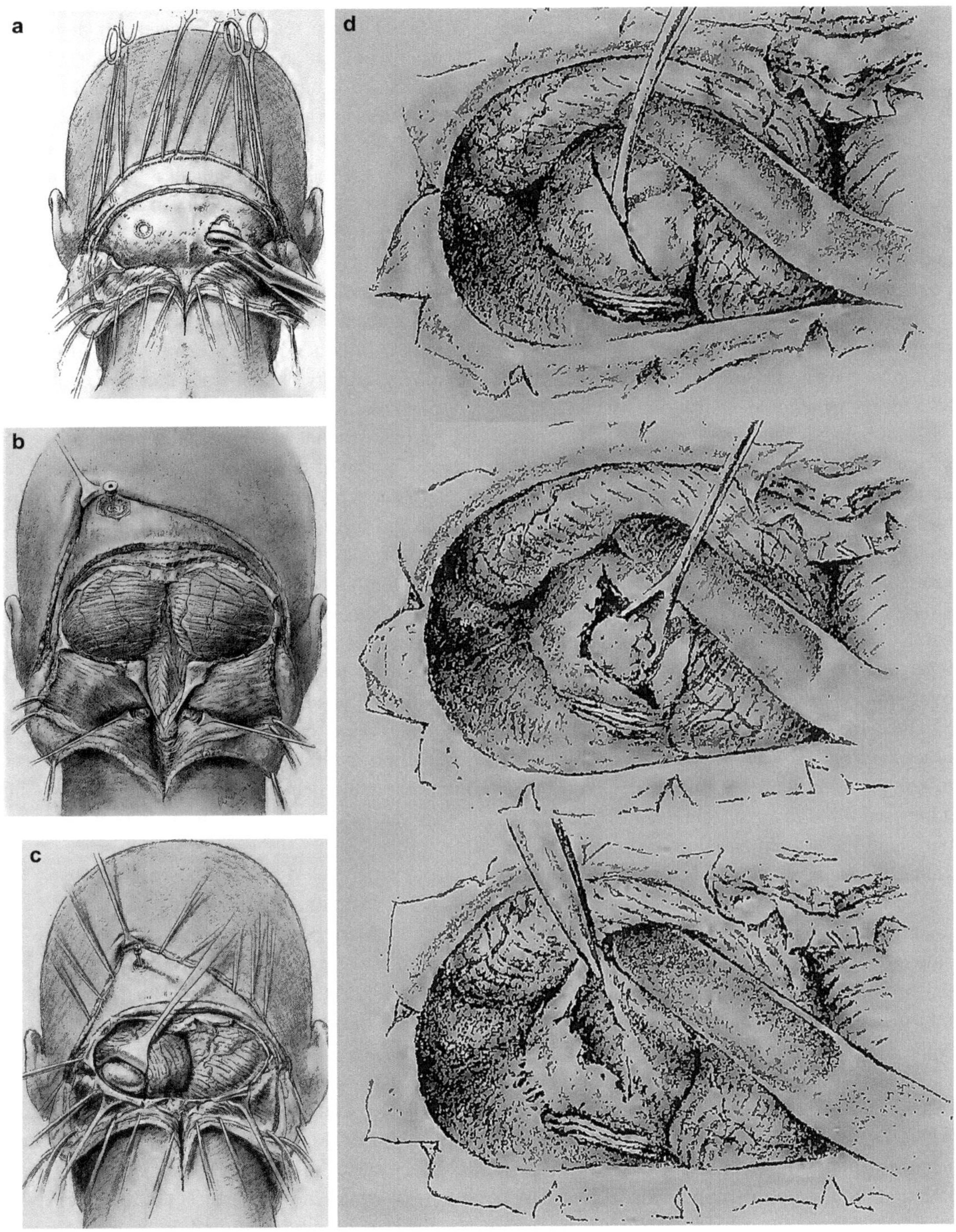

Fig. 4.6 Bilateral suboccipital osteoclastic approach and internal decompression of a vestibular schwannoma. (**a**) Denudation of the suboccipital region; exposure of the foraminal field by reflection of flaps; primary bone opening; (**b**) Extreme foraminal herniation (pressure cone) in a case in which tension was so great as to necessitate removal of the laminae of the atlas and carrying the dural incision to the atlas. (**c**) Exposure of encysted fluid within the arachnoid overlying a tumor. (**d**) The method of treating the tumor by intracapsular enucleation. (Reproduced from Cushing [2])

disseminated his reflections, technical improvements, refinements, and results in three scientific papers published in 1925, 1934, and 1941, consistently highlighting the advantages of his strategy in comparison to Cushing's [3–5].

Dandy asserts that the bilateral approach does not enhance the outcomes in the intracranial surgical domain relative to the unilateral approach, and that it is more exhausting for the surgeon and poses greater risks for the patient. He asserts that the methodology should mirror that employed for neurectomies of the trigeminal, vestibular, and glossopharyngeal nerves, which were performed to address trigeminal neuralgia, Ménière's disease, and glossopharyngeal neuralgia as standard surgical interventions at that time. The issue of elevated intracranial pressure caused by the tumor must be addressed, for which he recommends a ventricular puncture in cases of large tumors, as the ventricle is consistently dilated, along with the evacuation of cerebrospinal fluid from the cisterna magna and, when necessary, resection of the cerebellar hemisphere portion overlying the tumor. It commends the utilization of Avertin (tribromoethanol) as an adjunct to other anesthetics. The issue regarding the safety of preoperative awareness of tumor laterality was addressed through advancements in clinical diagnosis and the implementation of preoperative air ventriculography, a technique invented by Dandy in 1918. The tumor was completely excised following internal decompression with a spoon and subsequent extracapsular dissection of the residual tumor. Dandy reports a perioperative death rate of 10.87% among 46 patients who underwent full tumor excision, with no recurrences observed throughout the follow-up period. He clarifies that all his mortality cases were patients who were operated on while comatose, asserting that it is impossible to preserve the lives of these individuals due to permanent damage to their brain stems.

Subsequently, Dandy expresses concern with the functionality of the facial nerve, which he has had to sever in all instances except for two patients with small tumors. Dandy methodically conducted accessory-facial nerve neurorrhaphy for facial nerve recovery between 10 days and 2 weeks post-tumor excision. It emphasizes the significance of the tumor segment that persists within the internal auditory canal and its contribution to recurrences, prompting him to consistently excise this intracanalicular segment of the tumor so that "... it is necessary to chisel away the outer lip of the acoustic foramen in order to gain access to this hidden retreat of the final fragments of the tumour."

The academic rivalry between Cushing and Dandy culminated in the predominance of Walter Dandy's strategy, which was adhered to until the late twentieth century. The advent of noninvasive diagnostic means, in particular magnetic resonance imaging, has allowed a safe diagnosis of vestibular schwannoma and allows its early diagnosis and follow-up by imaging in cases where a microsurgical resection is not performed. Additionally, the emergence of stereotactic radiosurgery has enabled nonsurgical intervention for vestibular schwannoma. Significant advancements in surgical techniques have also occurred, including the adoption of the surgical microscope, bipolar coagulation, high-speed motors, ultrasonic aspiration, and microsurgical instrumentation, alongside notable modifications to the lateral suboccipital retrosigmoid approach.

4.3.5 Modern Retrosigmoid Approach

Historically, the evolution of neurosurgical access to the cerebellopontine angle has demonstrated that, despite the current universal adoption of a unilateral retrosigmoid approach, significant variability exists among neurosurgeons, surgical teams, and academic institutions. Numerous technique variations are published, many of which merely resurrect outdated proposals that can only be identified through a thorough examination of the scientific literature.

Our proposal for cranial opening via the retrosigmoid approach to the cerebellopontine angle is predicated on the following principles: supine positioning; a subtly curved retro-auricular skin

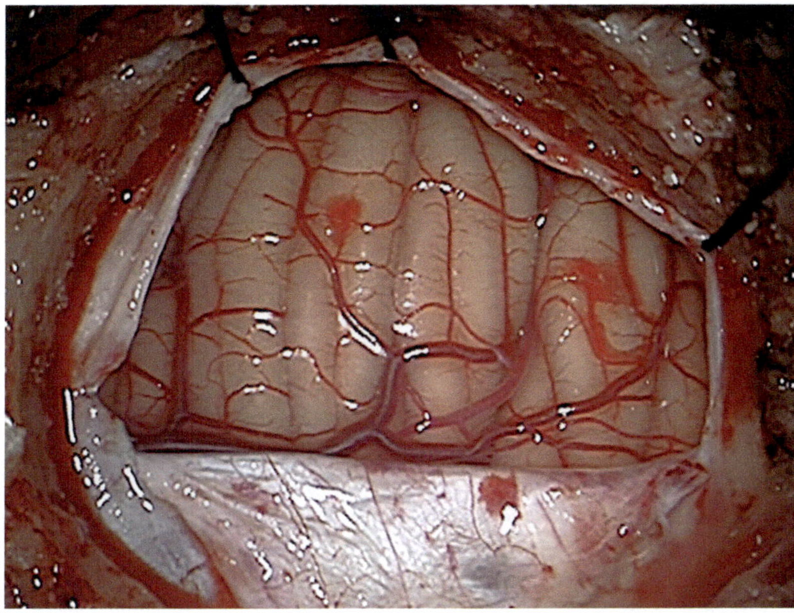

Fig. 4.7 Intraoperative image depicting the contemporary right retrosigmoid craniectomy and dural incision, positioned caudal to the transverse sinus and medial to the sigmoid sinus

incision; an initial perforation of the bone utilizing a 4–6 mm drill to access the dura mater with a high-speed motor; expansion of the opening with a 4 mm drill to delineate the lower third of the transverse sinus cranially, the border of the sigmoid sinus laterally, and extending medially and caudally as required; and, ultimately, a dural incision of approximately 2–3 mm along the trajectory of the dural sinuses (Fig. 4.7). Currently, certain authors advocate for the retention of a semi-seated position during cerebellopontine angle surgery, contending that this posture facilitates the caudal displacement of the cerebellar hemisphere upon accessing the cerebellopontine angle and mitigates the accumulation of cerebrospinal fluid, serum, blood, and bone debris at the base of the surgical field. Some suggest a curvilinear incision encircling the ear, which facilitates the positioning of soft tissue retractors and expands the angle of access to the deepest region of the operative field. Bone excision may be performed using a trephine hole centered on the asterion, occasionally supplemented by additional holes, with bone being excised between them using a vertical saw along the contours of the dural sinuses, facilitating repair of the bone defect without necessitating any cranioplasty procedure. It has recently been suggested to extensively skeletonize the dural sinuses to enhance dura retraction and broaden the approach angle (*extended retrosigmoid approach*). The asterion can be challenging to identify in the surgical field, prompting some to advocate for the utilization of a neuronavigator to accurately position the craniotomy.

The dura mater is closed using loose nonabsorbable sutures, incorporating a segment of dura mater substitute. Subsequently, the open mastoid cells are sealed with bone wax, and the bone defect is filled with surgical cement, helping to occlude the mastoid cells, secured with low-profile miniplates. Some practitioners weakly approximate the dura mater without replacements and fill the cranial defect with bone sawdust taken from the aperture, or they cover the bone window with a titanium mesh secured by low-profile miniplates. Alongside these minor adjustments that do not substantially alter the retrosigmoid approach, recent years have witnessed the use of expanded approaches (far-lateral approach), reintroduction of cerebellopontine angle endoscopy, and also minimally invasive techniques according to the principles of keyhole surgery.

4.4 Key Messages

- *The vestibular schwannoma is the most common tumor of the cerebellopontine angle, and the retrosigmoid approach is the predominant technique utilized by neurosurgeons for microsurgical resection, establishing a significant correlation among the cerebellopontine angle, vestibular schwannoma, and retrosigmoid approach.*
- *Since the early twentieth century, when neurosurgery first developed, significant breakthroughs have been achieved in the contemporary microneurosurgical technique treating vestibular schwannomas of the cerebellopontine angle.*
- *The bilateral suboccipital approach and internal tumor decompression, pioneered by Harvey Cushing, significantly reduced surgical mortality rates during that period.*
- *Walter Dandy enhanced the unilateral suboccipital approach, resulting in reduced mortality and increased rates of total tumor excision.*

References

1. Cruveilhier J. Anatomie pathologique du corps humain. Paris: B Baillière; 1835–1842.
2. Cushing H. Tumors of the nervus acusticus and the syndrome of the cerebelopontile angle. Philadelphia/London: BW Saunders; 1917.
3. Dandy WE. An operation for the total removal of cerebellopontile (acoustic) tumors. Surg Gynec Obst. 1925;41:129–48.
4. Dandy WE. Removal of cerebellopontile (acoustic) tumors through a unilateral approach. Arch Surg. 1934;29:338–44.
5. Dandy WE. Results of removal of acoustic tumors by unilateral approach. Arch Surg. 1941;42:1026–33.
6. Fraenkel J, Hunt J, Woolsey G, et al. Contributions to the surgery of neurofibroma of the acoustic nerve with remarks on the surgical procedure. Ann Surg. 1904;40:293–319.
7. Krause F, Heymann E. Surgical operations of the head. New York: Allied Book Co; 1919.
8. Murri A. An address upon diagnosis of tumour of the cerebellum. Lancet. 1897;30:291–5.
9. Oppenheim H. Über mehrere Fälle von endocraniellem Tumor, in welchen es gelang, eine genauere Lokaldiagnose zu stellen. Berl Klin Wochenschr. 1898;27:38–40.
10. Samii M, Gerganov V. Surgery of cerebellopontine angle lesions. Berlin/Heidelberg: Springer-Verlag; 2013.
11. Von Monakow C. Über Neurofibrome der hinteren Schädelsgrube. Berl Klin Wchnschr. 1900;37:721–4.

5 Vestibular Schwannoma

5.1 Introduction

Vestibular nerve schwannoma is the most prevalent and characteristic tumor of the cerebellopontine angle. It constitutes approximately 10% of all cerebral tumors, comprises one-third of posterior fossa tumors, and represents over 90% of cerebellopontine angle tumors. Consequently, it is the quintessential tumor of the cerebellopontine angle, and numerous neurosurgeons have devoted their expertise solely to its microneurosurgical management. The fight has been immense because of the benign tumor's growth within a confined volume, complicated by intricate anatomical linkages and significant risks of neurological morbidity.

While the histopathology of vestibular schwannomas is comparable, they differ in location, growth pattern, and size. Imaging diagnosis is straightforward and reliable, exhibiting minimal variability, and their clinical manifestations are often dull and unremarkable compared to the prominence of imaging diagnostics. The size of the lesion dictates the varying treatment recommendations, the challenges of microneurosurgical intervention, and the associated morbidity and mortality of the procedure [4, 20]. We have structured the analysis of vestibular schwannoma according to its dimensions. In this chapter, we will outline the general characteristics of vestibular schwannoma, followed by a detailed examination of small-sized, medium-sized, and large and giant tumors in subsequent chapters, concluding with a distinct analysis of cystic schwannomas.

5.1.1 History of the Neurosurgical Management of the Vestibular Schwannoma

The argument between Walter Dandy and Harvey Cushing concerning the treatment of these tumors in neurosurgery is legendary. Cushing's proposed partial resection resulted in a significant recurrence risk among survivors, while Dandy advocated for complete excision to prevent the recurrence of a histologically benign tumor. Moreover, Dandy's surgical approach was considerably less aggressive, as the excision was performed via a unilateral suboccipital approach. Dandy validated the potential diagnosis of hydrocephalus linked to substantial tumors and identified the tumor's location by ventriculography, which he developed. Consequently, years later, this treatment approach was implemented to counteract Cushing's dogmatism, resulting in a postoperative mortality rate reduction to 10%, albeit at the expense of hearing loss in all patients and facial paralysis in 95% of them. Subsequently, the trans-labyrinthine and middle fossa techniques were developed, focusing on the anatomical and functional preservation of the facial nerve. The treatment's evolution had various

J. M. González-Darder, *Microneurosurgery of Cerebellopontine Angle*,
https://doi.org/10.1007/978-3-032-03091-7_5

challenges until a significant advancement emerged with Theodore Kurze's introduction of the surgical microscope in 1957, followed by otologist William House's treatment of vestibular schwannoma through trans-labyrinthine and middle fossa approaches a few years later, using a microsurgical technique. Due to these advancements, postoperative mortality in the 1960s decreased to around 5%.

Nonetheless, numerous advancements have been achieved since that time, enhancing the outcomes of microneurosurgical intervention for vestibular schwannoma, hence diminishing morbidity, mortality, and recurrence rates. The diagnostic field has evolved from conventional X-ray with targeted projections and petrosal bone tomography to computed tomography (CT), developed by Godfrey Hounsfield in 1972, and magnetic resonance imaging (MRI), which was introduced for neurological diagnosis in the end of the twenty century. Alongside the surgical microscope, bipolar coagulation, the renowned Midas Rex high-speed motor, and the ultrasonic aspirator were incorporated into the neurosurgical repertoire in the 1980s, while microneurosurgical instruments and devices have undergone continuous enhancement. Electrophysiological investigations, which served as the foundation for detecting vestibular schwannomas for decades, were introduced into the operating room in the 1990s, subsequently abandoned for diagnostic purposes, and repurposed for intraoperative monitoring of cranial nerves and long sensory, auditory, and motor pathways (SSEP, BAEP, and TcMMEP). Ultimately, advancements in anesthetic and postoperative care have also exerted a considerable influence. In accordance with the idea of continuous progress, it is important to emphasize the contribution of neurosurgeons who are primarily focused on treating this condition, exemplified by Madjid Samii and his protégés in Germany. Ultimately, an enhanced comprehension of the surgical microneuroanatomy of the cerebellopontine angle, particularly through laboratory investigations utilizing fixed and injected anatomical specimens while simulating operating room conditions in accordance with Albert Rothon's philosophy, culminates in a series of measures that have augmented the possibilities for complete resection, concomitant with elevated rates of preservation of the involved cranial nerve functions, accompanied by minimal mortality. Furthermore, VS is a surgical domain of interest in otology, employing particular techniques or integrating with neurosurgery methods. The advent of stereotactic radiosurgery, developed by Lars Leksell in Sweden during the 1960s and later used extensively, now concludes the available therapeutic options for vestibular schwannomas [4, 11, 20].

5.1.2 Semantic Considerations

Vestibular nerve schwannoma is also referred to as *acoustic neuroma* in English, and this interchangeability occurs in other languages as well. In German, the terms *Vestibularisschwannom* or *Akustikusneurinom* are used indistinctly, and the same is in Spanish, where the terms *Neurinoma del acústico* and *Schwannoma del nervio vestibular* are used. Outdated names for this tumor are peripheral glioma, peripheral neuroglioma, neuroschwannoma, schwannoglioma, or neuroma, and it should not be conflated with neurofibroma. The term *vestibular schwannoma* has been selected for this book, referring to a benign tumor arising from the Schwann cells of the vestibular segment of the eighth cranial nerve.

5.2 Anatomical Considerations

Vestibular schwannoma initially fills the internal auditory canal and subsequently expands to the cerebellopontine angle cisterns, progressively occupying the cerebellopontine angle while engaging all anatomical structures of the auditory canal and the cerebellopontine angle as it develops [13, 19]. Ultimately, the tumor compresses the brainstem, middle cerebellar peduncle, cerebellum, and fourth ventricle in accordance with its dimensions. In each chapter, we shall delineate the specific microneurosurgical anatomy pertinent to the microneurosurgical management of each tumor category based on its size.

5.3 Pathology

Vestibular schwannoma is a benign neoplasm arising from Schwann cells that envelop nerve fibers and constitute their myelin sheath. Consequently, its origin in cranial nerves, particularly in the vestibular nerve, takes place outside the designated *root entry zone*, a region several millimeters from the apparent exit of the nerve from the brainstem, where the myelin sheath is supplied by oligodendroglia rather than Schwann cells [15, 20].

5.3.1 Histopathology

Schwannomas develop as well-defined masses with rounded boundaries, encapsulated to isolate the tumor from the arachnoid and pia mater. Their surface may be crossed by irregularly organized veins and tiny arterioles that branch from the anterior inferior cerebellar artery (AICA) as it courses along the surface or originate from the dura mater encasing the internal auditory meatus. Histologically, two distinct zones are identified, termed Antoni A and Antoni B, each exhibiting a markedly different histological pattern. The distinctive structure of schwannoma was delineated over a century ago by Danish pathologist Nils R.E. Antoni, forming the foundation for the histological diagnosis of schwannoma. In his 1917 monograph, Harvey Cushing characterized these tumors as exhibiting a combination of fibrous regions where nuclei are typically arranged in palisades or whorls (Antoni A zones), alongside areas of a loose reticular architecture (Antoni B zones), often accompanied by adipose or hyaline alterations. Antoni A regions exhibit elevated cellularity characterized by fusiform nuclei. Occasionally, the cells aggregate in a manner that the nuclei create palisades, resulting in interspersed regions devoid of nuclei. This configuration is referred to as Verocay bodies. Antoni B zones are characterized by hypocellularity and disorganization, accompanied by an infiltration of macrophages. The Antoni A and B zones alternate inside the tumor, exhibiting a gradual disruption of the cellular architecture in the transition from the Antoni A zone to the Antoni B zone, accompanied by an increase in macrophages. In these transitional zones, the tumor activity of the cells in the Antoni A region is heightened. The cellularity of the Antoni B zone is sparse, disordered, and diverse, comprising tumor Schwann cells, macrophages, and other inflammatory cells, including T lymphocytes. These cells are abundant in lysosomes and contain myelin remains in their cytoplasm, indicating phagocytic activity. Schwannomas may exhibit regions of degeneration, fatty and hyaline metaplasia, or cysts of varying sizes. The tumor exhibits limited vascularization with an uneven pattern, occasionally displaying hyalinized arteries and perivascular hemosiderin deposits. Malignant transformation is rare. The tumor is encased by a delicate capsule composed of several layers of collagen. The primary immunohistochemical markers that differentiate schwannoma are the S100 protein and the SOX10 protein, both of which identify Schwann cells. Tumor cells also exhibit positivity for VEGF (*Vascular Endothelial Growth Factor*). There may also be positivity for EMA (*Epithelial Membrane Antigen*) and for markers of reticulin or collagen IV in the tumor cells. The limited neurofilaments of the viable axons within the vestibular nerve, encased by the tumor, can be distinctly identified. There exist two diagnostic variations of schwannoma. Cellular schwannoma is distinguished by hypercellularity and the majority or exclusive presence of an Antoni A pattern, lacking well-defined Verocay bodies. Melanotic schwannoma is an uncommon, highly pigmented tumor that has melanotic characteristics and carries a risk of malignant development.

5.3.2 Molecular Biology

Sporadic vestibular schwannoma results from the loss or mutation of the *NF2* tumor suppressor gene located on chromosome 22q12. The inactivation of the *NF2* gene is not present in all sporadic vestibular schwannomas; thus, in 40% of instances, the tumorigenesis may be attributed to alternative epigenetic pathways, as changes in numerous genes have been identified in schwannoma. Conversely, mutations in the *NF2* gene have been identified in 50% of spontaneous meningiomas and in several ependymomas. The *NF2* gene comprises 17 exons and encodes a protein known as merlin (moesin-ezrin-radixin-like) or schwannomina. The merlin protein exists in two forms: the phosphorylated form, which lacks tumor suppressor action, and the nonphosphorylated form, which triggers a metabolic pathway that leads to cancer suppression. This suppressor role is executed via many intracellular and extracellular routes. The inhibitory influence of merlin on cell proliferation is triggered by increased cell density, hence regulating the aberrant development of the associated cell lines. Consequently, when modifications arise in this pathway or there is aberrant phosphorylation of merlin, it fosters an environment conducive to unregulated cell proliferation and the subsequent formation of a tumor. The merlin protein is additionally implicated in various mechanisms that regulate cell development. Patients with neurofibromatosis type 2, exhibiting bilateral schwannomas, demonstrate identical genetic abnormalities and disruptions in the regulation of cell proliferation control. The etiology of *NF2* gene mutation remains unclear. While ionizing radiation is recognized as an oncogenic factor in sporadic vestibular schwannoma, no correlation has been established with nonionizing radiation, specifically exposure to electromagnetic fields produced by mobile phones, which have seen widespread use in recent decades.

Neurofibromatosis type 2 is an autosomal dominant condition resulting from a mutation in the *NF2* gene on chromosome 22q12, which produces the neurofibromin 2 protein, also known as merlin or schwannomina. The diagnosis is established either through the identification of the gene mutation or by fulfilling a set of clinical criteria, the most significant of which is the presence of bilateral vestibular schwannomas (Fig. 5.1). Neurofibromatosis type 2 is characterized by an inherited mutation in the *NF2* gene, following a Mendelian autosomal dominant pattern with high penetrance, resulting in over a 95% likelihood of the patient developing bilateral vestibular schwannomas. Nevertheless, approximately 50% of individuals with neurofibromatosis type 2 lack a familial history of the disorder or detectable gene mutations, suggesting these cases arise from de novo mutations accompanied by loss of heterozygosity. In 25% of cases, segmental or regional mosaicism occurs, affecting only a specific area of the patient's body due to the change of the *NF2* gene. If the genetic abnormality is inherited, it will affect all the organism's cells, but if the alteration is the consequence of a mutation during advanced stages of embryonic development, it will affect part of the organism's cells. Should the mutation happen early, bilateral vestibular schwannomas may manifest; con-

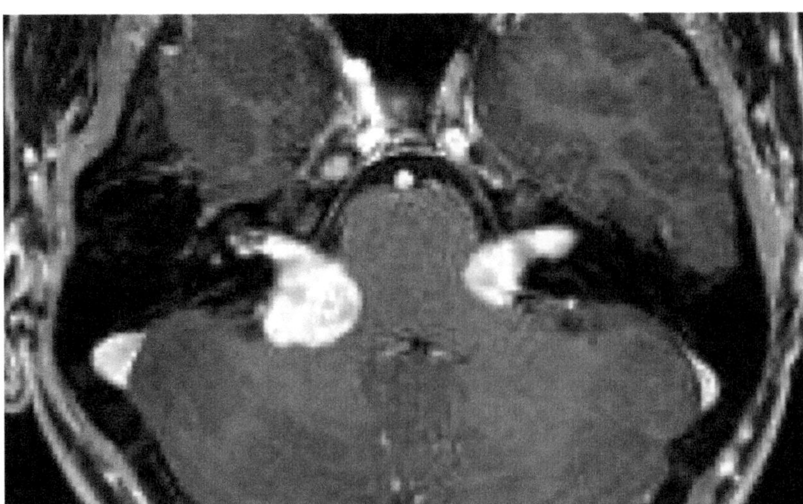

Fig. 5.1 Bilateral vestibular schwannomas in a patient with neurofibromatosis type 2

versely, if the mutation occurs later, the patient may present with a unilateral vestibular schwannoma and an ipsilateral intracranial neoplasm of a different type, typically a meningioma.

From a genetic perspective, various subtypes of neurofibromatosis type 2 can be identified:

- Familial neurofibromatosis type 2: the mutation is inherited from a parent; it impacts all of the patient's cells; it affects 50% of the kids; it constitutes approximately 50% of the cases.
- Sporadic neurofibromatosis type 2: the mutation arises at conception (prezygotic mutation in the parental germ line); it impacts all of the patient's cells; it affects 50% of the progeny; it constitutes around 20% of cases.
- Mosaic neurofibromatosis type 2: the mutation arises postconception (mutation in postzygotic cells); it impacts only a subset of the patient's cells, contingent upon the mutation's occurrence; it influences a portion of the germ cells, resulting in a probability of less than 50% for offspring inheritance; it also affects certain somatic cells, elucidating the varied clinical manifestations among patients, where mutations may be undetectable in standard genetic analyses (lymphocytes) and only identifiable in tumor cells and specific clinical presentations; it constitutes the remaining 30% of cases.

Neurofibromatosis type 2 must not be confused with *neurofibromatosis type 1*, wherein the tumor suppressor gene *NF1* on chromosome 17 is mutated, leading to a distinctly different clinical presentation. While the majority of individuals with neurofibromatosis type 2 exhibit bilateral vestibular schwannomas upon diagnosis, there exists a significant possibility that an individual with neurofibromatosis type 2 and a solitary unilateral vestibular schwannoma may subsequently acquire a contralateral one after many years. In the pediatric population, the interval until the emergence of the second vestibular schwannoma is reduced.

Finally, *schwannomatosis* should be contemplated, a condition characterized by several schwannomas and meningiomas, although vestibular schwannomas are uncommon. Schwannomatosis is a hereditary disorder caused by mutations in at least two tumor suppressor genes (*SMARCB1, LZTR1*) on chromosome 22; however, the presence of a change in the *NF2* gene appears to be requisite for disease manifestation. There exist hereditary instances exhibiting an autosomal dominant pattern of low penetrance, with several sporadic cases.

5.3.3 Growing Patterns

Schwann cells, from which the tumor originates, envelop the nerve fibers in the distal segment of the cranial nerve roots before they escape from the intracranial area. Between this section and the root entrance zone, where oligodendrocytes supply the myelin sheath, is the *Obersteiner–Redlich transition zone*, an area of several millimeters where the central myelin sheath given by oligodendroglia is substituted by that of Schwann cells. The origin of schwannomas is more frequently found in the transition zone than in the distal zone of the nerve, which accounts for the tumor's relatively distal positioning along the nerve root, as the transition zone is situated at a variable distance from the nerve's exit from the brainstem. The genesis of the tumor in the vestibular nerve rather than the cochlear nerve remains unknown. Traditionally, it was asserted that vestibular schwannomas predominantly arise from the superior vestibular nerve; however, evidence suggests that the tumor occurs with equal frequency in both segments of the nerve. The true origin of the tumor can only be definitively established in very small tumors, typically identified solely through targeted autopsy research.

Consequently, the tumor typically initiates in the segment of its intracanalicular trajectory from which it expands towards the cerebellopontine angle cistern and, to a lesser degree, towards the fundus of the internal auditory canal. A minor proportion of tumors originate in the cisternal segment of the nerve root and do not possess an intracanalicular component, while, in rare instances, some may arise from the brief segment of the nerve extending from the fundus of the internal auditory canal to the vestibule or semicircular canals, exhibiting intra-labyrinthine growth. The typical tumor that arises in the internal auditory canal extends into the cistern and, despite its soft consistency, can alter the internal auditory canal and meatus, resulting in their expansion or erosion due to its generally gradual growth.

The average growth rate of vestibular schwannoma is sluggish, although it is not uniformly consistent across time, exhibiting phases of accelerated growth and intervals of dormancy. When evaluating the growth rate of indolent tumors, it is essential to consider the measurement technique and the interval between assessments. MRI pictures and software measurements possess a measurement error, which may mislead the viewer into believing that a tumor's size is consistent with the previous scan, despite evident differences when compared to an earlier examination. Certain tumors have rapid proliferation alongside swift symptom progression, exemplified by cystic schwannoma. Others may have spontaneous involution attributed to extensive necrosis resulting from a vascular disorder. Consequently, average growth rates should be interpreted with caution, as it is unfeasible to ascertain the specific behavior of an individual tumor. The acknowledged average growth rate for solid tumors is 1–2.5 mm annually, but for cystic tumors, it is 3.5 mm each year.

Schwannoma is a benign, slowly proliferating tumor. The proportion of tumors exhibiting active growth is contingent upon the duration of follow-up. Imaging studies demonstrate a significant variety, revealing that 5–75% of tumors exhibit growth. The growth rate varies, averaging 1–2 mm annually for slow-growing species and 2–4 mm for fast-growing species. Nevertheless, due to the nonlinear nature of growth, forecasting the future size of a tumor cannot be accurately derived from the average growth documented in the literature or from the established growth of an individual tumor. No indicators of quick development exist; nevertheless, data indicate that smaller tumors tend to grow more frequently than larger ones, and it is a well-established fact that cystic tumors exhibit more rapid growth than solid tumors.

5.3.4 Dimensions at Diagnosis

While the statistical distribution curve of vestibular schwannoma sizes in the general population remains inadequately defined, it is evident that the sizes of tumors identified in population studies at the time of diagnosis, when symptomatic, or when treated with otological, microneurosurgical, or stereotactic radiosurgery techniques, exhibit significant variability. It may be observed that tumors managed with microsurgery tend to be larger, those treated with stereotactic radiosurgery are often smaller, averaging 25 mm, while those under observation are the smallest.

The dimensions of the vestibular schwannomas are the metrics most closely associated with clinical complaints, surgical complexity, and treatment outcomes. The assessment of tumor size has been extensively studied to identify the most accurate and pertinent measurement technique, focusing on the distinction between linear and volume measurements. In this context, various classifications have been established by surgeons, primarily focused on the microneurosurgical management of this condition. Aside from stereotactic radiosurgery treatment, where lesion volume is a critical metric, microneurosurgery classifications rely on assessing the greatest linear diameter of the tumor, measured across any of the three axes. Schwannomas can be categorized by size into small (<15 mm), medium (15–25 mm), large (25–40 mm), and giant (>40 mm), as well as by grades (I: 1–10 mm; II: 11–20 mm; III: 21–30 mm; IV: 31–40 mm; V: >40 mm). Intracanalicular tumors are defined as small, measuring less than 10 mm, which corresponds to the average length of the internal auditory canal. The Hannover or Matties and Samii classification, published in 1997, is one of the most well-recognized classifications due to the influence of its authors and is based exclusively on the criterion of tumor growth extent. The classification delineates five degrees of extension that can be associated with the linear measures of the lesion, encompassing both the intracanalicular and cisternal segments (Fig. 5.2):

- Grade T1: Pure intracanalicular tumor (measuring less than 11 mm in length and 8 mm in width).
- Grade T2: Intra-extrameatal tumor, devoid of contact with the brainstem (about 21 mm in length and 15 mm in width).
- Grade T3: A cisternal tumor that occupies the cerebellopontine angle cistern; however, it does not make contact with the brainstem (T3a), or that reaches the brainstem without causing compression or displacement (T3b), measuring approximately 31 mm in length and 23 mm in width.
- Grade T4: Tumor that compresses the brainstem (T4a) or severely compresses the brainstem (T4b), displacing the brainstem or the fourth ventricle and associated with hydrocephalus (about 45 mm in length and 38 mm in width).
- Grade T5: A large tumor that spreads past the midline.

The Koos classification of 1998 categorizes tumors based on size into four distinct degrees.

- Grade I: Minor intracanalicular neoplasm (according to grade T1 of Samii).
- Grade II: Small tumor with protrusion in the cerebellopontine angle, although without contact with the brainstem (corresponding to grade T2 of Samii).
- Grade III: Tumor that fills the entire cerebellopontine angle cistern without displacing the brainstem (equal to grade T3 of Samii).
- Grade IV: Significant tumor causing displacement of the brainstem and cranial nerves (comparable to Samii grades T4 and T5).

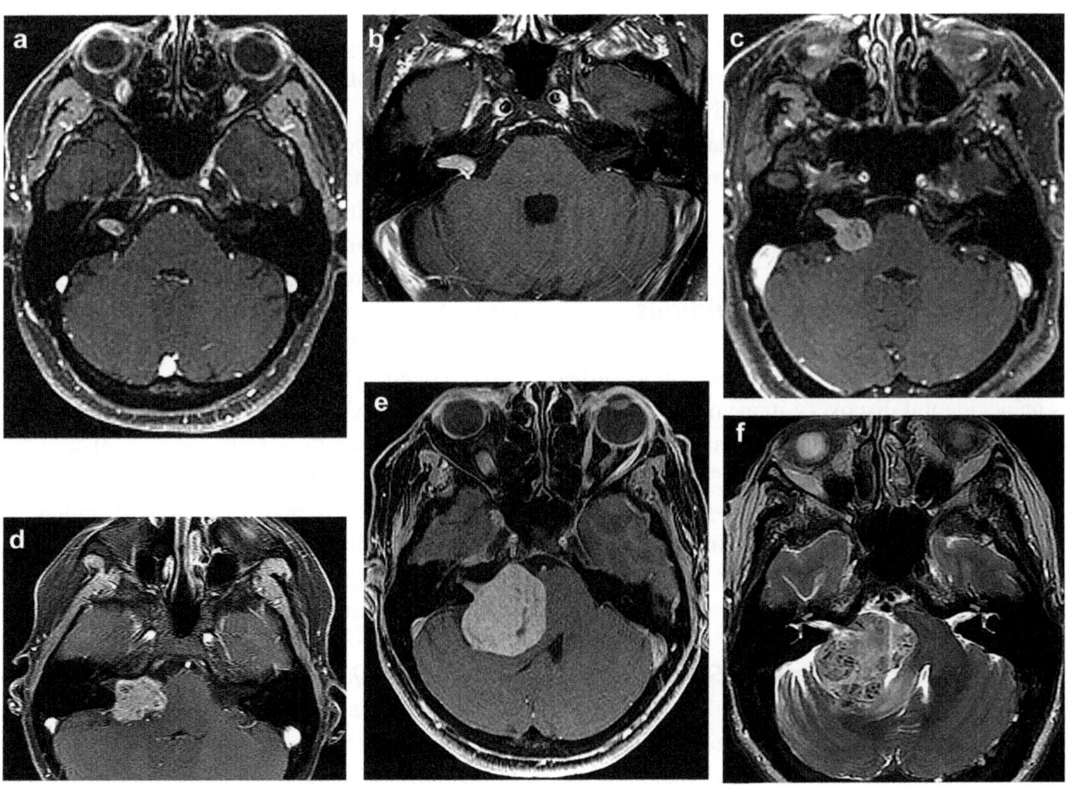

Fig. 5.2 Classification of vestibular schwannomas based on size, adhering to the Matties and Samii scale. (**a**) Grade T1. (**b**) Grade T2. (**c**) Grade T3a. (**d**) Grade T3b. (**e**) Grade T4. (**f**) Grade T5

5.4 Clinical Considerations

5.4.1 Epidemiology

Vestibular schwannoma exhibits an incidence of 1.5 new cases per 100,000 inhabitants annually, reflecting an increase in recent decades likely attributable to enhanced diagnostic capabilities via MRI and improved accessibility of this imaging modality to the population, which may elucidate disparities among countries or racial and cultural groups within nations. The prevalence of vestibular schwannoma, determined through autopsy examinations of temporal bones, ranges from 1% to 2.5%. The prevalence established from population MRI studies is significantly lower, at 0.02%. A separate concern is the occurrence of incidental cases identified in neurosurgical series, which happens in a significant proportion exceeding 10% of cases. In almost 95% of instances, sporadic vestibular schwannomas are unilateral, whereas bilateral occurrences are associated with people diagnosed with neurofibromatosis type 2. The mean age of onset occurs during the fourth and fifth decades of life, with a lower incidence in men compared to women, and it is rare in children. Vestibular schwannoma occurs more frequently in women than in males [20, 22].

5.4.2 Asymptomatic Individuals

Vestibular schwannoma is increasingly identified as an accidental discovery in asymptomatic individuals receiving imaging examinations for unrelated conditions. Numerous asymptomatic tumors monitored with imaging will remain static or asymptomatic, thus necessitating no treatment whatsoever.

5.4.3 Patients Exhibiting Symptoms

A series of clinical stages corresponding to the growth of a typical vestibular schwannoma has been delineated, following the standard progression from the internal auditory canal, through the occupation of the cerebellopontine angle cistern, leading to varying degrees of compression of the brainstem and cerebellum, and the displacement of the fourth ventricle, which may result in hydrocephalus. These clinical stages were pertinent historically, when the diagnosis of vestibular schwannomas was mostly clinical, thus rendering the systematic categorization of growth degrees in relation to lesion size significant. Conversely, clinical experience indicates that first symptoms exhibit considerable variability, and not all patients present the anticipated clinical manifestations corresponding to each growth stage. Ultimately, as is presently true for nearly all neurosurgical conditions, the neurosurgeon evaluates the diagnosed patient solely by examining the symptoms pertinent to the treatment indication and modality, with a focus on prognostic outcomes regarding the anticipated results. It is crucial for the neurosurgeon to be aware of this clinical sequence, as the correlation between symptoms and size is not unequivocal.

Typically, four clinical phases are defined. The initial stage is the intracanalicular phase, wherein the tumor is confined to the internal auditory canal, resulting in symptoms associated with vestibulocochlear dysfunction, hence its traditional designation as the *otological phase*. It would align with Samii-grade T1 and T2 tumors, with a maximum size of 20 mm. The facial nerve is located in the internal auditory canal, but its clinical involvement is rare. During this period, the canal and the internal auditory meatus will also expand. The second phase is the cisternal stage, during which the tumor resides in the cerebellopontine angle cistern until it encroaches upon the brainstem and cerebellum, typically at the level of the middle cerebellar peduncle. In this growth phase, the tumor can theoretically impair the function of any cranial nerve within the cerebellopontine angle, from the fourth to the twelfth, hence its classical designation as the *neurological phase*. This pertains to Samii-grade T3 tumors, measuring approximately 20–40 mm. The third phase involves the compression of the brainstem and cerebellum, potentially resulting in symptoms related to long pathways or cerebellar function. It would pertain to Samii-grade T4a tumors exceeding 40 mm in size. The fourth stage pertains to the emergence of obstructive hydrocephalus resulting from the displacement of the fourth ventricle, historically referred to as the *neurosurgical phase*. It pertains to Samii-grade T4b and T5 tumors, characterized by their enormous dimensions.

Cushing delineated these growth stages of vestibular schwannomas in his 1917 book, stating: "They seem to originate, as a rule, in the distal portion of the nerve within the auditory canal and consequently may cause, through pressure absorption, a dilatation of the porus acusticus internus. From this point, the tumors spread inward throughout the nerve until it becomes completely enveloped. The adjoining structures in the cerebellopontile angle suffer from secondary compression effects. Ultimately, an internal hydrocephalus is produced, and the general pressure phenomena of an intracranial tumor rapidly supervene."

5.4.4 Clinical Manifestations

In the subsequent chapters, we shall categorize the tumors by size and provide a detailed explanation of the symptoms pertinent to each group. We shall now conduct a comprehensive evaluation of the symptoms and diagnosis of vestibular schwannoma as a whole. In a study of 1000 patients operated on by Samii [16], cochlear function was compromised in over 90% of cases, vestibular function in 50–60%, trigeminal nerve involvement in 10–20%, and facial nerve involvement in 5–15%. Additionally, lower cranial nerve or oculomotor involvement with diplopia was observed in less than 5% of patients, based on both subjective symptoms and clinical examination findings.

The predominant cochlear malfunction is hearing loss, although deafness is comparatively rare. Subjective hearing loss impacts 95% of patients, characterized by patients as hypoacusis in over half of instances or cophosis in the remainder. Hearing loss may be gradual or abrupt, and deafness can arise from either progressive hearing loss or occur suddenly. Auditory symptoms develop gradually over a duration of 3 to 5 years. Hearing loss is the symptom with the most prolonged interval between manifestation and diagnosis. Tinnitus occurred in 63% of patients, whether coupled with hearing loss or deafness, is more prevalent in smaller tumors, and had an average duration of 3.1 years before diagnosis. Vestibular symptoms were observed in 61% of patients and exhibit considerable variability, encompassing vertigo, dizziness, positional dizziness, and gait instability, which may manifest individually or in conjunction, with varying intensity and effects on the patient's quality of life. The interval from presentation to diagnosis is approximately 2.1 years. Distinguishing vestibular symptoms from cerebellar symptoms is crucial, as the former are indicative of tiny tumors, while the latter are associated with large tumors. Symptoms associated with the malfunctioning of other cranial nerves exhibit significant variability, contingent upon the tumor's size and predominant development direction, and manifest a shorter period before diagnosis. Trigeminal nerve abnormalities, often manifesting as facial hypoesthesia, occur in 24% of patients, typically lasting approximately 1 year. Facial paranesthesia occurs infrequently, impacting 6.3% of patients for approximately 0.7 years. Trigeminal neuralgia is exceedingly uncommon, occurring with a prevalence of 5.6% with an average duration of approximately 2 years. Diplopia may also occur due to the involvement of the sixth cranial nerve. Facial paresis manifested in 5.2% of patients, with a symptom duration of 1.9 years, although it was identified during clinical examination in 17% of patients. Glossopharyngeal paresis occurred in a mere 2% of patients and hypoglossal paresis in 1% of patients, exclusively in cases of medium and large tumors, or type T3 and T4 tumors, when vestibular schwannoma expands caudally.

Cerebellar signs were observed in over 20% of patients, including ataxic gait, intentional tremor, and abnormal cerebellar examination, whereas long-tract involvement and symptoms of intracranial hypertension due to obstructive hydrocephalus are few. Numerous patients with vestibular schwannoma experience headaches in the ipsilateral occipital region, sometimes accompanied by muscle tension, nausea, or vomiting. Individuals with neurofibromatosis type 2 exhibit bilateral schwannomas in over 95% of instances, presenting symptoms akin to those previously mentioned. Neurofibromatosis type 2 must be contemplated in young individuals presenting with unilateral vestibular schwannoma, particularly when accompanied by another sporadic schwannoma at any site or a meningioma.

5.4.5 Patients with Neurofibromatosis Type 2

Various forms of genetic alteration yield distinct clinical presentations, categorized into three types:

- Gardner type, characterized by bilateral vestibular schwannomas occurring in young adults (third decade of life), often as the sole finding.
- Wishart type, marked by multiple aggressive tumoral lesions in the central nervous system alongside bilateral vestibular schwannomas, manifesting in childhood and associated with an elevated incidence of cutaneous and ocular manifestations.
- Congenital type, identified by bilateral vestibular schwannomas diagnosed within the first days or months of life.

The age of presentation is a significant prognostic indicator, as earlier disease onset correlates with a poorer prognosis. The condition clinically presents in all instances before the age of 60, and life expectancy is considerably reduced compared to the general population and unaffected relatives. The rise in mortality is linked to tumor proliferation, associated neoplasms, malignant transformation of tumors, and treatment-related effects. From a neurosurgical perspective, it is crucial to note that the majority of patients with neurofibromatosis type 2 exhibit bilateral vestibular schwannomas, as this is the primary clinical characteristic that characterizes the disorder. Nonetheless, certain patients are diagnosed with a solitary vestibular schwannoma and exhibit supplementary clinical characteristics that raise a strong suspicion of neurofibromatosis type 2, including meningiomas, gliomas, posterior subcapsular opacities in the lens, familial history, and an age of less than 30 years.

5.5 Diagnostic Considerations

The diagnosis of vestibular schwannoma is predominantly established using MRI, although supplementary testing provides critical insights for determining the optimal surgical indication and method, as well as the tailored surgical strategy for each patient. Diagnostic methods encompass imaging, electrophysiological, otological, and vestibular procedures.

5.5.1 Imaging Modalities

The majority of patients receive a diagnosis by MRI and present at the neurosurgeon's office without undergoing supplementary tests, such as a CT scan. MRI delivers highly accurate details regarding the characteristics of the lesion, including its internal structure, dimensions, volume, extent, and its relationship with the cranial nerves, cerebellum, and brainstem. In contrast, CT offers insights into the osseous components of the petrosal bone, particularly the deformation of the internal auditory canal, the integrity of the inner ear, the extent of the mastoid and petrosal cells, and the positioning of the jugular bulb, all of which are essential for microneurosurgical intervention.

The characterization of the lesion is highly precise with CT and MRI. Vestibular schwannoma is a well-circumscribed lesion that exhibits significant enhancement following contrast injection. When small, it resides in the internal auditory canal, whereas upon enlargement, it occupies the cerebellopontine angle cisterns and exerts a mass effect on the cerebellar peduncle. In the initial scenario, Vestibular schwannoma has a nodular morphology; however, in the subsequent circumstance, it assumes the shape of an ice cream scoop atop a cookie cone. Vestibular schwannoma is typically unilateral, though it may be bilateral in cases of neurofibromatosis type 2. On CT, vestibular schwannoma presents as a slightly hyperdense rounded mass in the cerebellopontine angle, exhibiting hyperdensity upon contrast administration (Fig. 5.3). Typically, there are no calcifications, and the meatus and/or the internal auditory canal are dilated, facilitating the differential diagnosis from meningioma. The T1-weighted MRI sequence exhibits an intermediate signal with pronounced gadolinium enhancement in all instances. This augmentation may manifest throughout the tumor in a homogenous or heterogeneous manner or exhibit regions devoid of enhancement in cystic tumors. In T2-weighted sequences, vascular structures exhibit an intermediate signal between cerebrospinal fluid and brain parenchyma, appearing as a defect within the uniform brightness of the cerebrospinal fluid-filled cisterns. In the advanced T2-weighted FIESTA (*Fast Imaging Employing Steady-state Acquisition*) sequence, the relations with cranial nerves can be identified in small lesions (Fig. 5.4). Complex lesions, including intratumoral hemorrhaging, are infrequent. The differential diagnosis of vestibular schwannoma encompasses schwannomas originating from other cranial nerves, meningioma, arachnoid cysts, metastases, and other uncommon tumors of the cerebellopontine angle, which will be examined in subsequent chapters. A crucial factor in diagnosing nature is that vestibular schwannoma is the predominant lesion of the cerebellopontine angle. While the analysis of morphological sequences is typically adequate, spectroscopy or perfusion may be employed to enhance the differential diagnosis of malignant tumors or metastases.

A relevant question is the measurement of the size of the vestibular schwannomas, since it is related to clinical symptoms, indication for surgery, clinical results after surgery, and dosage for stereotactic radiosurgery treatment. The simplest

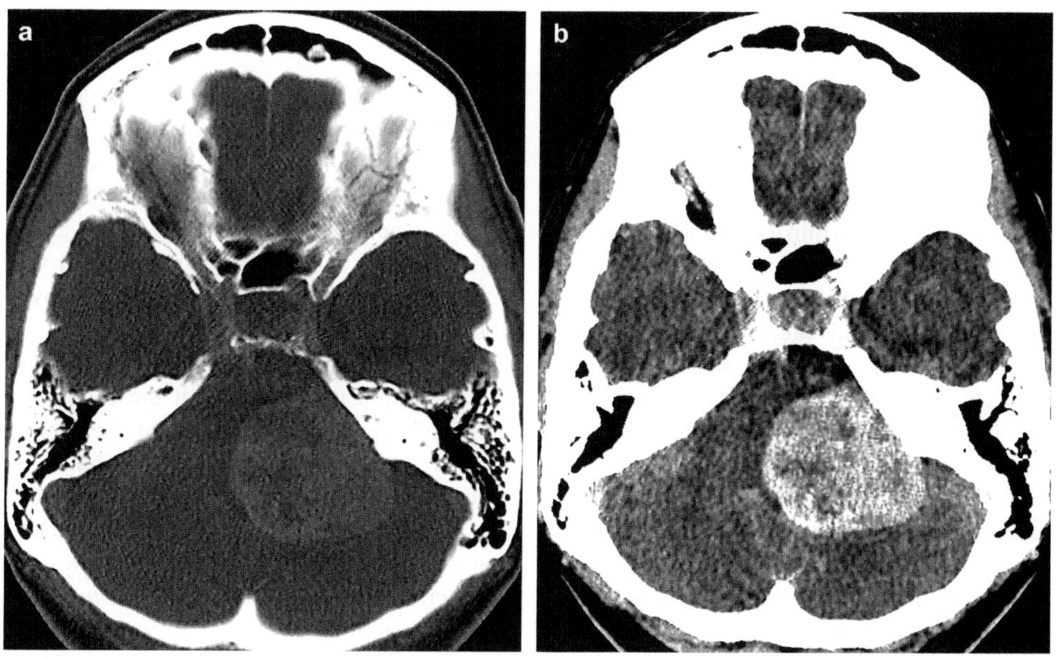

Fig. 5.3 CT diagnosis of vestibular schwannoma. (**a**) Axial section with a bone window revealing a somewhat hyperdense mass situated in the left cerebellopontine angle. (**b**) Following the administration of contrast, pronounced augmentation with an uneven pattern is noted

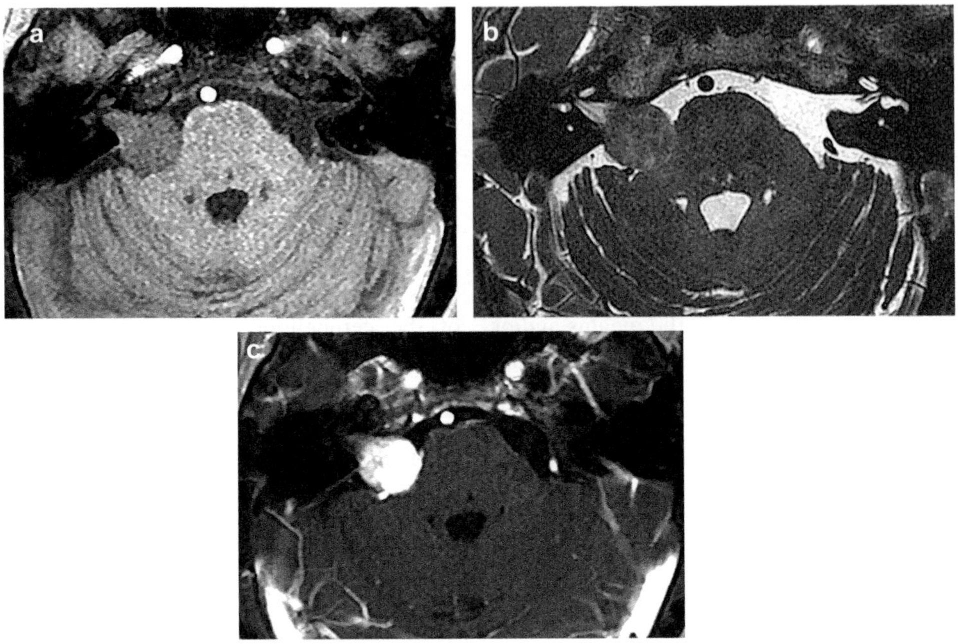

Fig. 5.4 MRI diagnosis of vestibular schwannoma. (**a**) Axial slice at the level of the auditory canal in T1-weighted sequence, displaying a tumor occupying the auditory canal and the cerebellopontine angle cistern, accompanied by an enlargement of the internal acoustic meatus. (**b**) Axial section at the auditory canal level in T2-weighted FIESTA sequence, displaying a tumor occupying the cerebellopontine angle cistern and partially encroaching upon the internal auditory canal, while preserving the fundus. (**c**) Axial section at the level of the auditory canal in a T1-weighted sequence post-gadolinium administration, exhibiting a pronounced signal enhancement attributable to significant contrast uptake in the cisternal segment of the tumor

measurement method is the linear one (mm), where the maximum measurement of the tumor in the axial plane is taken from its deepest limit in the internal auditory canal. Sometimes, more interesting is the determination of the volume of the tumor (cc). The simplest volumetric calculation method is to assimilate the shape of the tumor to an ovoid and calculate the volume with the approximate formula of its volume ($v = [a.b.c]/2$), where a, b, and c are the maximum measurements of the tumor in the axial, coronal, and sagittal planes. Many authors exclude the intracanalicular component of the tumor from the measurement for volume calculation, since if it is included, the calculated volume increases significantly in lesions of intermediate size, with the error being smaller in small and very large lesions. Current imaging equipment is outfitted with software for calculating volumes by semiautomatic segmentation, where the operator draws the outline of the tumor in several slices or determines representative regions of interest (ROIs) of the tumor, so that the computer application automatically calculates the volume. Any measurement method used must be well defined to analyze results and allow comparisons, although there is always an element of error due to variability in measurements made by an observer or among different observers.

Imaging studies also provide information about complications, although these complications are rare. The most important are compression of the brainstem and hydrocephalus. The gradual growth of most vestibular schwannomas and the persistent preservation of the arachnoid layers result in the tumor displacing the brainstem, creating a discernible *cleavage plane*, especially prominent in the T2-weighted MRI sequence. In large tumors, there may be findings of displacement or vasogenic edema in the white matter, but seldom abnormalities that suggest tumor invasion. Hydrocephalus linked with vestibular schwannoma occurs at a variable rate, contingent upon the tumor size and patient age. A recent meta-analysis revealed that 70% of hydrocephalus cases are communicative, whereas the remaining 30% are obstructive. The former is notably more prevalent in elderly individuals (60 years compared to 44 years) and is associated with bigger tumors (4.6 cm versus 3 cm). The data indicate that a significant portion of hydrocephalus linked with vestibular schwannoma is likely pre-existing chronic adult hydrocephalus in older individuals resulting from various etiologies, whereas genuinely obstructive hydrocephalus is attributed to large tumors in younger people. In numerous instances, distinguishing between communicative and obstructive hydrocephalus proves challenging, impacting therapy and prognosis (Fig. 5.5).

The thin-section CT imaging study with a bone window also reveals alterations caused by the tumor in the temporal bone, manifested as expansion of the meatus or the internal acoustic canal. The evaluation of the measurements of this anatomical structure reveals variations linked with sex, side, and age; nonetheless, it has been demonstrated that the extent of neurological impairment and tumor size is typically correlated with the degree of bone damage. The axial section with a bone window of the CT at the level of the internal auditory canals allows for the measurement of the maximal diameter of the meatus and the length of the posterior wall of the canal. The normal meatus measures 7.9 mm in diameter on the healthy side; however, it is markedly larger at 11.6 mm in average on the affected side. Additionally, the canal length is considerably shorter on the affected side in people with deafness, measuring 10.4 mm compared to 11.2 mm on the healthy side. Additional valuable aspects for planning and executing the microneurosurgical approach, including access and excision of the lesion, can be derived from the CT imaging with a bone window. The degree and volume of mastoid pneumatization should be evaluated, as

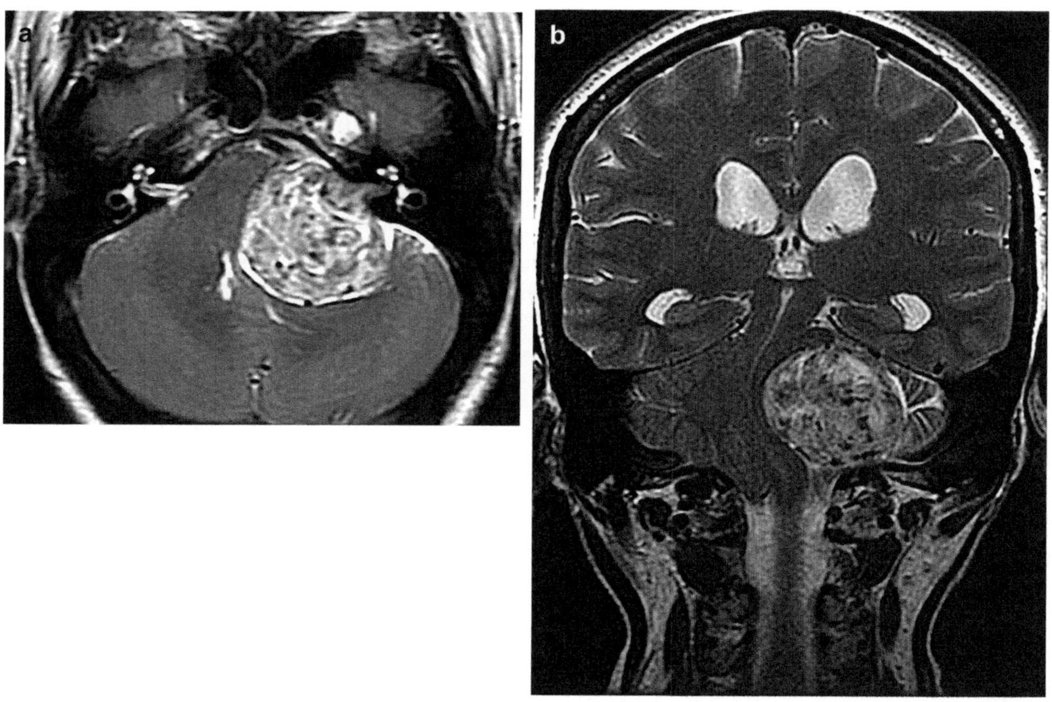

Fig. 5.5 MRI diagnosis of a large vestibular schwannoma. (**a**) Axial section in T2-weighted sequence, illustrating the displacement of the brainstem, cerebellum, and fourth ventricle. A hypointense region exists between the tumor and the nerve tissue, exhibiting a density akin to cerebrospinal fluid or a cleavage plane. (**b**) Coronal section illustrating the displacement of the brainstem and the dilation of the supratentorial ventricular system

it is significant for retrosigmoid craniectomy and is often more pronounced in males. Pneumatization of the petrosal bone is lacking in over 50% of the patients. Pneumatized cells, if identified, must be positioned concerning the transmeatal access. Another point of interest is to identify the most superior position of the jugular bulb in the coronal examination, which is found in 15% of cases at the level of the internal auditory canal, in 15% at the canal's floor, and, thankfully, far from the canal in the remaining 60% of patients. In the transmeatal approach, it is crucial to identify the locations of the lateral and posterior semicircular canals within the petrosal bone to avoid damaging them during bone excision, especially in patients with functional hearing that must be preserved (Fig. 5.6).

Consequently, the essential imaging studies required for a secure microneurosurgical resection of vestibular schwannoma include a thin-section bone assessment via CT in both axial and coronal planes, as well as an MRI examination in three planes, incorporating T1-weighted sequences both pre- and post-gadolinium administration, T2-weighted sequences, and highly T2-weighted sequences with thin sections (FIESTA).

5.5.2 Otologic and Vestibular Tests

Otologic and vestibular assessments were crucial for diagnosing vestibular schwannoma before the introduction of imaging modalities, particularly MRI. Relevant otologic assessments include *pure tone audiometry* and *speech discrimination evaluation*. The initial assessment evaluates the hearing threshold in each ear across various frequencies of the audible range. Sound is delivered via headphones (air conduction) or a vibrator positioned against the mastoid (bone conduction), and the minimum audible level (threshold) is assessed for each frequency. The outcome is documented in a graph displaying the frequency and threshold for each frequency, or as a number representing the average of the thresholds for the evaluated auditory spectrum. In nearly all individuals with vestibular schwannoma, there is a gradual and asymmetric loss of high-frequency hearing on the affected side. The *verbal speech discrimination test* assesses the percentage of words comprehended by the patient in each ear when presented at an easily audible volume. Verbal speech discrimination is significantly compromised in retrocochlear lesions, such as vestibular schwannomas. Another verbal assessment is the *word perception threshold*, a form of audiometry involving words that determines the volume at which the patient can accurately repeat 50% of the presented words. All these tests are pertinent in the differential diagnosis of many otological issues; nevertheless, their specificity for diagnosing vestibular schwannoma is significantly lower than that of imaging tests.

Vestibular assessments were beneficial before the advent of more precise imaging techniques. The most significant are *caloric stimulation electronystagmography* and *evoked vestibular myogenic potentials*. Caloric stimulation electronystagmography evaluates ocular movements triggered by stimuli that elicit nystagmus, including caloric stimulation of the tympanic membrane via the introduction of hot or cold water or air into the external auditory canal. The reflex is facilitated by the stimulation of the lateral semicircular canal, which is innervated by the superior vestibular nerve. Consequently, in addition to the diagnostic suspicion of a vestibular schwannoma, the lack of response to caloric stimulation when a vestibular schwannoma is already identified suggests that it likely originates from the upper vestibular nerve. Myogenic muscle potentials are elicited by high-frequency auditory stimuli directed at the ear while simultaneously recording the electromyographic activity of the sternocleidomastoid muscle, as the investigation focuses on the vestibular–cervical reflex that activates cervical muscles in response to sound stimuli. The initial element of the record is an inhibitory potential transmitted via the saccular route of the superior vestibular nerve. These tests facilitate the detection of selective involvement of the upper or lower vestibular nerve in diminutive vestibular schwannomas and other otological conditions.

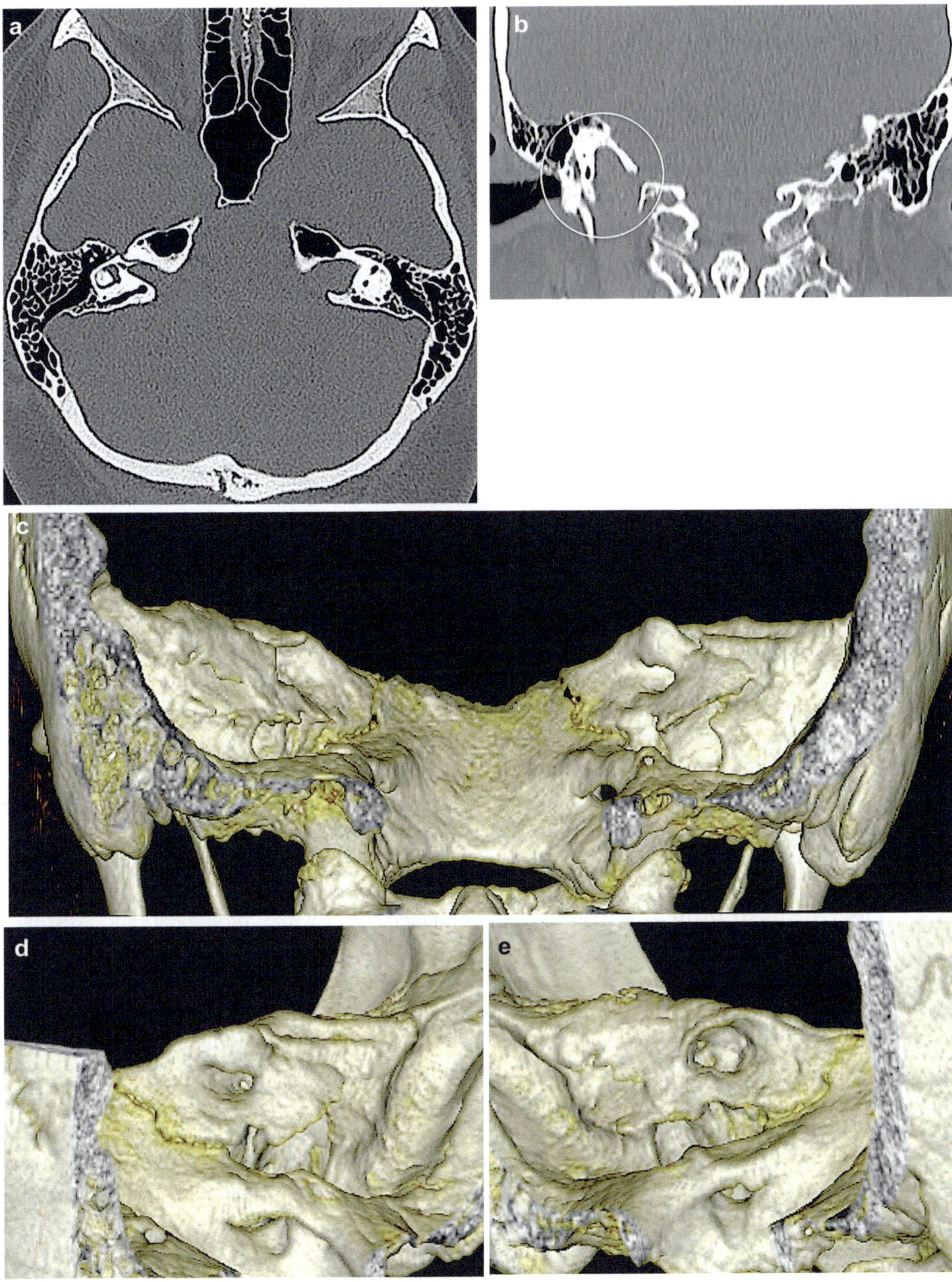

Fig. 5.6 Findings in the thin-section CT examination of the temporal bone utilizing a bone window for the diagnosis of vestibular schwannoma: (**a**) Axial section demonstrating enlargement of the left meatus and auditory canal relative to the right. Pneumatized cells are present on both sides of the posterior surface of the petrosal bone, adjacent to the posterior wall of the internal auditory canal. Pneumatized cells are present on both sides near the apex of the petrosal bone. (**b**) Coronal section displaying the cast of the jugular bulb positioned exceptionally high on the right side. (**c–e**) Three-dimensional reconstruction of the petrosal bone illustrating the asymmetry of the internal acoustic meatus in a case of left vestibular schwannoma, presented in a posterior view and in a Stenvers radiological projection of both sides

5.5.3 Functional Auditory Perception

The present neurosurgical application of otological tests is to assess functional hearing (*useful hearing*). Useful hearing is pertinent for determining treatment indications and modalities, as well as for comparing auditory outcomes pre- and post-microneurosurgical and otological intervention. Various measures have been developed for evaluating functional hearing by audiometry and word discrimination. The *Gardner–Robertson scale* adheres to the 50/50 rule, wherein useful hearing is defined as an audiometric average below 50% of the maximum, coupled with recognition of more than 50% of words (grade II). Alternative classifications employ different criteria, such as the AAO-HNS (*American Association of Otolaryngology-Head and Neck Surgery*) scale, which adheres to the 50/70 rule for identical assessments. A subjective evaluation of functional hearing can be conducted by inquiring directly with the patient regarding their experiences in daily-life scenarios (such as using the telephone or identifying the source of ambient sounds) or in their typical work environments or recreational activities.

5.5.4 Electrophysiological Studies

Among electrophysiological studies, the *auditory brainstem evoked potentials* (BAEPs) are the most specific for diagnosing vestibular schwannomas, as the prolongation of latency between the peaks of waves I-III and I-V is highly indicative of vestibular schwannoma, despite the study's sensitivity not exceeding 90% of cases.

5.5.5 Screening

Patients exhibiting the aforementioned symptoms consult their family physician, who subsequently sends them to an otologist. The primary objective of the otologist is to conduct a clinical differential diagnosis and commence the etiological diagnosis. The diagnosis of vestibular schwannoma is not conducted by a neurosurgeon; therefore, other professionals must perform diagnostic evaluations among the numerous patients exhibiting non-specific symptoms, within which individuals with vestibular schwannomas are concealed, utilizing existing diagnostic methods judiciously. To develop a diagnostic algorithm for a specific geographic region or territory, it is essential to identify the at-risk population to be studied, assess the available diagnostic tools and their reliability, evaluate the financial resources allocated for the project, and establish the acceptable number of undiagnosed patients, referred to as false negatives. The population at increased risk of developing vestibular schwannomas should include those with unilateral hearing loss, according to the significant prevalence of cases in which patients report hearing loss as their initial symptom. The sensitivity and specificity for diagnosing vestibular schwannomas of any size using MRI exceed 95% and improve with dual observer assessment, establishing it as the most reliable method. BAEPs exhibit exceptional sensitivity, exceeding 95% for detecting retrocochlear abnormalities; however, they possess low specificity, evidenced by a 25% false negative rate in diagnosing vestibular schwannomas. CT yields inferior results, with false negatives surpassing 25%, even with contrast enhancement, while otological and vestibular assessments demonstrate an even higher incidence of false negatives. Several decades ago, when MRI was either inaccessible or too expensive, diagnostic algorithms were developed by rationally correlating the various studies available at that time. An illustration of this approach is as follows, enabling the identification of the five vestibular schwannomas that an adult cohort of 100 patients with unilateral hearing loss may exhibit. Initially, radiological and otological examinations would be conducted, resulting in 72 patients exhibiting entirely normal findings, hence allowing for the preliminary exclusion of vestibular schwannoma. Of the remaining 28 patients, one or more tests would yield abnormal results, necessitating a CT study to diagnose four cases of VS. To identify the fifth case, a cisternography should be conducted on the remaining 24 patients, of which 23 would present normal results. The subsequent diagnostic algorithm utilizing the same diagnostic methods would be more efficient and cost-effective. The initial diagnostic method employed for at-risk patients would have been BAEPs, which would have yielded normal results in 88 cases in whom vestibular schwannoma was conclusively excluded. The remaining 12 would undergo radiological and otological examination, revealing normal findings in five and abnormalities in seven. The patients will be examined using CT, which will reveal four tumors, while the remaining three patients will undergo cisternography with CT to identify the last patient with vestibular schwannoma. Currently, it is evident that the preferred first-line diagnostic method for screening the population at potential risk of incidental vestibular schwannoma is MRI utilizing T1-weighted sequences, T1 with gadolinium, T2-weighted, and T2-FIESTA sequences.

5.6 Surgical Categories

In microneurosurgical therapy of vestibular schwannomas, the primary factor to consider is the linear dimension of the tumor. Consequently, we have categorized tumors into small-sized or canalicular tumors, encompassing Samii grades T1 and T2, Koss grades I and II, measuring less than 20 mm; medium-sized or cisternal tumors, comprising Samii grade T3 and Koss grade III, with a size under 30 mm; and, finally, large and giant tumors, represented by Samii grades T4 and T5 or Koss grade IV, exceeding 40 mm in size. In the subsequent chapters, we shall examine vestibular schwannomas individually based on these three sizes. The second criterion of interest is the tumor's internal structure, which enables differentiation between solid and cystic consistencies. A chapter exclusively dedicated to cystic schwannomas is reviewed. Additionally, factors to consider include the number of tumors, typically singular and notably bilateral, the correlation with hydrocephalus, and the recurrence of tumors following therapy with microneurosurgery or stereotactic radiosurgery.

5.7 Microneurosurgical Management

Treatment modalities for vestibular schwannoma encompass microneurosurgical excision and stereotactic radiosurgery [4, 6, 7, 9, 13, 20]. The criteria for patient selection for imaging surveillance or treatment recommendations, as well as the treatment methodology, will be addressed thereafter. The objective of microneurosurgery is to safely excise the lesion, aiming for a total resection (GTR: *Gross Total Resection*) while retaining facial nerve function and functional hearing. Various microneurosurgical therapy techniques have been suggested over time. The microneurosurgical intervention should be tailored for the complete excision of the lesion, ensuring a cure for the condition while preserving the anatomical and functional integrity of the associated neurological structures, thus facilitating symptomatic relief for the patient and minimizing morbidity and mortality risks. Alternative solutions have been suggested in reaction to the notion of GTR. One century ago, Dandy introduced two-stage resection, which has since been intermittently advocated for substantial tumors. Following the implementation of stereotactic radiosurgery, intracapsular tumor excision has been suggested to subsequently administer stereotactic radiosurgery to the capsule. It has been proposed that tumor remnants be deliberately retained to safeguard the functionality of the facial nerve and then managed with stereotactic radiosurgery. In clinical practice, each patient requires a tailored solution; thus, the objectives of microneurosurgery must be personalized. Consequently, there exists a diverse array of options: radical resection with no collateral damage; radical resection with minimized collateral damage; radical resection with acceptance of collateral damage, which will be subsequently repaired; *subtotal resection* (STR) to reduce collateral damage while monitoring the remnants or completing treatment with stereotactic radiosurgery; and, finally, resection solely aimed at obtaining diagnostic material or alleviating brainstem compression or hydrocephalus, without any intention of lesion excision.

Concerning the choice of surgical approach, there are three alternatives: the trans-labyrinthine approach, the middle fossa approach, and the retrosigmoid approach. The *trans-labyrinthine approach* is the quintessential otological technique, facilitating the removal of tumors of any dimension; nonetheless, it necessitates the removal of the inner ear and precludes the preservation of hearing in patients with functional hearing capacity. The advantage is in its provision of early access to the facial nerve at the fundus of the internal auditory canal, which is traced to the brainstem along the anterior margin of the tumor. Furthermore, it does not necessitate the engagement of the cerebellum or the temporal lobe. The *middle fossa approach* is advantageous for tiny tumors, facilitating the preservation of the middle and inner ear, hence protecting residual hearing. This is a middle fossa extradural approach occasionally employed by otologists and neurosurgeons. The *retrosigmoid approach* uniquely facilitates the resolution of cerebellopontine angle vestibular schwannomas of any dimension while preserving the integrity of the inner ear's auditory structures, making it a standard technique for neurosurgeons. The retrosigmoid approach offers distinct advantages over the trans-labyrinthine and middle fossa techniques and is a mile-stone neurosurgical method; thus, it will be the focus of this section for the resection of typical vestibular schwannomas. However, the retrosigmoid approach exhibits a greater incidence of tumor remnants at the fundus of the internal auditory canal compared to the trans-labyrinthine route. The retrosigmoid approach for vestibular schwannoma does not differ from the general strategy outlined in the chapter concerning the position, incision, craniotomy, and dura mater opening, as described in Chap. 2. It is important to note that, concerning the methods for microvascular decompression of cranial nerves in the absence of structural pathology in the cerebellopontine angle, the craniotomy should be as extensive as feasible to provide multiple access points to the lesion, especially in the case of large tumors.

5.7.1 Retrosigmoid Approach with Transmeatal Access

The fundamental concepts of microneurosurgical intervention for vestibular schwannomas focus on achieving gross total resection of the tumor while preserving the anatomical and functional integrity of the cranial nerves (Fig. 5.7). The conventional method is retrosigmoid craniectomy, as detailed in the chapter on surgical technique. The intracanalicular component of the tumor is resected via transmeatal access, facilitated by the drilling of the posterior wall of the internal auditory canal. The strategy for resecting the extracanalicular segment, irrespective of its dimensions, involves the internal decompression of the tumor using an ultrasonic aspirator. This process should be methodical and incremental, followed by the organized removal of small sections of the capsule to preserve the cleavage plane with the neurovascular structures. The arteries exhibit significant diversity, yet they are meticulously preserved, with only the minor branches supplying the tumor being coagulated and severed. The veins must be retained to the greatest extent feasible. The cranial nerve roots possess certain anatomical places and interactions with the tumor, necessitating their active identification using anatomical references and verification through direct electrical stimulation. The deliberate sacrifice of the vestibulocochlear nerve is permissible solely when hearing is irretrievably lost, as the tumor arises from the vestibular nerve, and the cochlear nerve is typically integrated into the tumor in instances of auditory impairment. To ensure the morphological and functional preservation of the cranial nerve roots, they must be meticulously separated from the tumor using a refined microneurosurgical technique; if necessary, retaining a minor remnant of the tumor is acceptable in order to safeguard its function. Intraoperative electrophysiological monitoring, encompassing direct electrical stimulation, is beneficial in attaining these goals. The excision of the tumor from the brainstem and cerebellum

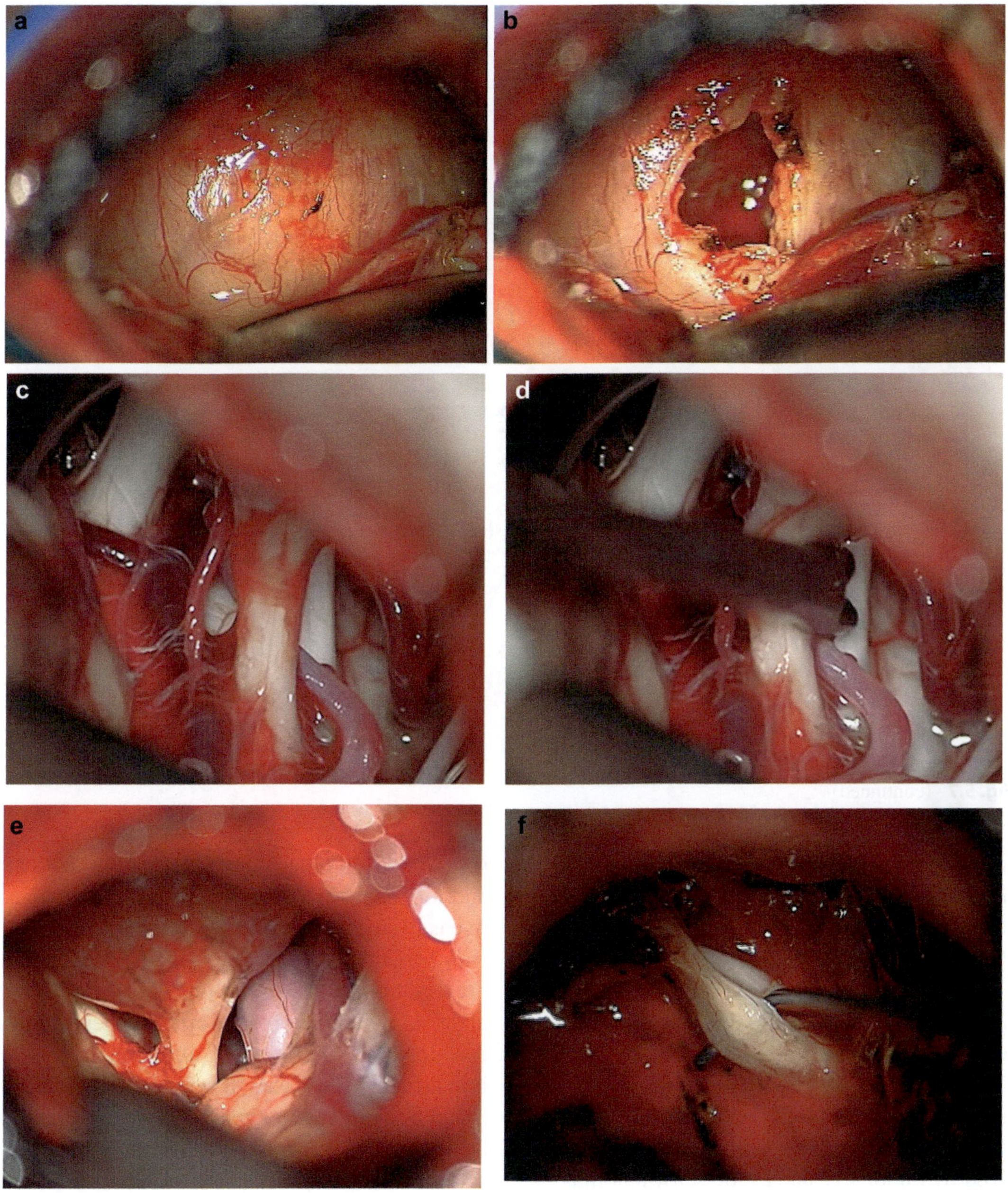

Fig. 5.7 Surgical pictures displaying the microneurosurgical intervention for a right vestibular schwannoma. (**a**) Image of the tumor revealed following arachnoid dissection, cerebrospinal fluid evacuation, and cerebellar retraction. (**b**) Image of the tumor following capsule incision and initiation of internal decompression utilizing an ultrasonic aspirator. (**c**) A picture displaying the neurovascular linkages in the cerebellopontine angle, illustrating, from left to right, the trigeminal nerve, vestibulocochlear nerve, and facial nerve, adjacent to the anterior inferior cerebellar artery. (**d**) Illustration displaying direct electrical stimulation of the facial nerve. (**e**) The picture depicts the vestibulocochlear nerve's entry into the tumor, with the vertebral artery visible on the right and the facial nerve on the left. (**f**) Dissection of the vestibulocochlear nerve from the facial nerve utilizing a nerve hook. (**g–h**) Image displaying the internal auditory canal post-drilling of its posterior wall, illustrating the condition before and after the complete excision of the tumor while preserving the facial nerve. (**i**) Conclusive picture of the cerebellopontine angle post-tumor excision, illustrating from left to right the cisternal trajectory of the trigeminal, facial, and abducens nerves

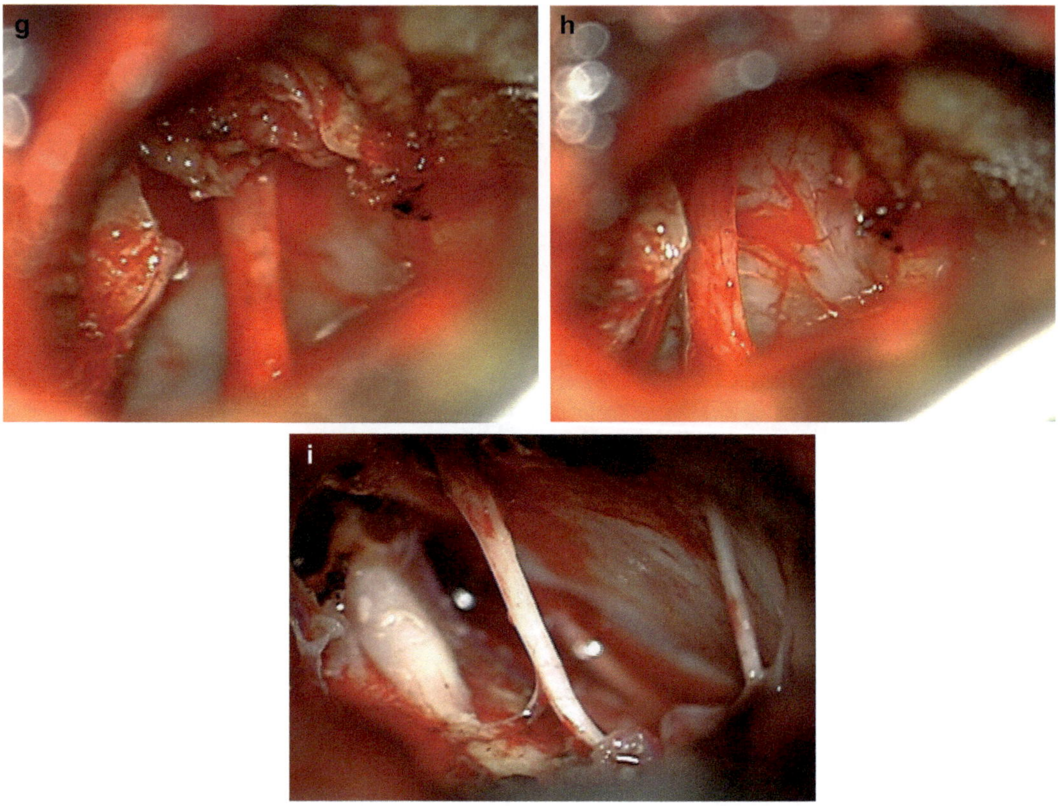

Fig. 5.7 (continued)

must be conducted meticulously, minimizing the use of bipolar coagulation. Separation is feasible due to the existence of an arachnoid layer between the tumor and the pia mater or cleavage plane. Following the entire excision of the lesion, meticulous hemostasis is required, and all measures to avert cerebrospinal fluid fistula must be executed during closure. The subsequent chapters will delineate the nuances of microneurosurgical resection of vestibular schwannomas, categorized by tumor size and cystic schwannomas.

5.8 Vestibular Schwannomas that Require Specific Treatment

5.8.1 Patients with Type 2 Neurofibromatosis

The treatment recommendations and objectives for vestibular schwannoma in patients with neurofibromatosis type 2 depend upon the patient's auditory capacity. The primary therapeutic objective is to sustain functional hearing in one or both ears for an extended duration, prioritizing the preservation of hearing in one ear while eventually safeguarding other critical neurological functions or life, even if it compels hearing impairment in both ears. If both ears exhibit functional hearing and methods exist to preserve this hearing post-surgery, the smaller vestibular schwannoma should be prioritized for early intervention. If the tumors are of identical dimensions, it is advisable to commence with the side exhibiting superior auditory perception. Ultimately, when the vestibular schwannomas are of the same dimensions and auditory function is comparable, electrophysiological parameters are employed to determine the optimal side. If functional hearing is present in only one ear, the tumor on the deaf side is excised, and further therapy for the contralateral side, where hearing is still present, is contemplated. In instances where both vestibular schwannomas are diminutive and auditory function is preserved, the alternative of bilateral excision may be presented, even at the expense of bilateral hearing loss. For individuals unwilling to assume this risk, or in cases where the size of the vestibular schwannoma precludes the possibility of preserving hearing post-resection, monitoring is advised until significant hearing loss manifests. If a vestibular schwannoma is quite big and exhibits signs of brainstem compression, the tumor should be removed or an internal decompression should be performed to attempt to preserve any existing usable hearing. Similar to sporadic schwannomas, it is the responsibility of the neurosurgeon to advise the patient about the likelihood of preserving usable hearing based on their experience and to present this choice only when a genuine possibility exists. The published surgical outcomes demonstrate that approximately 50% of patients retain useful hearing, while over 75% maintain functional integrity of the facial nerve postoperatively. However, these statistics are less favorable in standard neurosurgical practice and should be regarded as those specific to the neurosurgeon performing the procedure. Even under optimal conditions, the clinical outcomes of vestibular schwannoma excision in patients with neurofibromatosis type 2 are inferior to those in those with sporadic vestibular schwannomas, due to the more pronounced invasion of the nerve bundle by the tumor. One approach is to observe the clinical progression of lesion growth and auditory impairment, advising microsurgery solely in the presence of significant neurological complaints.

An additional issue with vestibular schwannomas in patients with neurofibromatosis type 2 is their occurrence in younger individuals and their more erratic behavior compared to sporadic VSs; the development rate is more unpredictable, and the progression is less predictable. Moreover, stereotactic radiosurgery is an inadequate choice as, aside from the inherent limits of this treatment for sporadic vestibular schwannoma, it also appears to be less effective in long-term tumor development management. Consequently, growth control in sporadic vestibular schwannomas is 90% at 5 years, in contrast to about 75% in individuals with neurofibromatosis type 2. Moreover, it is concerning because 50% of malignancy cases in vestibular schwannomas treated with stereotactic radiosurgery, as reported in the literature, arise in patients with neurofibromatosis type 2, despite this group constituting less than 10% of the overall patient population treated. The enhanced ability to generate malignancy is predicated on the concept that radiation serves as a secondary factor, augmenting the pre-existing genetic changes in the patient, so predisposing them to malignant transformation (two-hit hypothesis). Based solely on size, it is generally advised to reserve stereotactic radiosurgery for intracanalicular or tiny tumors, whereas larger tumors or those exhibiting rapid growth should not undergo stereotactic radiosurgery treatment [8].

A palliative microneurosurgical treatment for patients with neurofibromatosis type 2 has recently been suggested, involving indirect decompression of the tumor by enlarging the internal auditory canal through drilling the upper and posterior surfaces of the canal via a middle fossa approach without attempting tumor resection. The external decompression of the tumor facilitates temporary enhancement or stabilization of hearing as the tumor progresses and the patient experiences hearing loss; however, the tumor will likely necessitate microneurosurgical resection ultimately [5].

Exceptionally, in instances of uncontrollable progression of recurrence, the administration of antiangiogenic agents, specifically Bevacizumab, has been suggested. This treatment results in partial regression of the lesion in 40% of cases and enhances auditory function in 20% of patients, albeit with significant complications associated with prolonged use of the medication. This treatment is predicated on the aberrant regulation of VEGF in schwannomas, which promotes vascular proliferation within the tumor to sustain its viability via capillary and vessel development.

5.8.2 Microneurosurgical Management of Tumors Treated with Stereotactic Radiosurgery

Stereotactic radiosurgery is an efficacious treatment for clinical control and growth control of vestibular schwannomas. Nonetheless, in a minority of instances, subsequent microneurosurgical rescue procedures may be required due to radiation-induced adverse effects, tumor growth resulting from disease progression or malignant transformation, or the development or enlargement of cysts within the tumor (refer to case 2 in Chap. 21) [7].

Adverse effects of radiation by stereotactic radiosurgery manifest in fewer than 10% of treated individuals, occurring more frequently in cases with big tumors and with elevated marginal radiation doses. They often manifest between 6 and 18 months posttreatment and resolve autonomously within weeks, either naturally or with corticosteroid medication. Early tumor growth following radiosurgery, typically observed between 6 and 18 months but potentially apparent within the first 3 years, is generally attributable to reversible factors, particularly intratumoral edema and necrosis. This phenomenon occurs in over 20% of cases and can augment tumor volume by as much as 40%; hence, it is designated in the literature as *pseudoprogression*. Symptoms of brainstem compression and hydrocephalus can be alleviated with the implementation of an external ventricular or ventriculoperitoneal shunt. If tumor excision is necessary, extensive decompression of the posterior fossa and subtotal intracapsular tumor resection are advised, including a trans-labyrinthine approach for deaf patients.

The expansion of the irradiated vestibular schwannomas after an extended time of stability post-therapy with stereotactic radiosurgery happens in 10% of instances, typically after 3–4 years of treatment. Slow development may indicate a recurrence, whereas rapid expansion compels suspicion of malignant change. Another manifestation of tumor proliferation following stereotactic radiosurgery is the development of cysts, or the accelerated expansion of pre-existing cysts. Retreatment of the irradiated tumor should be considered when tumor development is associated with new symptoms. One alternative is to administer stereotactic radiosurgery again, which may be advised for patients exhibiting delayed growth. The optimal choice is salvage therapy with microneurosurgical resection. The objectives of microneurosurgical intervention today encompass, alongside the preservation or enhancement of neurological function and alleviation of brainstem compression, the acquisition of specimens to exclude malignant transformation and diminish the likelihood of recurrence. The objective of microneurosurgical approach should be the complete excision of the irradiated tumor. The achievement of these objectives is obstructed by the adherence of the tumor to the arachnoid, brainstem, cerebellum, and other neurovascular structures, complicating the dissection and separation of these functional entities from the tumor. Furthermore, radiation-induced devascularization of the cranial nerves renders them more susceptible to microneurosurgical intervention injury. Consequently, in numerous instances, the cranial nerves, especially the facial nerve, should be preserved alongside a portion of the tumor capsule to prevent inducing a total and irreversible anatomical loss or functional impairment. Frequently, these remains are so inconspicuous that they are overlooked in postoperative control tests, and the majority will never proliferate. The clinical outcomes of microneurosurgery in vestibular schwannomas treated with stereotactic radiosurgery that exhibit growth are marginally inferior compared to those that are non-irradiated, and the complication rate is somewhat elevated.

5.8.3 Recurrence Following Microneurosurgery

The recurrence rate of vestibular schwannomas excised via microneurosurgery is minimal, under 10% in instances of gross total resection, typically occurring after an interval of many years. It is essential to distinctly separate recurrence following complete excision from the regrowth of tumor remnants purposely or unintentionally retained during a STR. Recurrence is more prevalent following STR and increases in frequency with the size of the residual tumor volume post-microsurgery (refer to case 1 in Chap. 21). Recurrence does not necessitate urgent and mandatory retreatment; the lesion may be monitored through imaging until retreatment is considered appropriate, which can be performed via microneurosurgery or stereotactic radiosurgery.

Microneurosurgery encounters increased challenges compared to the initial approach, primarily due to scar adhesions that form in the surgical region, complicating the identification of the separation planes between tumor regrowth and the brainstem, as well as the cranial nerve roots, especially the facial nerve. This also elevates the danger of increased morbidity from the involvement of more cranial nerves, and the incidence of general problems associated with the approach is heightened, including cerebrospinal fluid fistula. However, the choice of a STR is inadvisable, as the inherent dangers of the STR are comparable to those associated with a GTR or NTR (*Near Total Resection*), and it will only yield transient control until tumor regrowth becomes highly probable.

In the absence of functional cochlear or facial function following the initial intervention, microneurosurgery is the preferred option, as it facilitates a safe gross total resection of the recurrence. Nonetheless, if functional cochlear or facial nerve activity remains, it must be acknowledged that preserving it will be exceedingly challenging; hence, stereotactic radiosurgery would be a superior alternative to microsurgery. In cases of significant recurrence or a pertinent cystic component exerting pressure on the brainstem, accompanied by new neurological symptoms or hydrocephalus, microneurosurgical intervention is advised [17].

Limited studies examine the outcomes of microneurosurgical intervention for recurrences, but there is greater experience with stereotactic radiosurgery treatment. Microsurgery reports an intraoperative anatomical loss of 50% of the facial nerve after reintervention. Conversely, stereotactic radiosurgery demonstrates a permanent loss of facial nerve function that does not exceed 5%, which is far lower than that associated with microneurosurgery, albeit somewhat greater than when stereotactic radiosurgery is administered as the initial treatment. This is ascribed to the compromised microvasculature of the facial nerve resulting from the surgical scar of the initial procedure and the challenges of accurate stereotactic radiosurgery dosimetry in a previously operated area. The control of tumor growth with stereotactic radiosurgery is approximately 90% at 5 years, albeit lower than the initial treatment efficacy. This is once again ascribed to the challenge of executing a strategy customized to the tumor, as the enhancement caused by the scar from the prior operation may be indistinguishable from the tumor's own augmentation.

5.9 Complications, Prevention, and Management

Complications of vestibular schwannoma microneurosurgery can be categorized into two primary groups: those arising from the approach and those stemming from the treatment of the tumor [13, 25]. Complications arising from the approach encompass cerebrospinal fluid leak, meningitis, venous sinus thrombosis, and headache, as discussed in the chapter on the retrosigmoid route (refer to case 3 in Chap. 21). Complications arising from tumor excision encompass vascular complications and cranial nerve impairment. Vascular complications include bleeding in the surgical site and complications arising from ischemia secondary to section, coagulation, or spasm of the arteries. Postoperative hematoma is infrequent, occurring in under 3% of instances, and is typically well tolerated by patients, managed symptomatically (refer to case 4 in Chap. 21). Ischemia of the internal auditory or labyrinthine artery results in ischemia of the inner ear, leading to cochlear and vestibular symptoms, along with those previously experienced by the patient. The loss of this artery in the event of anatomic loss of the vestibulocochlear nerve is clinically insignificant. Ischemia of the major arteries, especially the anteroinferior cerebellar artery, which is most vulnerable during surgical procedures, results in various brainstem ischemic syndromes. The most notable is the Marie-Fox lateral pontine syndrome, characterized by a diverse clinical presentation including dysarthria, ipsilateral facial paralysis and hypoesthesia, dysphagia, Horner syndrome, conjugate ocular movement disorders, contralateral hypoesthesia, vestibular symptoms, and hearing loss. The most common consequences of microneurosurgery for vestibular schwannoma are associated with acute or permanent impairment, or complete loss of function, of the cranial nerves. All individuals with vestibular schwannoma have varying degrees of compromised vestibular function, and when sectioning the vestibular nerve, there is an irreversible loss of any remaining ipsilateral vestibular function. Due to the gradual nature of vestibular functional loss, numerous people establish compensation before surgery and manage the nerve loss very successfully. Over 50% of individuals necessitate a prolonged adaptation time, during which symptoms of dizziness and instability endure, and may gain from vestibular rehabilitation programs. The objective for patients with functional hearing is to preserve it; however, this is not a primary concern for most patients, excepting for those with neurofibromatosis type 2. In small tumors, the preservation of functional hearing in patients with preoperative useful hearing can occur in 50% of instances. The preservation of functional hearing correlates with the tumor's size, the level of preoperative hearing, and the neurosurgeon's proficiency. The procedure involves the anatomical identification of the auditory nerve, its separation from the tumor originating from the vestibular nerve, and the preservation of the cochlear nerve roots. The trans-labyrinthine method precludes the preservation of hearing, whereas the middle fossa approach facilitates it.

A primary goal of microneurosurgery for vestibular schwannomas is the preservation of facial nerve function, as it is infrequently affected before surgery, even in substantial tumors. The facial nerve predominantly transmits motor fibers but also includes sensitive fibers (e.g., cutaneous regions of the external ear), sensory fibers (e.g., gustatory), and autonomic fibers (e.g., regulating lacrimal secretion). To assess the severity of facial nerve impairment, the House–Brackmann (HB) scale, which exclusively evaluates motor function, has been globally recognized. The scale comprises six severity degrees and assesses the overall function of the nerve trunk, rendering it ineffective for branch lesions [14].

- Grade I, normal: facial function is intact throughout all regions.
- Grade II, modest dysfunction: grossly, slight weakening is discernible upon careful examination, potentially accompanied by minimal synkinesis; at rest: normal symmetry and tone; forehead motion exhibits moderate to good function; eyes demonstrate entire closure with minimal effort; and the mouth displays slight asymmetry.
- Grade III, moderate dysfunction: a pronounced yet non-disfiguring asymmetry between the two sides, accompanied by noticeable but not severe synkinesis, contracture, and/or hemifacial spasm; at rest, symmetry and tone are normal; forehead movement exhibits slight to moderate motion, eye closure is complete but requires effort, and mouth movement is slightly weak despite maximum effort.
- Grade IV, fairly severe dysfunction: pronounced weakness and/or disfiguring asymmetry; at rest: normal symmetry and tone; absent motion of the forehead; inadequate closure of the eye and mouth with asymmetry despite utmost effort.
- Grade V, severe dysfunction: gross, with minimal discernible motion; asymmetry at rest; absent brow movement, incomplete eyelid closure, and only slight oral movement.
- Grade VI, or total paralysis, signifies the absence of movement entirely.

The preservation of the facial nerve's anatomy and function is correlated with the tumor's size and the neurosurgeon's expertise. In skilled hands, the functional preservation of the facial nerve (HB grades I-III) achieves 90% in unselected tumor series utilizing a retrosigmoid technique, showing no significant differences compared to excision by trans-labyrinthine or middle fossa procedures. From a technical perspective, it is crucial to achieve maximal volumetric reduction of the tumor through internal decompression and resection of parts of the capsule before initiating the dissection of the facial nerve root. The proximal segment at its egress from the brainstem and the distal segment within the internal auditory canal are recognized either by direct vision or electrical stimulation. Once the leftover tumor mass is reduced, its dissection commences using a fine, sharp dissector or a blunt needle-shaped dissector, adhering to the orientation of the nerve. It is prudent to vary the dissection direction to prevent excessive stress on the nerve fibers, which could result in rupture, thereby dispersing the stretching more evenly. These maneuvers are executed based on the data obtained from the intraoperative electromyographic recording. Neurotonic discharges indicate that the nerve must remain undisturbed for a period, halting the dissection from the remainder of the tumor capsule. It may be judicious to retain a minor remnant of tumor or capsule affixed to the nerve rather than compromise its anatomical integrity. Postoperative facial paralysis is total if the nerve is not structurally preserved (*neurotmesis*); nevertheless, certain patients, especially younger individuals, may retain muscular tone for several days. Upon successful physical preservation of the facial nerve, evidenced by an intraoperative electromyographic response to direct stimulation, immediate paralysis may manifest, or it may arise subsequently, within days or even weeks; however, entire or partial functional recovery should be anticipated. The recovery of facial nerve function is variable; however, in instances of late paralysis, the prognosis is highly favorable since it is associated with the activation of specific viruses that may induce transitory facial nerve neuritis. The fundamental principles of facial nerve rehabilitation and various neurosurgical procedures for its restoration will be addressed in another context.

The engagement of additional cranial nerves in the posterior fossa results in issues of differing clinical significance. Alteration of the fourth or sixth cranial nerves results in temporary diplopia. Manipulation of the trigeminal nerve results in various sensory disturbances in the face, typically hypoesthesia accompanied by neuropathic pain. The most severe condition is hypoesthesia or anesthesia of the first branch of the trigeminal nerve, resulting in corneal anesthesia. This, when coupled with facial nerve paralysis, markedly elevates the risk of corneal ulceration and its complications, potentially resulting in corneal opacity and necessitating corneal transplantation. Impairment of the lower cranial nerves results in dysphagia and vocal cord paralysis, which collectively elevate the risk of tracheal aspiration and pneumonia. Nutrition delivered by a nasogastric tube or gastrostomy mitigates the risk of this severe consequence, as well as tracheostomy. The involvement of the accessory or hypoglossal nerve is anecdotal.

From a technical perspective, optimal prevention involves the meticulous handling of all cranial nerve roots during the dissection of the tumor capsule, accompanied by continuous electromyographic monitoring to detect neurotonic discharges. A frequently overlooked stressful factor is extensive wall aspiration during surgical procedures. Upon isolating any cranial nerve, the separation must be preserved by placing a soft material imbued with saline, which is then removed at the conclusion of the surgery. The positioning of patties should be avoided since they often cling to tissue and can damage nerves upon removal or may be unintentionally displaced during surgery.

5.10 Results, Prognosis, and Follow-Up

5.10.1 Imaging Surveillance of Tumors Treated with Microsurgery

Patients who have had vestibular schwannoma excision are monitored by imaging studies, specifically contrast-enhanced T1-weighted MRI [12]. The recommendation is to conduct a study 6 months post-surgery, as the inflammatory changes that enhance with gadolinium that can be confused with tumor remnants are diminished or stabilized during this period. This mitigates patient uncertainty regarding the final outcome of the resection and prevents potentially detrimental decisions by the surgeon regarding retreatment with stereotactic radiosurgery or microneurosurgery. This six-month postoperative study should be standard for patients with GTR, characterized by the surgeon's assessment of no residual tumor, and NTR, where the surgeon perceives an insignificant amount of residual tumor, less than 5% of the initial volume. When the objective of surgery is a STR or small resection, an MRI can be conducted at any time to advance the treatment strategy for the residual lesion, as the remaining tumor will be readily identifiable in the MRI examination.

Six months post-GTR or NTR, various patterns of gadolinium enhancement may be observed in the MRI (Fig. 5.8). The lack of enhancement indicates the absence of any residual lesion. Linear enhancement, perhaps located in the walls of the internal auditory canal, at the canal's fundus, or externally on the surface of the brainstem or cerebellum, indicates a likelihood of scar-type enhancement with a minimal possibility of recurrence. Nonetheless, it is true that within the enhancement area, especially if it is substantial or occupies the fundus of the auditory canal, where the distal segment of the vestibular nerve was severed, there may be remnants that permit recurrence. In these patients, a new imaging study at 5 years may be adequate, or, if hearing is preserved, when hearing declines.

The third form of enhancement is nodular, located either within or outside the internal auditory canal, a finding that strongly indicates the presence of a tumor remnant with a significant probability of recurrence. In the absence of neurofibromatosis type 2, the residual tumor volume is the primary risk factor for recurrence. The existence of a residual nodule increases the likelihood of regrowth, and when it exceeds 2.5 cc, regrowth is inevitable. Conversely, for diminutive nodules (< 0.5 cc), the likelihood of recurrence is minimal, often remaining inactive in numerous instances and ultimately resolving in others. Consequently, patients with nodules above 0.5 cc should undergo annual monitoring for a decade, followed by assessments every 5 years. In contrast, individuals with nodules smaller than 0.5 cc necessitate less rigorous monitoring, with evaluations every 5 years deemed enough.

A further concern pertains to the duration of follow-up. Patients undergoing surgery for vestibular schwannoma exhibit a highly favorable natural history with minimal anecdotal perioperative mortality; thus, surgical intervention does not significantly impact survival rates, which are nearly equivalent to those of the general population. Given that life expectancy in developed nations is approximately 80 years, the continual monitoring of patients can impose significant financial burdens on healthcare systems and frequently extend beyond the professional tenure of the neurosurgeon who operated, resulting in many individuals potentially losing follow-up care. The likelihood of late recurrences with new clinical symptoms necessitating retreatment is minimal, but certain clinical studies indicate that 50% of individuals who underwent surgery for vestibular schwannoma with GTR, as confirmed by early MRI, exhibit some degree of recurrence two decades post-operation. A further issue is that, in instances of hearing loss, there are no preliminary warning signs to notify the patient of a potential recurrence. Ultimately, every patient who has undergone microneurosurgery for vestibular schwannoma feels worry regarding the potential for recurrence, which, however unlikely, could necessitate further surgical intervention or the shocking reliving of the initial diagnosis. All these factors advocate for the necessity of continuous observation of all patients who have undergone surgery for sporadic vestibular schwannoma.

5.11 Management Modalities

Upon the identification of a sporadic vestibular schwannoma, three therapeutic management options are available: surveillance with imaging, microneurosurgical intervention, and stereotactic radiosurgery. The choice of treatment recommen-

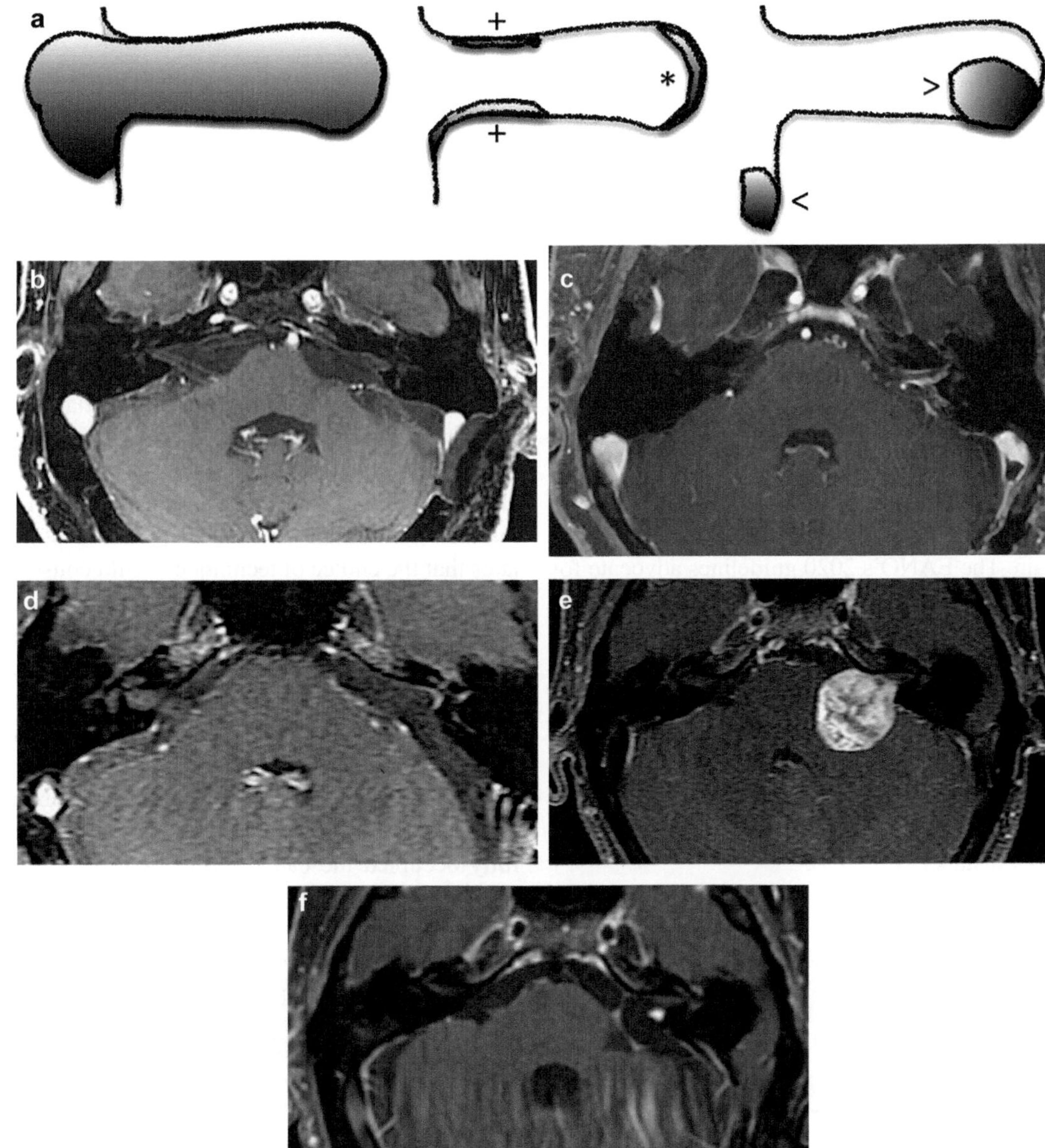

Fig. 5.8 Signal increase patterns in T1-weighted MRI following gadolinium injection in postoperative MRI, 6 months post vestibular schwannoma microneurosurgery. (**a**) Schematic representation of the patterns: left, displaying a tumor occupying the internal auditory canal and extending into the cistern; center, illustrating linear enhancement along the internal auditory canal walls (+) and a cupping shape at the fundus (*); right, showing a nodular remnant within the canal (>) and a new nodule unrelated to the excised tumor (<). (**b**) Axial MRI section without enhancement following gadolinium administration. (**c**) Axial section exhibiting a linear increase in the walls of the internal auditory canal. (**d**) Axial section exhibiting linear cupping enhancement. (**e**, **f**) Axial section of the tumor pre- and post-resection, demonstrating nodular enhancement indicative of a remnant as well as a linear enhancement in the middle cerebellar peduncle

dation is contingent upon numerous criteria, some of which have been previously addressed but will be reviewed comprehensively. In this context, factors pertaining to the tumor (dimensions, proliferation rate), the patient (clinical manifestations, functional hearing, age, and comorbidities; desires and anticipations), and healthcare (surgeon's expertise and institutional experience) must be taken into account. The amalgamation of these elements generates an unlimited array of distinct scenarios to recommend the optimal treatment solution for the patient.

5.11.1 Imaging Observation

Observation is the optimal strategy for a small tumor that exhibits no growth, preserves useful hearing, and presents no additional neurological symptoms, particularly in senior individuals with comorbidities and in those who do not express anxiety regarding the presence of a tumor in their brain. The EANO's 2020 guidelines advocate for surveillance through recurrent MRI examinations or otological assessments for incidentally identified or asymptomatic tumors [10]. It is acknowledged that 50% of individuals would exhibit either an enlargement of the lesion or a deterioration in auditory function within the subsequent 5 years [24]. Nevertheless, there are no factors that may forecast the specific progression in any given instance (Fig. 5.9).

5.11.2 Microneurosurgical Resection

Microneurosurgery is the optimal method for medium, large, or giant vestibular schwannomas exhibiting growth, accompanied by non-functional hearing and neurological symptoms, in patients of any age without comorbidities and those who are apprehensive about having a tumor in their cranium, provided the tumor is excised by a skilled neurosurgeon in a facility equipped with the requisite technology. EANO advocates for microsurgery in cases with Koos grade IV tumors that are symptomatic or pose a potential life-threatening risk due to brainstem compression, as well as for smaller tumors associated with cysts or where a gross total resection of the lesion is feasible with curative intent [10]. EANO stipulates that the choice of technique should consider auditory function, tumor characteristics, patient preferences, and the surgeon's expertise. The cumulative postsurgical death rate for the series is below 0.5%. The preservation of functional hearing exceeds 60%, with favorable prognostic markers including a tumor size of less than 1 cm, the presence of cerebrospinal fluid at the fundus of the canal, indicating that the tumor has not fully occupied the canal during its growth, and

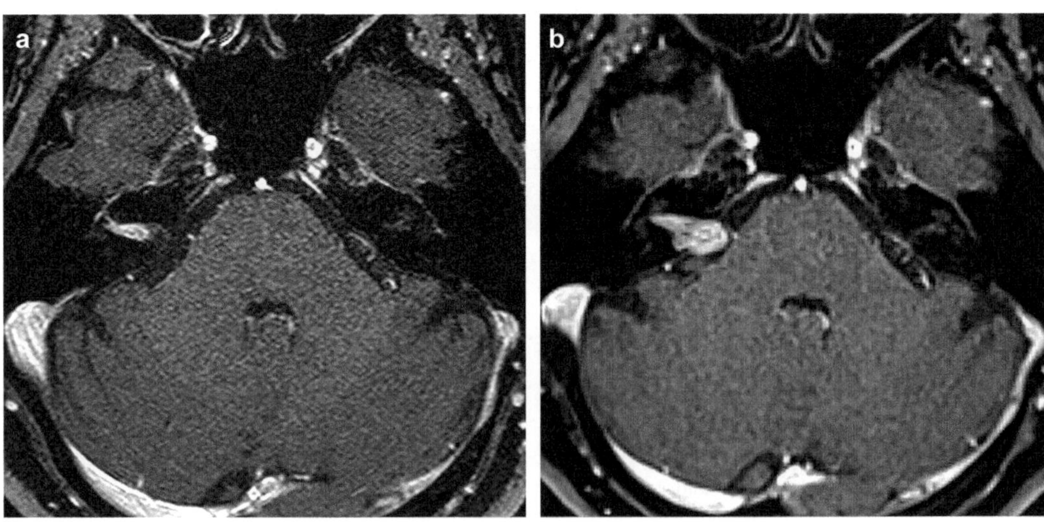

Fig. 5.9 Small-sized right vestibular schwannoma, monitored through imaging, exhibiting growth. (**a**) Axial T1-weighted picture with gadolinium at the time of diagnosis. (**b**) Subsequent MRI conducted 5 years later

adequate hearing function before microsurgery. The rates of satisfactory facial function post-surgery vary based on tumor size, averaging 30% in instances classified as HB grades I-III. The GTR of the tumor markedly diminishes the likelihood of recurrence in comparison to the STR, and the chance of recurrence is contingent upon the residual tumor volume (Fig. 5.10).

5.11.3 Stereotactic Radiosurgery

Stereotactic radiosurgery is the optimal method for a vestibular schwannoma of sufficient size for radiation treatment (typically <30 mm), exhibiting no evident growth, preserving useful hearing, and devoid of additional neurological symptoms, particularly in an older patient, preferably elderly, with comorbidities, who does not express anxiety regarding the presence of a tumor in the cranial cavity. The EANO recommendations specify that stereotactic radiosurgery is appropriate for tumors smaller than 30 mm and contraindicated for tumors exerting mass effect on the brainstem or classified as Koos grade IV [10]. Various prospective studies indicate that stereotactic radiosurgery is superior to microneurosurgery in preserving auditory and facial function for tumors measuring less than 30 mm. Nonetheless, there are no randomized and prospective trials that provide a dependable comparison of the two therapy alternatives. The tumor's persistence post-stereotactic radiosurgery treatment, despite a reduction in volume, necessitates continuous imaging follow-up to identify potential recurrences (Fig. 5.11) [1, 3, 21, 23].

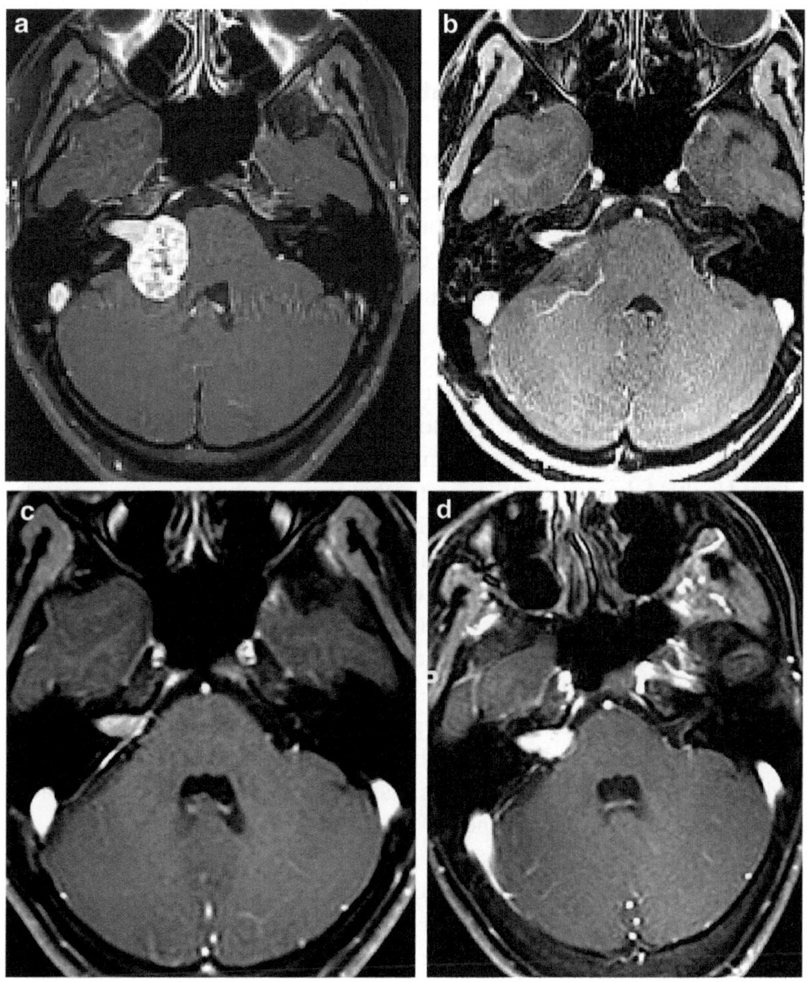

Fig. 5.10 Recurrence following subtotal resection of a right VS. (**a**) Axial T1-weighted MRI with gadolinium, displaying a Samii-grade T4a VS before surgery. (**b**) Axial T1-weighted MRI with gadolinium, displaying a nodular intracanalicular tumor remnant 6 months post-surgery. (**c**, **d**) Axial T1-weighted MRI sections with gadolinium, demonstrating tumor progression throughout consecutive annual evaluations

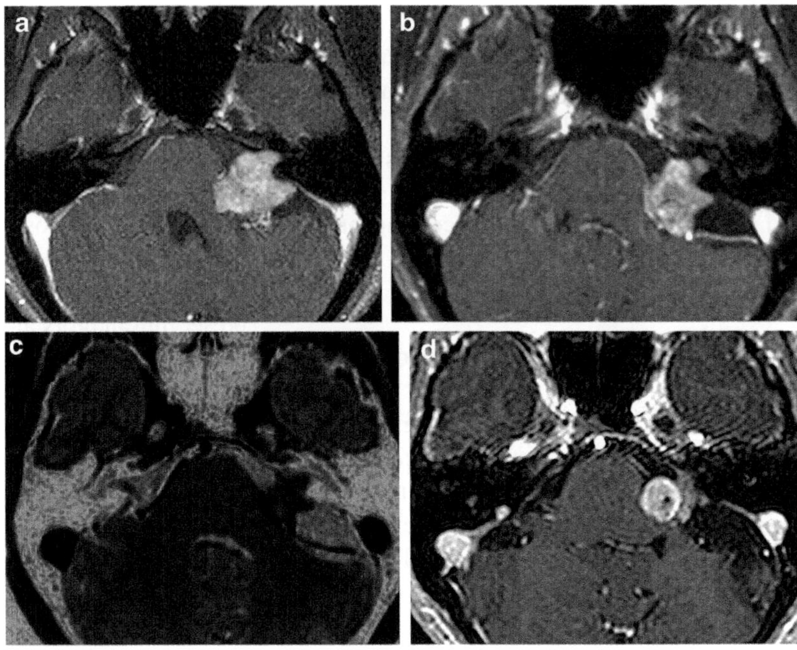

Fig. 5.11 Recurrence following stereotactic radiosurgery treatment of a left vestibular schwannoma. (**a**) Axial T1-weighted MRI with gadolinium, displaying a Samii-grade T3b tumor before stereotactic radiosurgery. (**b**, **c**) Axial MRI sections, demonstrating the decrease in tumor size at 3 and 5 years post-stereotactic radiosurgery treatment. (**d**) Axial T1-weighted MRI segment with gadolinium, demonstrating nodular tumor development 1 year later

5.12 Healthcare Organization

An agreement exists that, for neurosurgery procedures necessitating complex surgical treatments, such as vestibular schwannoma, a positive correlation exists among hospital, departmental, and surgeon workload and high quality of care measures [2, 18]. Epidemiological research over several decades indicates that postcraniotomy mortality rates are reduced in units and among surgeons with a substantial workload. A recent research study utilizing data from the United States Health Administration indicates that facilities performing a large volume of microneurosurgical treatment for vestibular schwannomas (> 30 cases annually) achieve considerably superior outcomes compared to those with a lower caseload (< 6 cases annually). The enhanced care indicators encompass reduced follow-up duration, diminished incidence of significant postoperative problems such as cerebrospinal fluid leaks or hydrocephalus, abbreviated hospital stays, decreased rates of facial nerve impairment, adverse events, and readmissions. Nonetheless, this overarching perception, bolstered by statistical evidence, must be moderated by examining certain individual factors. The data acquired for these studies originate from administrative databases of health organizations, typically accessible only in nations with advanced healthcare systems, rendering them extensive and dependable; thus, extrapolation to other healthcare organizational systems may be unrealistic. Administrative statistics differ from clinical data, which, despite potential bias from the surgeon's perspective, can provide a more comprehensive evaluation of outcomes, incorporating the patient's viewpoint. In this context, some patients endure a distressing existence due to the presence of a tumor in their head, while being informed that it is benign and manageable by imaging or stereotactic radiosurgery; they opt for resection even at the risk of morbidity. A further contentious aspect of this research pertains to the assessment of care volumes, which is achieved by computing the quartiles of the overall volume attended, resulting in significantly low care volumes that occasionally reflect merely anecdotal activity. Conversely, facilities and surgeons with a higher patient volume manage, accept, and perform surgeries on more intricate cases referred from other institutions or practitioners, hence elevating the likelihood of increased morbidity when addressing more complex tumors and patients. The total cost of care is elevated in larger, more sophisticated centers that accommodate a higher volume of intricate patients. The initial treatment cost, excluding follow-up, is more for microsurgery compared to stereotactic radiosurgery, with this disparity increasing as the tumor size increases. Ultimately, more research underscores the significance of the surgeon's technical proficiency. In major centers, numerous surgeons are present, resulting in the accumulation of complex cases among superspecialist surgeons, while less experienced surgeons manage routine cases and encounter difficulties with complex cases. Certain research indicates that the learning curve requires a minimum of 50 vestibular schwannoma cases to be performed. Currently, there are no studies indicating that an increase in care volume correlates with inferior clinical outcomes. However, it remains challenging to ascertain the threshold at which significant differences emerge, warranting a health policy focused on the redistribution of care and human resources, particularly regarding the centralization of microneurosurgical interventions for complex lesions such as vestibular schwannomas. This healthcare reorganization could be efficiently centralized in facilities equipped with dedicated personnel for vestibular schwannoma management, including neurosurgery, otology, and radiotherapy teams, alongside appropriate equipment such as microsurgical and stereotactic radiosurgery tools, as well as treatment protocols developed in accordance with scientific society recommendations. The actual healthcare model in our context relies on the management of patients referred to otology or neurosurgery by clinical otologists or neurologists, who have established diagnoses through imaging studies, frequently utilizing criteria influenced by tradition, personal connections, institutions, or commercial interests. As not all otology facilities conduct microsurgery for vestibular schwannomas, numerous patients are sent to alternative otology, neurosurgery, or stereotactic radiosurgery units. In the discipline of neurosurgery, all units are trained to perform microneurosurgical interventions for vestibular schwannomas; nevertheless, most of them may operate as low-volume units.

Nevertheless, a preliminary consideration must be addressed before arranging treatment for vestibular schwannoma. This pertains to the rationale for recommending and implementing treatment for a benign lesion characterized by a slow growth rate, which can be monitored in a straightforward, effective, and efficient manner within our context, and where a postponement of treatment, in the most adverse scenario, may yield equivalent detrimental outcomes that are highly probable to arise posttreatment. Studies indicate that in nations with advanced healthcare systems, there is an increasing diagnosis of vestibular schwannomas, whereas the number of patients receiving microneurosurgical therapy remains stable or is seeing a modest decline. This indicates that patients are progressively undergoing imaging surveillance or receiving stereotactic radiosurgery. This perspective is increasingly bolstered by enhanced understanding of the natural history of asymptomatic or small vestibular schwannomas; however, it must consistently be weighed against the evidence that the outcomes of microneurosurgical or stereotactic radiosurgery interventions deteriorate with larger tumor size and poorer neurological function of patients at the time of treatment.

5.13 Key Messages

- *Vestibular schwannoma is the predominant tumor of the cerebellopontine angle, and although it correlates with tumor size, its clinical manifestations exhibit considerable variability.*
- *From a microneurosurgical standpoint, vestibular schwannomas are categorized by size, with the Matties and Samii scale and the Koos scale being the most prevalent classifications.*
- *Due to the relatively high incidence and the documented correlation between case load and outcomes, a healthcare organization must be instituted for the microneurosurgical management of vestibular schwannomas.*

References

1. Aboukaïs R, Bonne NX, Touzet G, et al. Progression of vestibular schawnnoma after gamma knife radiosurgery: a challenge for microneurosurgical resection. Clin Neurol Neurosurg. 2018;168:77–82. https://doi.org/10.1016/j.clineuro.2018.03.006.
2. Andresen NS, Gourin CG, Stewart CM, et al. Hospital volume and failure to rescue after vestibular schwannoma resection. Laryngoscope. 2020;130:1287–93. https://doi.org/10.1002/lary.28174.
3. Bailo M, Boari N, Gagliardi F, et al. Gamma knife radiosurgery for residual and recurrent vestibular schwannomas after previous surgery: clinical results in a series of 90 patients and review of the literature. World Neurosurg. 2017;98:60–72. https://doi.org/10.1016/j.wneu.2016.10.066.
4. Bambakidis N, Megerian CA, Spetzler RF, editors. Surgery of the cerebellopontine angle. Cham: Springer Nature; 2028.
5. Bernardeschi D, Peyre M, Collin M, et al. Internal auditory canal decompression for hearing maintenance in neurofibromatosis type 2 patients. Neurosurgery. 2016;79:370–7. https://doi.org/10.1227/NEU.0000000000001125.
6. Carlson ML, Vivas EX, McCracken DJ, et al. Congress of Neurological Surgeons systematic review and evidence-based guidelines on hearing preservation outcomes in patients with sporadic vestibular schwannomas. Neurosurgery. 2018;82:E35–9. https://doi.org/10.1093/neuros/nyx511.
7. Lee CC, Wu HM, Chung WY, et al. Microsurgery for vestibular schwannoma after gamma knife surgery: challenges and treatment strategies. J Neurosurg. 2014;121(Suppl):150–9. https://doi.org/10.3171/2014.8.GKS141312.
8. Chung LK, Nguyen TP, Sheppard JP, et al. A systematic review of radiosurgery versus surgery for neurofibromatosis type 2 vestibular schwannomas. World Neurosurg. 2018;109:47–58. https://doi.org/10.1016/j.wneu.2017.08.159.
9. di Russo P, Fava A, Vandenbulcke A, et al. Characteristics and management of hydrocephalus associated with vestibular schwannomas: a systematic review. Neurosurg Rev. 2021;44:687–98. https://doi.org/10.1007/s10143-020-01287-2.
10. Goldbrunner R, Weller M, Regis J, et al. EANO guideline on the diagnosis and treatment of vestibular schwannoma. Neuro-Oncology. 2020;22:31–45. https://doi.org/10.1093/neuonc/noz153.
11. González-Darder JM. Trepanation, trephining, and craniotomy. History and stories. Cham: Springer Nature; 2019.
12. González-Darder JM, Capilla-Guasch P, Escartín FP. Magnetic resonance imaging surveillance for vestibular schwannoma after microneurosurgical resection using a retrosigmoid transmeatal approach. World Neurosurg. 2020;139:e585–91. https://doi.org/10.1016/j.wneu.2020.04.073.
13. González-Darder JM, Quilis-Quesada V, Capilla-Guasch P, de Oliveira E. Abordajes neuroquirúrgicos de la patología craneal y cerebral. 2nd ed. Barcelona: Elsevier España; 2020.
14. House JW, Brackmann DE. Facial nerve grading system. Otolaryngol Head Neck Surg. 1985;93:146–7. https://doi.org/10.1177/019459988509300202.
15. Magro G, Broggi G, Angelico G, et al. Practical approach to histological diagnosis of peripheral nerve sheath tumors: an update. Diagnostics (Basel). 2022;12:1463. https://doi.org/10.3390/diagnostics12061463.
16. Matthies C, Samii M. Management of 1000 vestibular schwannomas (acoustic neuromas): clinical presentation. Neurosurgery. 1997;40:1–9. https://doi.org/10.1097/00006123-199701000-00001.
17. Perry A, Graffeo CS, Copeland WR 3rd, et al. Microsurgery for recurrent vestibular schwannoma after previous gross total resection. Otol Neurotol. 2027;38:882–8. https://doi.org/10.1097/MAO.0000000000001402.
18. Rezaii E, Li D, Heiferman DM, et al. Effect of institutional volume on acoustic neuroma surgical outcomes: state inpatient database 2009-2013. World Neurosurg. 2019;129:e754–60. https://doi.org/10.3390/diagnostics12061463.
19. Rhoton AL Jr. The cerebellopontine angle and posterior fossa cranial nerves by the retrosigmoid approach. Neurosurgery. 2000;47(Suppl 3):S93–129. https://doi.org/10.1097/00006123-200009001-00013.
20. Samii M, Gerganov V. Surgery of cerebellopontine angle lesions. Berlin-Heildelberg: Springer; 2013.
21. Savardekar AR, Terrell D, Lele SJ, et al. Primary treatment of small to medium (<3 cm) sporadic vestibular schwannomas: a systematic review and meta-analysis on hearing preservation and tumor control rates for microsurgery versus radiosurgery. World Neurosurg. 2022;160:102–113.e12. https://doi.org/10.1016/j.wneu.2021.11.083.
22. Schmidt RF, Boghani Z, Choudhry OJ, et al. Incidental vestibular schwannomas: a review of prevalence, growth rate, and management challenges. Neurosurg Focus. 2012;33:E4. https://doi.org/10.3171/2012.7.FOCUS12186.
23. Tosi U, Lavieri MET, An A, et al. Outcomes of stereotactic radiosurgery for large vestibular schwannomas: a systematic review and meta-analysis. Neurooncol Pract. 2021;8:405–16. https://doi.org/10.1093/nop/npab011.
24. Zanoletti E, Mazzoni A, d'Avella D. Hearing preservation in small acoustic neuroma: observation or active therapy? Literature review and institutional experience. Acta Neurochir. 2029;161:79–83. https://doi.org/10.1007/s00701-018-3739-x.
25. Zou P, Zhao L, Chen P, et al. Functional outcome and postoperative complications after the microsurgical removal of large vestibular schwannomas via the retrosigmoid approach: a meta-analysis. Neurosurg Rev. 2014;37:15–21. https://doi.org/10.1007/s10143-013-0485-7.

6 Small-Sized Vestibular Schwannoma

6.1 Introduction

This chapter will examine the features of small-sized vestibular schwannoma. This category encompasses grade T1 and T2 tumors according to the Matties and Samii classification, as well as grades I and II of the Koos classification, which concern lesions with a maximum axial plane size, including the intracanalicular part, of less than 20 mm. These are tumors that partially or wholly fill the internal auditory canal and may or may not extend into the cerebellopontine angle cistern. These diminutive vestibular schwannomas are not in contact with the brainstem; thus, some are entirely intracanalicular, while others are both intra- and extracanalicular. We categorize all these lesions collectively due to their analogous challenges in treatment recommendation and modality, their exclusively otological clinical symptoms, and their microneurosurgical treatment, which employs transmeatal access via a retrosigmoid approach. In our clinical practice, the incidence of patients with intracanalicular vestibular schwannomas referred for microneurosurgical intervention is minimal, as they are typically managed by clinical otologists for imaging surveillance or by surgical otologists via translabyrinthine microsurgical excision when hearing is nonfunctional, or they are directed towards stereotactic radiosurgery if hearing is preserved.

Currently, transmeatal access is the epicenter of all treatments for microneurosurgical resection of vestibular schwannomas via the retrosigmoid approach, particularly in small-sized tumors, where it is a crucial phase of the procedure. Rand and Kurze presented this access in 1964 as an alternative to the prevailing methods of that era, including the traditional retrosigmoid route by Dandy, the translabyrinthine technique utilized by otologists, and the middle fossa approach delineated a few years prior by Kurze and Doyle. Rand and Kurze characterized the technique as an adaptation of Dandy's retrosigmoid method, involving the enlargement of the internal acoustic meatus and the utilization of diamond bur drilling on the posterior wall of the internal auditory canal, extending to the opening to the fundus of the auditory canal. The objective was to safeguard hearing by maintaining the labyrinthine system and excising the tumor from unaffected nerve roots and arteries within the auditory canal with a microsurgical approach. The authors asserted that this access, in contrast to the translabyrinthine and middle fossa approaches, offered an expansive surgical field, direct visualization of the anterior inferior cerebellar artery, secure dissection of the tumor's entire surface, the ability to identify all cranial nerves and the brainstem's surface, and, ultimately, direct access to the facial nerve for immediate repair via end-to-end suture or nerve graft in the event of

J. M. González-Darder, *Microneurosurgery of Cerebellopontine Angle*,
https://doi.org/10.1007/978-3-032-03091-7_6

anatomical injury during microsurgical resection of the tumor.

6.2 Anatomical Considerations

The microneurosurgical treatment of small vestibular schwannomas relies on the transmeatal approach to the tumor; thus, we will provide a detailed description of the surgical anatomy of the internal auditory canal and its components.

6.2.1 Internal Auditory Canal and Meatus

The internal auditory canal is a bony tunnel that connects the inner ear to the posterior fossa. The structure possesses a truncated conical shape, featuring an opening to the posterior fossa or meatus that is broader than its deepest section, the fundus. The fundus is penetrated by several bone canals that allow the nerve filaments of the seventh and eighth cranial nerves to exit the skull. The fundus is segmented into quadrants, with a horizontal or falciform bony crest that divides it into two halves, along with a vertical crest that further splits the upper half into two sections. The internal auditory canal is approximately 10 mm long and 5 mm in diameter. The bony surface is enveloped by the dura mater originating from the posterior fossa, which is inserted into the canal resembling a glove finger. The adjacent bone is typically dense but may contain pneumatized petrosal cells; it is laterally related to the semicircular canals, and its posterior face can be in proximity to the jugular vein bulb when positioned superiorly. All these relations are readily identifiable in computed tomography (CT) thin-sliced bone imaging studies [7].

6.2.2 Neurovascular Elements of the Internal Auditory Canal

The internal auditory canal has five nerve trunks: the facial nerve, cochlear nerve, superior vestibular nerve, inferior vestibular nerve, and the intermediate nerve of Wrisberg. Despite the relatively stable positioning of the nerve roots, they consistently penetrate the bone in the fundus in a precise manner. The facial and superior vestibular nerves enter above the horizontal crest at the canal's base, with the facial nerve positioned anterior to the vertical crest and the superior vestibular nerve posterior to it; conversely, the cochlear and inferior vestibular nerves enter below the horizontal crest, with the cochlear nerve situated beneath the facial nerve and the inferior vestibular nerve located beneath the superior vestibular nerve. The structure and anatomical relationships of the intermediate nerve exhibit considerable variability, although it often associates with the cochlear nerve upon exiting the brainstem before ultimately merging with the facial nerve in the internal auditory canal. The labyrinthine artery, a branch of the anterior inferior cerebellar artery, is consistently located in the internal auditory canal. The canal may also encompass the loop of the anterior inferior cerebellar artery, observed in 50% of anatomical studies. This loop often resides posterior to the nerve roots; however, it may also be situated between or anterior to them. All neurovascular components are encased by an arachnoid layer that extends into the internal auditory canal, filled with cerebrospinal fluid (CSF), and connects to the cistern of the cerebellopontine angle. The dura mater, situated outside the arachnoid layer, attaches to the bone and merges with its periosteum, subsequently loosely encasing the nerve filaments that leave through the fundus, thereby generating the epineurium [5, 7].

6.3 Pathology

The etiopathogenesis, histology, and growth pattern of small-sized vestibular schwannomas are identical to those of bigger vestibular schwannomas, as they are merely tumors identified at an earlier stage of development. Small tumors rarely possess a cystic component. The small size does not imply that growth will not occur; however, it is accurate that small schwannomas in old people may experience minimal growth for the remainder of their lives, which does not preclude the necessity for monitoring. Histological examinations of autopsy results facilitate the incidental identification of tiny vestibular schwannomas, wherein their precise origin is traced to a branch of the vestibular nerve before encroaching upon the whole vestibular nerve or cochlear nerve. This condition persists for a time, and if the tumor is identified at an early stage, it is feasible to excise the tumor while selectively sectioning the damaged vestibular branch, preserving both the cochlear nerve and the unaffected vestibular branch. While it is widely acknowledged that the origin of vestibular schwannomas lies in the superior vestibular nerve, incidental schwannomas identified in autopsy studies exhibit a highly variable distribution, with comparable percentages among those situated in the superior vestibular nerve, inferior vestibular nerve, vestibular nerve trunk, and even the cochlear nerve trunk.

6.4 Clinical Considerations

Clinically, the symptoms of small-sized vestibular schwannomas may solely result from the involvement of the cranial nerves within the internal auditory canal, specifically the vestibulocochlear and facial nerves, aligning with the traditional otological stage. In their surgical series reviewing 1000 cases, Matties and Samii found that grade T1 intracanalicular tumors presented with deafness in 7% of instances, an average hearing loss duration of 3.6 years, tinnitus lasting 2.5 years, facial nerve dysfunction in 3% of cases, and, unexpectedly, facial hypoesthesia in 4% of cases. In intra-extracanalicular T2 tumors, deafness occurred in 17% of patients with a mean duration of hearing loss of 3.4 years and tinnitus lasting 2 years. Clinical involvement of the facial nerve was observed in 10% of cases, while trigeminal involvement was noted in 5% of patients [6].

6.5 Diagnostic Considerations

The diagnosis of small-sized vestibular schwannomas is precisely established using magnetic resonance imaging (MRI) examinations (Fig. 6.1). Nonetheless, in the case of millimetric lesions, false positives may occur, encompassing the intracanalicular positioning of the anterior inferior cerebellar artery loop, arachnoiditis, neuritis of the vestibulocochlear or facial nerve, and nonspecific lesions of an inflammatory or hyperemic origin. Consequently, these lesions warrant study, as many will resolve spontaneously due to their inherent characteristics; in such cases, otological, vestibular, and electrophysiological evaluations are crucial to validate the diagnostic hypothesis.

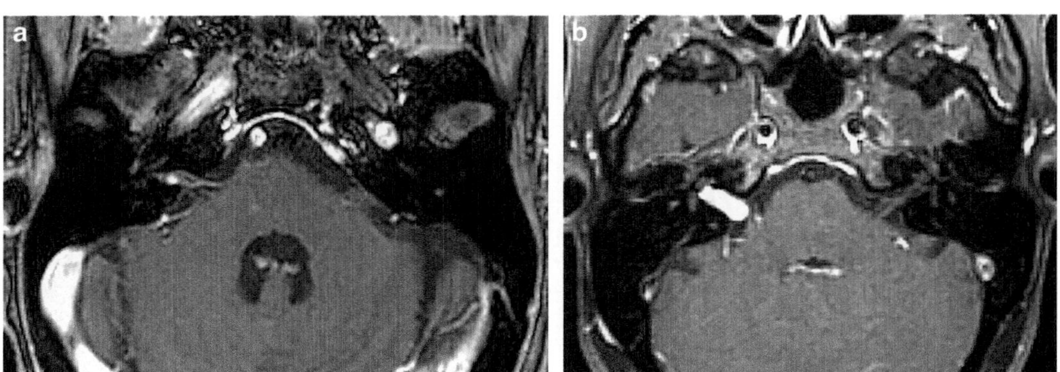

Fig. 6.1 Small-sized right vestibular schwannoma. (**a**) Axial T1-weighted MRI with gadolinium reveals a pure intracanalicular vestibular schwannoma, classified as Samii grade T1 and Koos grade I. (**b**) Axial T1-weighted MRI with gadolinium demonstrating a vestibular schwannoma encroaching into the cerebellopontine angle cistern, classified as Samii grade T2 and Koos grade II

The essential imaging studies required for microneurosurgical treatment of vestibular schwannoma include a thin-section bone study via computed tomography (CT) in axial and coronal planes, as well as an MRI study in all three planes, incorporating T1-weighted sequences both with and without contrast, T2-weighted sequences, and highly T2-weighted sequences with thin sections (FIESTA: *Fast Imaging Employing Steady-state Acquisition*).

6.6 Surgical Categories

While pure intracanalicular vestibular schwannomas can be distinguished from those that protrude into the cerebellopontine angle cistern (Fig. 6.2), there are no variations in the technical aspects of resection from a microneurosurgical perspective; the procedure is consistently executed by a retrosigmoid approach with transmeatal access.

6.7 Microneurosurgical Management

This section outlines the phases for the resection of typical small-sized vestibular schwannomas, namely those classified as T1 and T2 according to Matties and Samii, as well as Koos grades I-II, with a maximum size of 20 mm, inclusive of the intracanalicular component [1, 5, 8]. The retrosigmoid approach outlined in earlier chapters exhibits no specific nuances when executed for the excision of tiny vestibular schwannomas. Upon dura mater incision, cerebrospinal fluid is evacuated from the caudal cisterns, and the cerebellum is retracted to reveal the posterior aspect of the petrosal bone.

6.7.1 Pure Intracanalicular Vestibular Schwannoma

Pure intracanalicular vestibular schwannomas are classified as Matties and Samii grade T1 and Koos grade T1 tumors, measuring less than 11 mm in size. In pure intracanalicular tumors, the normal anatomy of the cerebellopontine angle is discernible following the incision of the dura mater and medial retraction of the cerebellum, allowing for the anatomical and electrophysiological identification of the facial, cochlear, and vestibular nerve roots, as well as the localization of the Tübingen line (Fig. 6.3a) [2]. The posterior aspect of the internal auditory canal is removed, revealing the tumor and neurovascular structures.

The dura mater is coagulated above the Tübingen line, and a flap is cut with a fine knife, thereafter elevated towards the meatus using a

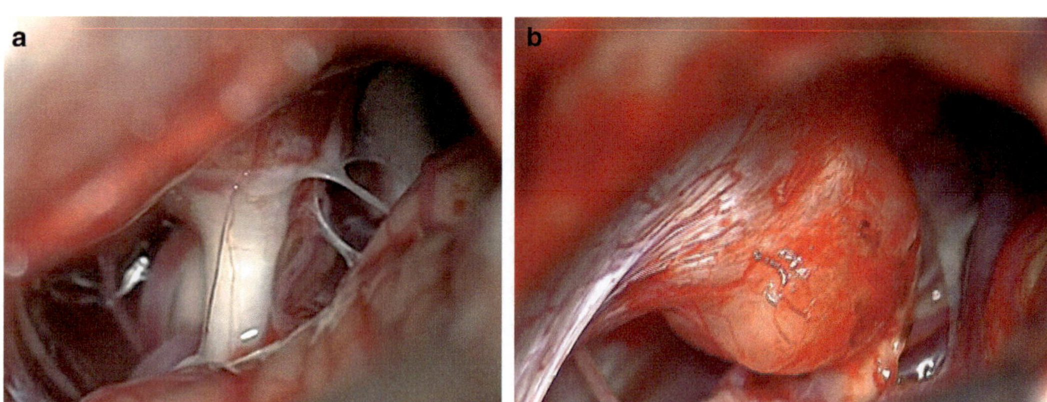

Fig. 6.2 Intraoperative views of a vestibular schwannoma encroaching upon the left cerebellopontine angle cistern. (**a**) Vestibular schwannoma exhibiting a little intracisternal protrusion. (**b**) Vestibular schwannoma exhibiting significant intracisternal bulging

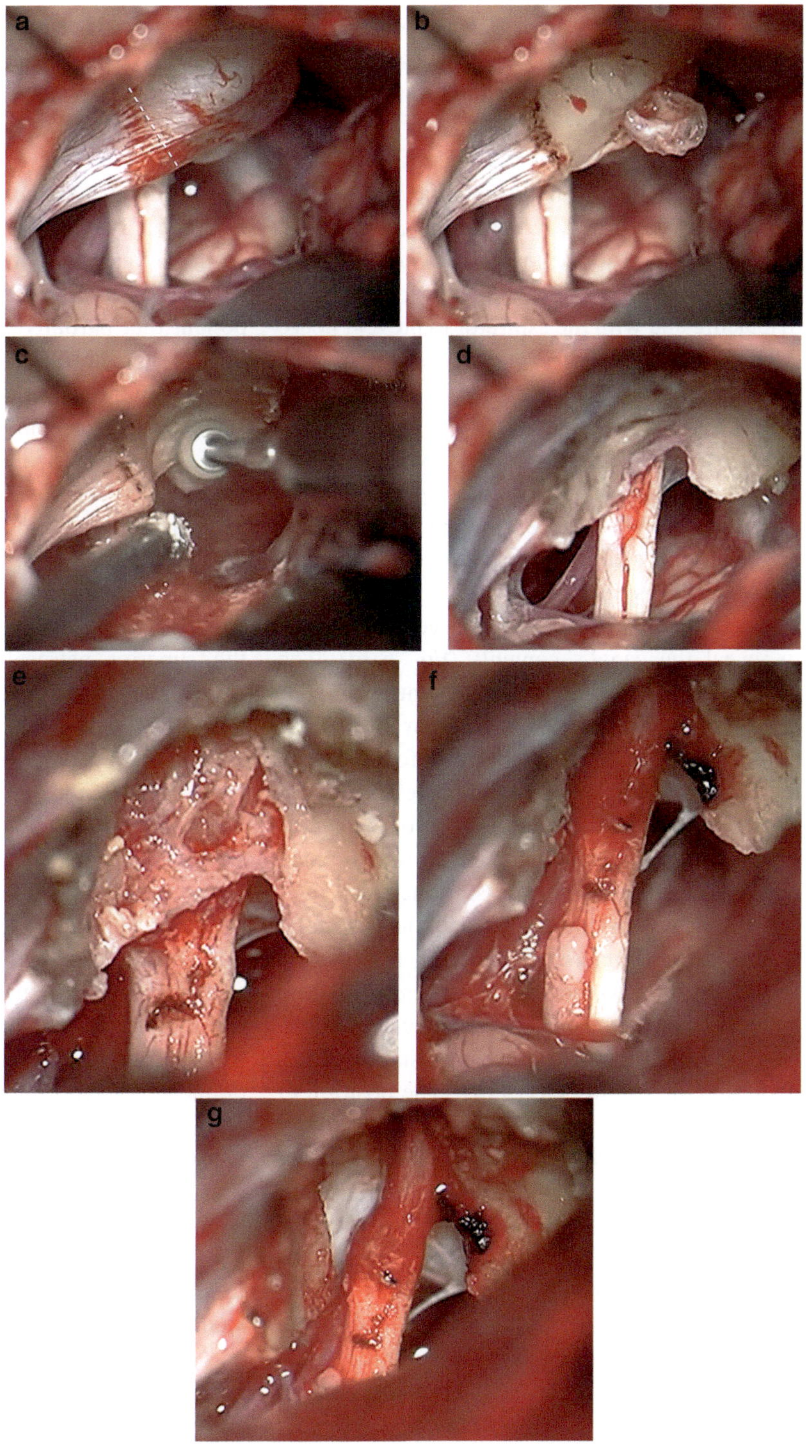

Fig. 6.3 Pure intracanalicular left vestibular schwannoma. (**a**) Intraoperative picture displaying the typical anatomy of the cerebellopontine angle. The Tübingen line is identifiable by the transition from the convoluted caudal dura mater to the smooth cranial dura mater. The vestibulocochlear and facial complexes are in a deeper anatomical plane, adjacent to the caudal boundary of the anterior inferior cerebellar artery loop. (**b**) Separation of the dura mater superior to the Tübingen line. (**c**, **d**) Illustrations of the thick osseous structure of the auditory canal wall during drilling. (**e**) Upon dura mater incision, the intrameatal vestibular schwannoma is observed. (**f**) Illustration of the stump of the vestibular nerve following its proximal transection at the point of emergence from the brainstem. (**g**) A conclusive picture displaying the total excision of the tumor, with the auditory canal exposed and including the cochlear and facial nerve roots within

sharp dissector and retained as a protective barrier for the nerves (Fig. 6.3b). A 1–3 mm drill powered by a high-speed motor is utilized for drilling, continuously irrigated with cold saline (Fig. 6.3c). It is recommended to position a substance on the floor of the surgical field to capture the sawdust generated by the drilling, preventing its dispersion throughout the subarachnoid region. Exercise caution with the drill to avoid displacing and with the aspirator to prevent nerve damage. The drill is positioned near the bone when stationary and is retracted only after it has fully ceased operation. The typically compact bone may exhibit mild bleeding, which is managed using bone wax. Upon entering a pneumatic cell, it is imperative to close it with muscle tissue and biological sealing material to avert a postoperative cerebrospinal fluid fistula. The dura mater of the canal is subsequently incised and excised to reveal the canal's contents (Fig. 6.3d). The canal must be exposed for a minimum of 180° posteriorly and, longitudinally, from the meatus to the inner boundary of tumor proliferation or to the fundus, if the tumor encompasses the whole canal. The anatomical configuration of the nerves indicates that the vestibular nerves are situated posteriorly; thus, when accessing the canal interior via the retrosigmoid approach, the vestibular nerves are encountered first. Given that tumors typically originate from these nerves, upon dura mater incision, the vestibular schwannoma is identified, with its proximal and distal boundaries visible depending on its size. The position of the facial nerve is verified with direct electrical stimulation, typically located in a more anterior and superior position inside the canal. The tumor is subsequently excised, preferably isolating the neoplastic tissue from the auditory nerve, the facial nerve, and the vascular structures present inside the canal. The tumor is often excised in small segments using highly precise forceps and micro-scissors (Fig. 6.3e, f). In certain instances, if the tumor is diminutive, it may be enucleated en-bloc (Fig. 6.4). The vestibulocochlear nerve or vestibular nerve root is severed proximally and, if required, distally.

6.7.2 Vestibular Schwannoma Abutting in the Cerebellopontine Angle Cistern

These are intra-extracanalicular tumors classified as grade T2 according to Matties and Samii, and grade II according to Koos, measuring up to 21 mm. In tumors with an extracanalicular component that partially occupies the cerebellopontine angle cistern, the normal architecture of the cerebellopontine angle may typically be discerned after dura mater incision. The configuration of neurovascular cerebellopontine angle components surrounding the tumor is organized in a clockwise direction for right-sided tumors and counterclockwise for left-sided tumors, commencing at the tumor: suprameatal eminence, superior petrosal venous channel draining into the superior petrosal sinus, trigeminal nerve, anterolateral surface of the brainstem and middle cerebellar peduncle, exit points of the facial nerve and vestibulocochlear nerve roots from the brainstem, choroid plexus, lower cranial nerve roots with their upper boundary delineated by the glossopharyngeal nerve, anterior inferior cerebellar artery with variable trajectory and associations, posterior surface of the petrosal bone with the dura mater folds indicating the Tübingen line, and ultimately, the smooth dura mater of the posterior surface of the internal auditory canal above the Tübingen line. The facial nerve must now be delineated via morphological criteria and electrophysiological methods employing direct electrical stimulation. The origin of the vestibular nerve must be recognized and distinguished from the cochlear nerve to facilitate its preservation (Fig. 6.5a). The vestibular nerve penetrates the tumor shortly after its emergence from the brainstem. The tumor may exhibit a fusiform or eccentric growth pattern and is excised in fragments, ensuring the nerve root remains free of tumor (Fig. 6.5b, c). The tumor displaces both the facial nerve and frequently the cochlear nerve roots, resulting in a more or less pronounced banding effect. The vestibulocochlear nerve, or vestibular

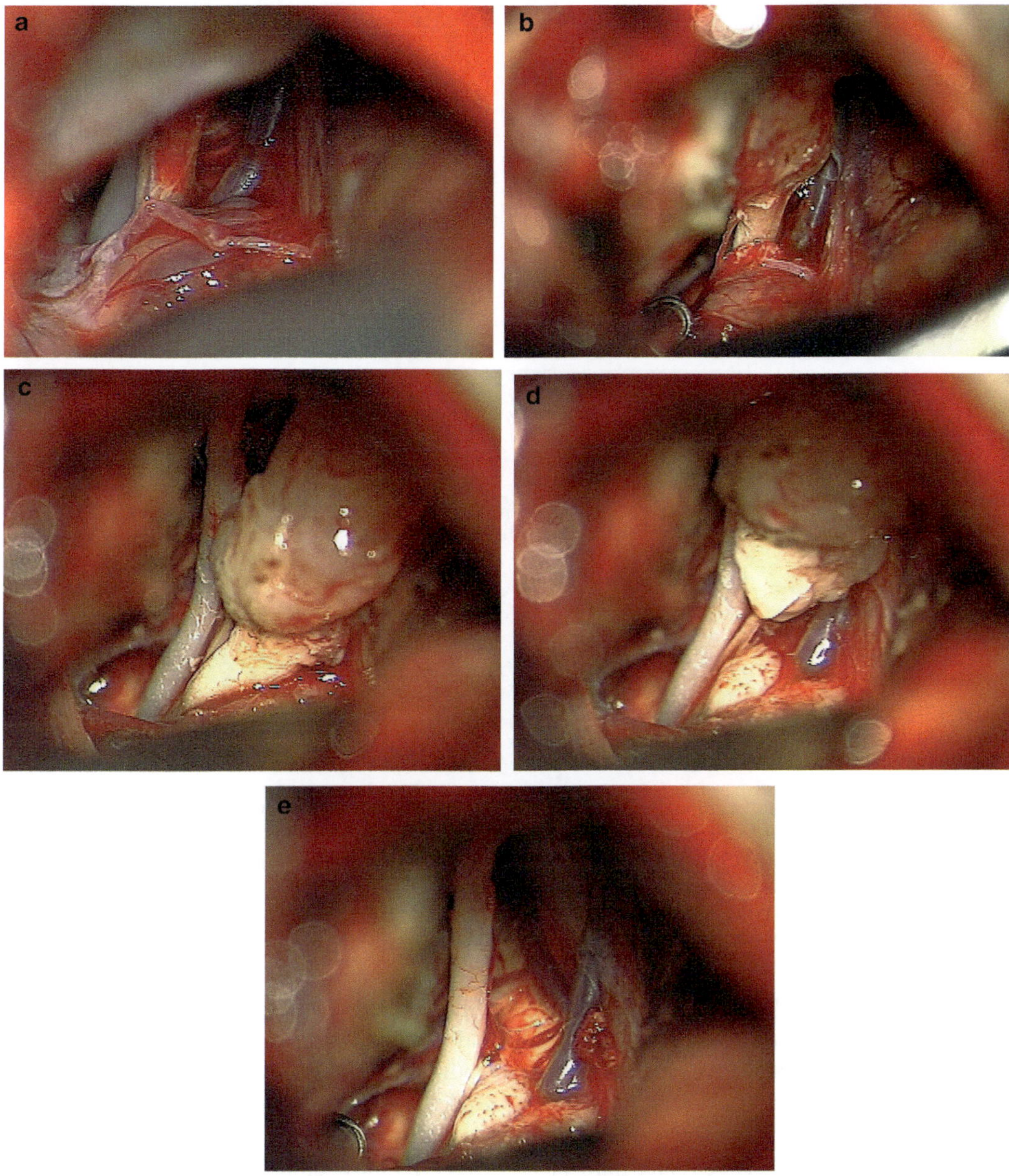

Fig. 6.4 Pure intracanalicular left vestibular schwannoma (**a**) Intraoperative picture displaying the typical building of the cerebellopontine angle. (**b**) Image subsequent to the exposure of the internal auditory canal. (**c**, **d**) Images following en-bloc removal of the tumor, prior to and subsequent to the proximal cutting of the vestibulocochlear nerve. (**e**) The final picture depicts the facial nerve beside the proximal stump of the vestibulocochlear nerve

nerve root, is transected proximally and, if required, distally. In this dissection, it may be beneficial to open the capsule and do internal decompression of the tumor, utilizing fine dissectors rather than the ultrasonic aspirator to attain a more precise and delicate decompression. Transmeatal access is performed as previously described, and the tumor is entirely excised in minute fragments, detaching it from the neurovascular structures of the internal auditory canal.

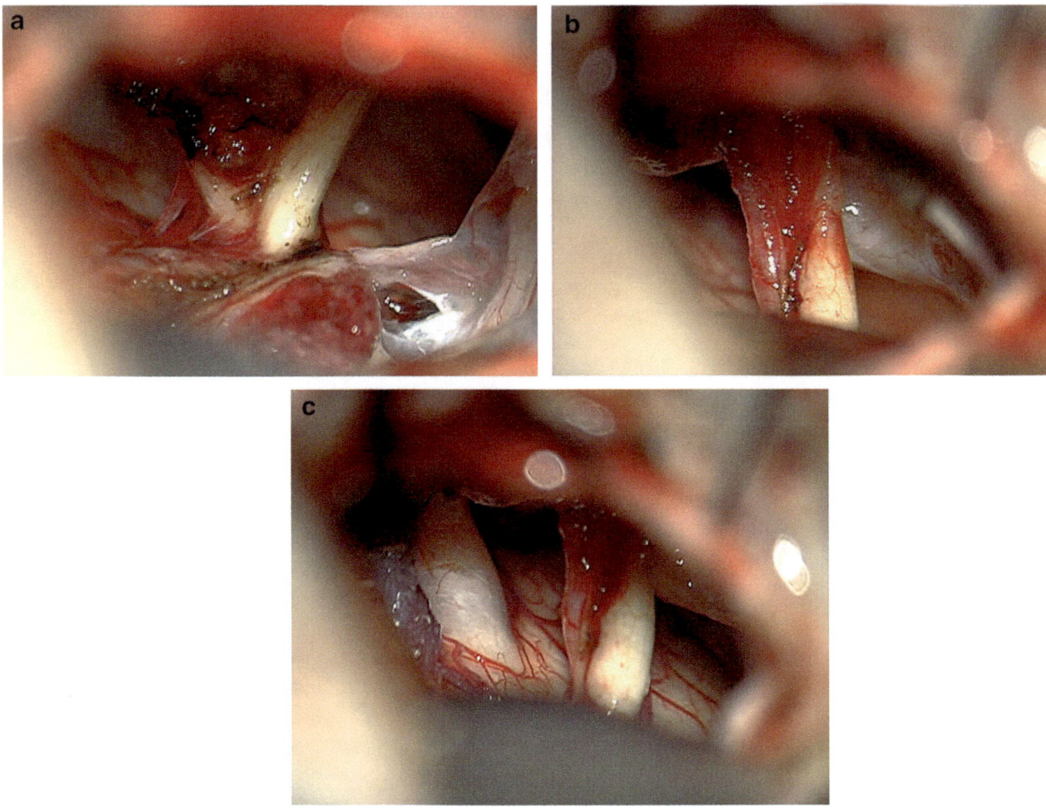

Fig. 6.5 Intracanalicular right vestibular schwannoma projecting into the cistern. (**a**) Intraoperative picture displaying the tumor situated between the vestibulocochlear and facial nerves, which arise concurrently from the brainstem. (**b**) Image displaying the excision of the tumor's cisternal and intracanalicular components following the incision of the internal auditory canal, showcasing the facial nerve and vestibulocochlear nerve. (**c**) Conclusive picture displaying the superior petrosal vein, trigeminal nerve root, and the facial and vestibulocochlear nerves as they exit the brainstem via their cisternal pathway

6.8 Small-Sized Vestibular Schwannomas That Require Specific Treatment

As stated, there are no distinctions in the microneurosurgical treatment between pure intracanalicular cases and those with an extracanalicular component that protrudes into the cerebellopontine angle cistern.

6.9 Results, Prognosis, and Follow-Up

The prognosis for microneurosurgical intervention in tiny vestibular schwannomas is highly favorable, achieving tumor control in over 90% of instances, with 80% of patients retaining functional hearing 5 years post-surgery, provided they had effective hearing prior to the procedure. Optimal facial nerve function (House–Brackmann grades I-III) is attained in 90% of individuals. Morbidity is rare, and fatality is occasional. The imaging follow-up protocol has been outlined in the preceding chapter and consists of regular MRI assessments typically conducted every 6 months, followed by a 5-year follow-up or an advanced MRI if there is a decline in hearing.

6.10 Management Modalities

The objective of therapeutic care for small vestibular schwannomas is to preserve hearing and, in cases of microsurgical resection, to achieve full tumor removal. Treatment alternatives encompass imaging surveillance, stereotactic radiosurgery, and microsurgery [3, 4, 9, 10]. All vestibular schwannomas exhibit a phase of asymptomatic proliferation, during which they may be diagnosed incidentally, typically at a diminutive size, followed by a symptomatic phase, wherein diagnosis can occur at any moment, with size varying significantly. It is acknowledged that all vestibular schwannomas exhibit growth, although the particular rate and velocity of growth for an individual tumor remain uncertain. It is also shown that in patients exhibiting symptoms such as hearing loss, this condition will advance to deafness over time, regardless of tumor growth. The functional prognosis of hearing post-treatment is contingent upon the tumor's size and the extent of otological involvement at the time of intervention. The objective is to ascertain the optimal therapy recommendation for a particular patient.

It is advisable to monitor very small lesions, as they may yield false positive results. Observation is advised for patients with unilateral hearing loss or deafness who do not suffer a decline in their occupational or social quality of life, a scenario likely to arise with untreated vestibular schwannoma. In contrast, patients with tinnitus or vertigo present distinct circumstances; while tinnitus may not significantly impair quality of life, it is distressing and tends to exacerbate over time. Conversely, vertigo adversely affects quality of life but tends to diminish as vestibular function deteriorates. The benefit of conservative treatment lies in its seamless transition to definitive intervention through stereotactic radiosurgery or microneurosurgery in the event of hearing degradation, concerning tumor growth, or a change in patient preference. The economic cost of surveillance is less than that of stereotactic radiosurgery or microneurosurgery, in addition to avoiding possibly unneeded procedures, even in the absence of complications. Conservative treatment enhances the quality of life for patients, with the exception of the phase of reconciling with the prospect of living permanently with a tumor that may necessitate treatment at some point in the future. Ultimately, surveillance is advised for little incidental tumors, as many remain static, others diminish in size, and any intervention entails risks of morbidity and mortality. Conversely, given the assertion that vestibular schwannoma is likely to progress and requires lifelong management and that while auditory function aids in diagnosis, it will inevitably decline, an alternative is to advocate tumor treatment via stereotactic radiosurgery or microneurosurgery.

In individuals with pure intracanalicular vestibular schwannomas and preserved hearing, a decision may be taken between surveillance and microneurosurgery, aiming for total resection while preserving hearing. If hearing is no longer beneficial at diagnosis, observation may continue; nevertheless, microsurgical excision can be recommended without the objective of preserving hearing by a translabyrinthine approach, which presents a lower risk compared to transcranial methods.

In the remaining intermediate scenarios, characterized by functional or marginally modified hearing, elevated surgical or anesthetic risk, or patient refusal of operation, the recommendation is once again observation or stereotactic radiosurgery. For tiny vestibular schwannomas, stereotactic radiosurgery preserves usable hearing in over 50% of patients at the time of treatment, accompanied by a minimal complication rate.

In 2017, the Congress of Neurological Surgeons (CNS) released evidence-based guidelines about hearing preservation across three treatment modalities for vestibular schwannomas, which offer the following recommendations pertaining to tumor-related criteria [3]:

- Observation: The most reliable prognostic indicators for preserving functional hearing include favorable outcomes in the preoperative word recognition test and/or the pitch threshold test, together with the absence of tumor progression. The size of the tumor upon diagnosis, age, and sex do not serve as predictors for the eventual onset of nonfunctional hearing during observation.
- Stereotactic radiosurgery: The primary prognosis indicators for preserving functional hearing include favorable word recognition test results and/or pure tone threshold scores, reduced tumor size, a marginal tumor dose of

≤12 Gy, and a cochlear dose of ≤4 Gy. Age and sex are not significant factors of hearing preservation outcomes.

- Microsurgery: The primary prognostic indicators for preserving functional hearing postoperatively include favorable preoperative word recognition and/or pure tone threshold scores, small tumor size typically under 10 mm, and the presence of a cerebrospinal fluid layer at the base of the internal auditory canal. Age and sex are not significant factors of hearing preservation outcomes.

6.11 Key Messages

- *Small vestibular schwannoma may be managed with stereotactic radiosurgery, microneurosurgical excision, or observation, subject to many factors.*
- *The transmeatal access serves as the basis for microneurosurgical resection* via *a retrosigmoid approach.*
- *The objective of treatment is to maintain effective hearing; all treatment modalities possess a reasonable functional prognosis.*

References

1. Bambakidis N, Megerian CA, Spetzler RF, editors. Surgery of the cerebellopontine angle. Chaim: Springer Nature; 2018.
2. Campero A, Martins C, Rhoton A Jr, et al. Dural landmark to locate the internal auditory canal in large and giant vestibular schwannomas: the Tübingen line. Neurosurgery. 2011;69(Suppl Operative 1):99–102. https://doi.org/10.1227/NEU.0b013e31821664c6.
3. Carlson ML, Vivas EX, McCracken DJ, et al. Congress of Neurological Surgeons systematic review and evidence-based guidelines on hearing preservation outcomes in patients with sporadic vestibular schwannomas. Neurosurgery. 2028;82:E35–9. https://doi.org/10.1093/neuros/nyx511.
4. Goldbrunner R, Weller M, Regis J, et al. EANO guideline on the diagnosis and treatment of vestibular schwannoma. Neuro-Oncology. 2020;22:31–45. https://doi.org/10.1093/neuonc/noz153.
5. González-Darder JM, Quilis-Quesada V, Capilla-Guasch P, de Oliveira E. Abordajes neuroquirúrgicos de la patología craneal y cerebral. 2nd ed. Barcelona: Elsevier España; 2020.
6. Matthies C, Samii M. Management of 1000 vestibular schwannomas (acoustic neuromas): clinical presentation. Neurosurgery. 1997;40:1–9. https://doi.org/10.1097/00006123-199701000-00001. PMID: 8971818
7. Rhoton AL Jr. The posterior fossa: microsurgical anatomy & surgical approaches. Neurosurgery. 2000;47(Suppl 3):S1–S279. https://doi.org/10.1097/00006123-200009001-00013.
8. Samii M, Gerganov V. Surgery of cerebellopontine angle lesions. Berlin/Heidelberg: Springer-Verlag; 2013.
9. Savardekar AR, Terrell D, Lele SJ, et al. Primary treatment of small to medium (<3 cm) sporadic vestibular schwannomas: a systematic review and meta-analysis on hearing preservation and tumour control rates for microsurgery versus radiosurgery. World Neurosurg. 2022;160:102–113.e12. https://doi.org/10.1016/j.wneu.2021.11.083.
10. Zanoletti E, Mazzoni A, d'Avella D. Hearing preservation in small acoustic neuroma: observation or active therapy? Literature review and institutional experience. Acta Neurochir. 2019;161:79–83. https://doi.org/10.1007/s00701-018-3739-x.

Medium-Sized Vestibular Schwannoma

7

7.1 Introduction

This chapter delineates the specific characteristics of vestibular schwannomas that neurosurgeons most commonly encounter, specifically medium-sized tumors classified as Matties and Samii grade T3 cisternal tumors that occupy the cerebellopontine angle cistern without reaching the brain stem (T3a) or that contact the brain stem without causing compression or displacement (T3b) and Koos grade III (tumors that fill the entire cerebellopontine angle cistern without displacing the brain stem), measuring between 20 and 30 mm, including the intracanalicular segment.

7.2 Anatomical Considerations

Given that these tumors reside in the cerebellopontine angle cistern, it is essential to examine the neurovascular structures of the cerebellopontine angle, which Rhoton categorized into three groups [5, 7]. The *superior neurovascular complex* comprises the trochlear nerve, the trigeminal nerve, the superior cerebellar artery (SCA), and its branches. The trochlear nerve arises from the posterior region of the brainstem, situated inferior to the inferior colliculus, and traverses the posterolateral margin of the midbrain, proceeding towards the free edge of the tentorium, positioned between the posterior cerebral artery superiorly and the superior cerebellar artery inferiorly. The trochlear nerve is the smallest cranial nerve and is situated within the arachnoid of the tentorial notch. The trigeminal nerve's apparent origin is located on the anterolateral aspect of the brainstem, immediately medial to the middle cerebellar peduncle, near the midpoint between the upper and lower borders of the pons, extending on an anterior–superior–lateral trajectory to enter Meckel's cave. The trigeminal nerve is the most substantial of all the nerves in the posterior fossa. The trigeminal nerve's interior structure consists of a large sensory root (*pars major*), a diminutive motor root (*pars minor*), and a variable quantity of aberrant rootlets. The superior cerebellar artery originates at the bifurcation of the basilar artery and has four segments: the anterior pontine-mesencephalic segment, the lateral pontine-mesencephalic segment, the cerebellar-mesencephalic segment, and the cortical segment. The superior cerebellar artery bifurcates into cranial and caudal branches at a variable distance from its origin, which are dispersed across the surface of the cerebellar vermis and hemisphere. The superior cerebellar artery is anatomically associated with the trochlear nerve on the lateral aspect of the tentorial notch, where the artery courses posterior to the nerve, perhaps establishing areas of contact between the two structures. The superior cerebellar artery is thereafter associated with the superior aspect of the trigeminal nerve. The principal venous structure

J. M. González-Darder, *Microneurosurgery of Cerebellopontine Angle*,
https://doi.org/10.1007/978-3-032-03091-7_7

in the upper region of the cerebellopontine angle is the superior petrosal venous complex, which empties into the superior petrosal sinus. A singular drainage channel, known as Dandy's vein, typically results from the confluence of two or more veins originating from the surface of the cerebellum and brain stem. Occasionally, multiple separate trunks converge into the superior petrosal sinus. The pontine-trigeminal vein, which concludes in the superior petrosal complex, may also have a close association with the trigeminal root.

The *middle neurovascular complex* comprises the abducens nerve, facial nerve, vestibulocochlear nerve, and the anterior inferior cerebellar artery (AICA). The abducens nerve originates visibly in the medullary-pontine sulcus, situated above the pyramid, and travels superior-laterally to Dorello's canal. The facial and vestibulocochlear nerves arise laterally in the medullary-pontine sulcus, situated above the supra-olivary fossa. The origin of the facial nerve is positioned somewhat anterior and inferior to the outlet of the vestibulocochlear nerve. The intermediate nerve of Wrisberg consists of a variable number of rootlets that arise and are situated between the two nerves, exhibiting adhesions to both. The intermediate nerve consists of sensory fibers integrated into the facial nerve, with its ganglionic neuronal cell bodies located in the geniculate ganglion. The facial–vestibulocochlear–intermediate complex is traveling superior-laterally to the internal auditory meatus. The anterior inferior cerebellar artery arises from the basilar artery stem and has four segments: the anterior pontine segment, the lateral pontine segment, the floccular-peduncular segment, and the cortical segment. The lateral pontine segment aligns with the trajectory of the anterior inferior cerebellar artery along the cerebellopontine angle, where the artery may interact with the facial and vestibulocochlear nerves, potentially contacting, deforming, or distorting these nerve roots. The anatomical connections and branches of the anterior inferior cerebellar artery in this segment are intricate and diverse. The artery's trunk typically courses anterior–inferior to the nerves, and in two-thirds of instances, an arterial loop extends to the internal auditory meatus. The arterial segment typically traverses the space between the facial and vestibulocochlear nerves and may be positioned medial to the meatus, extend to it, or perhaps penetrate the internal auditory canal. The meatal segment of the artery generates the labyrinthine, or internal auditory artery, which penetrates the internal auditory canal, providing minor branches to the bone, dura mater, and inner ear. Subsequent to the meatal loop, the artery reverts medially to supply blood to the brainstem and cerebellum while again associating with the facial and vestibulocochlear nerves. The venous drainage of the middle level of the cerebellopontine angle is primarily facilitated by the vein of the cerebellopontine fissure, which is formed by the confluence of multiple small veins and ascends towards the superior petrosal venous complex. The vein of the middle cerebellar peduncle is another venous channel that originates in the medullary-pontine sulcus and ascends cranially towards the superior petrosal complex.

The *lower neurovascular complex* comprises the glossopharyngeal nerve, vagal nerve, spinal or accessory nerve of Willis, hypoglossal nerve, and the posterior inferior cerebellar artery (PICA). The hypoglossal nerve, the final cranial nerve, is constituted by many small branches that emerge from the anterolateral or pre-olivary sulcus of the medulla oblongata, situated between the pyramid and the inferior olive. The remaining fibers originate from neurons placed in the anterior horn of the upper cervical spinal cord, in a varied number of rootlets that arise from the lateral surface of the medulla oblongata, namely in the posterolateral or retro-olivary sulcus, situated between the lateral edge of the inferior olive and the cuneate fasciculus. The glossopharyngeal nerve is composed of one or, less commonly, two rootlets. Following a brief segment, many rootlets arise across a few millimeters, constituting the vagal nerve and, further distally, the cranial segment of the accessory nerve. All of these rootlets extend laterally towards the jugular foramen, beneath the choroid plexus that projects from the fourth ventricle through the foramen of Luschka. The cervical segment of the accessory nerve is constituted by the convergence of many rootlets that arise from the cervical spinal cord, ascend through the foramen magnum, adhere to the interior surface of the jugular tubercle, and extend to the jugular foramen. The cervical segment of the accessory nerve traverses posteriorly to the dentate ligaments, vertebral artery, and hypoglossal nerve. The posterior inferior cerebellar artery exhibits significant variability and complexity in its origin, trajectory, and associations from its origin in the vertebral artery. The posterior inferior cerebellar artery is segmented into five components: anterior bulbar segment, lateral bulbar segment, tonsillar-bulbar segment, telo-velo-tonsillar segment, and cortical segment. The anterior bulbar segment is related to the roots of the hypoglossal nerve, while the lateral bulbar segment is variably associated with the roots of the lower cranial nerves, consistently positioned caudally to the facial and vestibulocochlear nerves. The venous drainage of the inferior compartment of the cerebellopontine angle occurs via tiny veins that empty into the inferior petrosal sinus.

The vestibular schwannoma expands into the *cerebellopontine angle cistern*, which is delineated superiorly from the cisterna ambiens by the lateral pontine-mesencephalic membrane, posteriorly from the cerebellar-medullary cistern by the lateral pontine-medullary membrane situated between the vestibulocochlear and glossopharyngeal nerves, and medially from the prepontine cistern by the anterior pontine membrane. The cerebellopontine angle cistern houses the superior and medium neurovascular complexes. The cerebellar-medullary cistern extends to the foramen magnum and spinal canal, housing the inferior neurovascular complex.

7.3 Pathology

The etiopathogenesis, histology, and growth patterns of medium-sized vestibular schwannomas are identical to those of other schwannomas. Similar to smaller tumors, they typically lack degenerative alterations, hemorrhages, or cysts. As they enlarge, they may erode the meatus or the internal auditory canal while increasingly occupying the cerebellopontine angle cistern.

7.4 Clinical Considerations

In theory, the clinical manifestations of medium-sized vestibular schwannomas would arise from the involvement of cranial nerves located in the internal auditory canal, as well as those in the cerebellopontine angle, corresponding to the traditional neurological phase. In the analysis conducted by Matties and Samii of 1000 cases within their surgical series, grade T3 tumors occupying the cerebellopontine angle cistern underwent surgical intervention, presented with deafness in 21% of patients, with an average hearing loss duration of 3.7 years and tinnitus lasting 1.9 years. Additionally, facial nerve dysfunction was observed in 13% of cases, alongside facial hypoesthesia in 13% of cases [6].

7.5 Diagnostic Considerations

The diagnosis of vestibular schwannoma is currently established using computed tomography (CT) and magnetic resonance imaging (MRI), which, for medium-sized vestibular schwannomas, exhibit all the defining criteria of the lesion. Medium-sized vestibular schwannomas are clearly delineated lesions that occupy either a portion or the entirety of the internal auditory canal and the cerebellopontine angle cistern until they make contact with the brainstem and cerebellum. These tumors exhibit substantial enhancement following gadolinium injection. The differential diagnosis included schwannomas originating from other cranial nerves, meningioma, arachnoid cyst, metastases, and other uncommon tumors of the cerebellopontine angle. The essential imaging studies required for a secure microneurosurgical intervention on a medium-sized vestibular schwannoma include a thin-section bone assessment via CT in both axial and coronal planes, as well as MRI in three planes, utilizing T1-weighted sequences with and without gadolinium, T2-weighted sequences, and highly T2-weighted sequences with thin sections (FIESTA: *Fast Imaging Employing Steady-state Acquisition*).

7.6 Surgical Categories

In microneurosurgical intervention for vestibular schwannomas, the primary determinant is the linear dimension of the tumor. However, there are no variations in the technical execution of the resection, whether the tumors partially or fully occupy the cerebellopontine angle cistern and make contact with the brainstem, as the resection is consistently performed via a retrosigmoid approach with transmeatal access. The second criterion of interest is the internal structure of the tumor, which may be cystic in certain instances. Cystic tumors are examined in a designated chapter below.

7.7 Microneurosurgical Management

We will now outline the stages for the removal of a typical medium-sized vestibular schwannoma that resides in the cistern without exerting pressure on the brainstem (Fig. 7.1). The tumors are classified as T3 according to Matties and Samii, and grade III according to Koos, with dimensions ranging from 20 to 30 mm, encompassing the intracanalicular segment. We shall proceed in a detailed and sequential manner, as this tumor size is the most commonly presented criterion for microneurosurgical intervention (Fig. 7.2) [1, 5, 8].

7.7.1 Position and Craniotomy

The chapter on the retrosigmoid approach reviews the position, anatomical references, incision, craniotomy, and dural opening. The dimensions of the cranial aperture are inconsequential for microneurosurgical resection of the vestibular schwannoma; the paramount consideration is the alignment of the craniotomy and dural incision with the inferior margin of the transverse sinus and the posterior boundary of the sigmoid sinus.

7.7.2 Cisternal Navigation

Upon incising the dura mater, access is obtained to drain cerebrospinal fluid, alleviate pressure in the posterior fossa, mobilize the cerebellum using a spatula, and delineate pertinent neurological structures within the cerebellopontine angle. The vestibular schwannoma typically expands to fill the superior segment of the cerebellopontine angle, with tumoral proliferation extending caudally from the tentorial plane to the medullary-pontine sulcus, the origin point of the facial and vestibulocochlear nerve roots from the brainstem. Consequently, it is recommended to decompress the cerebellar-medullary cistern and lower cranial nerves through the drainage of cerebrospinal fluid from the caudal cisterns. This enables the cerebellum to be retracted using a spatula, so revealing the tumor's surface, which in medium-sized vestibular schwannomas is obscured behind the cerebellum, distant from the brainstem in grade 3a tumors (Fig. 7.2a), and in proximity to the cerebellar peduncle and brainstem in grade 3b tumors (Fig. 7.2b).

7.7.3 Dissection of the Caudal Pole of the Tumor and Inferior Neurovascular Complex

After the cisterns posterior to the tumor have been evacuated, the arachnoid is excised to locate the caudal pole of the tumor and to detach it from the rootlets of the glossopharyngeal and vagal nerves. The rootlets are diminutive, and their quantity fluctuates, necessitating meticulous separation from the tumor. Upon achieving this, a pliable, damp material is inserted to facilitate separation and to later identify the nerves, cir-

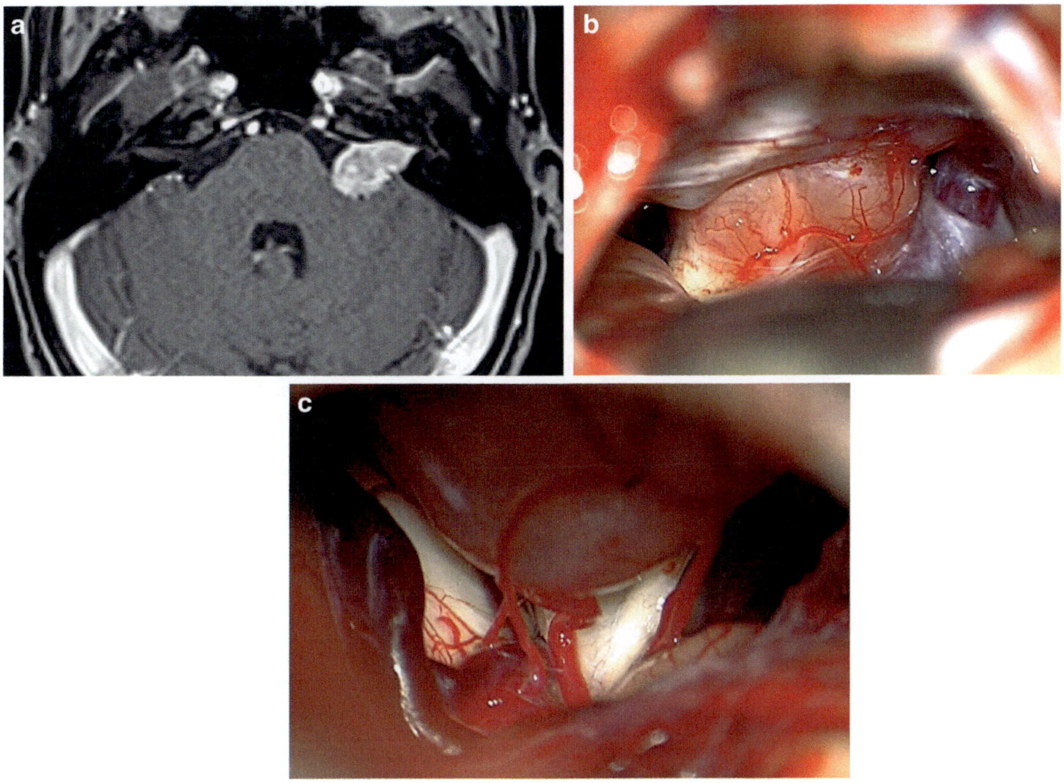

Fig. 7.1 Left medium-sized vestibular schwannoma (Matties and Samii grade T3a). (**a**) Axial T1-weighted slice following gadolinium administration. (**b**) Intraoperative imaging of the tumor in contact with the cerebellum before the removal of the arachnoid. (**c**) A picture displaying the growth pattern of the tumor, which bifurcates the vestibulocochlear nerve

cumventing the use of patties that are excessively thick and rigid, as they attach to the nervous tissue over time and cause injury upon removal. The accessory nerve creates a distinct trunk associated with the dura mater of the jugular tubercle, facilitating its identification. The anterior inferior cerebellar artery and, less frequently, the posterior inferior cerebellar artery may traverse this region, exhibiting highly varied associations with the cranial nerves and the caudal pole of the tumor. During the procedure, arteries traversing the tumor capsule may yield tiny arterioles that require coagulation and transection to facilitate the mobilization of the arterial trunks, which are additionally maintained apart using a moistened soft material (Figs. 7.2c, d).

7.7.4 Dissection of the Cranial Pole of the Tumor and Superior Petrosal Venous Complex

Focus is now on the cranial pole of the tumor, which varies in proximity to the tentorium based on its size, typically displacing the superior petrosal venous complex. The ascending cerebellopontine venous trunk, a component of the venous complex, is particularly noteworthy since it typically traverses the space between the external surface of the tumor and the middle cerebellar peduncle when the tumor is sufficiently enough to exert pressure on the cerebellum and brainstem. In smaller tumors, the upper pole can be dissected until the incisure border of the tento-

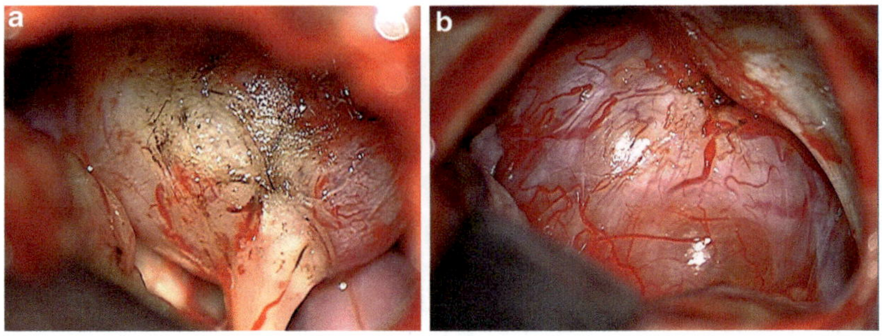

Fig. 7.2 Surgical pictures displaying the microneurosurgical intervention for medium-sized right vestibular schwannomas. (**a**) The picture illustrates a grade 3a vestibular schwannoma following the separation of the cerebellum. (**b**) Image displaying a grade 3b vestibular schwannoma following the separation of the cerebellum. (**c, d**) Illustration of the excision of the arachnoid and the exposure of the caudal cisterns for cerebrospinal fluid outflow. The lower cranial nerves, in their cisternal trajectory, are directed towards the jugular foramen. (**e**) Image following the removal of the arachnoid at the cranial pole of the tumor, allowing visualization of the tentorium, trochlear nerve, superior cerebellar artery, and superior petrosal vein complex. (**f**) Image of the tumor following internal decompression. (**g**) Following internal decompression and planned retraction of the capsule, the tumor volume has been diminished to aid in the dissection of neurovascular elements. (**h**) A picture displaying the trigeminal nerve positioned posterior to the tumor at a deeper anatomical level, adjacent to the brainstem. (**i, j**) Various phases of the tumor dissection from the vestibulocochlear nerve, which is flattened. (**k**) The internal auditory canal has been accessed, and its dura mater and tumoral capsule have been detached. (**l, m, n**) Images displaying the successive separation and dissection of the vestibulocochlear nerve. (**o**) A picture displaying the cerebellopontine angle post-tumoral excision, illustrating the trigeminal, facial, and lower cranial nerves closely together from left to right. The sixth pair is visible in the background. (**p**) Details of a case in which the proximal stump of the vestibulocochlear nerve is observed in contact with the facial nerve

rium is located, beneath which the trajectory of the trochlear nerve and the superior cerebellar artery can be discerned. Once identified, these structures are maintained separate from the capsule (Fig. 7.2e).

7.7.5 Internal Decompression and Debulking of the Tumor

After controlling the cranial and caudal poles of the tumor, the lateral aspect of the tumor and its entry into the internal auditory meatus are progressively revealed. The dura mater and arachnoid typically exhibit significant vascularization that supplies the tumor capsule, necessitating complete coagulation. At this stage, an assessment of the lateral aspect of the tumor capsule can be conducted using direct electrical stimulation to locate the facial nerve as it traverses the superficial surface of the tumor. Following the coagulation of the superficial veins associated with the tumor, a window is created in the capsule using a bipolar coagulator, and intracapsular debulking is performed with an ultrasonic aspirator (Fig. 7.2f, g). The ultrasound and aspiration power must be minimal. The resection is intermittently halted to attain hemostasis through bipolar coagulation of the irregular intratumoral vessels that may emerge. The excision is performed uniformly in all directions to excise the tumor methodically. Resection may be facilitated by compressing the tumor capsule inward with the wall aspirator and excising the underlying intracapsular segment with the ultrasonic aspirator. It is crucial to avoid perforating the capsule at any stage to prevent damage to concealed structures and to maintain the dissection plane. Internal decompression is a protracted and laborious process that necessitates precision and must be comprehensive to achieve true efficacy.

7.7.6 Dissection of the Tumoral Capsule

As the tumor is excised, the capsule is retracted using bipolar coagulation to retain its integrity

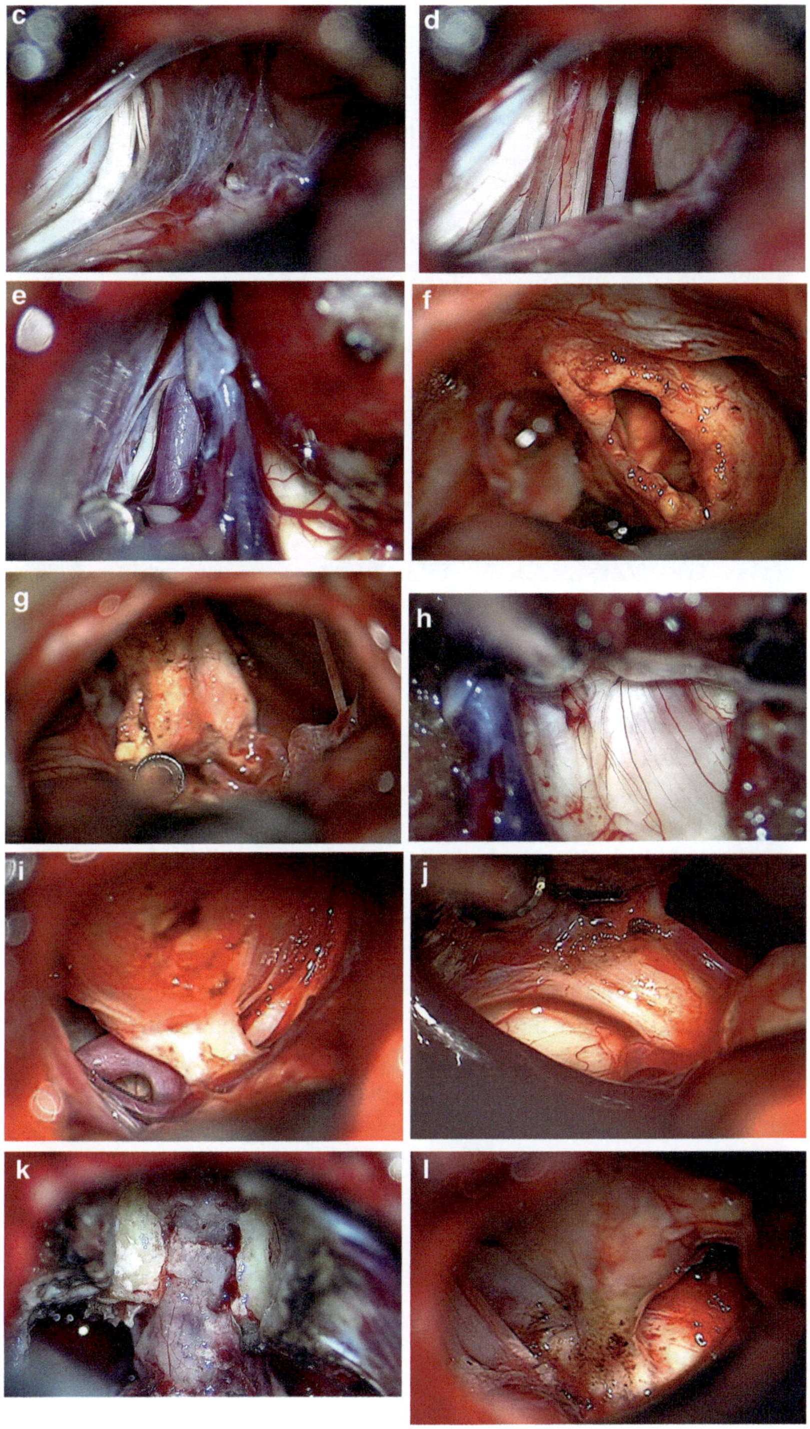

Fig. 7.2 (continued)

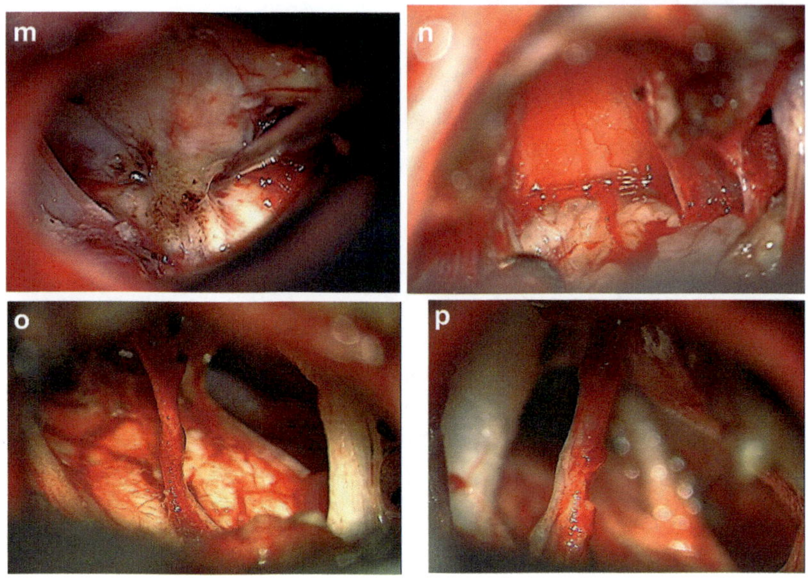

Fig. 7.2 (continued)

and preserve the cleavage plane. After securing the cranial nerves both caudal and cranial to the tumor, the capsule is released from the anterolateral region of the pons and lateral to the cerebellopontine vein, extending to the anterior part of the middle cerebellar peduncle, from which it must be meticulously detached. Attention should now be directed towards locating the trigeminal nerve, situated in a deep plane between the tumor and the pons, posterior and inferior to the tumor. The tumor compresses and displaces the trigeminal nerve significantly, although does not infiltrate the nerve fibers. The trigeminal nerve is frequently amalgamated inside the brainstem; however, it does not require disengagement from the pons to prevent damage (Fig. 7.2h).

7.7.7 Dissection of the Cisternal Segments of the Vestibulocochlear and Facial Nerves

Capsule retraction diminishes the tumor's bulk and facilitates the identification of the vestibulocochlear nerve at its entry point in the most caudal region of the tumor. To accomplish this, it is essential to elevate the tumor capsule at its most caudal region. At this stage, a segment of the vestibulocochlear nerve may be partially discernible before it enlarges and becomes enveloped by the tumor capsule (Figs. 7.2i, j). At the egress of the nerve trunk from the brainstem, there typically exists an irregularly formed venous plexus that must be meticulously coagulated. The facial nerve trunk must now be distinctly defined and acknowledged, based on three criteria. Anatomically, the facial nerve is situated in the retrosigmoid approach, posterior to the vestibulocochlear nerve, thereby residing in a deeper plane. Its appearance is distinct, exhibiting a whiter, brighter, and pearlescent quality compared to the vestibulocochlear nerve. Ultimately, it can be identified with direct electrical stimulation because of its unequivocal electromyographic response.

7.7.8 Dissection of the Tumoral Capsule from the Brainstem

The gradual excision of the capsule and detachment of the tumor capsule from the brainstem has now been accomplished, preserving the integrity of the facial nerve. The vestibulocochlear nerve is preserved intact to aid in orienting and microsurgical manipulation of the tumor. The tumor and capsule are resected in minute fragments using delicate forceps and sharp curved or straight microscissors (piecemeal resection), ensuring the preservation of the cleavage plane and the continuity of the capsule still connected to the cranial nerves.

7.7.9 Opening of the Internal Auditory Canal

After a substantial volumetric resection and extensive removal of the capsule, focus shifts to the internal auditory canal, which is accessed by drilling the posterior surface of the canal, utilizing Tübingen's line as a reliable anatomical reference (Fig. 7.2k). The specifics of this transmeatal approach have been showed in the chapter focused on small-sized vestibular schwannoma. The initial drilling of the bone reveals the dura mater, which enters the canal resembling a glove finger; thus, it must be longitudinally sectioned or resected to access the intracanalicular portion of the tumor [2].

7.7.10 Gradual Extirpation of the Tumor and Preservation of the Facial Nerve

The resection of the tumor and capsule is performed in increasingly smaller fragments while maintaining the tumor's remains anchored proximally and distally to the vestibulocochlear nerve, progressively isolating the facial nerve from the tumor in both its proximal and distal segments. As the facial nerve progressively broadens and becomes subtly incorporated into the tumor capsule, there may eventually be a point at which safe dissection is no longer feasible. Neurotonic discharges of the facial nerve and the heightened degree of direct stimulation parameters required to elicit an electromyographic response are definitive indicators of facial nerve distress or injury.

7.7.11 Proximal and Distal Section of the Vestibulochoclear Nerve and Resection of the Tumor

The proximal end of the vestibulocochlear nerve is now transected near the brainstem. A microhook is inserted between the vestibulocochlear and facial nerves, after which the former is severed with microscissors, typically resulting in a flattened facial nerve. On the proximal side, the nerve consists of a singular trunk; however, on the distal side, within the auditory canal, the vestibular and cochlear trunks can be discerned in occasions where the tumor has not fully infiltrated the auditory canal to the fundus. The vestibulocochlear nerve is also transected distally within the canal, isolating the residual tumor, which must be meticulously separated from the facial nerve, which follows a deeper trajectory. The dissection should now be performed bluntly, in both proximal and distal directions, utilizing a fine dissector and excising the small tumor nodules with fine, sharp, curved microscissors. The utilization of an aspirator or bipolar coagulation poses significant risks to the anatomical and functional integrity of the facial nerve. The neurosurgeon must now determine whether to proceed with the excision of the tumor remnants or to cease, weighing the preservation of the facial nerve's anatomical and functional integrity against its functional viability, even if it necessitates leaving a tumor remnant.

7.7.12 Final Overview

Following meticulous hemostasis, a last examination of the surgical field (Figs. 7.2p) and the final direct electrical stimulation of the monitored cranial nerves are conducted. The dura mater, craniotomy, and soft tissues are closed in accordance with the procedures outlined in the chapter on the retrosigmoid approach.

7.8 Medium-Sized Vestibular Schwannomas That Require Specific Treatment

There are no significant differences in the microneurosurgical treatment of medium-sized vestibular schwannomas occupying the cistern (Matties and Samii grade 3a) compared to those in touch with the brain stem (Matties and Samii grade 3b). Remarkably, a vestibular schwannoma can be enucleated en bloc when it is diminutive, exhibiting eccentric and predominantly extracanalicular growth while preserving the integrity of the vestibulocochlear nerve (Fig. 7.3).

7.9 Results, Prognosis, and Follow-Up

A recent meta-analysis of the literature examines the progression of patients who received microneurosurgical resection of small- to medium-sized vestibular schwannomas, defined as smaller than 30 mm. The research demonstrates that 56% of patients maintain functional hearing post-surgery, following an average follow-up period of 5.3 years. Over time, a decline in residual hearing is noted; however, distinguishing treatment-related deterioration from age-related physiological hearing loss may prove challenging. Tumor growth control is attained in 98% of cases over 5.8 years, resulting in a mere 2% recurrence rate. In the immediate postoperative period, good facial function (House-Brackman (HB) grade I-III) is observed in 90% of patients. Impairment in facial nerve function may represent either a new occurrence or an exacerbation of pre-existing facial nerve dysfunction before surgery. It is widely recognized that the evaluation of facial nerve function should occur no sooner than 6 months post-surgery, as spontaneous recovery is expected, provided that the anatomical integrity of the facial nerve has been maintained and that there is functional nerve transmission at the conclusion of the procedure, evidenced by low-intensity direct electrical stimulation.

7.10 Management Modalities

Medium-sized vascular malformations are the most commonly recommended for microneurosurgical intervention. In recent years, there has been a rise in radiation therapies, particularly stereotactic radiosurgery. Following the diagnosis of a sporadic vestibular schwannoma, there are three therapeutic management options: surveillance with imaging modalities, microneurosurgical intervention, and stereotactic radiosurgery [3, 4, 9, 10]. The choice of treatment recommendation is contingent upon various factors. In this context, factors pertaining to the tumor (dimen-

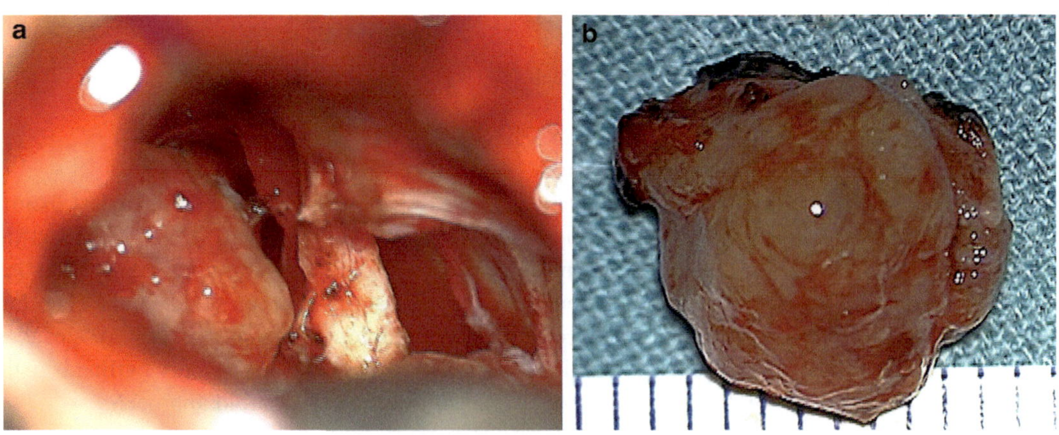

Fig. 7.3 Surgical pictures of the micro-neurosurgical treatment of a right vestibular schwannoma, displaying the enucleation and en bloc resection of the tumor. (**a**) Operative area. (**b**) Tumor

sions, growth rate), the patient (clinical manifestations, auditory function, age, comorbidities, desires, and anticipations), and healthcare (surgeon's expertise and institutional reputation) must be taken into account. The amalgamation of these elements generates a multitude of distinct scenarios to recommend the optimal treatment approach.

7.10.1 Imaging Observation

Observation would be the optimal strategy for a medium-sized vestibular schwannoma, exhibiting no evident growth, for patients possessing functional hearing and lacking further neurological symptoms and in elderly patients with comorbidities who express no anxiety regarding the presence of a tumor in the cranial cavity. The 2020 guidelines from the European Association of Neuro-Oncology (EANO) encourage monitoring through serial MRI examinations or otological assessments for incidentally identified or asymptomatic vestibular schwannomas. It is acknowledged that 50% of patients would exhibit either an enlargement of the lesion or a deterioration in auditory function within the subsequent 5 years. Consequently, the suggestion of observation is especially inadvisable for young patients, where tumor size escalation has been evidenced, and for those expressing concern regarding their tumor [4, 10].

7.10.2 Microneurosurgery

Microneurosurgery is the optimal method for a medium-sized vestibular schwannoma exhibiting growth, accompanied by hearing loss and neurological symptoms, in a patient of any age without comorbidities who is apprehensive about living with an intracranial tumor and if it is treated by a skilled surgeon in a facility with appropriate resources (Refer to case 8 in Chap. 21). EANO advocates for microsurgery in symptomatic Koos grade II–III tumors, particularly when cysts are present or where complete resection of the lesion is feasible with curative intent, as total tumor removal markedly diminishes the likelihood of recurrence [4, 9].

7.10.3 Stereotactic Radiosurgery

Stereotactic radiosurgery is the optimal method for a suitably sized tumor (typically under 30 mm), exhibiting no evidence of growth, in patients preserving functional hearing and absent additional neurological symptoms, in patients of any age, preferably older individuals with comorbidities, who do not express anxiety regarding the presence of a tumor in their cranial cavity (Refer to case 6 in Chap. 21). The EANO guidelines stipulate that stereotactic radiosurgery is appropriate for tumors measuring less than 30 mm in size [4]. Various prospective studies indicate that stereotactic radiosurgery is superior to microneurosurgery in preserving auditory and facial function for tumors smaller than 30 mm. A meta-analysis of the aforementioned literature examined the outcomes of individuals receiving stereotactic radiosurgery treatment for small or medium-sized vestibular schwannomas, defined as those measuring less than 30 mm. The study reveals that 59% of patients maintain functional hearing post-irradiation, with an average follow-up duration of 5.5 years, displaying no significant changes when compared to microneurosurgery outcomes. Tumor growth control is attained in 92% of cases after 6.2 years, resulting in an 8% recurrence rate, which significantly contrasts with microsurgery's 2% recurrence rate. Conversely, the tumor never completely vanishes, which may heighten concerns among many patients over potential recurrence. Concerning the decline in facial nerve function, facial function at or exceeding HB grade III is observed in merely 2% of instances during the immediate postoperative period, which is much lower than that of patients undergoing microsurgery. Nonetheless, in the absence of randomized and prospective studies that facilitate a dependable comparison of the two therapeutic options, stereotactic radiosurgery is advised as an alternative for patients unable to undergo surgery due to concurrent pathology, those hesitant to pursue microsurgery, and individuals indifferent to retaining a tumor within their skull over time [9].

7.11 Key Messages

- *Medium-sized vestibular schwannomas may be managed with stereotactic radiosurgery, microneurosurgical excision, or monitoring, contingent upon many factors.*
- *Microneurosurgical excision is done through a retrosigmoid approach and transmeatal access.*
- *Medium-sized vestibular schwannomas are the most prevalent tumors excised by microneurosurgery using the retrosigmoid approach.*
- *The objective of treatment is to preserve facial nerve function, and any treatment modality offers a good functional prognosis.*

References

1. Bambakidis N, Megerian CA, Spetzler RF, editors. Surgery of the cerebellopontine angle. Cham: Springer Nature; 2018.
2. Campero A, Martins C, Rhoton A Jr, et al. Dural landmark to locate the internal auditory canal in large and giant vestibular schwannomas: the Tübingen line. Neurosurgery. 2011;69(Suppl Operative 1):99–102. https://doi.org/10.1227/NEU.0b013e31821664c6.
3. Carlson ML, Vivas EX, McCracken DJ, et al. Congress of Neurological Surgeons systematic review and evidence-based guidelines on hearing preservation outcomes in patients with sporadic vestibular schwannomas. Neurosurgery. 2028;82:E35–9. https://doi.org/10.1093/neuros/nyx511.
4. Goldbrunner R, Weller M, Regis J, et al. EANO guideline on the diagnosis and treatment of vestibular schwannoma. Neuro-Oncology. 2020;22:31–45. https://doi.org/10.1093/neuonc/noz153.
5. González-Darder JM, Quilis-Quesada V, Capilla-Guasch P, de Oliveira E. Abordajes neuroquirúrgicos de la patología craneal y cerebral. 2nd ed. Barcelona: Elsevier España; 2020.
6. Matthies C, Samii M. Management of 1000 vestibular schwannomas (acoustic neuromas): clinical presentation. Neurosurgery. 1997;40:1–9. https://doi.org/10.1097/00006123-199701000-00001. PMID: 8971818
7. Rhoton AL Jr. The posterior fossa: microsurgical anatomy & surgical approaches. Neurosurgery. 2000;47(Suppl 3):S1–S279. https://doi.org/10.1097/00006123-200009001-00013.
8. Samii M, Gerganov V. Surgery of cerebellopontine angle lesions. Berlin/Heidelberg: Springer-Verlag; 2013.
9. Savardekar AR, Terrell D, Lele SJ, et al. Primary treatment of small to medium (<3 cm) sporadic vestibular schwannomas: a systematic review and meta-analysis on hearing preservation and tumour control rates for microsurgery versus radiosurgery. World Neurosurg. 2022;160:102–113.e12. https://doi.org/10.1016/j.wneu.2021.11.083.
10. Zanoletti E, Mazzoni A, d'Avella D. Hearing preservation in small acoustic neuroma: observation or active therapy? Literature review and institutional experience. Acta Neurochir. 2019;161:79–83. https://doi.org/10.1007/s00701-018-3739-x.

8 Large and Giant Vestibular Schwannoma

8.1 Introduction

This chapter will examine the characteristics of huge vestibular schwannomas. This category includes T4 and T5 grade tumors as classified by Matties and Samii, as well as grade IV according to Koos, with a maximum axial plane size, including the intracanalicular part, exceeding 40 mm. These are tumors that partially or completely occupy the internal auditory canal and the entire cisterns of the cerebellopontine angle, displacing the brainstem, middle cerebellar peduncle, and cerebellum, as well as the fourth ventricle, leading to some cases of obstructive hydrocephalus. We classify large and giant vestibular schwannomas together due to their analogous challenges in microneurosurgical therapy via a retrosigmoid approach. All patients exhibit symptoms related to otological, cranial nerve, and, in numerous instances, cerebellar, long pathway, or intracranial hypertension. In our clinical practice, nearly all patients with big or huge schwannomas are referred for microneurosurgical intervention, regardless of whether they are diagnosed by otologists or neurologists, as stereotactic radiosurgery is not an option for treatment.

8.2 Anatomical Considerations

As these tumors encompass the entire cerebellopontine angle, they impact all the neurovascular groups delineated by Rhoton [9]. The neurovascular groups have been comprehensively examined in the preceding chapter on medium-sized vestibular schwannoma. As transmeatal access is necessary to finalize resection via a retrosigmoid approach, all anatomical details concerning the meatus and internal auditory canal outlined in the chapter on small-sized schwannomas are equally relevant to large and giant vestibular schwannomas.

8.3 Pathology

The etiopathogenesis, histology, and growth pattern of large or giant vestibular schwannomas are identical to those of smaller schwannomas, as they are merely tumors identified at a later stage of development. A large size does not necessarily indicate rapid growth, malignancy, or an inability to grow further. Numerous large or giant vestibular schwannomas have cystic characteristics, which will be examined in the subsequent chapter.

J. M. González-Darder, *Microneurosurgery of Cerebellopontine Angle*,
https://doi.org/10.1007/978-3-032-03091-7_8

8.4 Clinical Considerations

Clinically, the symptoms of large and giant vestibular schwannomas may arise from the involvement of cranial nerves within the cerebellopontine angle, alongside symptoms resulting from brainstem and cerebellar compression, as well as hydrocephalus; this aligns with the traditional neurosurgical phase. In the analysis conducted by Matties and Samii of 1000 cases in their surgical series, grade T4 tumors with brain stem compression presented with deafness in 42% of instances, accompanied by an average duration of 3.6 years of hearing loss and 1.6 years of tinnitus. In 26% of cases, they were linked to a dysfunction of the facial nerve, and in 32% of cases, to trigeminal hypoesthesia [8].

8.5 Diagnostic Considerations

The diagnosis of large or giant vestibular schwannomas is established using computed tomography (CT) and magnetic resonance imaging (MRI) tests, with the lesions exhibiting characteristics akin to those of smaller variants (Fig. 8.1). Interestingly, the meatus and/or internal auditory canal should not be anticipated to be dilated in proportion to the tumor's size, as once the tumor grows in the cerebellopontine angle cistern, it may not induce further alterations in the bone. These tumors are more prone to exhibit internal alterations in imaging tests, including the regions of acute, subacute, or chronic hemorrhage; hypointense or hyperintense regions in T1 and T2-weighted sequences; uneven contrast enhancement; or cystic formations. The tumor, as it enlarges, displaces and compresses the brain stem, middle cerebellar peduncle, and cerebellum, with identifiable regions of edema (Fig. 8.2). In some instances, even in the biggest tumors, a thin hypointense halo may be shown between the tumor and the nerve tissue, indicating the presence of an arachnoid plane that separates the tumor from the pia mater (cleavage plane). The tumor may significantly displace the fourth ventricle and occasionally cause obstructive hydrocephalus or supratentorial communicating hydrocephalus, each presenting distinct semiology in imaging examinations. Electrophysiological studies are pertinent to the examination of the functionality of the auditory (BEAPs) and long tracts (SSEPs).

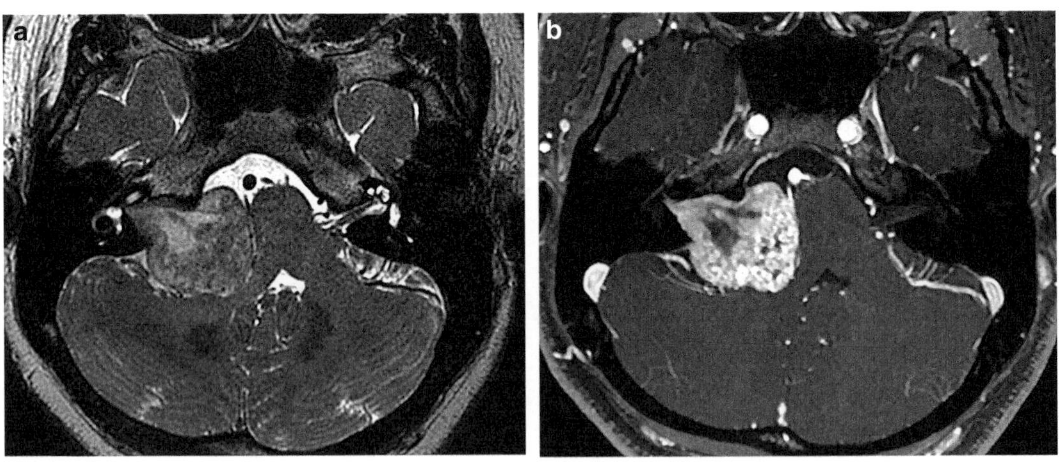

Fig. 8.1 Large Matties and Samii grade T4 right vestibular schwannoma. (**a**) Axial slice of T2 FIESTA MRI. (**b**) Axial slice of T1 MRI following gadolinium administration. Both sequences reveal a significant tumor that markedly compresses the cerebellar peduncle and brainstem. The meatus and internal auditory canal are significantly enlarged. The tumor exhibits internal abnormalities in both sequences, indicative of degenerative alterations. No evidence of edema or signal alterations in the brainstem is present

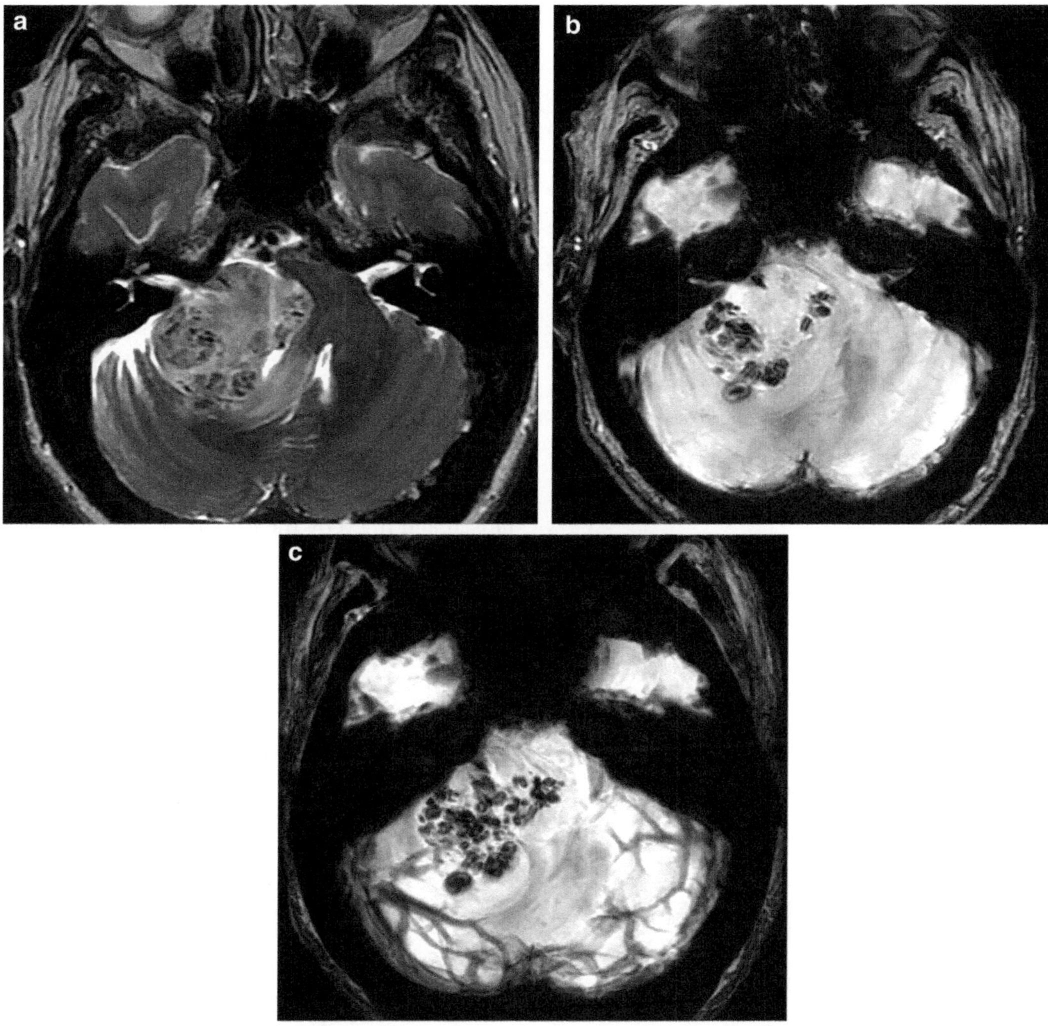

Fig. 8.2 Giant Matties and Samii grade T5 right vestibular schwannoma. (**a**) Axial MRI slice with T2 weighting. (**b**) Axial MRI slice of T2-GRE. (**c**) Axial MRI slice of T2-SWAN. The imaging studies reveal a substantial tumor that exerts a significant pressure on the brainstem, cerebellar peduncle, and cerebellum. The meatus and the internal auditory canal are not dilated. The tumor exhibits internal signal abnormalities. These alterations are associated with intratumoral microbleeds and hemosiderin, identifiable in the T2-GRE (*Gradient Echo*) sequence and particularly in the T2-SWAN (*Star Weighted Angiography*) sequence. Prominent signal alterations are observed in the cerebellar peduncle, accompanied by a halo of separation between the tumor and the brainstem, indicating the preservation of an arachnoid cleavage plane

8.6 Surgical Categories

Only two categories of large or giant vestibular schwannomas necessitate particular microsurgical intervention. The first type is cystic tumors, which will be addressed in the subsequent chapter. A distinct circumstance is the association of ventricular dilatation, necessitating specific considerations for the treatment method, but the microneurosurgical resection technique remains identical to that employed for tumors without hydrocephalus.

8.7 Microneurosurgical Management

We will now delineate the stages for the resection of large or giant vestibular schwannomas, specifically those classified as grade T4 and T5 according to Matties and Samii, as well as Koos grade IV. We shall address this comprehensively, as these are the tumors requiring microneurosurgical intervention due to the absence of alternative effective treatments [1, 2, 6, 7, 10].

8.7.1 Approach and Surgical Exposition of the Tumor

The retrosigmoid approach resembles that outlined in prior chapters; however, it may be beneficial to enhance its size by extending to the margins of the transverse and sigmoid sinuses, medially resecting a substantial portion of the occipital bone's squama, and caudally extending to the horizontal segment of the occipital bone's squama. Upon opening the dura mater, it is imperative to obtain significant cerebrospinal fluid (CSF) drainage from the caudal cisterns, the sole accessible sources, which is aided by the caudal extension of the craniotomy. Upon separation of the cerebellum, the tumor is observed to encompass the whole surgical field, with only the tentorium visible cranially, the cerebellum medially and caudally, and the posterior side of the petrosal bone at the caudal extremity. The arachnoid enveloping the tumor is excised and repositioned across the tumor's surface to reveal the maximum extent of the tumor (Fig. 8.3a). To enhance the visibility of the tumor, one may open the petrosal fissure of the cerebellum; however, in the case of large tumors, this fissure is often collapsed and filled by the tumor, making it difficult to identify.

8.7.2 Tumor Debulking

After exposing the tumor and delineating its margins, the superficial veins are coagulated, and an incision is created for internal decompression

a

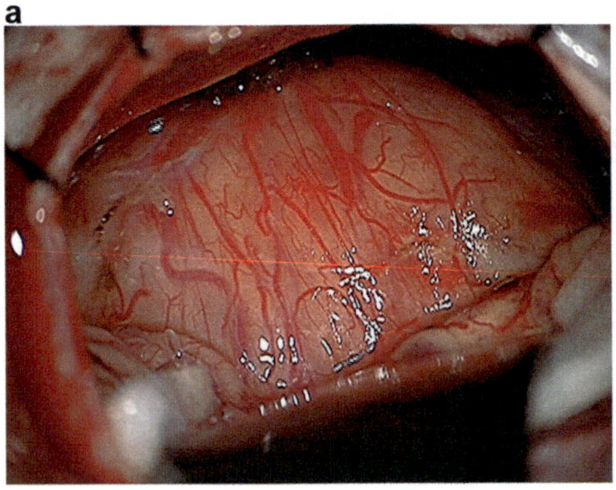

b

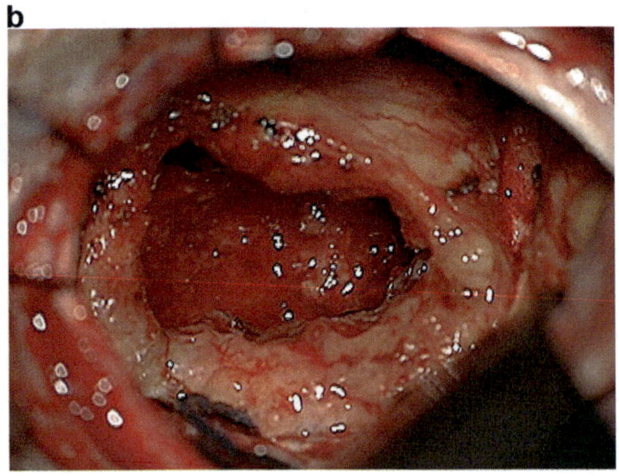

Fig. 8.3 Intraoperative pictures displaying the microneurosurgical removal of a large right vestibular schwannoma using a retrosigmoid approach. (**a**) Picture illustrating the tumor's complete occupation of the surgical field following the separation of the cerebellum. (**b**) Image following internal decompression of the tumor using the ultrasonic aspirator. (**c**) Following tumor removal, the integrity of the trigeminal nerve and the surface of the brainstem, along with maintained pial vascularization, can be detected. (**d**) A more caudal perspective reveals the trigeminal nerve, brainstem, and facial nerve on route to the auditory canal, with the sixth cranial nerve in the background

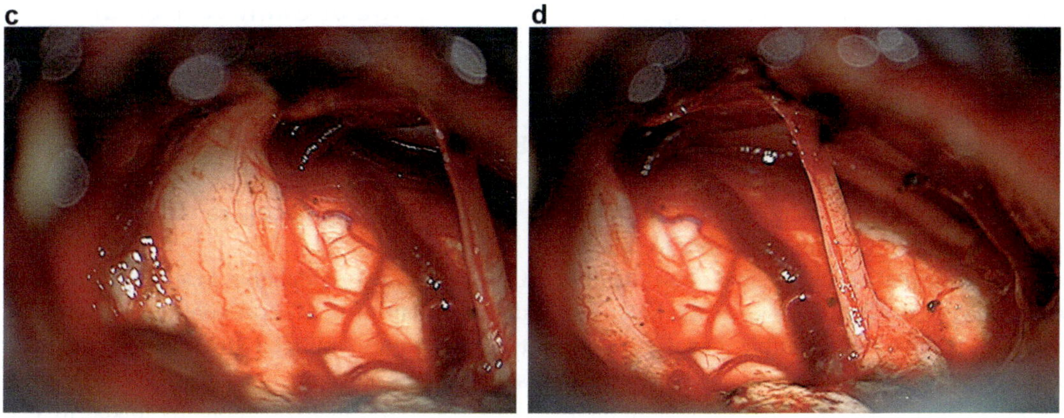

Fig. 8.3 (continued)

using the ultrasonic aspirator. Internal decompression aims to reduce a large tumor to a smaller size by evacuating its contents while maintaining the integrity of its capsule. The ultrasonic aspirator's power should not be significantly elevated, as the vestibular schwannoma is a delicate tumor. The capsule must remain intact to retain the cleavage plane with the neural structures and prevent unintentional damage to concealed structures that may otherwise be safeguarded. The debulking of these huge tumors is a laborious endeavor that must be periodically paused for the coagulation of hemorrhagic sites (Fig. 8.3b). Certain bleeding locations may resist bipolar coagulation due to vascular retraction, necessitating the application of a soft hemostatic agent for several minutes. The waiting period for internal hemostasis is utilized to delineate the tumor capsule and gradually reveal the neurovascular structures of the cerebellopontine angle: superiorly, the petrosal vein complex, followed by the trochlear nerve and the superior cerebellar artery (SCA); inferiorly, the lower cranial nerve roots and the anterior inferior cerebellar artery (AICA); posteriorly, the trigeminal nerve and the brainstem surface. Upon achieving a substantial decrease in tumor volume, the residual capsule may become wrinkled, resulting in the loss of the cleavage plane. Consequently, at this moment, sections of the capsule may be excised, increasing the initial aperture created for the internal decompression of the tumor.

8.7.3 Identification of Neurovascular Elements

The vestibulocochlear nerve, infiltrated by the tumor, can typically be identified as a small segment of nerve between the brainstem and the tumor. The facial nerve must now be identified using anatomical or electrophysiological references through direct electrical stimulation, as described in the previous chapter. The gradual and meticulous excision of tumor capsule segments facilitates the continuous decompression and delineation of the lower nerves, brainstem, trigeminal nerve (Fig. 8.3c, d), and the anterior inferior cerebellar artery.

8.7.4 Resection of Tumor and Nerve Management

Upon conclusion of this procedure, the large or giant tumor has been transformed into a significantly more manageable medium-sized tumor, and its extrameatal and intrameatal excision proceeds as delineated in the prior chapters. The facial nerve is typically significantly distended and weakened, complicating its anatomical and functional preservation. Nonetheless, if anatomical preservation has been accomplished in the final stages of resection, with or without the maintenance of nerve conduction through direct electrical stimulation, it is justifiable to retain a residual tumor portion rather than incur the anatomical loss of the facial nerve, as the latter will inevitably result in irreversible facial paralysis requiring subsequent management. Anatomical loss of the facial nerve is more prevalent upon its entry into the auditory meatus, perhaps due to the acute angle at this location, which necessitates traction that may sever the nerve fibers from the remaining tumor remains. Conversely, if there has been an anatomical loss of the facial nerve, resection of the intrameatal segment of the tumor can be conducted more aggressively and radically with a spoon or ultrasonic aspirator, as there are no neurological structures to preserve.

8.8 Large or Giant Vestibular Schwannomas that Require Specific Treatment

8.8.1 Large Schwannomas Associated with Hydrocephalus

Obstructive hydrocephalus resulting from the displacement of the fourth ventricle is a characteristic feature utilized to define vestibular schwannoma at its maximal size across all classes (Fig. 8.4). Not all hydrocephalus linked to vestibular schwannoma is obstructive; it is thought that only 30% are obstructive, while the remaining 70% are communicative hydrocephalus. A meta-analysis indicates that obstructive hydrocephalus manifests in somewhat younger patients (40–45 years) compared to communicative hydrocephalus (60 years) and is associated with bigger tumors (45 mm versus 30 mm). Conversely, when analyzing protein concentrations in the

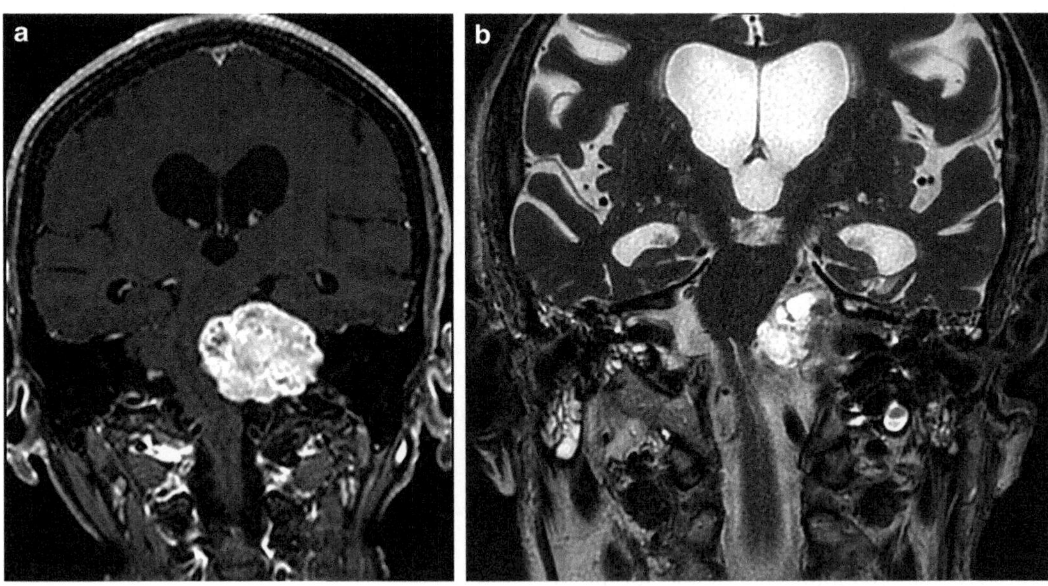

Fig. 8.4 Hydrocephalus linked to significant vestibular schwannomas. (**a**) Coronal T1-weighted picture with gadolinium demonstrating important enhancement and ventricular system dilatation, indicative of triventricular hydrocephalus, accompanied by a flattened subarachnoid space, suggesting obstructive hydrocephalus in a patient in his forties. (**b**) Coronal T2-weighted picture revealing a cystic tumor in an octogenarian patient, accompanied by ventricular dilation, significant cortico-subcortical atrophy, and expansion of the subarachnoid space, indicating dilation likely due to involutional changes, with an ambiguous contribution of the tumor to the development of ventriculomegaly

cerebrospinal fluid of patients with communicative hydrocephalus, levels are markedly elevated (350 mg/dL) compared to obstructive hydrocephalus (150 mg/dL) and in both instances exceed physiological values. The data indicate that vestibular schwannoma likely elevates cerebrospinal fluid protein levels that large tumors contribute to hydrocephalus through an obstructive mechanism, and that elderly patients contribute to hydrocephalus due to the physiological enlargement of the ventricular system. Elevated cerebrospinal fluid protein levels would promote communicative hydrocephalus due to the occlusion of the Pacchioni granulations in the dural venous sinuses, where cerebrospinal fluid absorption occurs. Consequently, the etiology of hydrocephalus linked to vestibular schwannoma is multifactorial.Tumor removal addresses both pathophysiological processes of hydrocephalus by removing the restriction of cerebrospinal fluid circulation pathways and the release of proteins into the cerebrospinal fluid by the tumor; thus, the optimal treatment for hydrocephalus associated with vestibular schwannoma is tumor excision. Resection of vestibular schwannoma alleviates 90% of hydrocephalus cases, with just a small proportion (5%) needing ventriculoperitoneal shunting as a conclusive intervention. In cases where hydrocephalus persists post-resection, the interim insertion of a lumbar or external ventricular shunt is advised, as definitive ventriculoperitoneal shunting is frequently circumvented. The advantageous function of external ventricular shunting is similarly noted when implemented before microneurosurgery, decreasing the proportion of patients necessitating ventriculoperitoneal shunting post-resection. It is posited that external shunting would eliminate proteins generated by the tumor from the cerebrospinal fluid and diminish the probability of hydrocephalus following tumor resection. Consequently, the insertion of a ventriculoperitoneal shunt before microsurgery is unwarranted and would only be permissible for symptomatic patients suffering from hydrocephalus when there are compelling reasons for a prolonged postponement of tumor microneurosurgical intervention, when resection surgery is inadvisable, or for patients who decline microneurosurgery as a treatment alternative [4].

8.9 Results, Prognosis, and Follow-Up

Fortunately, large or giant vestibular schwannomas are infrequent in neurosurgical practice within countries possessing robust healthcare systems, typically comprising fewer than 5% of surgical cases, resulting in limited surgical series. Conversely, due to the severity of these lesions and the challenges associated with surgical intervention, the treatment results in significant morbidity and carries a risk of postoperative mortality. This indicates that the diffusion of results is limited, consists of brief series, and originates from highly specialized neurosurgeons, leading to biased outcomes. A recent meta-analysis examining the outcomes of microneurosurgical intervention for vestibular schwannomas exceeding 30 mm revealed that complete resection was accomplished in 80% of patients, with anatomical preservation of the facial nerve in 90% of instances; however, only 60% of patients demonstrated favorable functional assessment (House Brackmann grades I-III). Clinical reality evidently yields inferior outcomes compared to those reported in the literature, due to the biases identified in these publications.

8.10 Management Modalities

Microsurgical intervention is the sole option for big or giant vestibular schwannomas, as the goal is to decompress the brainstem, achievable solely through tumor removal [3, 4, 5, 11–13]. Microneurosurgery aimed at complete resection is associated with elevated morbidity and mortality rates, prompting the frequent consideration of subtotal tumor excision. One hundred years ago, internal decompression of the tumor was conducted, accompanied by external decompression with a broad unilateral or bilateral suboccipital craniectomy. Fifty years ago, decompression involved a subtotal excision of the tumor, followed by a complete resection in a subsequent surgical procedure aimed at preserving facial nerve function; however, this two-stage resection approach did not yield superior outcomes. Subsequently, subtotal resection has been advised to alleviate pressure on the brainstem and preserve facial nerve function, followed by stereotactic radiosurgery for the residual tumor. This method facilitates effective management of the residual tumor's growth and the preservation of neurological function post-microneurosurgery. Some studies indicate the advantages of utilizing various modalities of ionizing radiation, apart from stereotactic radiosurgery, for tumors above 25–30 mm, which is the traditional size threshold for exclusive treatment with stereotactic radiosurgery. In this context, both single-session stereotactic radiosurgery and fractionated stereotactic radiosurgery have been employed. A meta-analysis indicates that both radiation therapy modalities and microneurosurgery followed by stereotactic radiosurgery achieve short-range growth control in around 90% of patients, with a microsurgical rescue treatment rate of under 10%.

8.11 Key Messages

- *Large and giant vestibular schwannomas necessitate microneurosurgical excision to alleviate the pressure on the brainstem.*
- *The retrosigmoid approach and transmeatal access are employed for microneurosurgical excision.*
- *There are two types of hydrocephalus associated with vestibular schwannoma: non-communicant, caused by obstruction of the fourth ventricle, and communicant, resulting from the release of proteins to cerebrospinal fluid. Complete excision of the tumor is the optimal course of action.*
- *The majority of patients receiving microneurosurgical excision exhibit a positive vital prognosis and a favorable functional outcome.*
- *The treatment objectives are to preserve facial nerve function, decompress the brainstem, and save lives.*

References

1. Bambakidis N, Megerian CA, Spetzler RF, editors. Surgery of the cerebellopontine angle. Chaim: Springer Nature; 2018.
2. Campero A, Martins C, Rhoton A Jr, et al. Dural landmark to locate the internal auditory canal in large and giant vestibular schwannomas: the Tübingen line. Neurosurgery. 2011;69(Suppl Operative 1):99–102. https://doi.org/10.1227/NEU.0b013e31821664c6.
3. Carlson ML, Vivas EX, McCracken DJ, et al. Congress of Neurological Surgeons systematic review and evidence-based guidelines on hearing preservation outcomes in patients with sporadic vestibular schwannomas. Neurosurgery. 2028;82:E35–9. https://doi.org/10.1093/neuros/nyx511.
4. di Russo P, Fava A, Vandenbulcke A, et al. Characteristics and management of hydrocephalus associated with vestibular schwannomas: a systematic review. Neurosurg Rev. 2021;44:687–98. https://doi.org/10.1007/s10143-020-01287-2.
5. Goldbrunner R, Weller M, Regis J, et al. EANO guideline on the diagnosis and treatment of vestibular schwannoma. Neuro-Oncology. 2020;22:31–45. https://doi.org/10.1093/neuonc/noz153.
6. González-Darder JM, Quilis-Quesada V, Capilla-Guasch P, de Oliveira E. Abordajes neuroquirúrgicos de la patología craneal y cerebral. 2nd ed. Barcelona: Elsevier España; 2020.
7. Kulwin CG, Cohen-Gadol AA. Technical nuances of resection of giant (> 5 cm) vestibular schwannomas: pearls for success. Neurosurg Focus. 2012;33:E15. https://doi.org/10.3171/2012.7.FOCUS12177.
8. Matthies C, Samii M. Management of 1000 vestibular schwannomas (acoustic neuromas): clinical presentation. Neurosurgery. 1997;40:1–9. https://doi.org/10.1097/00006123-199701000-00001.
9. Rhoton AL Jr. The posterior fossa: microsurgical anatomy & surgical approaches. Neurosurgery. 2000;47(Suppl 3):S1–S279. https://doi.org/10.1097/00006123-200009001-00013.
10. Samii M, Gerganov V. Surgery of cerebellopontine angle lesions. Berlin/Heidelberg: Springer-Verlag; 2013.

11. Jung S, Kang SS, Kim TS, et al. Current surgical results of retrosigmoid approach in extralarge vestibular schwannomas. Surg Neurol. 2000;53:370–7. https://doi.org/10.1016/s0090-3019(00)00196-8.
12. Starnoni D, Giammattei L, Cossu G, et al. Surgical management for large vestibular schwannomas: a systematic review, meta-analysis, and consensus statement on behalf of the EANS skull base section. Acta Neurochir. 2020;162:2595–6217. https://doi.org/10.1007/s00701-020-04491-7.
13. Starnoni D, Daniel RT, Tuleasca C, et al. Systematic review and meta-analysis of the technique of subtotal resection and stereotactic radiosurgery for large vestibular schwannomas: a "nerve-centered" approach. Neurosurg Focus. 2018;44:E4. https://doi.org/10.3171/2017.12.FOCUS17669.

9 Cystic Vestibular Schwannoma

9.1 Introduction

The predominant tumor of the cerebellopontine angle is the vestibular schwannoma, which has been thoroughly examined in the prior chapters, focusing on its most pertinent characteristic for microneurosurgical management: its size. These tumors can be categorized, in addition to their size, as solid or cystic, which is significant as it has long been established that the natural history, microneurosurgical treatment, and prognosis differ between the two types. In comparison to solid tumors, numerous studies indicate that cystic vestibular schwannomas exhibit a more rapid growth rate, greater size upon diagnosis, and a briefer clinical history, including instances of abrupt decline resulting from the unanticipated enlargement of the tumor's cystic component. The epidermoid cyst is the most distinctive cystic lesion of the cerebellopontine angle and ranks as the third most prevalent tumor in this region. Nonetheless, numerous cystic lesions of various origins inhabit the cerebellopontine angle, presenting specific challenges, including cystic vestibular schwannoma.

Microneurosurgical treatment for cystic tumors is traditionally regarded as more challenging than for solid tumors, yielding a less favorable prognosis, particularly with the functional outcome of the facial nerve.

9.2 Anatomical Considerations

Cystic vestibular schwannomas are typically large, encompassing nearly the whole cerebellopontine angle and impacting all neurovascular groups delineated by Rhoton, as discussed in the chapter on medium-sized vestibular schwannomas. The transmeatal approach required for microneurosurgical resection makes all anatomical considerations regarding the meatus and internal auditory canal, as discussed in the chapter on small-sized schwannomas, also relevant to cystic vestibular schwannoma.

9.3 Pathology

The majority of vestibular schwannomas are solid, but the prevalence of cystic vestibular schwannomas varies by study, accounting for 20–30% of instances. Various explanations have been proposed concerning the pathophysiology of cyst formation and growth. The creation of cysts was once attributed to the rapid proliferation of the tumor. Nevertheless, a greater cell proliferation rate has not been evidenced in cystic vestibular schwannoma relative to solid vestibular schwannoma, and it is now believed that cystic tumors exhibit accelerated growth specifically due to the formation of cysts. The subsequent development of cysts was

J. M. González-Darder, *Microneurosurgery of Cerebellopontine Angle*,
https://doi.org/10.1007/978-3-032-03091-7_9

associated with an atypical ratio of type A to type B Antoni cells within the tumor, suggesting that type B cells generate a myxomatous secretion responsible for cyst formation, a notion that remains unverified. The potential for recurrent microhemorrhages, accompanied by reparative processes and the creation of neocapillaries that may subsequently rupture, leading to more micro-hemorrhages, culminating in cyst formation, has also been proposed. The expansion of the original cyst is attributed to the influx of water into the cyst due to the hyperosmolarity of its contents. MMP-2 (*Matrix Metalloproteinase-2*) has recently been implicated. MMP-2 are proteolytic enzymes that degrade collagen and other proteins inside the intercellular matrix, facilitating tissue fragmentation and dissolution, as well as the development and proliferation of cysts.

9.4 Clinical Considerations

The epidemiological characteristics and clinical presentation of cystic vestibular schwannoma resemble those of solid vestibular schwannoma; however, the natural history is typically shorter and more accelerated. Instances of abrupt onset and quick progression have been reported due to the swift enlargement of the cyst. The mean size of the tumor upon diagnosis is greater than that of solid tumors; however, the differences are not statistically significant (refer to case 10 in Chap. 21).

9.5 Diagnostic Considerations

Diagnosis by computed tomography (CT) presents challenges. Cystic vestibular schwannoma typically appears on a CT scan as a hypodense region in the cerebellopontine angle, with uneven contrast enhancement. Changes in the diameter of the meatus or the internal auditory canal may occasionally be observed, suggesting that cystic vestibular schwannoma could be a solid tumor of prolonged evolution that has suddenly become cystic, as it is otherwise challenging to account for the resultant alterations in the bone (Fig. 9.1).

The imaging diagnosis is established with magnetic resonance imaging (MRI), revealing a

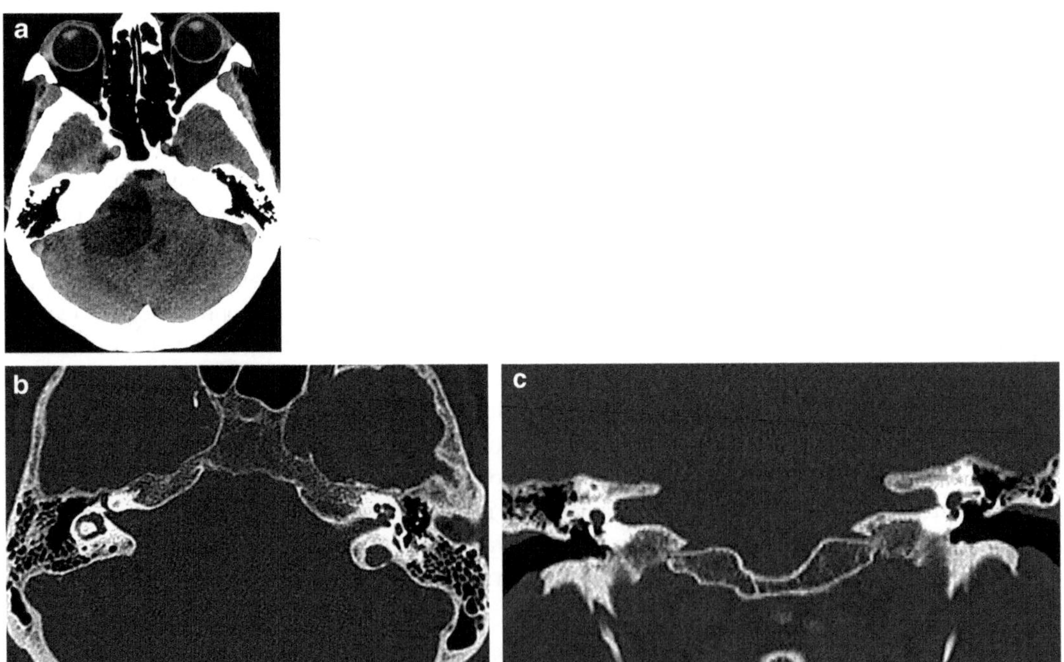

Fig. 9.1 CT diagnostic of a cyst vestibular schwannoma. (**a**) Axial CT scan without contrast reveals a hypodense lesion in the right cerebellopontine angle. (**b**, **c**) Thin CT sections of axial and coronal sections of the petrosal bone demonstrate the enlargement of the meatus and internal auditory canal

lesion comprising both solid and cystic components in the cerebellopontine angle. The cystic content exhibits iso- or hyposignal in T1-weighted sequences and hypersignal in T2-weighted sequences, whereas the solid component displays the characteristic features of vestibular schwannoma, demonstrating enhancement in T1-weighted sequences following gadolinium administration. The cyst may exhibit a level if it has recently hemorrhaged. The tumor's solid component is consistently associated with the trajectory of the vestibulocochlear nerve or the internal auditory canal. In substantial tumors, the lesion may significantly displace the brainstem, cerebellum, or fourth ventricle and may occasionally induce obstructive hydrocephalus (Fig. 9.2) [1].

9.6 Surgical Categories

The primary issue in defining and categorizing the various forms of cystic vestibular schwannoma is the absence of a universally agreed criterion for labeling a vestibular schwannoma as cystic. Confirmation of cysts observed in imaging tests is imperative during surgical procedures, as pictures exhibiting diminished signal or the absence of contrast enhancement in T1-weighted MRI sequences may be misinterpreted as cysts when they are, in fact, regions of degenerative alterations inside the tumor. Second, it is mandatory to verify the diagnosis of schwannoma by exhibiting positive for the S-100 protein in the cyst membrane. In imaging studies, it is essential to quantify the cystic component of the tumor, typically in the sections with the greatest diameter, or to determine the percentage of cyst volume relative to the total tumor volume. Most writers classify a vestibular schwannoma as cystic if the cyst(s) comprise over two-thirds of the maximum tumor diameter on MRI.

The basic classification categorizes cystic vestibular schwannoma into three types: type A, characterized by a single big cyst with a thin wall; type B, including a single cyst with a thick wall; and type C, consisting of several cysts. A comprehensive classification considers the cyst's overall location and wall thickness, categorizing cystic vestibular schwannomas into two primary types: type A, characterized by a central cyst with a thick wall, and type B, defined by a peripheral cyst with a thin wall. Type A lesions are classified into three subtypes based on the cyst and wall characteristics: subtype 1, polycystic with numerous small intratumoral cysts and a thick cyst wall; subtype 2, polycystic with several moderate-sized intratumoral cysts and a thick cyst wall; and subtype 3, monocystic with a single large cyst that may have either a thick or thin cyst wall. Type B lesions are classified into four subgroups according to the cyst's direction and location relative to the internal auditory canal: subtype 1, anterior; subtype 2, medial; subtype 3, posterior; and subtype 4, a combination of the aforementioned orientations. Others categorize cystic vestibular schwannoma into four groups: type A1, partial monocystic, featuring a solitary cyst within the tumor; type A2, partial multicystic, containing multiple cysts within the tumor; type B1, pure monocystic, characterized by a single large cyst encased in a thin wall; and type B2, pure multicystic, consisting of numerous cysts. All the categories possess a subjective element and exhibit considerable heterogeneity depending on the observer, rendering their clinical utility rather limited and erratic (Figs. 9.2 and 9.3).

9.7 Microneurosurgical Management

The diagnosis of cystic vestibular schwannoma and the treatment indications are fundamentally identical to those for solid vestibular schwannoma; however, the microsurgical technique and outcomes differ significantly [2]. Paradoxically, cystic vestibular schwannoma is not simpler to excise than solid vestibular schwannoma, contrary to the belief that tumor decompression is more feasible. The fundamental concepts of microsurgical intervention for cystic vestibular schwannoma align with those for solid vestibular schwannoma, as detailed in earlier chapters, concerning positioning, monitoring, surgical technique, and lesion access. The primary

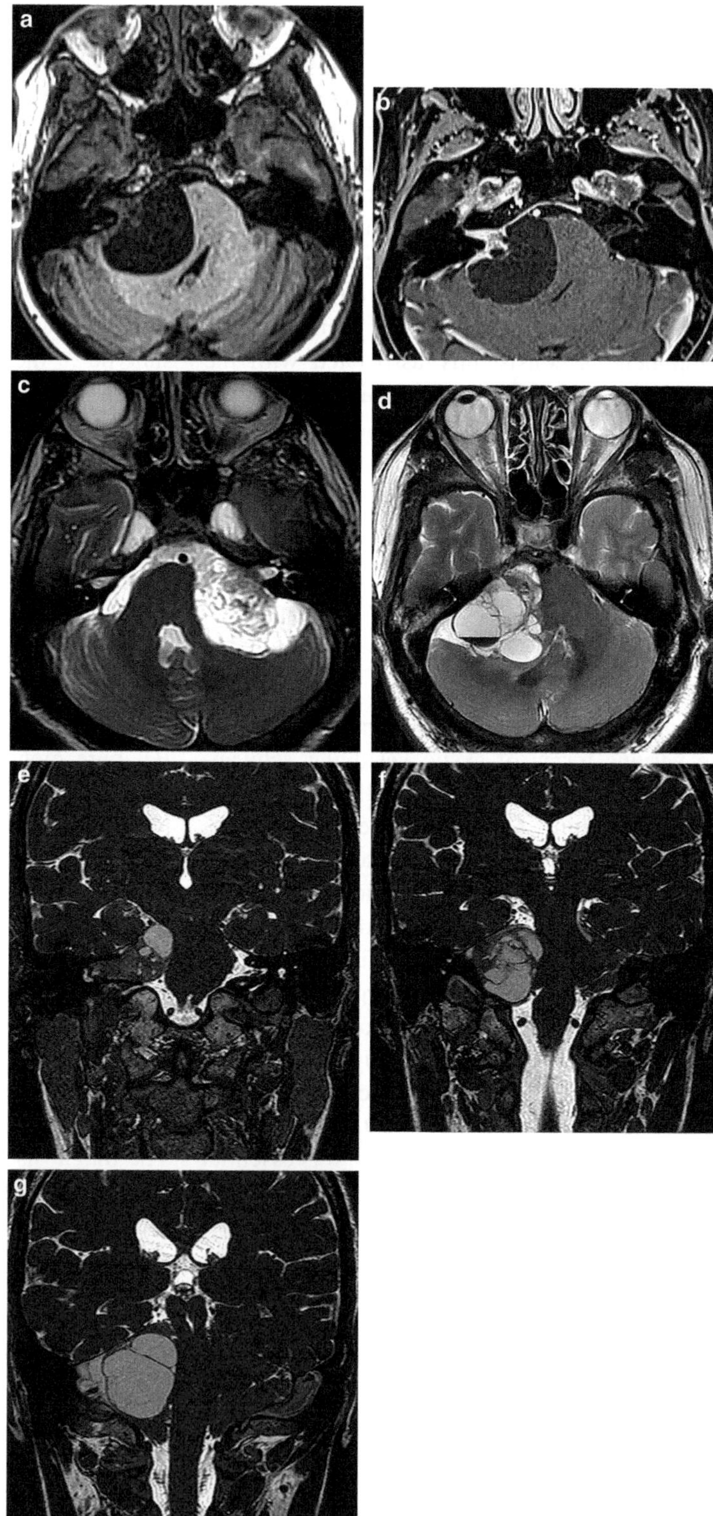

Fig. 9.2 MRI diagnoses indicate cystic vestibular schwannoma. (**a**) Axial MRI slice in T1-weighted sequence showing a cystic vestibular schwannoma. (**b**) Axial MRI slice in T1-weighted sequence following gadolinium administration demonstrates the enhancement of the solid intracanalicular component of the tumor. (**c**) Axial MRI slice of a cystic vestibular schwannoma in T2-weighted sequence, featuring several extremely thin-walled cysts. (**d**) Axial MRI slice of a cystic vestibular schwannoma in T2 sequence, exhibiting numerous thin-walled cysts of varying sizes, one of which has a discernible level. (**e–g**) Coronal MRI sections of a cystic vestibular schwannoma in T2 sequence, exhibiting numerous cysts. The content exhibits a reduction in signal relative to the cerebrospinal fluid, with the solid component primarily being intracanalicular

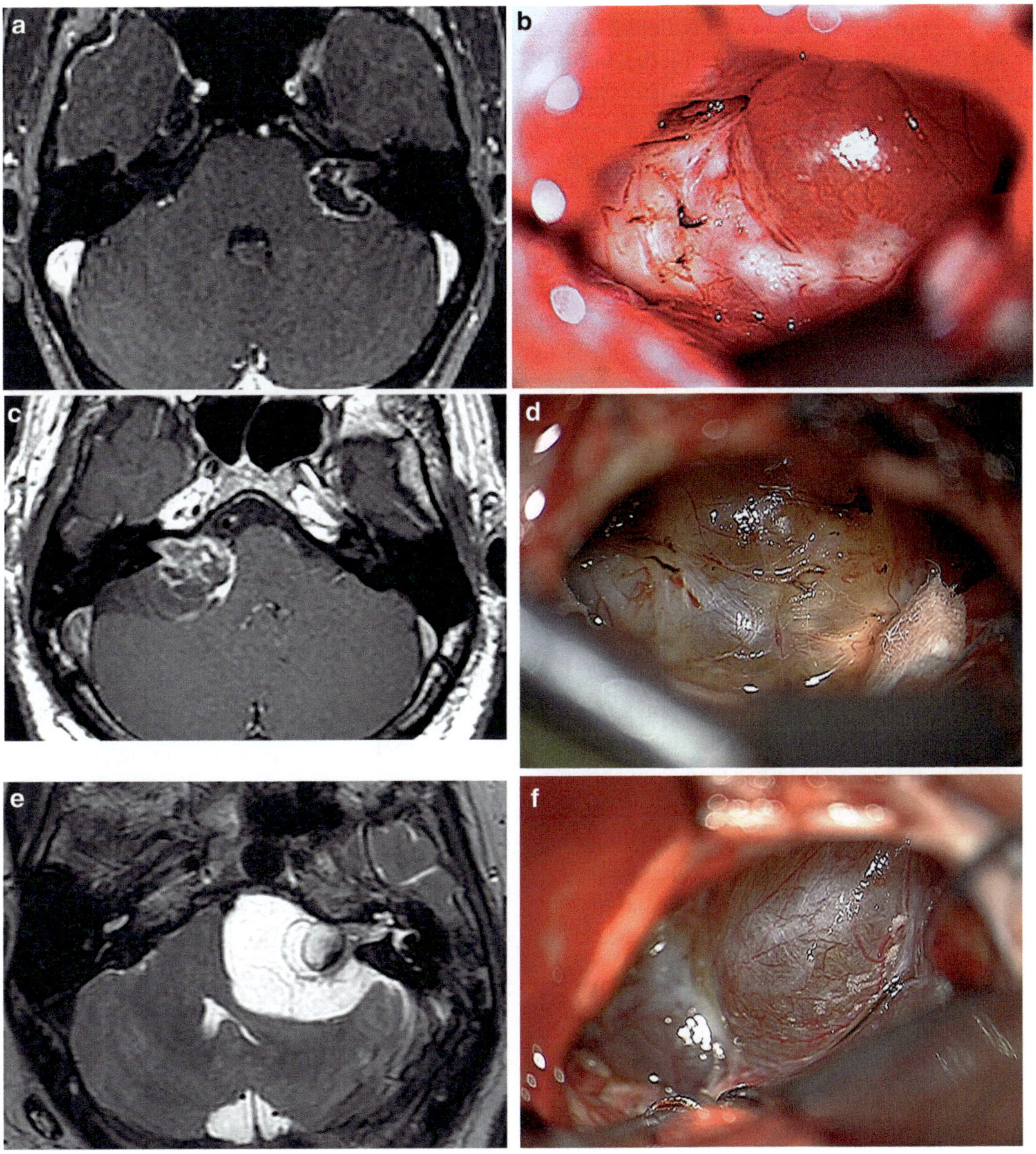

Fig. 9.3 Cystic vestibular schwannoma: concordance between imaging investigations and intraoperative findings. (**a**, **b**) Small left vestibular schwannoma with a solitary cyst. (**c**, **d**) Medium–large right vestibular schwannoma exhibiting several irregularly shaped cysts. (**e**, **f**) Giant left vestibular schwannoma accompanied by a solitary cyst

considerations for microsurgical intervention include the quantity, dimensions, and location of the cysts, the thickness of the cyst wall, and the adhesions of the cyst to neurological structures.

Large cysts can be first evacuated using puncture and aspiration; however, this may result in undesirable distortions of the tumor volume, potentially disrupting the interaction between the tumor wall and adjacent tissues or impairing the surgeon's orientation. Numerous cysts facilitate advancements in decompression; nevertheless, they should not usually be identified during surgery to inform the neurosurgeon about the extent of decompression or anatomical linkages. The delicate wall of the cyst poses a challenge in preserving the anatomical integrity of the tumor's capsule during arachnoid dissection. In instances of anteriorly located cysts, there exists a risk that the facial nerve is in close proximity to the membrane, increasing the likelihood of inadvertent injury despite attempts to locate it through direct electrical stimulation within the cyst wall. Similarly, medial cysts present challenges due to their proximity to the brainstem, complicating dissection when the wall is thin and adhesions exist between the wall and the pia mater, potentially compromising the safe dissection plane.

Upon identification of the neurovascular structures, they are stabilized using short sections of moistened material, while the tumor capsule and remnants of the cyst walls are retracted utilizing bipolar coagulation. The tumor is excised in small fragments utilizing forceps and fine microscissors while maintaining the cleavage plane and preserving the anatomical linkages with the nerve roots and arteries. Upon sufficient resection of the tumor, the procedure proceeds similarly to that of a medium-sized schwannoma, involving the separation of the tumor from the facial nerve, the opening of the internal auditory canal for the excision of the intracanalicular segment, and the transection of the vestibulocochlear nerve root both proximally and distally to achieve complete tumor resection (Fig. 9.4).

9.8 Cystic Vestibular Schwannomas that Require Specific Treatment

This is especially for large cystic vestibular schwannomas linked to hydrocephalus. The processes of hydrocephalus linked to vestibular schwannoma involve the restriction of the cerebrospinal fluid circulation channels and the release of proteins into the cerebrospinal fluid. Rapidly enlarging cystic vestibular schwannomas are more likely to induce obstructive hydrocephalus. In instances of acute hydrocephalus, a microsurgical tumor resection should be promptly arranged if the patient's clinical status permits surgery; otherwise, an external ventricular shunt may be contemplated.

9.9 Results, Prognosis, and Follow-Up

Review and meta-analysis of the published data indicate that, despite the aforementioned challenges, the extent of resection attained is comparable in cystic and solid vestibular schwannomas, with an 80% rate of gross total resection (GTR) in cystic tumors. Nonetheless, the functional outcome of the facial nerve is markedly inferior in cystic tumors, with favorable neurological function (House Brackmann grades I-III) observed in 50% of patients at 6 months, despite no significant differences in other clinical outcomes pertaining to morbidity and mortality. The likelihood of cystic vestibular schwannoma recurrence parallels that of solid tumors, and if recurrence occurs, it similarly tends to manifest as cystic in nature [3–5].

9.10 Management Modalities

The primary treatment for cystic vestibular schwannoma is microneurosurgical excision. The urgency for treatment indication is greater than in solid tumors due to the potential for rapid volumetric growth and clinical progression. Conversely, the indication for stereotactic radiosurgery is more limited, as instances of rapid growth and intratumoral hemorrhage have been reported post-treatment. For these same reasons, imaging observation is likewise not advised.

9.11 Key Messages

- *Cystic vestibular schwannoma is a distinct variant characterized by an erratic developmental natural history and clinical progression.*
- *Cystic vestibular schwannoma necessitates microneurosurgical resection* via *a retrosigmoid approach and transmeatal access.*

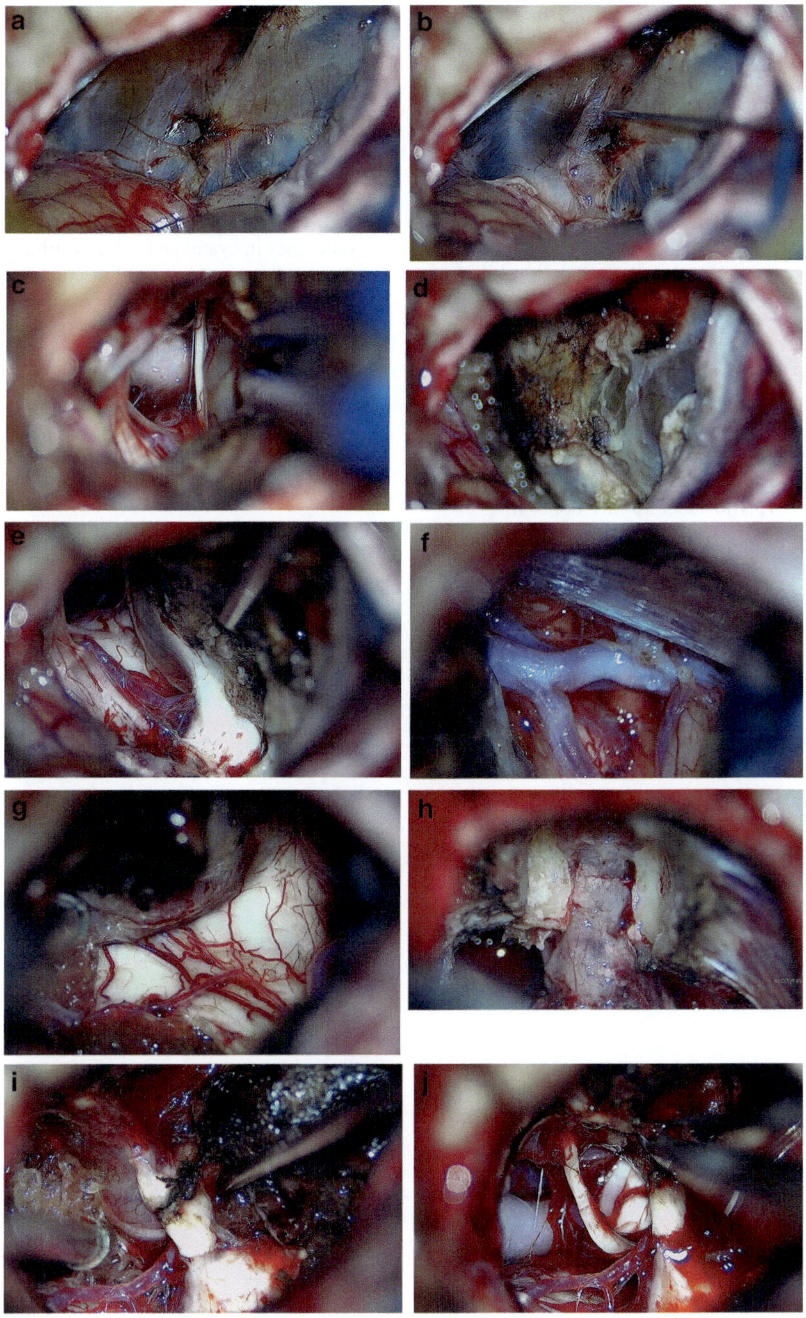

Fig. 9.4 Intraoperative pictures of a large cystic left vestibular schwannoma. (**a**) A picture displaying the tumor following the mobilization of the cerebellum. (**b**) Following the puncture of the cyst, the collapse of the tumor wall is observable. (**c**) Tumor decompression facilitates dissection of the caudal pole, enabling the identification of the lower cranial nerves and the trunk of the vertebral artery. (**d**) The evacuated tumor exhibits an uneven morphology. (**e**) The retraction of the tumor facilitates the identification of the vestibulocochlear nerve root in a caudal position. (**f**) Similarly, the cranial pole can be detached from the tentorium and the branches of the superior cerebellar artery. (**g**) Operative picture demonstrating the detachment of the tumor from the ventral aspect of the pons. (**h**) Illustration displaying the intracanalicular segment of the tumor following the incision of the internal auditory canal. (**i**) Image of the segment of the vestibulocochlear nerve root adjacent to the brainstem. (**j**) Image displaying the overall appearance post-tumor removal, demonstrating the anatomical preservation of the facial, abducens, and trigeminal nerves

- *The functional prognosis is optimistic, with the treatment objective being complete excision while preserving functional facial and auditory nerve functions.*
- *Recurrence is typically cystic again, and the rate is comparable to non-cystic vestibular schwannoma.*

References

1. Bonneville F, Savatovsky J, Chiras J. Imaging of cerebellopontine angle lesions: an update. Part 2: intra-axial lesions, skull base lesions that may invade the cerebellopontine angle region, and non-enhancing extra-axial lesions. Eur Radiol. 2007;17:2908–20. https://doi.org/10.1007/s00330-007-0680-4.
2. Samii M, Gerganov V. Surgery of cerebellopontine angle lesions. Berlin-Heidelberg: Springer-Verlag; 2013.
3. Thakur JD, Khan IS, Shorter CD, et al. Do cystic vestibular schwannomas have worse surgical outcomes? Systematic analysis of the literature. Neurosurg Focus. 2012;33:E12. https://doi.org/10.3171/2012.6.FOCUS12200.
4. Wu X, Song G, Wang X, et al. Comparison of surgical outcomes in cystic and solid vestibular schwannomas: a systematic review and meta-analysis. Neurosurg Rev. 2021;44:1889–902. https://doi.org/10.1007/s10143-020-01400-5.
5. Yashar P, Zada G, Harris B, et al. Extent of resection and early postoperative outcomes following removal of cystic vestibular schwannomas: surgical experience over a decade and review of the literature. Neurosurg Focus. 2012;33:E13. https://doi.org/10.3171/2012.7.FOCUS12206.

10 Other Schwannomas of the Cerebellopontine Angle

10.1 Introduction

Except for the first and second cranial nerves, which are extensions of the central nervous system, all other cranial and spinal nerves have their neuronal extensions encased by Schwann cells. The shift from the myelin sheath supplied by oligodendroglia to that supplied by Schwann cells occurs in the *transitional zone*, also known as the *Obersteiner–Redlich zone*. The transitional zone is a conical region measuring several millimeters that commences a few millimeters beyond the apparent exit of the nerve root from the pial surface of the brainstem. The portion of the nerve root extending from the brainstem pia mater to the transitional zone is referred to as the *root entry zone*. Consequently, all cranial nerves, except for the olfactory and optic nerves, are susceptible to the development of schwannomas. The cause is unidentified, but schwannomas exhibit a distinct propensity to proliferate more commonly in sensory fibers than in motor fibers. Generally, these tumors predominantly affect adult patients, are entirely benign, and are unrelated to neurofibromatosis, except for vestibular schwannoma. Vestibular schwannomas constitute over 90% of intracranial schwannomas, while among non-vestibular schwannomas, roughly 40% arise from the trigeminal nerve, 25% from the facial nerve, 10% from the lower cranial nerves, often referred to as jugular foramen schwannomas, with the remaining cranial nerves accounting for the rest of the cases. Schwannomas proliferate along the complete trajectory of the cranial nerves originating distal to the transitional zone. Cranial nerves can be divided into distinct segments: the cisternal segment, confined to the cisterns of the cerebellopontine angle; the foraminal segment, traversing the orifice or dural space through which they exit the cerebellopontine angle via the cranial base; and the extracranial course of the nerve. Schwannomas may develop in any of these segments and are classified as cisternal, foraminal, or extracranial schwannomas. Nonetheless, tumors frequently proliferate along the nerve, including many segments, hence exacerbating growth patterns, clinical manifestations, and microneurosurgical challenges for treatment. This chapter reviews cerebellopontine angle non-vestibular schwannomas, which are tumors that arise in the cisternal pathways of cranial nerves or at their exit points in the skull base. We shall delineate the pertinent anatomical features of each nerve concerning this pathology (Fig. 10.1), followed by an examination of its clinical, diagnostic, and therapeutic nuances, particularly microneurosurgical intervention [1, 17].

J. M. González-Darder, *Microneurosurgery of Cerebellopontine Angle*,
https://doi.org/10.1007/978-3-032-03091-7_10

10.2 Schwannomas of the Oculomotor Nerve

10.2.1 Anatomical Considerations

The apparent origin of the third cranial nerve, or oculomotor nerve, is situated in the most caudal region of the interpeduncular fossa, at the pontine-mesencephalic sulcus level. From this point, it traverses a slightly ascending and lateral pathway until it penetrates the cavernous sinus at the oculomotor triangle level (Fig. 10.1). The oculomotor nerve occupies the superior sector of the cerebellopontine angle along its cisternal trajectory. The oculomotor nerve, originating at the interpeduncular cistern and extending until it enters the roof of the cavernous sinus, is encased in its own cistern situated at the junction of the carotid, interpeduncular, prepontine, and cerebellopontine cisterns. The cisternal pathway of the oculomotor nerve is approximately 15 mm in length and consists of a singular trunk. The average distance of the central myelin covering of the oculomotor nerve to the Obersteiner–Redlich transitional zone is 1.5 mm. The oculomotor nerve comprises motor fibers originating from the oculomotor nucleus in the midbrain, which innervate the levator palpebrae muscle and several extraocular muscles (superior rectus, internal rectus, inferior rectus, and superior oblique).

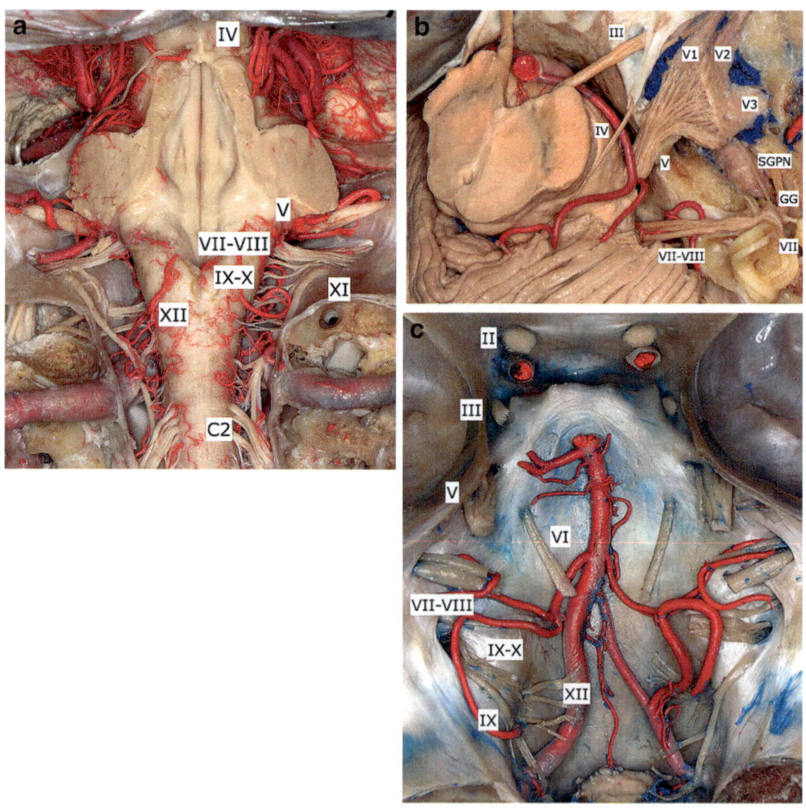

Fig. 10.1 Anatomical illustrations displaying the intracisternal trajectory of the cranial nerves. (**a**) An anatomical perspective of the posterior aspect of the brainstem following the resection of the cerebellum via the cerebellar peduncles. (**b**) Superolateral perspective of the right cerebellopontine angle. (**c**) Posterior perspective of the clivus and petrosal bones following the excision of the cerebellum and brainstem. The vessels have been positioned. (II optic nerve, III oculomotor nerve, IV trochlear nerve, V trigeminal nerve, VI abducens nerve, VII facial nerve, VII-VIII facial-vestibulocochlear complex, GG geniculate ganglion, GSPN greater superior petrosal nerve, IX-X glossopharyngeal and vagal nerves, XI accessory nerve, XII hypoglossal nerve, C2 second cervical posterior root)

Additionally, it contains parasympathetic fibers from the Edinger–Westphal nucleus, also situated in the midbrain, responsible for regulating pupillary function. Besides the cisternal section, the oculomotor nerve comprises two more segments. The cavernous segment traverses from its entry point in the ceiling of the cavernous sinus via the oculomotor triangle to its introduction in the orbit. It traverses this pathway along the lateral wall of the cavernous sinus. The final section pertains to the orbit, where it traverses the annulus of Zinn and thereafter bifurcates into branches [15].

10.2.2 Clinical, Diagnostic, and Treatment Considerations

A recent systematic analysis of the literature identified less than 90 documented occurrences of oculomotor nerve schwannomas, complicating diagnostic judgments and therapeutic suggestions [2, 4]. The average age of presentation is in the third decade, and there is a small predominance in women. Cisternal schwannomas of the third cranial nerve proliferate in the interpeduncular cistern, extending superiorly towards the retroinfundibular region and the floor of the third ventricle. When they attain a considerable size, they invade the cavernous sinus. Cisternal schwannomas include 40%, cisterno-cavernous schwannomas 10%, cavernous schwannomas 20%, cavernous-orbital schwannomas 10%, and orbital schwannomas the remaining 20%. The clinical manifestation includes diplopia and/or unilateral eyelid ptosis. A common symptom is ophthalmoplegic migraine, characterized by episodes of ptosis and diplopia, followed by a short duration of severe headache. In advanced tumors, symptoms and signs may arise due to compression of the brainstem or hydrocephalus. They are sometimes diagnosed inadvertently. Consensus exists in advocating for microneurosurgical intervention for big, symptomatic tumors or those exhibiting growth in imaging investigations; nevertheless, the challenge lies in the near certainty of full nerve injury and subsequent muscular paralysis following surgery. Consequently, following microsurgery, over 50% of patients experience deterioration, and more than 20% show no improvement. Consequently, stereotactic radiosurgery has been advised, as it is associated with reduced morbidity and the potential to enhance neurological function. Nevertheless, the issue lies in the fact that, despite magnetic resonance imaging (MRI) findings typically being indicative of schwannoma, the infrequency of the lesion renders preoperative diagnosis ambiguous and the recommendation for stereotactic radiosurgery precarious. Minor or asymptomatic lesions may be monitored through imaging and addressed when they enlarge or exhibit symptoms. Extensive tumors causing brainstem compression or hydrocephalus require microneurosurgical excision, followed by imaging surveillance and stereotactic radiosurgery of any residual tissue. The microneurosurgical procedure is typically conducted via a trans-sylvian or pretemporal pterional route.

10.3 Schwannomas of the Trochlear Nerve

10.3.1 Anatomical Considerations

The fourth cranial nerve, or trochlear nerve, originates in the posterior midbrain, in a point situated beneath the inferior quadrigeminal tubercle, approximately 5 mm from the midline. It traverses around the posterolateral margin of the midbrain, proceeding towards the free edge of the tentorium (Figs. 10.1). It is the sole cranial nerve that arises from the posterior aspect of the brainstem. It traverses within the arachnoid of the tentorial notch, initially in the quadrigeminal cistern and then in the ambiens cistern. The trochlear nerve is the smallest of the cranial nerves, measuring between 0.5 and 1 mm in diameter and comprising 1100 to 3000 nerve fibers. It is the nerve with the longest intracranial trajectory, approximately 25 mm, but not all of this trajectory is within the cistern. It is a purely motor nerve that innervates one muscle, the superior oblique. The nerve arises from a motor nucleus in the midbrain and, along its intra-mesencephalic trajectory, exhibits the distinctive feature of decussation, crossing fibers with the contralateral nerve and emerging on the opposing side. The trochlear nerve comprises several segments. Following its cisternal trajectory, the nerve penetrates the dura mater at the tentorium's margin to attach to the exterior surface of the cavernous sinus, traversing its cavernous portion. It has recently been noted that there exists a brief intratentorial or trigonal segment, approximately 4 mm in length, from the point where the nerve enters the dura mater in the posterior region of the oculomotor triangle to its position in the lateral wall of the cavernous sinus. The orbital segment is located farther distally, extending from the nerve's entry into the orbit outside the annulus of Zinn to the superior oblique muscle.

10.3.2 Clinical, Diagnostic, and Treatment Considerations

A recent systematic assessment of the literature identified merely 45 documented cases of trochlear schwannoma, complicating the ability to formulate diagnostic findings and therapeutic recommendations [13]. The typical age of onset is the fourth or fifth decade, with a somewhat higher prevalence in men. Tumors vary in type based on their growing site. Cisternal tumors develop from their emergence from the midbrain to their ingress into the cavernous sinus. This region encircles the midbrain, with tumors occurring more frequently in the ambiens and crural cisterns than in the quadrigeminal cistern. Rare tumors have been identified in both cisternal and cavernous parts (cisterno-cavernous), along with a singular occurrence of a pure intra-tentorial tumor. Ultimately, there are neoplasms situated in the cavernous sinus. The predominant presenting symptom is diplopia, observed in 60% of patients, resulting from paresis or paralysis of the superior oblique muscle. Headache is the second most prevalent symptom, occurring in 50% of patients, followed by ataxia and, subsequently, functional impairment of the trigeminal or oculomotor nerves. Large tumors exhibit symptoms indicative of long tracts and cerebellar involvement. The characteristic clinical triad of trochlear schwannomas includes diplopia, resulting from paralysis or paresis of the trochlear nerve, involvement of the long pathways, and headache. Certain patients do not report diplopia due to the occurrence of postural mechanisms or compensatory conjugate ocular mobility, attributed to the low involvement of the superior oblique muscle in overall ocular movement. Conversely, other individuals have intolerable diplopia that appears disproportionate to the restricted range of ocular worsened motions resulting from superior oblique muscle dysfunction. Tumors of the trochlear nerve are typically large at diagnosis, averaging about 30 mm in size. Cisternal schwannomas comprise 85%, while cisterno-cavernous schwannomas constitute the remaining 15%. Consensus exists in advocating for microneurosurgical intervention for large, symptomatic tumors or those exhibiting growth in imaging studies; however, the challenge lies in the fact that surgery almost invariably leads to total nerve damage and paralysis of the superior oblique muscle, occurring in over 80% of patients. The identification of the nerve trunk is exceedingly challenging during tumor dissection, even with the execution of an intracapsular resection. Consequently, numerous patients deteriorate while many others fail to show improvement. The primary benefit of the fourth nerve is its exclusive innervation of the superior oblique muscle, which significantly enhances the likelihood of spontaneous recovery following tumor resection with anatomical preservation of the nerve. This is also true for end-to-end suturing of the nerve with an interposed graft, provided the proximal and distal ends are maintained post-tumor excision. The majority of patients tolerate diplopia effectively, regardless of the use of corrective lenses. Ultimately, repair with ocular muscle reconstruction surgery demonstrates a favorable functional prognosis. The primary objective of microneurosurgical treatment is the full removal of the tumor, with the secondary aim of preserving the anatomical and functional integrity of the nerve. An alternative to microneurosurgical intervention is stereotactic radiosurgery, which necessitates similar considerations as those for schwannomas of the oculomotor nerve, due to the lesion's extreme rarity rendering accurate preoperative diagnosis uncertain and the indication for stereotactic radiosurgery precarious. Minor or asymptomatic lesions may be monitored through imaging and addressed upon growth or the onset of symptoms. Ultimately, large tumors causing brain stem compression, hydrocephalus, or affecting other cranial nerves necessitate microneurosurgical removal. In instances of incomplete resection, monitoring of the residual tumor via MRI is required, or the remnant should be addressed with stereotactic radiosurgery. When microneurosurgical intervention is warranted, the approach is predominantly supratentorial, particularly the subtemporal transtentorial technique. In the other instances, the tumor is excised via a conventional retrosigmoid infratentorial technique.

10.4 Schwannomas of the Trigeminal Nerve

10.4.1 Anatomical Considerations

The fifth cranial nerve, or trigeminal nerve, originates on the anterolateral surface of the pons, in a point situated just medially to the middle cerebellar peduncle and at the midpoint between the upper and lower boundaries of the pons. Upon departing, the nerve root proceeds in an anterior–superior–lateral trajectory to access Meckel's cave (Fig. 10.1). The trigeminal nerve's interior structure consists of a large sensory root (*pars major*), a diminutive motor root (*pars minor*), and a variable quantity of aberrant rootlets. Facial sensory fibers, exhibiting distinct somatotopic organization, penetrate the pons and are disseminated throughout the trigeminal nucleus, which extends caudally from the midbrain throughout the brainstem, whereas motor fibers emanate from the trigeminal motor nucleus situated in the pons. The trigeminal nerve is the biggest nerve in the posterior fossa, measuring around 5 mm in diameter. The investigations indicate variability in results; nonetheless, the total count of nerve fibers is approximately 25,000 in V1, 50,000 in V2, and 75,000 in V3, whereas the motor root contains around 7500 fibers. The sensory fibers are organized into approximately 50 fascicles, whereas the motor fibers are organized into around six. The average distance of central myelin covering for the trigeminal nerve to the Obersteiner–Redlich transitional zone is 4.2 mm, constituting approximately one-third of the root's intracranial length, which ranges from 8 to 15 mm.

After this cisternal segment, the nerve traverses to the Meckel's cave at a varied angle. The cave contains the most distal segment of the root, known as the *retrogasserian root*, together with the semilunar ganglion of Gasser, where the pars minor is situated in a deep anatomical plane. Meckel's cave, which exhibits varying diameters, contains the cerebrospinal fluid (CSF) dependent on an arachnoid expansion of the cerebellopontine angle cisterns. The gasserian ganglion generates the three branches of the trigeminal nerve, which exit the intracranial cavity via the superior orbital fissure (V1 branch or ophthalmic nerve), foramen rotundum (V2 branch or maxillary nerve), and foramen ovale (V3 branch or mandibular nerve, the sole branch containing motor fibers). Before exiting the cerebral cavity and becoming extracranial, each branch exhibits varying degrees of complexity in its interactions. The V1 branch traverses the lateral wall of the cavernous sinus, passes through the orbital fissure, proceeds into the orbit, and ultimately exits the skull via the supraorbital notch. The V2 branch proceeds directly to the foramen rotundum, thereafter traversing the pterygopalatine fossa and infraorbital fissure before ultimately exiting through the infraorbital foramen. The V3 branch exits the intracranial region straight into the infratemporal space via the foramen ovale, distributing its motor and sensory fibers along several branches.

10.4.2 Clinical, Diagnostic, and Treatment Considerations

Schwannomas of the trigeminal nerve are prevalent tumors, constituting 40% of non-vestibular intracranial schwannomas [8, 9, 14]. The typical age of onset is the third or fourth decade, with a little predominance in women. The varying anatomical relationships of the branches of the trigeminal nerve complicate the systematic classification of nerve segments in tumor categorization. Conversely, due to their asymptomatic characteristics in the clinical presentation of most patients, by the time they are detected, they have typically attained considerable size and extensive involvement throughout the nerve length, occupying many segments and anatomical regions inside the intracranial, skull base, and extracranial areas. In this regard, numerous classifications have been suggested. The quintessential classification is that of Jefferson from the 1950s, which categorizes them into four groups: type 1, primarily situated in the middle fossa; type 2, predominantly found in the posterior fossa; type 3, which proliferates in both regions, extending through the trigeminal foramen of Meckel's cave; and type 4, which pertains to tumors arising from the branches of the trigeminal nerve beyond the gasserian ganglion. The tumor distribution based on this classification is as follows: type 1 constitutes 40% of instances; type 2, 20%; type 3, 30%; and type 4, 10%. The acknowledgment that tumors frequently affect multiple segments of the nerve and anatomical regions, along with the capability of MRI to illustrate this, resulted in the suggestion, at the close of the last century, of a more intricate yet precise classification of trigeminal schwannomas into six categories, divided into two fundamental types. Tumors that exclusively impact a single compartment are classified as type P (posterior fossa and intradural), type M (middle fossa and interdural), and type E (extradural and extracranial), with E1 indicating involvement of the orbit and E2 indicating involvement of the infratemporal or pterygopalatine fossa. Tumors impacting multiple compartments include types MP (middle fossa and posterior fossa), ME (middle fossa and extradural or extracranial), and MPE (middle fossa, posterior fossa, and extradural or extracranial) (Figs. 10.2 and 10.3). Additional factors to consider in the classification of these tumors include the size and internal characteristics observed in imaging examinations, particularly the presence of cysts.

Clinically, trigeminal schwannomas manifest in patients with symptoms indicative of sensory nerve dysfunction affecting one or more branches. In 90% of cases, patients report tingling or paresthesia; 60% exhibit a diminished corneal reflex upon examination; and one-third experience atypical facial pain or secondary trigeminal neuralgia. Weakness of the masticatory muscles is observed in 50% of cases, although it must be determined through clinical examination. Other cranial nerves may also be implicated, or there may be compression of the brainstem; in certain instances, the diagnosis is entirely incidental. The tumor's varying extension in specific compartments enhances the clinical presentation, especially in instances involving the cavernous sinus or posterior fossa. The clinical history precedes the diagnosis, spanning several years. The imaging diagnostic reveals no distinct features compared to other cerebral schwannomas, other than their excessively large size and involvement of several compartments (Fig. 10.2). Their considerable size results in numerous tumors exhibiting a heterogeneous appearance in MRI examinations following gadolinium administration. Trigeminal schwannomas are mostly benign tumors, although instances of malignancy characterized by rapid growth and aggressive behavior have been documented. Only in a limited number of instances do people with neurofibromatosis type 2 present. Their substantial size at diagnosis results in imaging investigations indicating minimal or no growth over the observation period.

Consensus exists in advocating for microneurosurgical intervention for substantial, symptomatic tumors or those exhibiting growth in imaging examinations. Trigeminal schwannomas confined to the posterior fossa (type 2 or type P) or mostly situated in the posterior fossa are addressed via a traditional retrosigmoid craniotomy, typically resulting in total excision of the tumor. Trigeminal schwannomas confined to the middle fossa (type 1 or type M) or mostly situated in the middle fossa are addressed via a middle fossa pterional craniotomy with extradural access, typically resulting in total excision of the tumor. Trigeminal schwannomas that engage

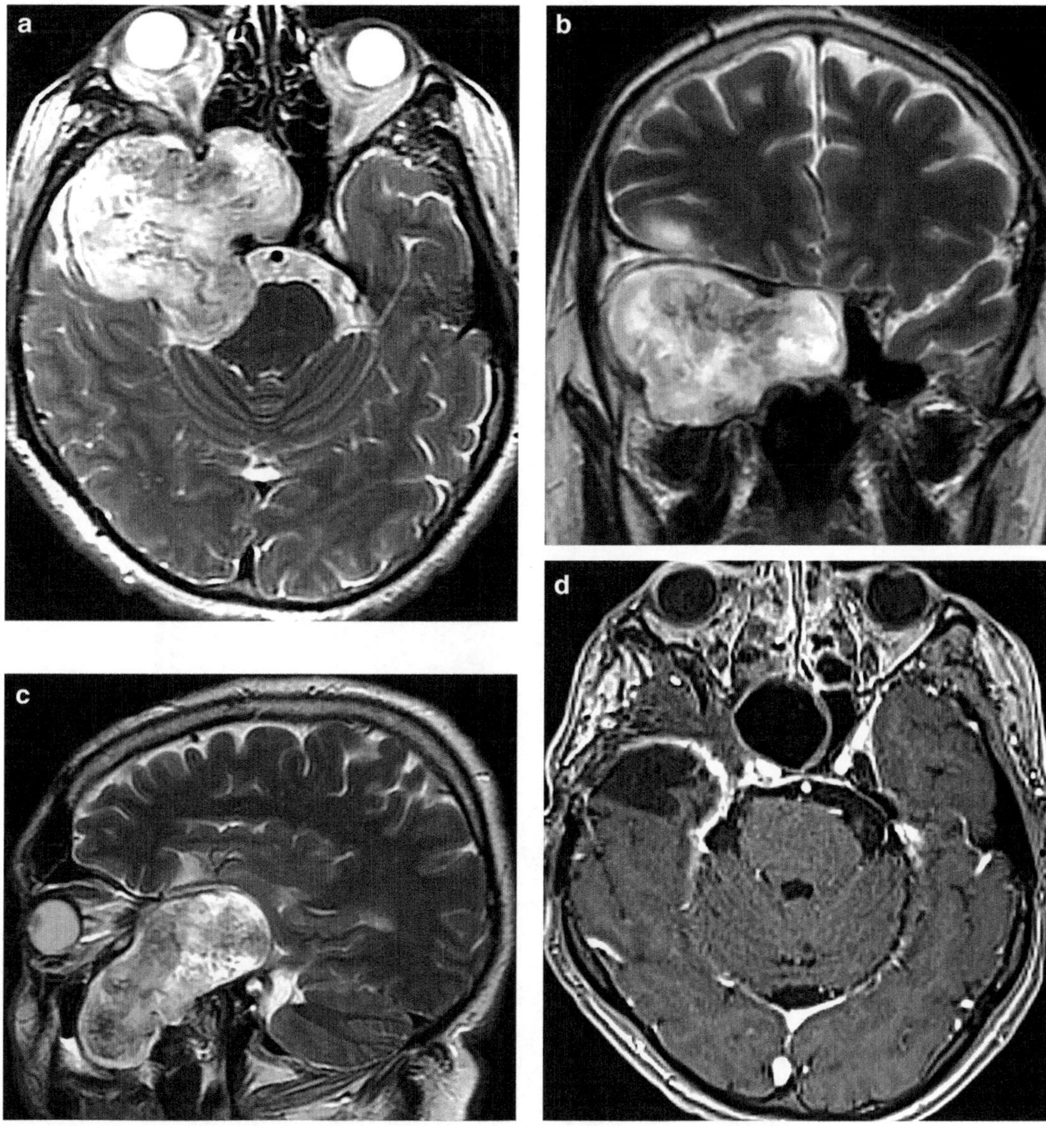

Fig. 10.2 Schwannoma of the right trigeminal nerve, encompassing the middle fossa, posterior fossa, and extradural space, with expansions into the infratemporal and sphenoidal sinuses (MPE type). (**a–c**) T2-weighted MRI pictures in the axial, coronal, and parasagittal planes. (**d**) Axial T1-weighted MRI with gadolinium, 6 months post-microneurosurgical resection

numerous compartments (type 3 or types MP, ME, MPE) exhibit increased complexity. Before the advent of microsurgery and MRI diagnostic imaging, the morbidity and mortality associated with the surgical management of trigeminal schwannomas were elevated, and partial or subtotal resections were commonplace. In addition to microsurgery and accurate anatomical diagnosis, the most significant advancement in the microneurosurgical management of trigeminal schwannomas, especially large ones located in the middle fossa, has been the introduction of the extradural approach to the middle fossa. In this region, the schwannoma is interdural, and the dissection of the dura mater from Meckel's cave and the lateral wall of the cavernous sinus,

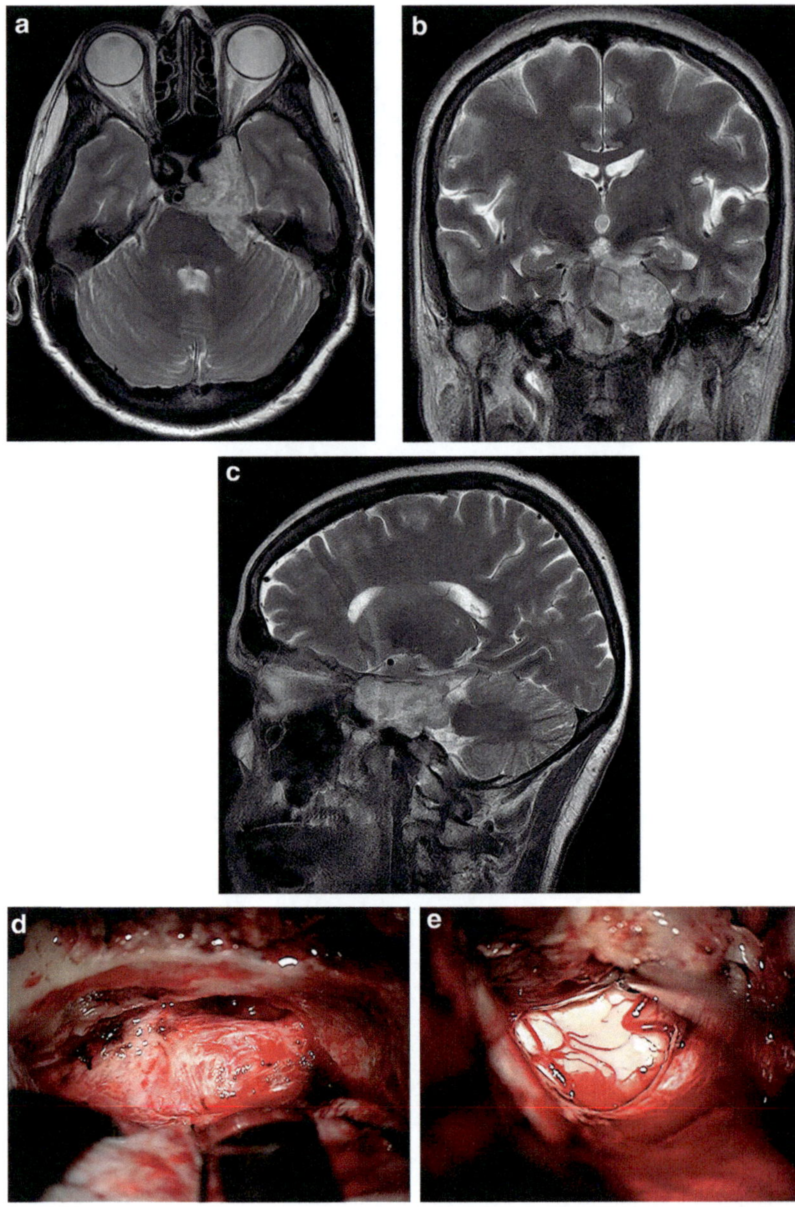

Fig. 10.3 Schwannoma of the left trigeminal nerve, involving the middle and posterior fossa (MP type). (**a**-**c**) T2-weighted MRI slices in the axial, coronal, and parasagittal planes. (**d**) Intraoperative picture displaying the extradural approach to the middle fossa following the peeling of the dura mater, illustrating the tumor alongside the V2 and V3 branches. (**e**) Image displaying the pons of the brainstem following the excision of the posterior fossa extension

accessed via a trans-zygomatic pterional approach, facilitates the exposure of a substantial portion of the capsule (Fig. 10.3). By executing a thorough internal decompression with an ultrasonic aspirator, all extensions can be traced to the posterior fossa or to the extradural or extracranial area. Schwannoma is a soft tumor characterized by minimal vascularization, allowing the compartments it invades to be readily and systematically evacuated, thus preserving the capsule that typically contains nerve fascicles. Upon achieving enough decompression, the fibrous capsule of the tumor is meticulously detached from the affected trigeminal nerve fascicles, including the root, ganglion, or peripheral branches. The considerable size of the trigeminal nerve facilitates the identification of intact fascicles during microneurosurgical excision. Neuroendoscopy facilitates dissection and excision, especially in areas obscured from the microscope's view. An alternative is to do a two-step or multi-stage surgical procedure, with each stage focused on the radical excision of individual compartments. Ultimately, schwannomas located peripheral to the ganglion of Gasser (type 4 or type E) necessitate tailored therapies for each instance.

Concerning the outcome, in all instances, even with complete resection, there may be a transient decline in sensory function, or the patient may not observe any improvement post-resection. Nonetheless, neuralgic face pain often resolves in most instances, whereas neuropathic pain either remains unchanged or may even manifest to some degree post-surgery. An alternative to microneurosurgical intervention is stereotactic radiosurgery, which necessitates the same precautions as those for schwannomas affecting other cranial nerves. Furthermore, tiny trigeminal schwannomas appropriate for stereotactic radiosurgery are not the rule. The outcomes of stereotactic radiosurgery cannot be juxtaposed with those of microneurosurgical resection due to the smaller size of the irradiated tumors compared to the resected ones. Minor or asymptomatic lesions may be monitored through imaging and addressed when they enlarge or exhibit symptoms. Ultimately, large tumors causing brainstem compression, neuralgic pain, or affecting other cranial nerves necessitate microneurosurgical removal. In instances of inadequate resection, it is imperative to monitor the residuals using imaging or adjunctive stereotactic radiosurgery subsequently.

10.5 Schwannomas of the Abducens Nerve

10.5.1 Anatomical Considerations

The apparent origin of the sixth cranial nerve, or abducens nerve, is situated in the medial region of the medullary-pontine sulcus, from which it proceeds on a cranial and slightly lateral trajectory until it reaches Dorello's canal (Fig. 10.1). This is the cisternal section of the nerve, located in the prepontine cistern at the cerebellopontine angle. This route is situated between the pons and the dural surface of the clivus and just medially to the basilar artery. The length of the cisternal segment is varied; however, it is rather lengthy, measuring approximately 15 mm, as it is the second cranial nerve in terms of length. The nerve consists of a singular trunk containing between 1600 and 7000 nerve fibers. The abducens nerve is a purely motor nerve, with its nucleus located in the deep region of the brainstem, adjacent to the fourth ventricle, and it innervates solely one muscle, the external rectus. The root entry zone has an average measurement of 1.5 mm extending to the Obersteiner–Redlich transitional zone.

In addition to the cisternal segment, the sixth pair comprises two additional segments. The intracavernous segment commences with its entry through the posterior wall of the cavernous sinus via Dorello's canal. After traversing beneath Gruber's petro-sphenoidal ligament, the nerve is situated on the lateral aspect of the intracavernous portion of the internal carotid artery. The nerve follows a slightly ascending and lateral trajectory, positioning itself on the medial aspect of the ophthalmic nerve, ultimately attaching to the lateral wall of the cavernous sinus before exiting through the superior orbital fissure. The nerve in this intracavernous segment may be singular or composed of two or more fascicles. The orbital segment extends from the point where the nerve traverses the annulus of Zinn to its termination in the lateral rectus muscle [15].

10.5.2 Clinical, Diagnostic, and Treatment Considerations

A recent thorough analysis of the literature identified merely 30 documented occurrences of abducens nerve schwannomas, complicating diagnostic judgments and therapeutic suggestions [2, 10]. The typical age of onset occurs in the fourth or fifth decade, with a little higher prevalence in males. Abducens schwannomas are classified into three distinct types: cisternal tumors that develop in the intracranial segment of the nerve, extending from its emergence from the brainstem to Dorello's canal; cavernous tumors that proliferate within the intracavernous segment of the nerve; and tumors that invade both regions (cisterno-cavernous). Only the first and the last groups proliferate in the cerebellopontine angle. Patients with isolated cavernous abducens schwannoma have paresis or paralysis of the lateral rectus muscle and report diplopia. Upon inspection, a diminished or absent ability to abduct the eye is observed, attributable to paresis or paralysis of the lateral rectus muscle. Cisternal and cisterno-cavernous tumors exhibit a more aggressive presentation linked to the involvement of more cranial nerves, compression of the brainstem, and hydrocephalus. The distinct clinical presentation of cisternal tumors arises from their initial growth in the prepontine cistern, which subsequently lateralizes toward the cerebellopontine angle, while cisterno-cavernous tumors occupy both compartments. Cisternal schwannomas comprise 50%, cisterno-cavernous tumors constitute 20%, and cavernous tumors represent the remaining 30%. Consensus exists in advocating surgical intervention for big, symptomatic tumors or those exhibiting growth in imaging investigations; however, the drawback is that surgery almost invariably leads to total nerve damage and subsequent muscle paralysis. This is due to the considerable challenge of identifying the nerve during tumor excision, even when just intracapsular debulking is conducted. Consequently, numerous patients deteriorate, while many others fail to improve following microneurosurgery. The primary benefit of the sixth cranial nerve is its exclusive innervation of a single muscle, the external rectus. Consequently, spontaneous recovery following resection, provided the nerve's anatomical integrity is maintained, is highly probable. This recovery is also likely after end-to-end suturing of the nerve or through the use of an interposed nerve graft, assuming the proximal and distal ends are preserved post-tumor excision. Ultimately, correction by ocular muscle reconstructive surgery yields favorable functional and aesthetic outcomes. An alternative to microneurosurgical intervention is stereotactic radiosurgery, which necessitates similar considerations as those for other cranial nerve schwannomas. The exceptional rarity of the lesion renders preoperative diagnosis uncertain, making the indication for stereotactic radiosurgery hazardous. Minor or asymptomatic lesions may be monitored through imaging and addressed when they enlarge or exhibit symptoms. Extensive tumors causing brain stem compression or affecting other cranial nerves necessitate microneurosurgical resection, followed by successive MRI assessments if resection is inadequate, or treatment of the residual tumor with stereotactic radiosurgery. The retrosigmoid technique is advantageous for addressing cisternal lesions in the microneurosurgical treatment of cerebellopontine angle tumors, while combined supra-infratentorial approaches, either in one or two stages, are effective for cisternocavernous lesions.

10.6 Schwannomas of the Facial Nerve

10.6.1 Anatomical Considerations

The seventh cranial nerve, or facial nerve, arises from the brainstem at the lateral aspect of the medullary-pontine sulcus, approximately 1–2 mm superior to the exit point of the vestibulocochlear nerve (Fig. 10.1). The motor nucleus of the facial nerve is situated in the pons, and the fibers constituting the nerve do not traverse ventrally to the anterior surface of the brainstem; instead, they course rostrally to the fourth ventricle, encircling the nucleus of the abducens nerve from the interior to the exterior, thereby forming a loop that is positioned superficially on the floor of the fourth ventricle. Following its exit, the facial nerve traverses a few millimeters in close proximity to the pons, subsequently diverging and associating with the vestibulocochlear nerve approximately 4 mm later, as well as with the intermediate nerve of Wrisberg in a considerably more variable manner, ultimately integrating into it. The egress of both nerve roots is anatomically related to the choroid plexus of the fourth ventricle, which emerges at the cerebellopontine angle via the lateral foramina of Luschka, as well as with the flocculus of the cerebellum. In the microneurosurgical technique utilizing the retrosigmoid approach, these structures are located in the deepest region of the petrosal fissure of the cerebellum. The cisternal trajectory of the facial nerve directs it to the internal acoustic meatus and thereafter via the internal auditory canal to the fundus of the canal. During this route, the nerve root is intradural, encased by the arachnoid matrix and cerebrospinal fluid. The length of the facial nerve in its cisternal portion is approximately 18 mm (the intracanalicular segment is around 11 mm), with an average diameter of 1.6 mm. The entry zone is notably short, averaging 2.9 mm in length to the Obersteiner–Redlich transitional zone. The facial nerve comprises roughly 10,000 axons, with around 6000 designated as motor fibers, while the remainder consists of sensory, parasympathetic, and gustatory fibers. The facial nerve constitutes a singular trunk until the geniculate ganglion, after which it assumes a fascicular pattern.

The facial nerve is anatomically segmented into six parts. The cisternal section traverses the cerebellopontine angle to the internal acoustic meatus. The intracanalicular segment extends via the internal auditory canal to its fundus, where it penetrates the bone above the horizontal crest and posterior to the vertical crest of Bell. The labyrinthine segment traverses an intraosseous path to the geniculate ganglion, with its entry constricted by the periosteum of the bone surrounding the nerve trunk. The segment is exceedingly tiny (<0.7 mm) and short (3–5 mm) and related with the cochlea and the superior semicircular canal. The geniculate ganglion is an enlargement of the facial nerve where the intermediate nerve fibers diverge, generating the greater superficial petrosal nerve (GSPN), which traverses the bony surface of the petrous bone via a fragile and susceptible bony canal. Traction on the petrosal nerve may damage the geniculate ganglion and, consequently, the facial nerve. The facial nerve traverses a petrosal bone canal alongside two other segments. The horizontal or tympanic segment leads to the stapes and, following a directional change of approximately 90°, transitions into the vertical or mastoid segment, measuring about 15 mm to the stylomastoid foramen. This portion of the nerve generates several branches, with the chorda tympani being the most significant. Ultimately, at the departure of the facial nerve through the stylomastoid foramen lies the extratemporal segment, which has a wider width (2–3 mm) and extends until it penetrates the parotid gland, where it bifurcates into two trunks in the *pes anserinus* [15, 23].

10.6.2 Clinical, Diagnostic, and Treatment Considerations

Facial nerve schwannomas are uncommon tumors that can develop at any location along the nerve's trajectory and often affect multiple anatomical segments. Tumors that arise in the cisternal and canalicular segments, as these are the sole types that proliferate at the cerebellopontine angle, may be mistaken for vestibular schwannoma. The relative frequency of involvement of these two segments fluctuates by series; however, it is estimated that merely 20–25% of facial nerve schwannomas originate in the cisternal or intracanalicular segment of the nerve. Some may extend to the geniculate ganglion, adopting an hourglass morphology characterized by a typically more dilated portion in the cistern and a smaller portion in the ganglion, adjacent to the middle cranial fossa (Fig. 10.4a). Tumors arising from the geniculate ganglion or the greater superficial petrosal nerve exclusively proliferate within the middle fossa.

Clinically, facial nerve schwannomas are anticipated to mostly cause paresis or paralysis of the face muscles due to dysfunction of the facial nerve. Nonetheless, the symptoms predominantly exhibit vestibulocochlear characteristics, as facial schwannomas in these regions also impact the vestibulocochlear nerve. This seemingly unforeseen circumstance also occurs in facial schwannomas originating in other intrapetrous segments of the nerve, as the facial schwannoma, despite not involving the vestibulocochlear nerve, impacts both the inner ear and the middle ear. Conversely, symptoms resulting from the direct involvement of the facial nerve correlate with the specific segment affected by the schwannoma: tumors in the cisternal or canalicular segment commonly manifest as sensorineural hearing loss or tinnitus; those in the labyrinthine segment exhibit facial paresis and sensorineural hearing loss; tumors in the geniculate ganglion and tympanic segment present with facial paresis and conductive hearing loss; those in the mastoid segment are characterized by facial paresis, otorrhea, and conductive hearing loss; and finally, extratemporal tumors appear as masses in the parotid gland. The imaging diagnostic relies on

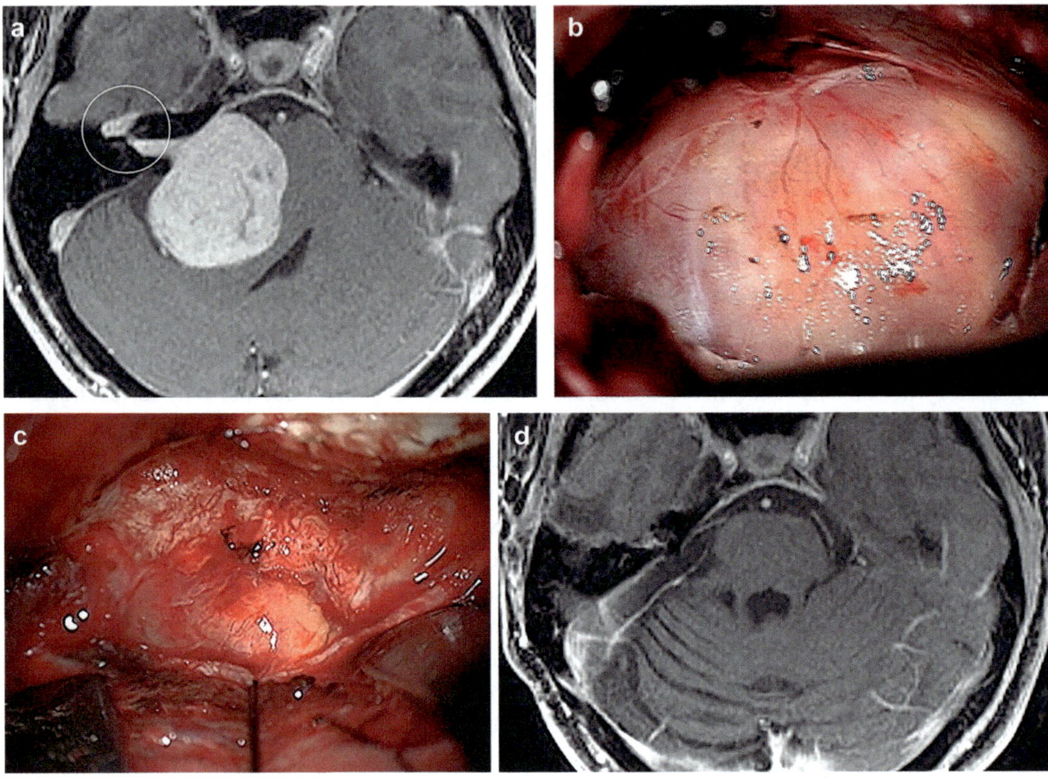

Fig. 10.4 Schwannoma of the right facial nerve. (**a**) Axial T1-weighted MRI with contrast revealing a lesion characterized by a large mass in the cerebellopontine angle, extending into the internal auditory canal, and a small petrosal mass located at the site of the geniculate ganglion (circle). (**b**) Intraoperative imaging of the retrosigmoid approach to the intracisternal and intracanalicular parts of the tumor. (**c**) Intraoperative imaging of the extradural access to the geniculate ganglion lesion through a subtemporal extradural middle fossa approach. (**d**) Axial T1-weighted MRI with contrast illustrating the final outcome of both resections

computed tomography (CT) and magnetic resonance imaging (MRI). Nonetheless, there are no distinct diagnostic differences between cisternal and/or intracanalicular facial nerve schwannomas and vestibular schwannomas. Pathognomonic signs of facial nerve schwannoma are evident when an intra-labyrinthine extension of a cisternal schwannoma is present (labyrinthine tail sign) or when the tumor involves the geniculate ganglion (Fig. 10.4a). Otological, vestibular, and electrophysiological examinations reveal no major discrepancies for differentiating between schwannomas of the facial and vestibular nerves; the sole distinction is that facial schwannomas better preserve auditory function compared to vestibular tumors. The presence of a tiny cisternal or intracanalicular tumor accompanied by facial paralysis strongly indicates facial nerve schwannoma.

The treatment modalities are identical to those for schwannomas of other cranial nerves: observation, microneurosurgical excision, and stereotactic radiosurgery [16, 21]. The guidelines for these treatments align with those provided for vestibular schwannoma and other intracranial schwannomas. The treatment modality is contingent upon the tumor's dimensions, clinical manifestations, functionality of the facial and auditory nerves, the neurosurgeon's expertise, and the patient's preferences. The challenge lies in the extreme difficulty of accurately diagnosing facial schwannoma preoperatively, except in the aforementioned unusual cases. Based only on the preoperative suspicion of facial nerve schwannoma, the following recommendations may be formulated. Small tumors measuring less than 30 mm and asymptomatic will be monitored via imaging, but symptomatic patients with House-Brackmann IV-V facial function will undergo stereotactic radiosurgery, and symptomatic tumors with poorer facial function will be subjected to microneurosurgical resection. Tumors above 30 mm in size should be excised to attain complete resection, particularly in instances with compromised facial function, while considering a facial nerve reconstruction treatment. In patients with adequate facial function, the objective would be to perform internal decompression of the tumor to maintain facial nerve function and thereafter address the residual tumor using stereotactic radiosurgery. A recent meta-analysis comparing the outcomes of microneurosurgical and stereotactic radiosurgery treatments revealed that facial nerve function improved in 25% of patients following microneurosurgery, stabilized in 40%, and deteriorated in 35%. In contrast, after stereotactic radiosurgery, facial function improved in 20% of patients, stabilized in 70%, and worsened in 10%. While these findings may indicate the advantages of stereotactic radiosurgery, this study is biased due to the lack of size comparisons; thus, they should be interpreted cautiously, as microneurosurgically treated tumors are typically larger and present in individuals with compromised facial nerve function. The retrosigmoid approach facilitates the excision of tumors of any size situated in the cisternal and/or intracanalicular segments, yet it does not provide access to the labyrinthine or geniculate portions of the tumor. Conversely, the translabyrinthine approach permits the removal of tumors in the labyrinthine and/or intracanalicular and/or cisternal segments, but is applicable solely to patients with non-functional hearing; it does not enable the resection of tumors located more distally unless accompanied by a petrosectomy. The middle fossa technique is optimal for tumors located in the tympanic segment, geniculate ganglion, and intracanalicular segment. Consequently, in some instances, a staged interventions for the cerebellopontine angle and petrosal or geniculate segments of the tumor becomes beneficial (Fig. 10.4).

10.7 Schwannomas of the Intermediate Nerve of Wrisberg

10.7.1 Anatomical Considerations

The intermediate nerve is constituted by the fusion of many rootlets that originate directly from the brainstem or are observed separately from the origins of the vestibulocochlear nerve or the facial nerve. During its cisternal trajectory, it traverses the space between the vestibulocochlear and facial nerve roots, creating one or more diminutive fascicles that are affixed to either nerve, rendering it typically unidentifiable during surgical procedures. The Obersteiner–Redlich transitional zone of the intermediate nerve is situated less than 1 mm from the nerve's egress from the brainstem. In the internal auditory canal, roughly 3 mm from the fundus, the intermediate nerve has been completely incorporated into the facial nerve. The intermediate nerve conducts parasympathetic fibers from the superior salivary parasympathetic nucleus to the lacrimal and salivary glands, conveys taste sensory information from the tongue to the solitary nucleus, and relays general cutaneous sensitivity from the Ramsay–Hunt skin zone to the spinal trigeminal nucleus. Upon integration into the facial nerve, it disseminates and assimilates its fibers initially via the great superior petrosal nerve and subsequently through the chorda tympani [15, 23].

10.7.2 Clinical, Diagnostic, and Treatment Considerations

Schwannomas arising from the intermediate nerve are exceedingly uncommon, with only 13 occurrences documented in the literature [3]. Given that the nerve regulates tear production, gustation, and cutaneous sensitivity in the

Ramsay–Hunt region and nasal mucosa, it is anticipated that patients may report symptoms such as crocodile tears, dry eye, hypogeusia, or Hitselberger's sign. Nonetheless, this is seldom in clinical practice. Furthermore, a certain percentage of vestibular or facial schwannomas are linked to one or more of the aforementioned symptoms or signs, but their delicacy often renders them unrecognized by both patients and clinicians. They are identified in 30% of small vestibular schwannomas, 60% of big vestibular schwannomas, and 80% of giant vestibular schwannomas. This prompts the inquiry of whether schwannomas of the nervus intermedius genuinely exist or if certain vestibular and facial nerve schwannomas are, in fact, schwannomas of the nervus intermedius that have assimilated one or both nerves into the tumor. This latter option is more probable. Identifying the origin of a schwannoma in the nervus intermedius is exceedingly challenging using imaging techniques and during surgical procedures, except in cases of very small tumors that distinctly separate the vestibulocochlear and facial nerve roots, which remain intact along their anatomical pathway.

10.8 Intralabyrinthine Schwannomas

10.8.1 Anatomical Considerations

Upon reaching the fundus of the internal auditory canal, the vestibulocochlear nerve bifurcates into three fascicles: the cochlear fascicle, which traverses the anteroinferior quadrant of the fundus beneath the transverse crest to reach the cochlea, and the superior and inferior vestibular fascicles, which ascend and descend across the posterior half of the fundus, above and below the transverse crest, respectively, to innervate the labyrinth. The superior vestibular fascicle innervates the utricle and the superior and lateral semicircular canals, whereas the inferior vestibular fascicle innervates the saccule and the posterior semicircular canal.

10.8.2 Clinical, Diagnostic, and Treatment Considerations

Approximately, 50 schwannomas have been documented along this brief stretch of the vestibulocochlear nerve, extending from the fundus of the internal auditory canal to its target organs [5, 11]. These are referred to as intralabyrinthine schwannomas. They arise from either the short portion of the nerves supplying the cochlea and labyrinth or from the nerve fibers situated within these sensory organs. The cases presented occur in adults, with equal prevalence in both sexes. The majority of patients exhibit hearing loss of various severity and progression; 70% experience tinnitus, and an additional 70% suffer from vertigo. Intralabyrinthine schwannomas are diminutive lesions that, prior to the advent of MRI, were incidentally discovered during otological procedures in individuals with Ménière's disease. MRI can detect these tumors preoperatively as small, well-circumscribed lesions that exhibit enhancement following gadolinium injection in T1-weighted sequences, situated intralabyrinthine, and without expansion into the internal auditory canal. The management of these tumors falls under the otological domain, as excision is performed by a translabyrinthine approach. This surgical method resulted in total hearing loss. Consequently, patients exhibiting symptoms of hypoacusis with functional hearing and without refractory vertigo may undergo imaging and get symptomatic management. Patients presenting with deafness and intractable vertigo are optimal candidates for resection, facilitating the verification of the lesion's origin. Another indication is the assessment of the lesion type in individuals exhibiting an increase in lesion size, especially if it encroaches upon the internal auditory canal, potentially jeopardizing the facial nerve. The correlation between functional hearing and persistent vertigo complicates therapeutic decision-making, as pharmacological labyrinthectomy may be employed to address vertigo, and if unsuccessful, the patient may undergo surgical resection, resulting in permanent deafness. The likelihood of impacting the facial nerve during the otological management of these schwannomas is negligible. There is no documented experience with stereotactic radiosurgery for intralabyrinthine schwannomas; however, the lesion's diminutive size, intraosseous positioning, and proximity to healthy neural structures present a risk of functional decline due to the irradiation or subsequent edema.

10.9 Schwannomas of the Glossopharyngeal Nerve

10.9.1 Anatomical Considerations

The apparent origin of the ninth cranial nerve, or glossopharyngeal nerve, from the brainstem occurs in the posterolateral or retrolivary sulcus of the medulla oblongata, manifesting as one or more rootlets situated below the choroid plexuses that exit the fourth ventricle via the lateral recesses of Luschka. These rootlets converge to form a single trunk a few millimeters later, en route to the jugular foramen. The jugular foramen functions as an outlet from the cerebral cavity for the glossopharyngeal, vagal, and accessory nerves via their neural compartments. A significant number of venous channels traverse the jugular foramen, organized into two clusters: an anterior, smaller group directed towards the inferior petrosal sinus, and a posterior, larger group leading to the sigmoid sinus, which extends into the bulb of the jugular vein. A fibrous band and/or a variably developed bony crest often separates the neural component from the sigmoid component. The glossopharyngeal nerve transmits motor fibers to the swallowing muscles from its motor nucleus, or nucleus ambiens, situated in the medulla oblongata, and sensory fibers from the posterior oral cavity and taste fibers from the posterior tongue to the nucleus of the solitary tract, in addition to visceral control fibers from the chemoreceptors and baroreceptors located in the carotid sinus. The mean length of the glossopharyngeal nerve in its cisternal trajectory is 16 mm, with an average diameter of 1.5 mm. The entry zone length to the Obersteiner–Redlich transitional zone is 1.5 mm. Besides this cisternal section, the nerve comprises two more anatomical segments [15]. The foraminal segment traverses the jugular foramen, with the nerve encased in the epineurium. Subsequently, in the extracranial portion, the nerve detaches from its association with the base of the skull.

10.9.2 Clinical, Diagnostic, and Treatment Considerations

Schwannomas of the glossopharyngeal nerve are infrequent tumors; however, examples are encountered despite the nerve being predominantly motor in function [20]. A recent comprehensive assessment of the literature identified just 42 documented occurrences, complicating the ability to formulate diagnostic judgments and therapeutic recommendations due to the shortness of the series. The mean age of onset is the third decade, with a little higher prevalence in women compared to men. Tumors are categorized into four groups based on their nerve growth and imaging study results: type 1, predominantly intradural tumors; type 2, primarily intraosseous tumors with or without intracranial extension; type 3, chiefly extracranial tumors; and type 4, hourglass-shaped intra-extracranial tumors. The literature indicates the following tumor distribution: type 1, 75%; type 2, 10%; type 3, 5%; and type 4, 10%. Only the initial two groups proliferate in the cerebellopontine angle, whereas the remaining groups also undergo microneurosurgical intervention via an approach to the skull base. The glossopharyngeal nerve function is disturbed in only one-third of individuals at the time of diagnosis. Injury to the glossopharyngeal nerve manifests as paralysis of the soft palate muscles, resulting in contralateral uvula deviation and impaired swallowing mechanics. The predominant symptoms are associated with vestibulocochlear dysfunction, present in 85% of patients, followed by symptoms resulting from intracranial hypertension and cerebellar compression, observed in 40% of patients at diagnosis. The remaining cranial nerves may be affected in several people, depending upon the tumor's size and its major cranial or caudal expansion. Glossopharyngeal schwannomas induce hearing loss primarily at intermediate frequencies, in contrast to vestibular schwannomas, which impact high frequencies. This results from the specific topographic arrangement of cochlear fibers in the nerve in accordance with tone frequency somatotopy. The imaging diagnosis is established using MRI, which reveals all the distinctive features of the schwannomas previously detailed (Fig. 10.5a). The jugular foramen may also host other rather common tumors, including meningioma and chemodectoma situated in the bulb of the jugular vein, necessitating differential diagnosis. In tiny tumors, the proximity of the tumor to the nerve fibers along their cisternal pathway is evident in high-weighted T2 imaging tests (FIESTA: Fast Imaging Employing Steady-state Acquisition). In CT imaging, the chemodectoma of the jugular glomus situated in the bulb of the jugular vein typically appears hyperdense and exhibits high contrast enhancement, resulting in decalcification and erosion of the bone around the jugular foramen or jugular bulb. In MRI, this tumor appears iso- or hypointense on T1-weighted sequences, exhibiting significant contrast enhancement, and is hyperintense on T2 sequences, with involvement of the venous vascular systems. In this context, digital subtraction angiography (DSA) is advised with two primary aims: to exclude chemodectoma due to its distinctive hypervascularization and to assess the tumor's relationship with the jugular vein bulb and the inferior petrosal sinus. Similar to other cerebellopontine angle schwannomas, a definitive referral for surgical intervention is indicated for big, symptomatic tumors or those exhibiting growth in imaging assessments. The aim of the surgery is the total excision of the lesion while preserving the anatomical and functional integrity of the glossopharyngeal nerve. The complete excision of the tumor is contingent upon its dimensions and is accomplished in the majority of instances (Fig. 10.5b). In certain instances, resection may be partial, necessitating imaging follow-up to detect potential recurrences. Following microneurosurgical tumor removal, an additional increase in cranial nerve deficit symptoms is typically observed; nevertheless, deterioration occurs in one-third of cases involving one or more cranial nerves. Concerning the function

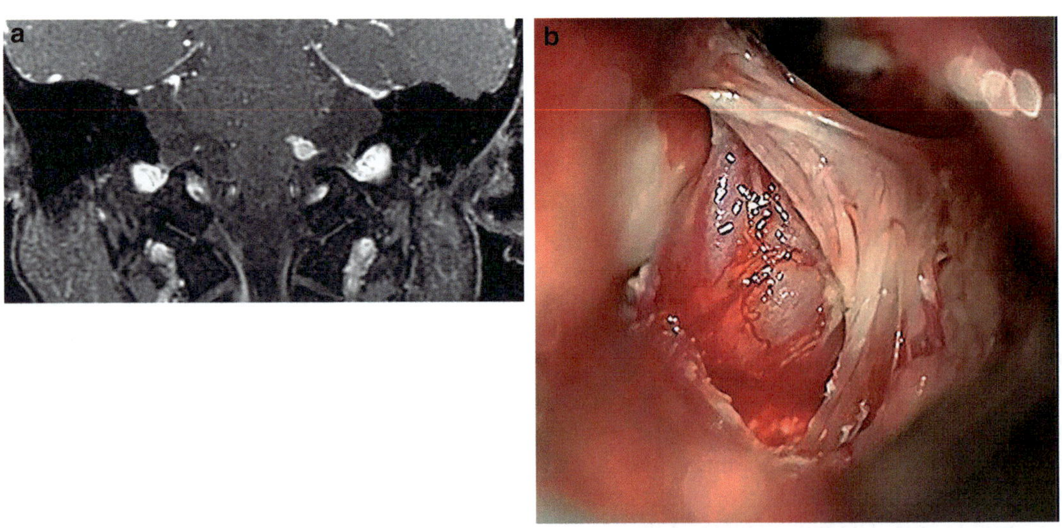

Fig. 10.5 Schwannoma of the left glossopharyngeal nerve. (**a**) Coronal section of T1-weighted MRI with contrast revealing a rounded lesion in the anterolateral region of the medulla oblongata, at the level of the medullo-pontine sulcus. (**b**) Intraoperative imaging of the retrosigmoid approach to the lesion

of the glossopharyngeal nerve, the principle is deterioration or total paralysis of the nerve in individuals who previously exhibited normal function prior to the resection. While many deficits are transient, the concurrent involvement of the glossopharyngeal and vagal nerves can lead to severe consequences, including potential bronchial aspiration and pneumonia. An alternative to microneurosurgical intervention is stereotactic radiosurgery, which necessitates similar considerations as those for other non-vestibular angle schwannomas due to the lesion's exceptional rarity, rendering preoperative diagnosis uncertain and the indication for stereotactic radiosurgery unwarranted. Minor or asymptomatic lesions may be monitored through imaging and addressed when they enlarge or exhibit symptoms. Ultimately, large tumors causing brain stem compression or affecting other cranial nerves necessitate microneurosurgical excision, and if resection is inadequate, should be supplemented with stereotactic radiosurgery subsequently or monitored through imaging for residuals. The strategy for a microneurosurgical approach to glossopharyngeal schwannomas depends upon the tumor's classification. Type 1 and 2 tumors located intracranially, with or without extension into the jugular foramen, may be excised via a conventional retrosigmoid technique. In other forms of tumor growth, an extensive retro and presigmoid infralabyrinthine approach with an appropriate cervical trajectory is required to gain control of the jugular vein caudally, the bulb of the jugular vein cranially, and the sigmoid sinus externally. This comprehensive method allows for the excision of the tumor in its extracranial segment, within the foramen, and any intracranial extension.

10.10 Schwannomas of the Vagal Nerve

10.10.1 Anatomical Considerations

The tenth cranial nerve, or vagal nerve, originates from the brainstem in the posterolateral or retrolivary sulcus of the medulla oblongata, displaying as multiple rootlets that extend toward the jugular foramen without converging into a single trunk. These rootlets emerge caudally to those of the glossopharyngeal nerve and cranially to those of the cranial portion of the accessory nerve (Fig. 10.1). The vagal nerve transmits fibers responsible for visceral parasympathetic regulation of cardiac and digestive functions. The mean length of the vagal nerve in its cisternal portion, extending from the brainstem to the jugular foramen, is 13 mm, with a diameter of 0.9 mm. The length of the entry zone to the Obersteiner–Redlich transitional zone measures 1.6 mm. Besides the cisternal section, the nerve comprises two additional anatomical segments [15]. The foraminal segment traverses the jugular foramen, with the nerve enveloped by the epineurium. Subsequently, in the extracranial portion, the nerve detaches from its association with the base of the skull.

10.10.2 Clinical, Diagnostic, and Treatment Considerations

Vagal nerve schwannomas are uncommon tumors, rendering it difficult to formulate diagnostic conclusions and therapeutic recommendations due to the limited number of documented solitary cases [6, 8]. A recent systematic examination of the literature identified merely seven cases of entirely intradural vagal schwannomas located in the cerebellopontine angle. In all instances, with one exception, the tumors were diminutive, allowing for a definitive determination of their origin in the nerve. Vagal nerve involvement manifests in patients with highly nonspecific symptoms, including hearing loss, vertigo, or ataxia, reminiscent of vestibular schwannoma symptoms. Certain instances have been documented in conjunction with paroxysmal arterial hypertension, akin to that observed in microvascular compression of the vagal nerve root or the rostral ventrolateral (RVL) region of the medulla oblongata, elucidated by analogous pathophysiological mechanisms. The MRI examination facilitates the diagnosis of the lesion associated with the lower cranial nerves and rules out vestibular schwannoma. The treatment involves microneurosurgical resection via a conventional retrosigmoid route. Microsurgery facilitates the confirmation of origin in the vagal nerve roots, enables the acquisition of materials for histological validation, and alleviates symptoms. In instances of paroxysmal hypertension, the risk of significant hypotension during the immediate postoperative phase following tumor excision must be observed.

10.11 Schwannomas of the Accessory Nerve

10.11.1 Anatomical Considerations

The eleventh cranial nerve, or auxiliary nerve, is unique since it is the sole cranial nerve that traverses the foramen magnum, originating at the confluence of ventral and dorsal rootlets of the first cervical medullary segments up to C7. The accessory nerve consists of a series of intracranial rootlets originating from the medulla oblongata, situated inferior to those of the vagal nerve (cranial portion), and additional rootlets emerging from the cervical spinal cord (cervical or spinal component). These rootlets, present in varying quantities, are integrated irregularly; the most cranial rootlets may independently reach the jugular foramen, while others connect with the caudal roots of the accessory nerve, creating a singular trunk, 1–2 mm in thickness, that ascends to the jugular foramen, adhering to the dura mater of the foramen magnum and the jugular tubercle (Fig. 10.1). The nerve has around 1700 to 2000 myelinated fibers, with the transitional zone situated in proximity to the exit of the rootlets from the medulla oblongata or spinal cord. Upon entering the jugular foramen, it resides with the glossopharyngeal and vagal nerves within the neural compartment. It is a purely motor nerve that innervates the sternocleidomastoid and trapezius muscles, along with a portion of the pharyngolaryngeal muscles. The motor neurons are situated in the caudal region of the medullary motor nucleus, also known as the ambiguous nucleus, and in the cervical nucleus. This specific constitution renders the length of the cisternal segment of the spinal nerve highly varied, yet invariably extensive. The accessory nerve comprises the cisternal segment, which includes the cervical and cerebellopontine angle parts, along with two additional segments: one associated with the jugular foramen and the other extracranial.

10.11.2 Clinical, Diagnostic, and Treatment Considerations

Schwannomas of the accessory nerve are rare tumors; however, isolated cases are infrequently observed despite their mostly motor function. A recent comprehensive assessment of the literature identified only 62 documented cases, complicating the ability to formulate diagnostic judgments and therapeutic recommendations due to the shortness of the series [22]. The mean age of onset is the fourth decade, with a little higher prevalence in women compared to males. Based on their growth patterns along the nerve and imaging study results, tumors are categorized into four classifications: type 1, intradural tumors located in the cisternal segment; type 2, tumors primarily situated in the jugular foramen; type 3, intraspinal tumors positioned in the initial segments of the cervical spine; and type 4, extracranial tumors. The literature indicates the following tumor distribution: type 1, 50%; type 2, 30%; type 3, 5%; and type 4, 15%. Tumors of the first and second groups proliferate in the cerebellopontine angle, while type 3 also undergoes microneurosurgical intervention via an approach to the skull base and cervical spine. Clinically, accessory nerve involvement is observed in a limited number of patients at the time of diagnosis. Injury to the accessory nerve is characterized by the paralysis of the sternocleidomastoid and trapezius muscles, resulting in impaired neck rotation and shoulder elevation, accompanied by notable muscular atrophy. The most common symptoms that result in diagnosis are headache, neck pain, or shoulder pain. Furthermore, each topography has a distinct and unique clinical condition. Cisternal tumors present with headaches and symptoms associated with the involvement of lower cranial nerves, including the hypoglossal nerve, as well as compression of the brainstem and cerebellum. Neoplasms of the jugular foramen induce a characteristic jugular foramen syndrome, accompanied or unaccompanied by symptoms associated with brainstem or cerebellar involvement. Cervical segment tumors manifest as discomfort and muscle contraction due to irritation of the cervical spinal nerve roots and dura mater, potentially leading to tetraparesis. Ultimately, tumors in the extracranial region manifest as latero-cervical masses characterized by slow growth, non-pulsatility, mobility, and varying degrees of tenderness upon palpation, with minimal muscular involvement. These tumors are often misidentified as cervical lymph nodes and are excised, leading to transection of the accessory nerve. The imaging diagnosis is established with MRI, which reveals all the diagnostic features of the schwannomas previously described. The jugular foramen may also host other very prevalent tumors, including meningiomas and, primarily, chemodectomas situated in the glomus of the jugular vein, necessitating differential diagnosis as previously discussed. In tiny brain tumors, the proximity of the tumor to the nerve fibers along their cisternal pathway is evident in significantly increased T2 imaging tests (FIESTA).

In all cases of cerebellopontine angle accessory schwannomas, surgical intervention is unequivocally advised for large, symptomatic tumors or those exhibiting growth in imaging examinations. The aim of the procedure is the total excision of the lesion while ensuring the anatomical and functional integrity of the accessory nerve. The complete excision of the tumor depends upon its size and is accomplished in the majority of instances. In a few instances, resection may be partial, necessitating imaging follow-up to detect potential recurrences, despite the low incidence. Following microneurosurgical tumor removal, an increase in cranial nerve deficit symptoms is typically observed; nevertheless, in certain instances, there may be a worsening of one or more lower cranial nerves. An alternative to microneurosurgical intervention would be stereotactic radiosurgery. Minor or asymptomatic lesions may be monitored through imaging and treated upon growth or the onset of symptoms. Ultimately, large tumors causing brainstem compression or affecting other cranial nerves necessitate microneurosurgical removal; if resection is inadequate, stereotactic radiosurgery should be employed for the remnants, or the residuals monitored via imaging. The methodology for microneurosurgical intervention of accessory schwannomas depends upon the tumor's location. Type 1 tumors situated intracranially with or without extension into the jugular foramen may be excised via a retrosigmoid technique. For foraminal tumors, an infralabyrinthine retro and presigmoid approach, continued in a cervical direction, is required to gain access to the jugular vein caudally, the bulb of the jugular vein cranially, and the sigmoid sinus externally. The tumor can be excised from its extracranial segment, within the foramen, and from any intracranial extension. A far-lateral approach to the foramen magnum without condylectomy is recommended for cervical segment tumors, in conjunction with an osteoplastic cervical laminectomy at specific levels, determined by the tumor's caudal extent. Ultimately, pure extracranial tumors are excised using a high latero-cervical approach, eliminating the necessity for bone resection.

10.12 Schwannomas of the Hypoglossal Nerve

10.12.1 Anatomical Considerations

The twelfth cranial nerve, or hypoglossal nerve, is constituted by multiple branches that arise from the anterolateral or preolivary sulcus of the medulla oblongata, situated between the pyramid and the inferior olive. These branches converge to create one or two distinct fascicles before exiting the intracranial cavity via the anterior condylar foramen or hypoglossal canal (Fig. 10.1). The occipital condyles are situated in the anterolateral region of the occipital foramen magnum's rim, possess an oval morphology measuring approximately 24 mm, and are orientated anteriorly and medially, making a 45° angle relative to the sagittal plane. The occipital condyle is traversed by the anterior condylar foramen, or hypoglossal canal, which extends anteriorly and laterally, producing an approximate 45° angle with the sagittal plane. Consequently, at its intracranial beginning, the hypoglossal canal is situated at the intersection of the posterior third and the anterior two-thirds of the condyle, and at its extracranial terminus, it is positioned at the junction of the posterior two-thirds and the anterior third. The hypoglossal canal has a measurement range of 18–24 mm. The hypoglossal canal accommodates the hypoglossal nerve, a meningeal arterial branch arising from the ascending pharyngeal artery, and a venous plexus. A depression on the rear aspect of the condyle houses the posterior condylar foramen, through which the condylar emissary vein traverses, linking the vertebral venous plexus to the sigmoid sinus. The nerve transmits motor fibers from the hypoglossal nucleus in the medulla oblongata to the majority of the tongue muscles. The cisternal section of the hypoglossal nerve is brief until the hypoglossal canal. The Obersteiner–Redlich transitional zone of the hypoglossal nerve is situated within the medulla oblongata, with the entry zone measuring less than 0.1 mm. Besides the cisternal segment, the hypoglossal nerve comprises two more anatomical segments [15]. The foraminal section traverses the hypoglossal canal, whereupon the nerve is enveloped with epineurium. Subsequently, in the extracranial section, the nerve detaches from its association with the base of the skull and forms new connections with the lower cranial nerves, namely the glossopharyngeal and vagal nerves.

10.12.2 Clinical, Diagnostic, and Treatment Considerations

Hypoglossal nerve schwannomas are uncommon tumors; however, they may be encountered despite the nerve's exclusive motor function. Hypoglossal schwannomas constitute around 1% of intracranial schwannomas. A recent systematic assessment of the literature identified merely 160 documented cases, including neurofibromas, complicating the ability to formulate diagnostic findings and therapeutic recommendations due to the brevity of the series [12]. The average age of presentation is in the fourth decade, with a little predominance in women compared to men. Based on their progression along the hypoglossal nerve and imaging study results, tumors are categorized into four groups: type 1, solely intradural tumors; type 2, intra-extradural or hourglass tumors; type 3, extracranial tumors impacting the base of the skull; and type 4, extracranial tumors devoid of bone involvement at the base of the skull. The literature indicates the following tumor distribution: type 1, 30%; type 2, 40%; type 3, 5%; and type 4, 25%. Only the initial two groups proliferate at the cerebellopontine angle, but individuals in the third group also have microneurosurgical intervention via an approach to the skull base.

The hypoglossal nerve is involved in nearly all patients at the time of diagnosis. Acute injury to the hypoglossal nerve is characterized by fast atrophy of the ipsilateral half of the tongue and resultant difficulties in swallowing, chewing, and articulating words. Nevertheless, when the involvement is subtle and chronic, these signs and symptoms remain undetected for an extended period. Consequently, numerous individuals receive incidental diagnoses during dental or otorhinolaryngological (ENT) evaluations for unrelated intercurrent conditions. Conversely, certain patients undergo prolonged examination for neurodegenerative illnesses until an imaging investigation is conducted. It is believed that the retention of a limited number of undamaged nerve fibers may be enough to sustain proper tongue functionality. This indicates that, at the time of diagnosis, tumors are sizable and identified by neurological symptoms that are more significant to the patient, particularly those resulting from the involvement of lower cranial nerves, the brainstem, or the cerebellum. A common symptom is headache, typically nuchal or occipital in nature. In instances of hydrocephalus resulting from brainstem compression, the characteristic symptoms and indicators of intracranial hypertension manifest. Each tumor type may exhibit specific characteristics in its clinical presentation. Extracranial tumors without bone involvement at the base of the skull may manifest as cervical lumps that vary in tenderness upon touch, and tongue atrophy is comparatively rare. The diagnosis is established using MRI imaging, which reveals all the diagnostic features of the schwannomas previously reported (Fig. 10.6a, b). A pathognomonic indicator of hypoglossal schwannoma is the enlargement of the hypoglossal canal shown in bone studies with thin-section CT, albeit this is only evident in tumors that develop entirely or partially within the canalicular segment of the nerve (Fig. 10.6c).

Consensus exists about the surgical intervention for big, symptomatic cerebellopontine angle schwannomas or those exhibiting growth in imaging studies. The aim of the surgery is the total excision of the lesion while preserving the anatomical and functional integrity of the hypoglossal nerve. The complete excision of the tumor depends upon its size and is accomplished in 80% of cases. In many instances, excision is incomplete owing to size, technical challenges, or the intent to anatomically maintain the hypoglossal nerve. In such patients, imaging surveillance is essential to detect any recurrences. Concerning the neurological function of the

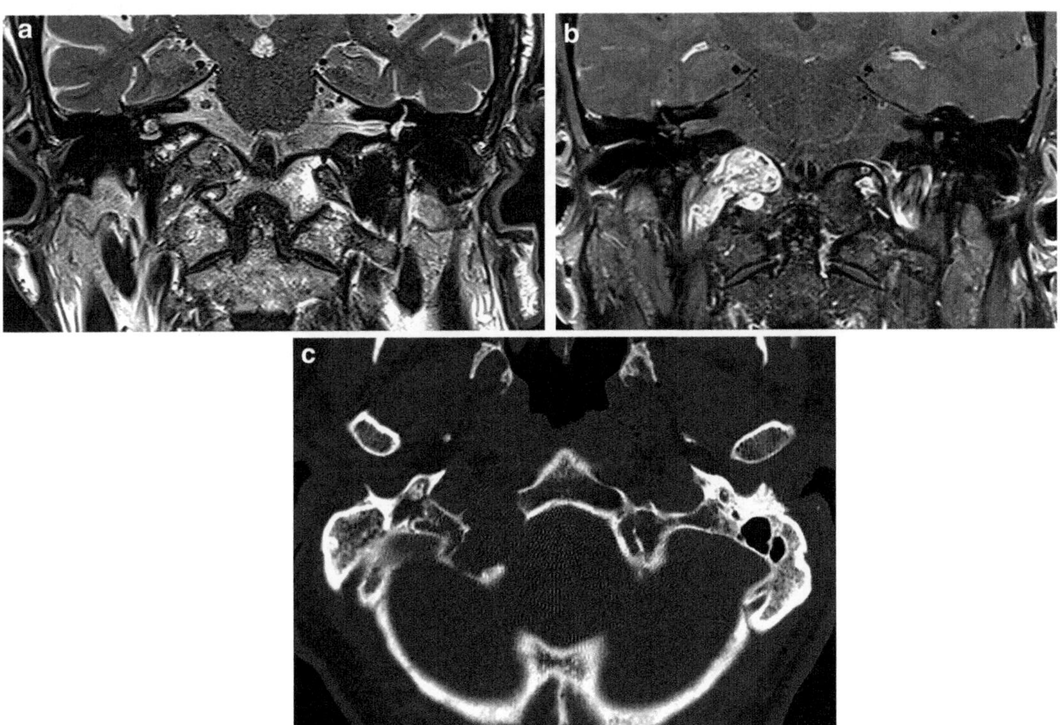

Fig. 10.6 Medium-sized type 2 schwannoma of the right hypoglossal nerve. (**a-b**) Coronal MRI sections weighted in T2 and T1 with gadolinium reveal a lesion partially involving the occipital condyle, characterized by a globular intracranial extension and a more linear extracranial extension. (**c**) An axial CT scan without contrast reveals destruction of the occipital bone near the foramen magnum

hypoglossal nerve, achieving improvement is challenging due to the typically apparent tongue atrophy at the time of diagnosis. Patients exhibiting partial functional impairment of the nerve during surgery typically experience deterioration post-resection, and it is not uncommon to develop new, often transitory, deficiencies in other cranial nerves, particularly the ninth and tenth. When proximal and distal stumps of the hypoglossal nerve can be acquired post-tumor excision and there is no significant atrophy of the tongue, an end-to-end anastomosis may be conducted, typically with an interposed saphenous nerve graft. This nerve graft has a diameter comparable to that of the hypoglossal nerve, and suturing is feasible if the proximal end of the hypoglossal nerve has already consolidated into a single fascicle, beyond the rootlets that constitute it at its exit from the medulla oblongata. An alternative to microneurosurgical intervention is stereotactic radiosurgery, which demands similar considerations as those for other non-vestibular cerebellopontine angle schwannomas. The extreme rarity of the lesion renders its preoperative diagnosis ambiguous, and the indication for stereotactic radiosurgery poses significant risks. Minor or asymptomatic lesions may be monitored through imaging and treated upon growth or the onset of symptoms. Ultimately, large tumors that compress the brain stem or affect other cranial nerves necessitate microneurosurgical excision, and if resection is insufficient, remnants should be followed by stereotactic radiosurgery or monitored with imaging. The microneurosurgical management of hypoglossal schwannomas is presently highly secure due to the implementation of the far-lateral approach since the 1980s, which has significantly diminished postoperative morbidity and mortality. Type 1 tumors that do not extend into the hypoglossal canal and are restricted to the cerebellopontine angle can be excised with a conventional retrosigmoid technique. When the tumor infiltrates the hypoglossal canal, as seen in types 2, 3, and 4, a far-lateral approach is suitable for accessing the tumor via a partial condylectomy and drilling of the posterior aspect of the condyle and the hypoglossal canal, along with resection of both the intracranial and extracranial segments (Fig. 10.7). A large drilling of the condyle can jeopardize occipito-cervical stability, demanding some form of instrumented stabilization. Ultimately, type 5 tumors are entirely extracranial and are excised using a high latero-cervical approach, eliminating the necessity for bone excision.

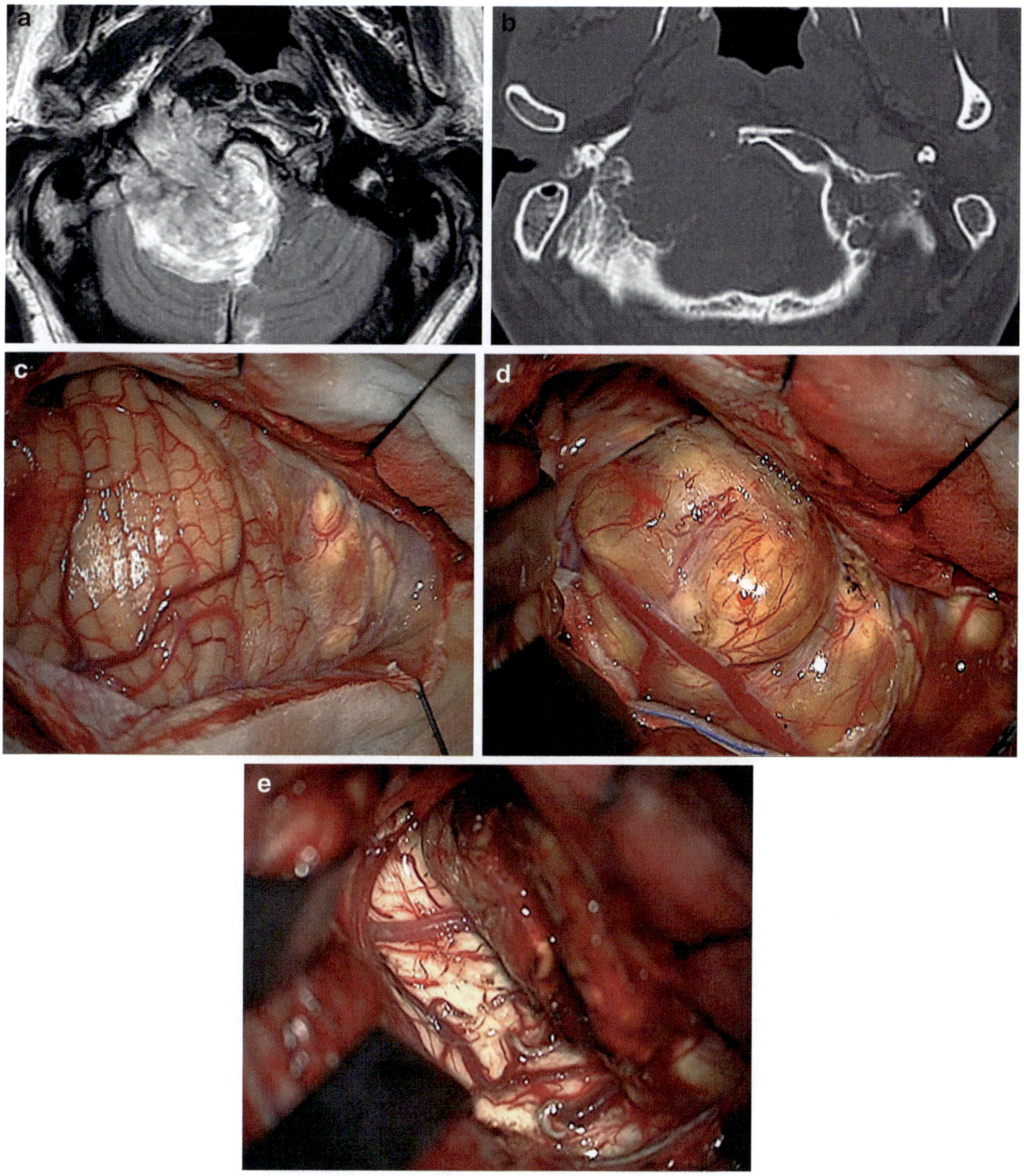

Fig. 10.7 Type 2 schwannoma of the right hypoglossal nerve. (**a**) An axial T2-weighted MRI reveals a huge lesion at the base of the skull and in the cerebellopontine angle, displacing the cerebellar hemisphere and medulla oblongata with extracranial extension. (**b**) Axial CT slice demonstrating extensive osseous destruction. (**c**–**e**) Intraoperative pictures displaying the far-lateral approach to the lesion, its exposure, and the final result following the excision of the intracranial segment of the tumor

10.13 Schwannomas of the Sympathetic Plexus of the Petrosal Internal Carotid Artery

Petrosal apex schwannomas are rare tumors [7, 18]. Schwannomas situated near the petrosal apex may originate from the abducens nerve, trigeminal nerve, greater superficial petrosal nerve, or sympathetic fibers of the internal carotid artery surrounding the petrosal portion of the internal carotid artery [18]. Only a limited number of schwannomas originating from the sympathetic internal petrosal carotid artery fibres have been documented. The cervical sympathetic plexus originates from the internal carotid nerve, a direct extension of the superior cervical ganglion. The internal carotid nerve ascends alongside the internal carotid artery, producing a lateral branch that forms the internal carotid plexus and a medial branch that generates the cavernous plexus. The internal carotid plexus connects with the tympanic plexus and, via the deep petrosal nerve, to the sphenopalatine ganglion, providing sympathetic innervation to several facial mucosal glands, including the lacrimal and parotid glands. The internal carotid plexus supplies fibers to the third, fourth, fifth, and sixth cranial nerves, as well as the ciliary ganglion.

Clinically, these rare tumors manifest with diplopia resulting from abducens nerve dysfunction, hearing loss, and, in rare cases, headache, atypical facial pain, and autonomic abnormalities. MRI diagnosis reveals no distinctive abnormalities, except for the position at the petrous apex and, notably, the displacement of the petrosal segment of the internal carotid artery (Fig. 10.8a, b). The surgical approach to the tumor is consistently supratentorial, accessing the lesion by a middle fossa extradural approach to the Kawase triangle. The tumor must be removed meticulously, given its proximity to the wall of the internal carotid artery, which may be compromised during resection (Fig. 10.8c, d). Alternative treatments include imaging observation or stereotactic radiosurgery; nevertheless, because of the limited number of cases, it is impossible to give recommendations.

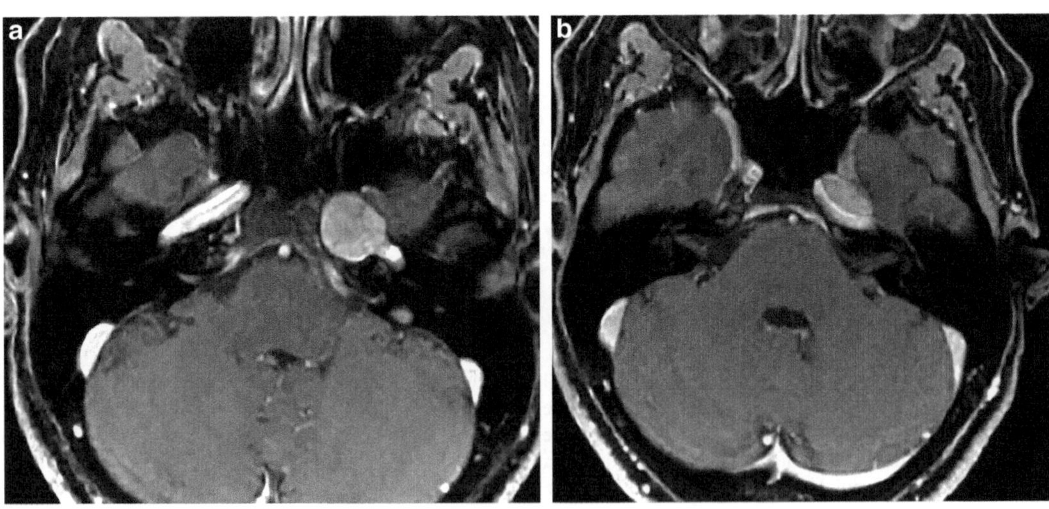

Fig. 10.8 Schwannoma of the sympathetic internal carotid artery nerve. (**a**, **b**) Axial T1-enhanced MRI slices post-gadolinium administration, illustrating the tumor and the displacement of the petrosal internal carotid artery. (**c**) Intraoperative picture displaying the extradural approach to the middle fossa targeting the Kawase triangle, illustrating the tumor before excision (from above to below: internal carotid artery, SGPN, V3, and V2 branches of the trigeminal nerve). (**d**) Image displaying the operative field after tumor excision

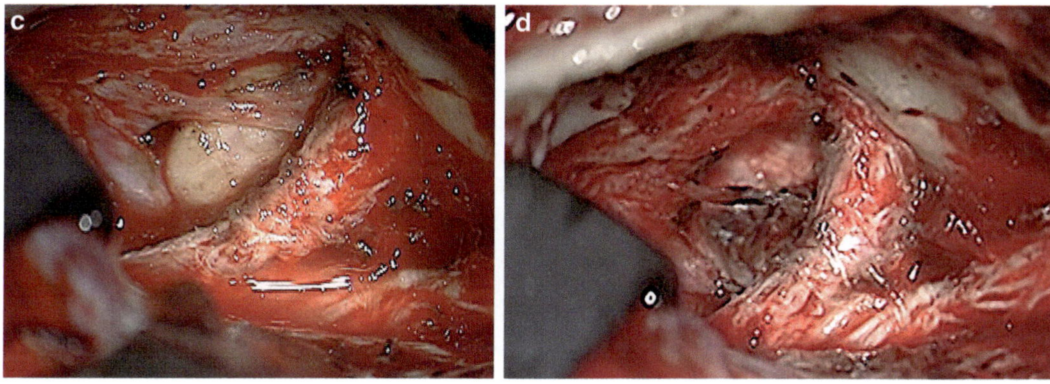

Fig. 10.8 (continued)

10.14 Key Messages

- *Schwannomas can develop in any cranial nerve, predominantly in sensory nerves, despite the absence of a discernible pattern in their relative frequency.*
- *Cranial nerve schwannomas may arise in the cisternal segment of the nerve and disseminate through the skull base foramina to multiple extracranial regions.*
- *Aside from topography and the extracranial development pattern, diagnostic imaging lacks distinctive features that would enable a definitive diagnosis of schwannoma in a particular cranial nerve.*
- *Preoperative diagnosis by imaging techniques is unreliable due to its rarity; hence, therapy is generally microneurosurgical, rendering stereotactic radiosurgery or surveillance potentially hazardous.*
- *The prognosis after removal is generally favorable; nonetheless, there is a considerable risk that complete excision may lead to the nerve's loss of functionality.*
- *Subtotal excision and postoperative imaging surveillance or stereotactic radiosurgery are recommended to maintain the neurological function of the nerve.*

References

1. Bambakidis N, Megerian CA, Spetzler RF, editors. Surgery of the cerebellopontine angle. Cham: Springer Nature; 2028.
2. Celli P, Ferrante L, Acqui M, et al. Neurinoma of the third, fourth, and sixth cranial nerves: a survey and report of a new fourth nerve case. Surg Neurol. 1992;38:216–24. https://doi.org/10.1016/0090-3019(92)90172-j.
3. Constanzo F, Teixeira BCA, Sens P, et al. Cerebellopontine angle schwannomas arising from the intermediate nerve: a scoping review. Neurosurg Rev. 2020;43:1431–41. https://doi.org/10.1007/s10143-019-01173-6.
4. Douglas VP, Flores C, Douglas KA, et al. Oculomotor nerve schwannoma: case series and literature review. Surv Ophthalmol. 2022;67:1160–74. https://doi.org/10.1016/j.survophthal.2021.11.008.
5. Frisch CD, Eckel LJ, Lane JI, et al. Intralabyrinthine schwannomas. Otolaryngol Clin N Am. 2015;48:423–41. https://doi.org/10.1016/j.otc.2015.02.004.
6. Gazzeri R, Galarza M, Costanzo de B, et al. Large pure intracranial vagal schwannoma. J Clin Neurosci. 2009;16:565–7. https://doi.org/10.1016/j.jocn.2008.05.008.
7. Goudihalli SR, Goto T, Bohoun C, et al. Sympathetic plexus schwannoma of carotid canal: 2 cases with surgical technique and review of literature. World Neurosurg. 2028;118:63–8. https://doi.org/10.1016/j.wneu.2018.06.244.
8. Guclu B, Sindou M, Meyronet D, et al. Cranial nerve vascular compression syndromes of the trigeminal, facial, and vagus-glossopharyngeal nerves: comparative anatomical study of the central myelin portion

and transitional zone; correlations with incidences of corresponding hyperactive dysfunctional syndromes. Acta Neurochir. 2011;153:2365–75. https://doi.org/10.1007/s00701-011-1168-1.
9. MacNally SP, Rutherford SA, Ramsden RT, et al. Trigeminal schwannomas. Br J Neurosurg. 2008;22:729–38. https://doi.org/10.1080/02688690802272172.
10. Nakamizo A, Matsuo S, Amano T. Abducens nerve schwannoma: a case report and literature review. World Neurosurg. 2019;125:49–54. https://doi.org/10.1016/j.wneu.2019.01.123.
11. Neff BA, Willcox TO Jr, Sataloff RT. Intralabyrinthine schwannomas. Otol Neurotol. 2003;24:299–307. https://doi.org/10.1097/00129492-200303000-00028.
12. Nonaka Y, Grossi PM, Bulsara KR, et al. Microsurgical management of hypoglossal schwannomas over 3 decades: a modified grading scale to guide surgical approach. Neurosurgery. 2011;69(Suppl Operative 2):ons121–40. https://doi.org/10.1227/NEU.0b013e31822a547b.
13. Ozoner B, Gungor A, Ture H, et al. Surgical treatment of trochlear nerve Schwannomas: case series and systematic review. World Neurosurg. 2022;162:e288–300. https://doi.org/10.1016/j.wneu.2022.03.006.
14. Pamir MN, Peker S, Bayrakli F, et al. Surgical treatment of trigeminal schwannomas. Neurosurg Rev. 2007;30:329–37. https://doi.org/10.1007/s10143-007-0093-5.
15. Rhoton AL Jr. The cerebellopontine angle and posterior fossa cranial nerves by the retrosigmoid approach. Neurosurgery. 2000;47(Suppl 3):S1–S297. https://doi.org/10.1097/00006123-200009001-00013.
16. Rotter J, Lu VM, Graffeo CS, et al. Surgery versus radiosurgery for facial nerve schwannoma: a systematic review and meta-analysis of facial nerve function, postoperative complications, and progression. J Neurosurg. 2020;135:542–53. https://doi.org/10.3171/2020.6.JNS201548.
17. Samii M, Gerganov V. Surgery of cerebellopontine angle lesions. Berlin-Heidelberg: Springer; 2013.
18. Takase H, Araki K, Seki S, et al. Unique diagnostic features and surgical strategy for intracranial carotid sympathetic plexus schwannoma: case report and literature review. World Neurosurg. 2017;98:876.e1–8. https://doi.org/10.1016/j.wneu.2016.11.105.
19. Tubbs RS, Veith P, Griessenauer CJ, et al. A new segment of the trochlear nerve: a cadaveric study with application to skull base surgery. J Neurol Surg B Skull Base. 2014;75:8–10. https://doi.org/10.1055/s-0033-1349787.
20. Vorasubin N, Sang UH, Mafee M, et al. Glossopharyngeal schwannomas: a 100-year review. Laryngoscope. 2009;119:26–35. https://doi.org/10.1002/lary.20045.
21. Xu F, Pan S, Alonso F, et al. Intracranial facial nerve schwannomas: current management and review of literature. World Neurosurg. 2017;100:444–9. https://doi.org/10.1016/j.wneu.2016.09.082.
22. Yan P, Wang P. Accessory nerve schwannoma: a new case report and systematic review. Interdiscip Neurosurg. 2020;19:100571. https://doi.org/10.1016/j.inat.2019.100571.
23. Yang SH, Park H, Yoo DS, et al. Microsurgical anatomy of the facial nerve. Clin Anat. 2021;34:90–102. https://doi.org/10.1002/ca.23652.

11 Meningioma

11.1 Introduction

Meningiomas are the third most prevalent form of intracranial tumor, following gliomas and metastases, and they account for approximately 20% of patients in surgical series. Meningiomas of the skull base account for approximately 50% of surgical cases, while those of the posterior fossa account for approximately 10% of all meningiomas. Nearly 50% of these are situated in the cerebellopontine angle, 40% in the tentorial or convexity aspect of the cerebellum, and less frequently in other locations. Nevertheless, the distribution of meningiomas of the posterior fossa is highly variable in the series as a result of the significant disparities in the classifications, which are typically topographical.

11.1.1 Classification of Meningiomas of the Cerebellopontine Angle

Intracranial meningiomas are classified according to the location of their implantation in the dura mater, despite the fact that they are derived from leptomeningeal cells rather than the dura mater. In an anatomical context, the cerebellopontine angle is a dihedral angle, with a medial plane formed by the brain stem, middle cerebellar peduncle, and petrosal surface of the cerebellum, and a lateral plane formed by the posterior surface of the petrosal bone. These planes converge toward the petroclival junction, the deepest portion of the cerebellopontine angle. In an anatomical condition, the cerebellopontine angle is extremely acute, almost a virtual space. It is occupied by the cerebellopontine angle cisterns, which are filled with cerebrospinal fluid (CSF). The cranial nerves traverse the angle on their cisternal journey from the brainstem to the foramina, where they cross the skull base. The arterial and venous vessels of the posterior circulation also traverse the cerebellopontine angle.

The cerebellopontine angle is enlarged and transformed into a significantly larger space by the retrosigmoid approach. The cerebellopontine angle is now characterized by an inverted truncated pyramid with a cranial base that is wider than the caudal base. Both bases have wide foramina for communication with the supratentorial and spine spaces (tentorial foramen and foramen magnum, respectively). The cerebellopontine angle has three sides: the medial side, which corresponds to the brain stem and cerebellum; the lateral side, which corresponds to the petrosal and mastoid portions of the temporal bone and the jugular part of the occipital bone; and the posterior side, which corresponds to the squama of the occipital bone. The dura mater covers the entire internal surface of the cerebellopontine angle, except for its medial aspect, which is why it can be the location of meningiomas. Conversely, the cerebellopontine angle is traversed by cranial nerves that pass through specific anatomical

J. M. González-Darder, *Microneurosurgery of Cerebellopontine Angle*,
https://doi.org/10.1007/978-3-032-03091-7_11

points, from their origin in the brain stem to the bony holes at the base of the skull that facilitate their exit to the extracranial space. The classification of cerebellopontine angle meningiomas is determined by these two elements: the anatomical points from which meningiomas develop and the cranial nerves of the posterior fossa that define the clinical expression, microneurosurgical strategy, and patient's morbidity.

In this regard, various classifications have been proposed, some of which are exceedingly restrictive, such as Samii's, which restricts the meningiomas of the cerebellopontine angle to those that settle on the posterior surface of the petrosal bone. Those that do so medially to the trigeminal nerve are classified as petroclival meningiomas. In his classification, meningiomas of the cerebellopontine angle are further subdivided into several subtypes based on their relationships with the internal acoustic meatus: meatal, which is centered on the internal acoustic meatus; premeatal, which is anterior to the meatus and extends to the trigeminal nerve; retromeatal, which originates behind the meatus and extends to the sigmoid sinus; suprameatal, which is above the meatus and extends to the tentorium; and inframeatal, which is located below the meatus and extends to the jugular foramen. This classification takes into account the potential for meningiomas to extend to the internal auditory canal, jugular foramen, Meckel's cave, supratentorial, medial, contralateral, or toward the foramen magnum [1].

Our proposed classification of cerebellopontine angle meningiomas is predicated on the selection of tumors that can be exposed and resected using the retrosigmoid and far-lateral approaches. This classification encompasses, in addition to those that are strictly associated with the cerebellopontine angle, other neighboring tumors that are accessible through those surgical approach. Therefore, the subsequent categories may be taken into account:

- Meningiomas of the convexity of the cerebellum or of the squama of the occipital bone. These are meningiomas that are implanted in the dura mater of the most lateral portion of the internal aspect of the occipital bone squama. They have the potential to extend to the sigmoid sinus in its most lateral portion and to the transverse sinus in its most cranial portion.
- Petrosal meningiomas. They are recognized as genuine meningiomas of the cerebellopontine angle, as they are developing from the dura mater of the posterior aspect of the petrosal bone. The following are divided into four locations:
  - Posterior petrosal meningiomas are located behind the internal acoustic meatus and are therefore found before the facial and vestibulocochlear cranial nerves in the standard retrosigmoid approach. They may be related to the sigmoid sinus in their most posterior portion.
  - Anterior petrosal meningiomas, which are situated in front of the internal acoustic meatus and may extend to the trigeminal nerve, are situated behind the facial and vestibulocochlear cranial nerves in the standard retrosigmoid approach.
  - Petrosal meningiomas of the internal auditory canal that develop in close proximity to the internal acoustic meatus or canal.
  - Petrosal meningiomas of the jugular foramen, which extend from the internal auditory meatus to the foramen magnum.
- Petroclival meningiomas. They originate from the dura mater of the upper two-thirds of the clivus and the petroclival junction, and as a result, they are located medial to the trigeminal nerve, or behind the nerve in the conventional retrosigmoid approach.
- Meningiomas of the foramen magnum. They are expanding in the dura mater that encompasses the caudal third of the clivus and the border of the foramen magnum.
- Meningiomas of the tentorium, which are initiated in the tentorium and are classified into two primary subtypes:
  - Meningiomas of the incisura, which are situated on the free margin of the tentorial meatus.
  - Meningiomas of the tentorium, which are situated on the caudal side of the tentorium surface.

- Extensions. Meningiomas of any topography may exhibit intraosseous extension, occupy the internal auditory canal, jugular foramen, or Meckel's cave, or expand toward the supratentorial space or spinal canal, either medially or contralaterally.

In the last 50 patients that we have operated on and used to select the figures and illustrative cases in this book, 10% of the meningiomas are of the convexity of the cerebellum, 50% are petrosal or of the cerebellopontine angle itself, 25% are petroclival, 10% are of the foramen magnum, and the remaining 5% are tentorial, according to the classification described. Although meningiomas that are centered on the internal acoustic meatus and the jugular foramen have been anecdotal, a certain number of cases have resulted in the meningioma reaching, entering, or growing within any of these orifices.

From a neurosurgical perspective, an alternative method of classifying cerebellopontine angle meningiomas is to consider their relationships with the cranial nerves in the retrosigmoid approach. In general, there are tumors that are situated before the seventh and eighth cranial nerves when approached, such as meningiomas of the convexity of the cerebellum and posterior petrosal. Alternatively, there are tumors that are situated behind these cranial nerves in the retrosigmoid approach, such as the anterior petrosal meningiomas, and others that are also anterior to the fifth nerve, such as the petroclival meningioma. Some tumors grow directly in relation to these cranial nerves, such as those of the internal acoustic canal and jugular foramen. Finally, there are tumors that have variable relationships with the lower cranial nerves, such as meningiomas of the foramen magnum. Lastly, there are other meningiomas that have a very anecdotal relationship with the cranial nerves, such as those of the tentorium or cerebellar convexity.

Despite the benefits of these classifications that are centered on the standard retrosigmoid approach, it is evident that certain large meningiomas or those situated at the limits of the cerebellopontine angle may benefit from extended approaches, such as the far lateral approach, combined approaches, such as the retro-presigmoid approach, or specific supratentorial or trans-petrosal approaches. These aspects will also be taken into account in this chapter when determining the most appropriate approach for each distinct type of meningioma.

11.2 Anatomical Considerations

The internal auditory and jugular foramina are prominently visible on the posteromedial surface of the petrosal and mastoid portions of the temporal bone, which is covered by the dura mater. This is the lateral surface of the cerebellopontine angle. The meatus and internal auditory canal, which are the entry points for the facial and vestibulocochlear nerves, are the most critical surgical components of this wall. The internal auditory meatus is a pertinent anatomical point because it is necessary to remove the posterior surface of the meatus and the internal auditory canal to access the contents of the internal auditory canal (*transmeatal access*). The posterior semicircular canal is situated laterally, and pneumatized petrosal cells may be present at the posterior margin of the canal. The subarcuate eminence is situated immediately above the meatus, while the endolymphatic duct is situated inferolateral to the meatus. Lastly, the jugular bulb may contact the posterior border of the meatus if it is elevated abnormally. The dura mater completely covers the internal surface of the internal auditory canal, and the arachnoid extends into the canal in a manner reminiscent of a glove finger. The suprameatal tubercle, which extends from the upper border of the meatus to the tentorium, is located above the acoustic meatus. When the distal trigeminal nerve root is obstructed by this suprameatal tubercle, it must be resected (*suprameatal access*).

The jugular foramen, also known as the posterior lacerum foramen, is a space located at the base of the skull between the temporal and occipital bones. It is situated approximately 5 mm below the internal auditory meatus, 5 mm above the hypoglossal canal, and 8 mm lateral to the jugular tubercle. The sigmoid sinus, jugular bulb, inferior petrosal sinus, and lower cranial nerves with the glossopharyngeal, vagal, and accessory nerves, as well as other anatomical elements of minor relevance, such as the Arnold or Jacobson nerves, the cochlear aqueduct, and some small arterial branches, all traverse the jugular foramen. Nevertheless, the dura mater obscures the majority of the foramen when the cerebellopontine angle is approached through the retrosigmoid approach, revealing only the cranial nerves' entrance. The inferior petrosal sinus is located in the anteromedial or petrosal compartment of the jugular foramen, which is divided into two compartments by dural bands. The sigmoid sinus is located in the posterolateral or sigmoid compartment. The neural compartment, which is situated between the two compartments, is divided into two sections: one section is dedicated to the glossopharyngeal nerve, and the other is dedicated to the vagal and accessory nerves. The dura mater also encompasses all other anatomical components of the lateral surface of the cerebellopontine angle. The sigmoid sinus is situated in a fissure that leads to the jugular foramen. The endolymphatic sac is situated between the layers of the dura mater, occupying the region inferolateral to the internal auditory meatus and extending toward the sigmoid sinus. The endolymphatic sac communicates with the vestibule of the inner ear via the endolymphatic duct. Lastly, the subarcuate fossa is situated lateral to the meatus, where the small subarcuate artery enters.

The dura mater covers the occipital bone that surrounds the foramen magnum, which forms the floor of the cerebellopontine angle. The most anterior portion is the clivus, while the jugular tubercle, a bony prominence that is continuous more laterally with the squamous portion of the occipital bone, is located laterally. The jugular tubercle is situated between the hypoglossal canal caudally and the jugular foramen cranially. The inner, endocranial, or concave surface of the occipital squama is characterized by a midline internal occipital protuberance, which is followed by a medial internal occipital crest that extends toward the foramen magnum. The internal crest forms the lateral borders of the foramen magnum by dividing into two powerful branches before the foramen magnum. The transverse sinuses are housed within the internal occipital protuberance, which is connected to the sigmoid sinus by two broad canals that are grooved into the bone. These canals extend laterally toward the jugular foramen. The internal occipital protuberance, also known as the cruciform eminence, is formed at the intersection of the grooves for the sagittal sinus, the lateral sinuses, and the internal occipital crest. It is anatomically equivalent to the press of Herophilus or torcula and is situated approximately 1 cm below the root of the external occipital protuberance. Cerebellar fossae are broad, concave depressions that are located on each side of the occipital bone, beneath the canals, and beyond the internal crest. The occipital condyles are ovoid in shape and approximately 24 mm in size. They are situated in the anterolateral portion of the rim of the occipital foramen magnum and are oriented medially and forwards at a 45° angle to the sagittal plane. The anterior condylar foramen, or hypoglossal canal, traverses the occipital condyle in a forward and outward trajectory, at an angle of approximately 45° with the sagittal plane. Consequently, the hypoglossal canal is situated at the junction of the posterior third and the anterior two-thirds of the condyle at its intracranial origin and at the junction of the posterior two-thirds and the anterior third at its extracranial end. The hypoglossal canal is approximately 18–24 mm in length. The hypoglossal canal is the site of the hypoglossal nerve, a meningeal arterial branch from the ascending pharyngeal artery, and a venous plexus. The bony border of the foramen magnum is situated above the occipital condyle. The clivus is the most anterior part of the foramen magnum, and the jugular tubercle, a bony prominence that continues laterally with the squamous portion of the occipital bone, is located laterally. The jugular tubercle is situated between the hypoglossal canal and the jugular foramen, as previously mentioned. The posterior condylar foramen is situated in a depression on the posterior part of the condyle. This foramen is the conduit for the condylar emissary vein, which connects the vertebral venous plexus to the sigmoid sinus.

The inferior or caudal surface of the tentorium corresponds to the roof of the cerebellopontine angle. The walls of the superior petrosal sinus are formed by the anterolateral portion of the tentorium, which is inserted into the upper border of the petrosal bone. The lateral part of the tentorial or Pacchioni foramen is formed by the most anterior and medial portions, which are free. The tentorium border is related to the ambiens cistern and, more posteriorly, to the quadrigeminal cistern. The cerebellopontine angle's deepest portion is narrow and corresponds to the petroclival fissure, which is covered by dura mater and marks the boundary between the sphenoidal clivus and the temporal bone. This fissure extends from the jugular foramen caudally to the apex of the petrosal bone cranially [2–4].

11.3 Pathology

Meningiomas are tumors that arise from clusters of leptomeningeal cells in the parietal arachnoid layer. Their limit is evident and typically exhibits nodular or globular growth and lacks a capsule. They have the potential to expand by invading the fibrous layers that comprise the dura mater and, as a result, the underlying bone. However, bone invasion is exceedingly uncommon in cerebellopontine angle meningiomas, as is hyperostosis or en-plaque growth. The tumor's edges may extend as it develops into or on the surface of the meningeal lining, resulting in the distinctive *dural tail* observed in imaging studies. The meningioma respects the visceral arachnoid as it develops, thereby enabling the preservation of a virtual space between the tumor and the pia mater that envelops the nervous tissue or neurovascular elements, which is referred to as the *cleavage plane*. This space enables the safe microneurosurgical dissection of the tumor. The tumor may only very rarely invade the arachnoid and the pia mater, thereby penetrating the nervous tissue. This is a common occurrence in high-grade meningiomas, exceptional in meningiomas that are located at the base of the skull and, as a result, in the cerebellopontine angle. The presence of two or more independent lesions at the time of diagnosis or during follow-up is a specific form of presentation of meningiomas (*meningiomatosis*). This occurs in the absence of other diseases that induce the development of multiple tumors of distinct histological origin [5, 6].

11.3.1 Molecular Biology

Meningioma is a usually benign and slow-growing tumor that accumulates a large number of genetic abnormalities, which multiplicate when it is malignant. However, the presence of these genetic abnormalities is not characteristic of the different histological types of meningioma or the degree of malignancy. The most frequent and characteristic chromosomal alteration of meningioma is monosomy 22 and allelic losses in the 22q12.2 region, a region ofchromosome 22 where the *NF2* gene that encodes the merlin protein, which is a tumor suppressor, is located. This loss of the *NF2* gene is characteristic of neurofibromatosis type 2, and, in fact, virtually all meningiomas in patientswith neurofibromatosis type 2 and 50 to 80% of sporadic meningiomas have deletions in this region. Among grade 1 meningiomas, there is a great variety in the finding of inactivation of the *NF2* gene, with 75% in fibroblastic ortransitional meningiomas, 25% in transitional meningiomas, and only 1% in secretory meningiomas. Interestingly, in atypical and anaplastic meningiomas, the frequency of inactivation of the *NF2* gene is similar to that of benignmeningiomas, suggesting that the inactivation of the *NF2* gene would have a predominant role in tumor formation but not in its progression.

The *NF2* gene codes for the schwannomin/merlin protein (moesin-ezrin-radixin-like protein), which is a part of the band 4.1 family of cytoskeleton-associated proteins. Small insertions or deletions of this gene produce nonsense mutations resulting in a nonfunctional merlin protein. Loss of the merlin protein results in decreased cell adhesion and tumorigenesis. A reduced expression of schwannomin/merlin has been demonstrated in sporadic meningiomas. In addition to the inactivation of the *NF2* gene, other suppressor genes are also inactivated in meningiomas, such as the *EPB41L3* or *DAL1* gene, located at 18p11.3 and encoding the protein 4.1B, a regulator of proliferation and apoptosis.

The malignant progression of meningiomas is associated with the accumulation of other genetic aberrations beyond chromosome 22, with losses in 1p, 10q, and 14q and less frequent losses in 6q and 18q. Higher degrees are also associated with chromosomal gains in 1q, 9q, 12q, 15q, 17q, and 20q. In addition to these genetic changes, anaplastic meningiomas exhibit more frequent losses in 6q, 10q, 14q, and 9p, with amplification in 17q23 [5, 6].

11.3.2 Histopathology

Meningiomas are classically classified based on two criteria: pathology and prognosis, from a histopathological perspective. The 2007 WHO (*World Health Organization*) classification differentiates 15 types of meningiomas based on pathology: anaplastic, meningothelial, fibroblastic, transitional, psammomatous, angiomatous, microcystic, secretory, lymphoplasmacytic, metaplastic, chordoid, clear cell, atypical, papillary, rhabdoid, and anaplastic. Meningiomas can be categorized into three grades in terms of prognosis: grade 1, which are low-growing, non-malignant tumors that are associated with a long survival; grade 2, which are relatively low-growing tumors that occasionally have recurrences of a higher grade and may be malignant or non-malignant; and grade 3, which are malignant tumors that frequently recur with a high grade. Each histological type can be graded; however, certain histological types must be classified as grade 2 tumors (atypical, chordoid, or clear cell meningioma) or grade 3 tumors (rhabdoid or papillary meningioma). Approximately 85% of skull base meningiomas are grade 1, 8% are grade 2, and the remaining 7% are grade 3. There are no significant differences between meningiomas that develop outside the skull base and those that grow within it. Nevertheless, skull base meningiomas typically exhibit a lower rate of aggressiveness and, as a result, a lower propensity to recur compared to convexity meningiomas.

Meningiomas are typically benign tumors; however, their growth is inconsistent with their grade (Fig. 11.1). According to observational studies, the average time required to double the volume of a meningioma is 1.2 years for grade 1 and 0.5 years for grades 2 and 3, despite the fact that the time range is extremely broad for all grades and there is significant individual variability. Furthermore, the growth pattern is unpredictable, with linear growth being prevalent in grade 1 tumors, while exponential growth is observed in all grades, with grades 2 and 3 being particularly susceptible. It has been suggested that meningiomas may exhibit a *Gompertzian* progression, in which the tumor's growth pattern over time is contingent upon its volume. In accordance with this paradigm, the tumor would initially expand exponentially, subsequently transition to linear growth, and ultimately reach a plateau phase in which it experiences minimal growth as a result of trophic issues. As the diameter and volume of meningiomas increase, this model predicts that they will grow at a slower rate. Lastly, some tumors do not exhibit any growth over extended periods of observation, such as calcified meningiomas, particularly in elderly people.

11.4 Clinical Considerations

Meningiomas of the cerebellopontine angle commonly manifest symptoms associated with cranial nerve dysfunction, compression of the brain stem, cerebellar peduncle, or cerebellar hemisphere. Alternatively, they may manifest as a syndrome of intracranial hypertension as a result of mass effect or hydrocephalus. The symptoms are dependent upon the tumor's size and location. Tumors are being diagnosed in patients with scarce or minor symptoms or symptoms unrelated to meningioma, which are sometimes true serendipitous events, as the population gains access to imaging studies with magnetic resonance imaging (MRI). This presents challenges in terms of the distinction between imaging observation and active treatment recommendations. In general, the most prevalent symptoms are of an otological character, manifesting as tinnitus or hearing loss in 75% of patients. Almost half of the patients experience symptoms of cranial nerve dysfunction, whether they are of the irritative or deficit variety.

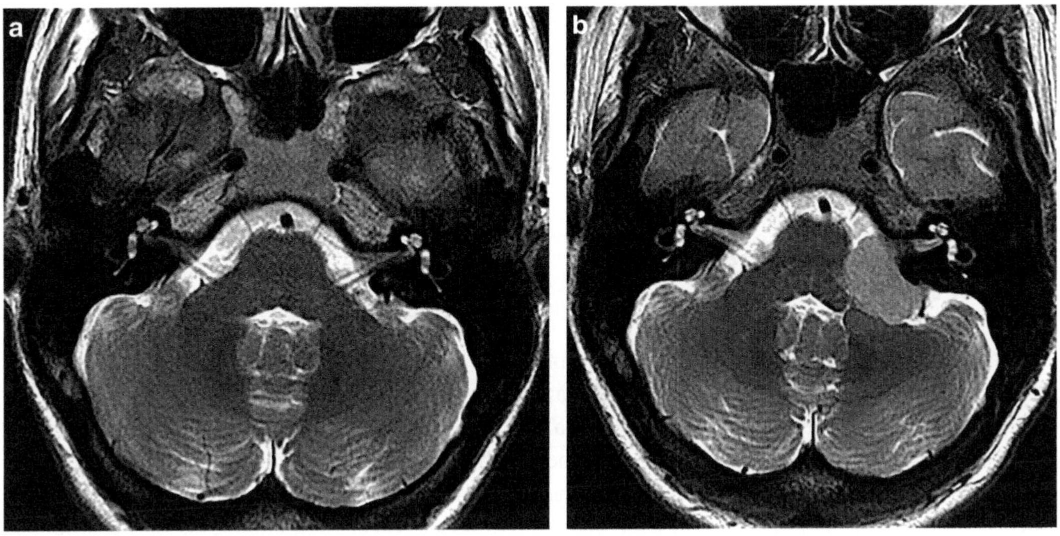

Fig. 11.1 Meningioma of cerebellopontine angle that grows. (**a**, **b**) Axial T2-weighted MRI sections from two investigations that were conducted 6 years apart, demonstrating the progression of a retromeatal meningioma

Cerebellar symptoms, such as ataxia or unsteady locomotion, are observed in one-third of patients as a result of compression of the cerebellar peduncle or cerebellum. The suboccipital region is the site of non-specific headaches in 25% of cases. Lastly, symptoms that are caused by intracranial hypertension or long pathways are significantly less common. Nevertheless, the clinical characteristics of each tumor location are unique.

11.4.1 Cerebellar Convexity Meningioma

These tumors are located in the dura mater, which extends from the interior surface of the occipital bone squama to the sigmoid sinus. They are related to the posterior surface or convexity of the cerebellar hemispheres. The symptoms are typically suboccipital headache and cerebellar symptoms or signs, or intracranial hypertension when they are large. They have a propensity to grow extremely huge and can either partially or completely obstruct the transverse or sigmoid sinus. Numerous tumors in this region are discovered incidentally during imaging investigations.

11.4.2 Petrosal Meningioma, Located Posterior to the Internal Acoustic Meatus

These meningiomas are usually paucisymptomatic, but when they grow, they can compress the cerebellum and displace the facial and vestibulocochlear nerves anteriorly or inferiorly. The symptoms are usually otological and vestibular. Occasionally, they enter the internal auditory canal, although this fact does not usually cause, contrary to what might be expected, a greater incidence or intensity of the clinical symptoms.

11.4.3 Petrosal Meningioma, Located Anterior to the Internal Acoustic Meatus

These meningiomas develop on the posterior surface of the petrosal bone, between the internal acoustic meatus and the cisternal course of the trigeminal nerve until the trigeminal root enters Meckel's cave. They are typically symptomatic and small in size, exhibiting symptoms that are associated with dysfunction or irritation of the neighboring cranial nerves. The symptoms are typically otological and vestibular, with secondary trigeminal neuralgia being a common occurrence. They occasionally penetrate the internal auditory canal or Meckel's cave.

11.4.4 Petrosal Meningioma of the Internal Acoustic Canal

These are exceptional lesions that develop within the internal auditory canal, similar to vestibular schwannomas. The seventh and eighth cranial nerves may be encircled or displaced by the tumor. They are clinically distinguished by the same symptoms as schwannoma, but they manifest earlier and with greater intensity. Therefore, severe hypoacusis or unilateral deafness is present in nearly all cases. Tinnitus is present in 50% of cases, and paresis or facial muscle paralysis is present in 25% of cases.

11.4.5 Petrosal Meningioma of the Jugular Foramen

These lesions are also uncommon, with just over 100 described cases. They develop within the jugular foramen and can extend to the cerebellopontine angle and the extracranial space. In the clinical setting, they initially manifest as a result of the lower cranial nerves' dysfunction, specifically the vagal nerve in 50% of cases, the glossopharyngeal nerve in 25%, and the accessory nerve in another 25% of patients. The majority of patients experience hearing loss, while a significant number of them experience tinnitus, vertigo, or instability [7–9].

11.4.6 Petroclival Meningioma

Unsteady gait and ataxia, headache, and involvement of the cranial nerves, including diplopia due to dysfunction of the sixth cranial nerve, are among the highly variable clinical symptoms. Cranial nerve involvement is observed in 90% of patients, with the trigeminal nerve being the most frequently affected. Hypoesthesia, paresthesia, or secondary neuralgia are present in over 60% of cases, followed by vestibulocochlear dysfunction [10–12].

11.4.7 Foramen Magnum Meningioma

Clinically, they exhibit an insidious course, with suboccipital headache being a frequent symptom. The intensity of the headache increases during exercise, Valsalva maneuvers, or specific head movements. Paresthesia or hyperesthesia may accompany the discomfort in the ipsilateral Arnold suboccipital nerve's territory. Progressive spastic tetraparesis may appear, which develops in a typically rotatory pattern, first ipsilaterally and then contralaterally. There are also disorders secondary to the involvement of the long sensory pathways, with Brown-Sequard syndrome. Horner syndrome or involvement of the cranial nerves is exceedingly uncommon [13, 14].

11.4.8 Tentorial Meningioma

The clinical presentation of these tentorial meningiomas is also variable due to the variability of their locations. Headache is the most prevalent symptom at the time of diagnosis, occurring in 80% of patients. Epileptic seizures are the second most common symptom in patients with cranially growing tumors, which are caused by the irritation of the temporal or occipital lobes. Less frequently, they exhibit gait disorders or disorders of higher functions. The eventual occlusion of the dural sinuses in those that grow in close proximity to them is well tolerated by patients, as it occurs at a gradual pace and enables the development of alternative venous drainage routes, even in the case of torcular meningiomas [15].

11.5 Diagnostic Considerations

Meningiomas are lesions that are easy to diagnose using imaging techniques. Meningiomas are extra-axial lesions with a typically globular morphology, although they may have a cake-like appearance (*plaque meningioma*), are in contact with the dura mater, and exhibit a brisk enhancement following contrast administration.

They are visualized as hyperdense masses in 75% of computed tomography (CT) studies, isointense in the remaining cases, and only in exceptional cases as hypointense. Intralesional calcifications may be present. The boundaries are uniform, with the exception of aggressive meningioma. Reactive hyperostosis may be observed in the underlying bone, which should be regarded as tumor infiltration from a surgical perspective. The majority of meningiomas develop contrast uptake in a consistent and intense manner, while others do so in a discontinuous or irregular manner. This latter condition is observed in meningiomas that are calcified and have necrosis, cysts, or intratumoral hemorrhage. The oedema in the adjacent nervous tissue may be more or less extensive. Meningiomas may be either solitary or multiple, and they can grow in locations that are not in contact with the dura mater, such as the ventricles, despite being free of arachnoid or meningothelial cells.

The diagnostic characteristics are even more pronounced in magnetic resonance imaging (MRI) investigations (Fig. 11.2). Unless necrosis, lesions, or hemorrhage are present, they are typically isointense with the brain parenchyma in the T1-weighted sequence. Unless there are intratumoral alterations, the administration of gadolinium results in a uniform increase in density for nearly all meningiomas. The limit of the tumor's implantation in the dura mater is typically abrupt; however, in certain instances, it becomes smooth, resulting in the formation of the *dural tail*, a feature that is highly indicative of meningioma. The T2-weighted sequence typically reveals a well-defined *cleavage plane* that distinguishes the meningioma from the nervous tissue. The T2 gradient is used to evaluate intratumoral calcifications in T2-weighted sequences. Vascular or flow sequences are employed to evaluate the potential invasion of the dural venous sinuses. MRIs are highly sensitive and specific in the diagnosis of meningioma. Furthermore, MRI enables the classification of tumors by defining the site of tumor implantation. MRI is capable of defining extensions beyond the cerebellopontine angle, including the petroclinoid, spinal, or supratentorial space, the cavernous sinus, or middle fossa, through orifices such as the Meckel's cave, internal auditory canal, and jugular foramen, and, finally, possibly, bone invasion.

Special consideration should be given to two locations of cerebellopontine angle meningiomas. Meningiomas of the internal auditory canal are nearly identical to tiny or small intracanalicular schwannomas of the auditory canal. The differential diagnosis of these lesions should also encompass other lesions, such as arachnoid cysts, lipomas, hemangiomas or hamartomas, and facial nerve schwannomas. The typical intracanalicular meningioma is a globular lesion that occupies the canal and bulges toward the cerebellopontine angle. It is isointense in the MRI sequence and exhibits an intense enhancement in density after gadolinium administration. Additionally, it may have a dural tail, calcifications, or a certain degree of bone invasion. Conversely, meningioma of the jugular foramen presents a differential diagnosis with chemodectoma and schwannoma. However, there is a lengthy list of lesions with this location, such as various bone tumors, metastases, or the invasion of parapharyngeal tumors. The invasive growth of the bone around the jugular foramen, which follows a centripetal expansion pattern in all directions, is the data that suggests a mass in the jugular foramen corresponds to a meningioma. This expansion pattern is extremely prevalent along the dura mater, resulting in a *plaque meningioma*, a tumor that is flattened. Globular varieties are exceedingly uncommon. Secondary changes in the bone of the base of the skull are also evident, including hyperostosis as a result of hypervascularization or infiltration.

Imaging studies also exhibit a highly distinctive pattern in aggressive meningiomas of WHO grades 2 and 3. In CT and MRI, they are depicted as masses with irregular boundaries, edema of

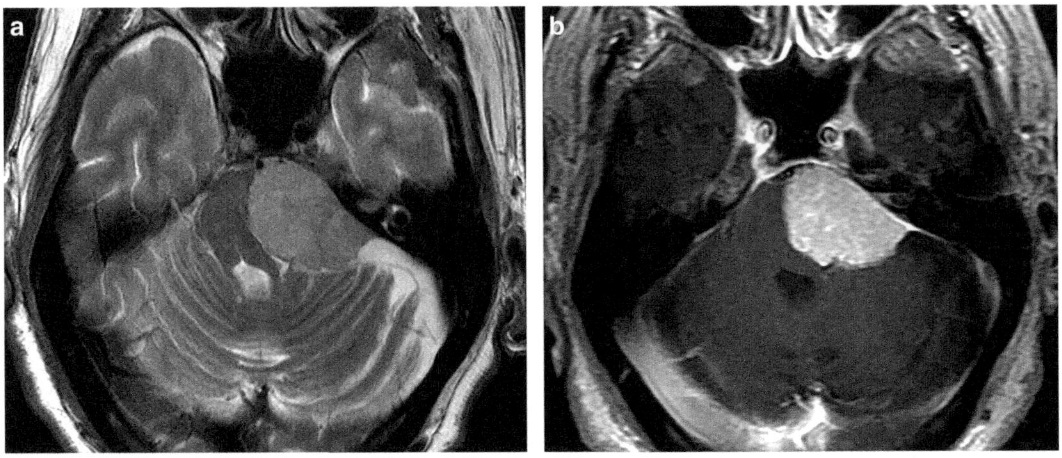

Fig. 11.2 Grade 1 meningioma of the left cerebellopontine angle. (**a**) Axial T2-weighted MRI section demonstrating a lesion with a signal intensity comparable to the parenchyma, which displaces the pons and cerebellum. A halo of hyposignal is present between the tumor and the nerve tissue, indicating a cleavage plane. (**b**) Axial T1-weighted MRI section following gadolinium administration, demonstrating the typical dural tail of the meningioma and an intense enhancement of the tumor

the perilesional nervous tissue, intense homogeneous or irregular contrast enhancement, osteolysis of the bone due to invasion of the underlying bone, and even extracranial growth (Fig. 11.3). In MRI, they are distinguished by their inadequately defined limits, irregular edges, or interdigitations that penetrate the nervous tissue. They are also accompanied by intense edema, which is evident in T2 and FLAIR (*Fluid Attenuated Inversion Recovery*) sequences. Their high cellularity may be reflected in a reduction in signal in ADC (*Apparent Diffusion Coefficient*) and an intense hyperintense state in the DWI (*Diffusion Weighted Imaging*) sequence.

Digital subtraction angiography (DSA) of cerebral vessels is employed only in rare cases for diagnostic purposes (Fig. 11.4). The vascular supply of these tumors is highly variable, as it originates from the ascending pharyngeal and occipital arteries, the vertebral artery, the anterior inferior cerebellar artery through the arcuate artery, and the internal carotid artery petrosal branches or the Bernasconi–Casignari artery from the cavernous segment. The arterial supplies are typically very fine, so preoperative embolization is not routinely employed, and hemorrhage can be controlled intraoperatively in all cases. The approach and surgical strategy for huge tumors with petroclival location are planned using angiography.

11.6 Surgical Categories

11.6.1 Cerebellar Convexity Meningioma

These are tumors that develop on the dura mater, which encompasses the interior surface of the occipital bone squama, with the exception of the rim of the foramen magnum, and extends to the sigmoid sinus. These tumors are concomitant with the posterior or suboccipital surface of the cerebellar hemispheres (Fig. 11.5). A retrosigmoid lateral suboccipital approach is used to remove meningiomas located more laterally in this broad area, while a paramedian or bilateral suboccipital approach is used to remove paramedian or medial meningiomas. Although they may be associated with the walls of the transverse, sigmoid sinuses, or torcula, these tumors are not related with the cranial nerves or the arteries of the posterior circulation.

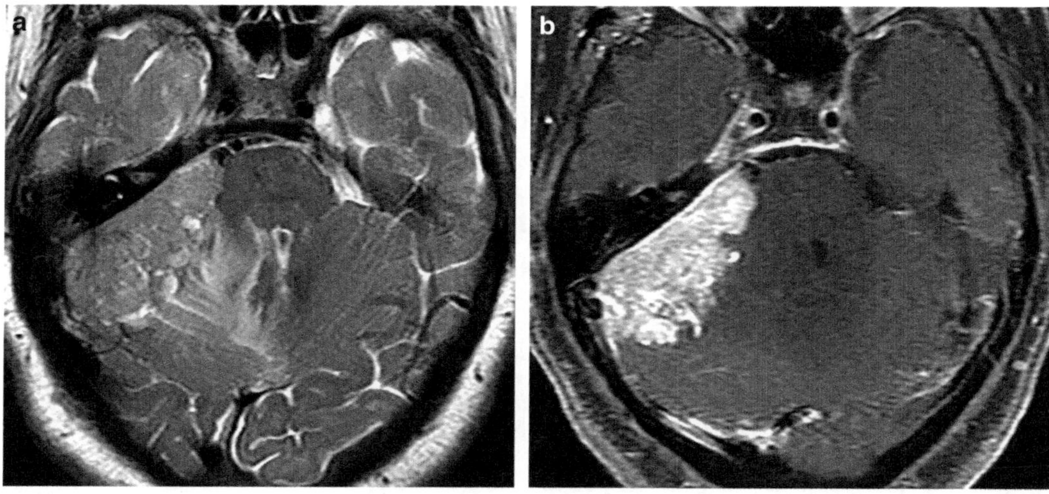

Fig. 11.3 Grade 3 meningioma of the right cerebellopontine angle. (**a**) An axial T2-weighted MRI section demonstrating a lesion with a signal intensity comparable to that of the parenchyma, which is poorly delineated and accompanied by edema. (**b**) An axial T1-weighted MRI section demonstrating an intense enhancement of the tumor following gadolinium administration, but with irregular boundaries and deficient delimitation with the cerebellum

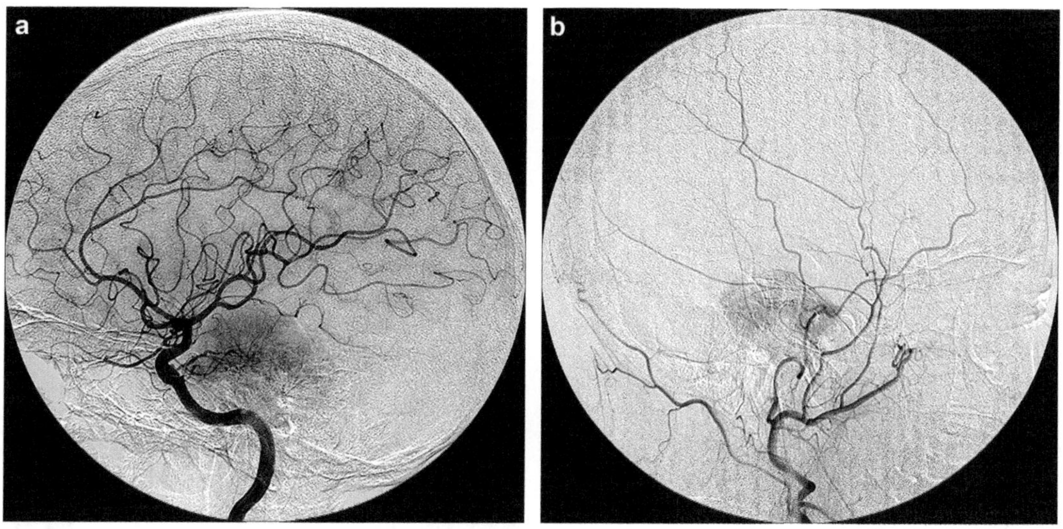

Fig. 11.4 Left petroclival meningioma. (**a**) DSA illustrating the vascularization of the tumor in the form of branches from the petrosal and cavernous segments of the internal carotid artery, specifically the Bernasconi–Casinnari artery. (**b**) Selective lateral DSA of the external carotid artery demonstrates minor vascularization through branches of the middle meningeal artery

11.6.2 Petrosal Meningioma, Located Posterior to the Internal Acoustic Meatus

These are meningiomas that develop on the posterior surface of the petrosal bone, between the internal acoustic meatus and the sigmoid sinus (retromeatal meningioma). They are associated with the petrosal surface of the cerebellum and cause the cranial nerves to be displaced anteriorly and inferiorly. Some of them grow to invade the sigmoid sinus, and they typically attain a large

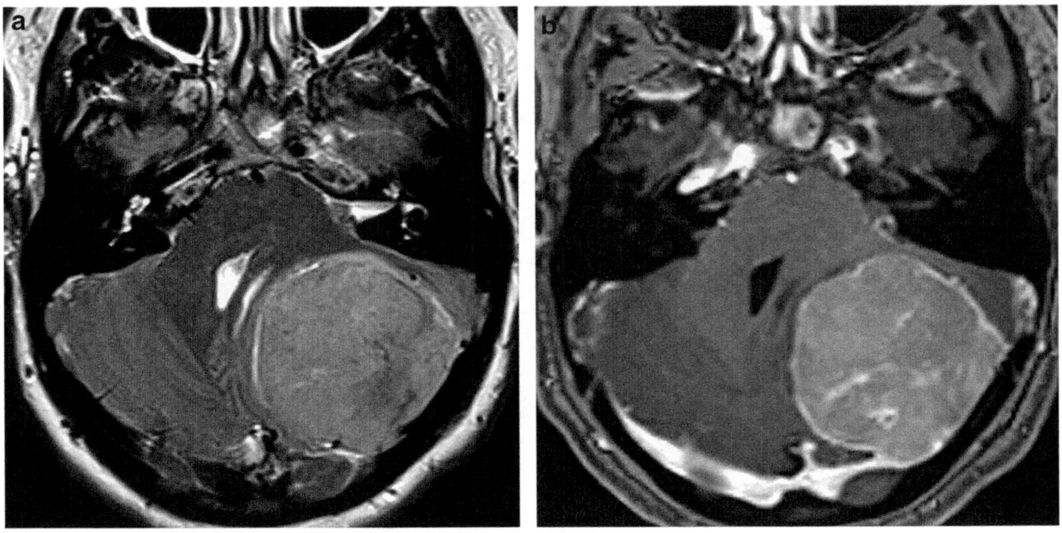

Fig. 11.5 Left cerebellar convexity meningioma. (**a**) Axial T2-weighted MRI section demonstrating a lesion with a signal intensity that is lower than the parenchyma, causing the pons, cerebellar peduncle, and cerebellum to be displaced. A halo of hyposignal between the tumor and the cerebellum suggests a cleavage plane. (**b**) Axial T1-weighted MRI section demonstrating an intense enhancement of the tumor following gadolinium administration. The transverse sinus is invaded by the tumor, despite the presence of flow in the sigmoid sinus from the superior petrosal sinus

size at the time of diagnosis. They have the potential to access the internal auditory canal or jugular foramen (Fig. 11.6).

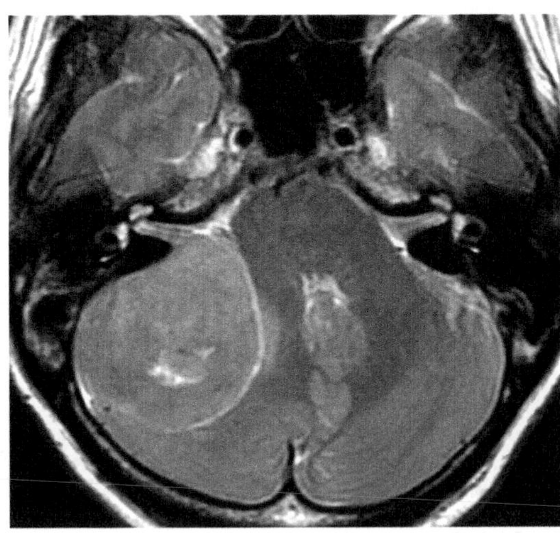

Fig. 11.6 Right retromeatal meningioma. Axial T2-weighted MRI section demonstrating a lesion with a signal comparable to the parenchyma, which displaces the pons, cerebellar peduncle, and cerebellum. A halo of hyposignal between the tumor and the cerebellum suggests a cleavage plane, and hyposignal is observed in the cerebellar peduncle

11.6.3 Petrosal Meningioma, Located Anterior to the Internal Acoustic Meatus

These are meningiomas that develop in the region immediately preceding the internal auditory meatus and behind the trigeminal nerve (premeatal meningioma). The trigeminal nerve is displaced superiorly or anteriorly, while the facial and vestibulocochlear nerves are displaced posteriorly or inferiorly. They are typically relatively small at the time of diagnosis due to their intimate relationship with the cranial nerves. They have the potential to access the internal auditory canal or jugular foramen (Fig. 11.7).

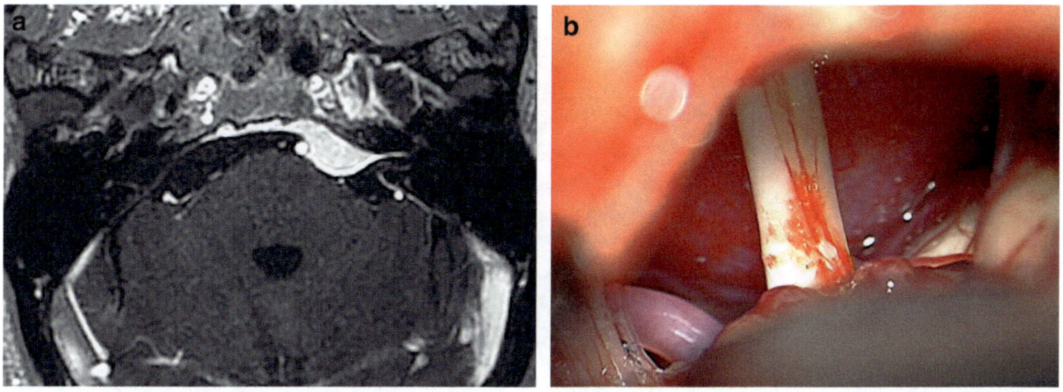

Fig. 11.7 Left premeatal meningioma. (**a**) Axial T1-weighted MRI section following gadolinium administration, demonstrating a significant increase in signal intensity from a small meningioma situated in front of the internal acoustic meatus. The dural tail extends extensively through the clival dura mater and insinuates itself into the internal auditory canal. (**b**) Intraoperative picture illustrating the tumor through a retrosigmoid approach, which is situated in a deeper plane than the facial–vestibulocochlear complex. The rootlets of the lower cranial nerves and the anteroinferior cerebellar artery are visible caudally

11.6.4 Petrosal Meningioma of the Internal Acoustic Canal

The clinical manifestations and imaging investigations of petrosal meningiomas of the internal auditory canal are indistinguishable from those of vestibular nerve schwannomas (refer to case 5 in Chap. 21). In comparison to schwannomas, the clinical symptoms are diagnosed at an early stage due to their severity. These are tumors that exhibit growth in the cistern of the cerebellopontine angle or that are exclusively intracanalicular (Fig. 11.8) [16].

11.6.5 Foramen Jugular Meningioma

Meningiomas of this location are uncommon; however, their growth pattern is highly variable due to their location in a foramen at the cranium base, which is typically caudal to the internal auditory meatus (infracanalicular meningioma) (Fig. 11.9). Meningiomas of the jugular foramen have been classified into four types: type 1, circumscribed to the jugular foramen; type 2, with a predominant extension toward the cerebellopontine angle (refer to case 12 in Chap. 21); type 3, with a predominant extension toward the extracranial space; and type 4, with an hourglass-shaped intra-extracranial extension. This classification is based on the potential for the tumor to extend through the jugular foramen and into neighboring structures. If the tumor extends intraosseously toward the middle ear, each of these varieties would have a distinct subtype. Growth within the cerebellopontine angle is typically flattened and extensive rather than highly globular [7–9].

11.6.6 Petroclival Meningioma

Petroclival meningiomas comprise approximately 2% of intracranial meningiomas. They are tumors that implant in the petroclival junction and the upper two-thirds of the clivus, medially to the trigeminal nerve. They are lesions that attain a significant size at the time of diagnosis, with an average maximum diameter of approximately 35 mm in surgical series. One-third of patients have tumors that exceed 45 mm in size (refer to case 13 in Chap. 21). The anatomical structures in the region are significantly displaced due to the enormous size of the lesions. Thus, they displace the basilar artery and the brainstem posteriorly and contralaterally, as well as the cranial nerves, from the third to the vestibulocochlear nerve. The tumor has the potential

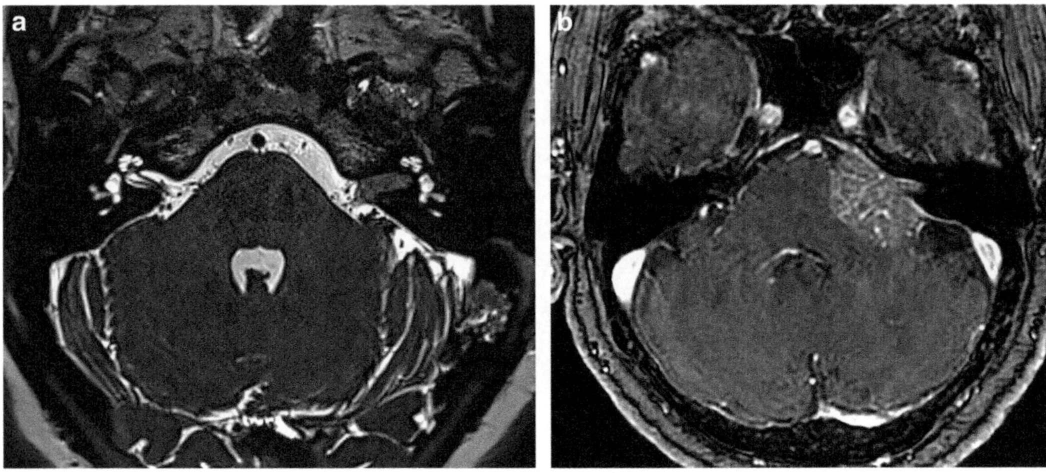

Fig. 11.8 Intracanalicular meningiomas. (**a**) Axial T2-weighted MRI section illustrating a lesion with a signal intensity comparable to that of the parenchyma, which is located in the left internal auditory canal. (**b**) Axial T1-weighted MRI section performed following gadolinium administration, demonstrating a tumor with irregular contrast enhancement, an intracanalicular and cisternal component, and the characteristic dural tail of meningiomas

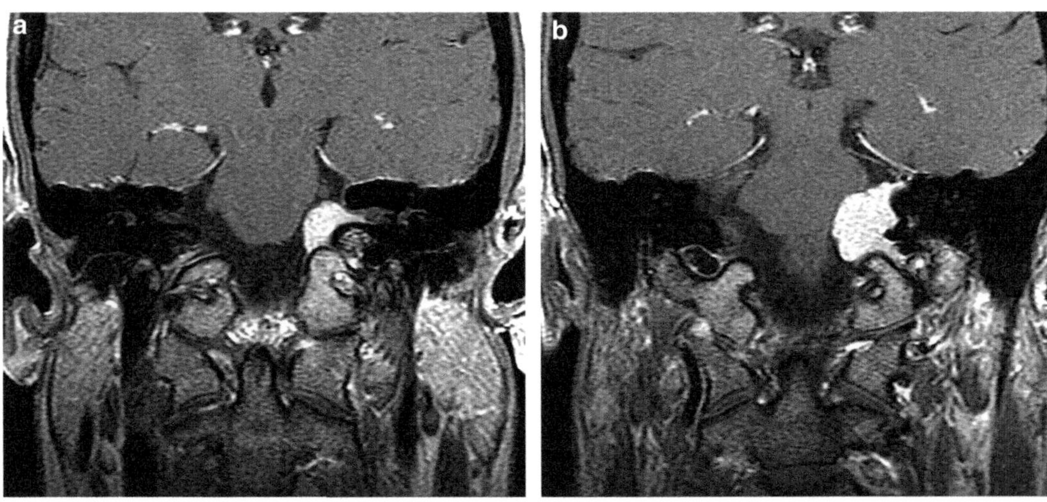

Fig. 11.9 Left infracanalicular jugular meningioma. (**a**) Coronal T1-weighted MRI section after the administration of gadolinium, displaying an intense increase in the intensity of the tumor signal, which grows in the cerebellopontine angle and within the internal auditory canal. (**b**) Coronal cut of the same tumor displaying a dural tail insinuating itself into the jugular foramen

to extend beyond the petroclival region to the contralateral side through orifices in the region, including the meatus of the Meckel's cave, internal acoustic meatus, jugular foramen, and Dorello's canal. Additionally, it has the potential to invade the ipsilateral cavernous sinus. The tumor compresses the brain stem at the level of the pons and causes the loss of the arachnoid layer that facilitates the recognition of the cleavage plane. In numerous instances, the brainstem exhibits symptoms of edema. The basilar artery is embedded in the tumor in some instances and is displaced in over half of the cases (Fig. 11.10).

In addition to these large and intricate petroclival meningiomas, there is an additional group of meningiomas in the same location that are

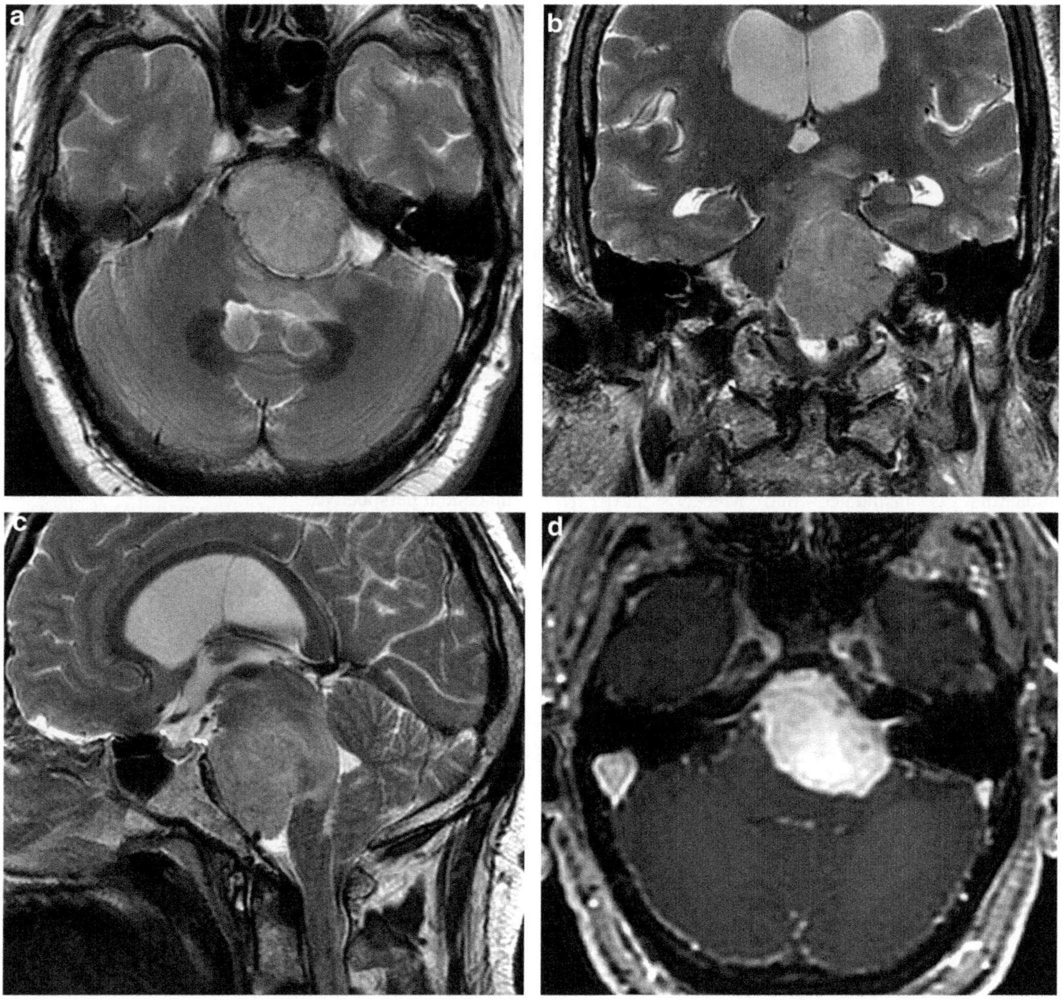

Fig. 11.10 Left large petroclival meningioma. (**a**) Axial T2-weighted MRI section displaying a lesion with lower signal intensity than the parenchyma, which displaces the pons and middle cerebellar peduncle, with a halo of hyposignal between the tumor and the nervous tissue, suggesting a cleavage plane. The basilar artery is displaced and embedded in the tumor. (**b**) Coronal T2-weighted MRI section displaying the tumor and ventricular dilatation. (**c**) Sagittal T2-weighted MRI section, which shows severe brain stem displacement. (**d**) Axial T1-weighted MRI section after administration of gadolinium, which shows an increase in the intensity of the tumor signal

more lateral and significantly smaller. These meningiomas are clinically evident with secondary trigeminal neuralgia and are identified at an early stage through imaging techniques due to the relevant clinical symptoms experienced by the patient. Clinicians can easily identify these meningiomas by conducting a rapid MRI examination of the patient (see case 28 in Chap. 21). These are tumors that are less than 10 mm in diameter and are located in the petroclival space, medially to the trigeminal nerve (Fig. 11.11). These petroclival meningiomas, which Al-Mefty refers to as *authentic*, are distinguished from other meningiomas in the same region that possess certain distinguishing characteristics. Consequently, *spheno-petroclival meningiomas* are significantly more extensive lesions, extending in plaque through the dura mater of the clivus

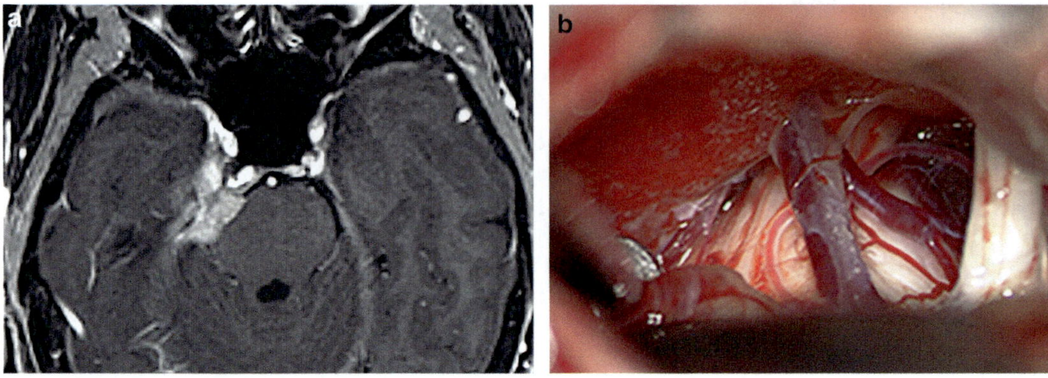

Fig. 11.11 Right small petroclival meningioma. (**a**) Axial T1-weighted MRI section following gadolinium administration, demonstrating a small petroclival meningioma that is insinuated into Meckel's cave. (**b**) Intraoperative picture illustrating the tumor through a retrosigmoid approach, which is situated in a deeper plane than the trigeminal nerve and the petrosal vein complex. The facial–vestibular–cochlear complex is visible from the caudal perspective

and both petrosal apexes and affecting both cavernous sinuses. Consequently, they are virtually unresectable. Some meningiomas are pure *clival meningiomas*, which originate in the middle third of the clivus and are therefore located in the midline. These meningiomas grow posteriorly, enclose the basilar artery, and progress to both sides, affecting the cranial nerves bilaterally [10–12].

11.6.7 Foramen Magnum Meningioma

Approximately 3% of intracranial meningiomas are foramen magnum meningiomas (Fig. 11.12). First, they are characterized by their growth in the intracranial and spinal spaces, and second, they can originate at any location in the vicinity of the foramen magnum. Their origin is in the dura mater that envelops the foramen magnum. They are further divided into anterior, lateral, and posterior, with the latter being situated behind the dentate ligament. It is estimated that 70% of the lesions are situated anterolaterally, 15% anteriorly, 10% posterolaterally, and the remaining 5% posteriorly.

In general, the meningioma located laterally grows between the hypoglossal nerve, which is deeper in the surgical approach, and the tenth and ninth nerves and medullary roots of the accessory nerve, which are displaced by the tumor in a posterior and superior direction, that is, superficial to the tumor in the surgical approach. The accessory nerve is displaced laterally and applied to the dura mater by the tumor (refer to case 11 in Chap. 21). The cranial and spinal nerve roots are displaced variably; however, the meningioma is generally located laterally. The tumor's relationship with the vertebral artery is also crucial, and in this regard, they are classified as tumors located cranially, caudally, or on one side or the other of the intradural V4 segment of the vertebral [13, 14].

11.6.8 Tentorial Meningioma

Tentorial meningiomas account for approximately 5% of intracranial meningiomas. The location, clinical presentation, and microneurosurgical approach of tentorial meningiomas are highly variable due to the tentorium's wide extension, its location separating the supratentorial space from the infratentorial space, its unique anatomy with the tentorial or incisural foramen through which both spaces communicate, and its relationship with the transverse dural sinuses, straight sinus, and Herophilus press. Approximately 50% of tentorial meningiomas direct their primary growth caudally, toward the posterior fossa, while the remaining 50% direct

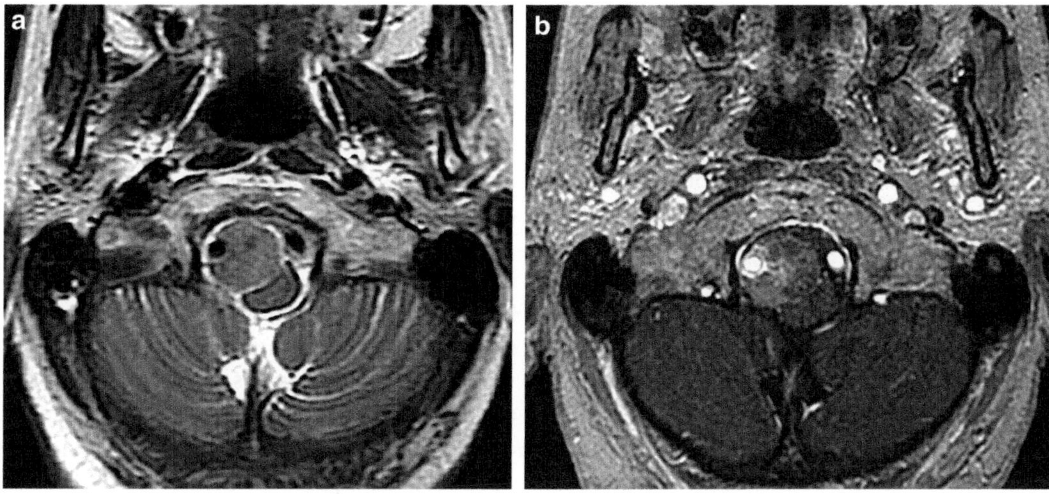

Fig. 11.12 Meningioma of the left foramen magnum. (**a**) Axial T2-weighted MRI section displaying tumoration of signal intensity similar to the parenchyma, which displaces the medulla oblongata, with a halo of hyposignal between the tumor and the brainstem, and which embeds the right vertebral artery. (**b**) Axial T1-weighted MRI section after gadolinium administration, displaying an irregular increase in tumor signal intensity

their primary growth cranially. The remaining 5–10% conduct their development in a manner that is consistent across both compartments (Fig. 11.13). The classification proposed by Yasargil, which considers the following categories, is typically followed in terms of their growth:

- Group 1: Medial or incisural meningioma, which develops on the free border of the tentorium and extends toward the midbrain.
- Group 2: Falcotentorial meningioma, which develops in the midline along the junction of the falx and the tentorium, following the straight sinus.
- Group 3: Paramedian meningioma, which develops on the tentorium's surface.
- Group 4: Torcular or peritorcular meningioma, which develops in the midline around the press of Herophilus.
- Group 5: Lateral tentorial meningioma, which develops on the most lateral portion of the tentorium's surface.

The distribution of the various topographies in surgical series is inconsistent; however, tumors from groups 1 and 5 are more prevalent, specifically those with incisural and lateral tentorial locations [15].

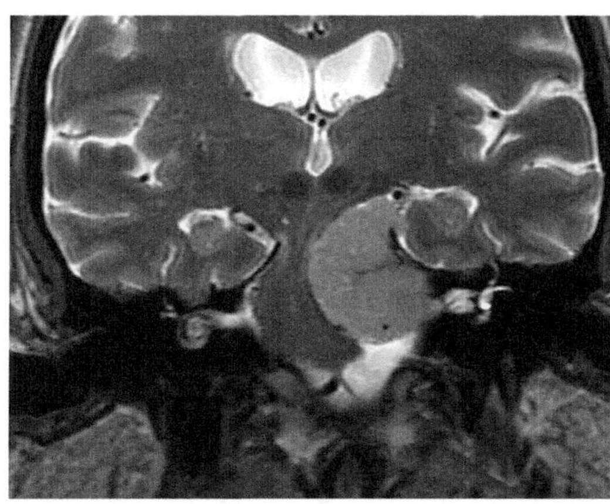

Fig. 11.13 Meningioma of the left tentorial incisure. A lesion with a signal intensity that is comparable to that of the brain is depicted in a coronal T2-weighted MRI section. The lesion displaces the midbrain and extends from the dura mater of the tentorium. The compression against the tentorial border results in a signal change on the contralateral peduncle

11.7 Microneurosurgical Management

11.7.1 Approach Selection

Regarding the selection of the approach, the neurosurgeon's confidence and expertise in each of the potential approaches, as well as the specific location of the tumor and its extension, determine the various options [1, 3, 17, 18]. Initially, the *bilateral medial suboccipital approach* and the *unilateral retrosigmoid approach* were the sole methods employed to treat the majority of meningiomas in the posterior fossa. However, certain tentorial lesions were resected using *supratentorial approaches* through the middle cranial fossa. A variety of practical strategies were devised for each of the lesions on an individual basis as a result of the advancements in microneurosurgery, intraoperative electrophysiological monitoring, imaging techniques, and skull base surgery. These were *transpetrosal* or *combined supra and infratentorial approaches*, which were highly technically demanding and complex. They resulted in a high morbidity and mortality rate in inexperienced hands or related to the technique itself, as they necessitated a long and lengthy learning curve. Consequently, and in accordance with the same rationale as the microsurgical treatment of brainstem cavernomas, there has been a disposition to revert to the *classic standard retrosigmoid approach* as the initial treatment option for these lesions. This approach is designed to optimize the microsurgical technique and incorporate specific access routes or modifications that are beneficial for the resolution of specific lesions. The retrosigmoid approach is a straightforward and secure method that is employed by all neurosurgeons for a variety of procedures. The retrosigmoid approach provides a comprehensive panoramic view of the cerebellopontine angle, encompassing the cisternal course of the cranial nerve roots from the oculomotor nerve to the hypoglossal nerve, as well as all relevant arteries of the posterior circulation and superior petrosal venous drainage, from the tentorium and tentorial notch to the foramen magnum. Rand and Kurze's *transmeatal approach* permits access to the internal auditory canal, while Samii's suprameatal approach permits access to the petrosal apex and Meckel's cave. Tentorial or tentorial notch meningiomas with supratentorial extension can be removed through partial resection of the tentorium (*transtentorial access*). In comparison to transpetrosal approaches, the retrosigmoid approach preserves the patient's hearing and has a lower morbidity rate in terms of complications, such as cerebrospinal fluid fistula, sinus thrombosis, or infections, than more complex approaches. In addition, the retrosigmoid approach can be readily expanded by combining it with the *presigmoid approach* or the *far-lateral approach*. Ultimately, in the event of giant petroclival meningiomas that have extensive and symptomatic extension to the supratentorial space in the middle fossa or cavernous sinus, it is always feasible to develop a stratified approach strategy over two *successive surgical procedures*. The first procedure will involve the complete resection of the infratentorial compartment, while the second will involve the resection of the supratentorial compartment.

11.7.2 Position and Craniotomy

There is no particularity in everything described in the chapters dedicated to surgical approaches to the cerebellopontine angle by a standard retrosigmoid approach regarding position, anatomical references, incision, craniotomy, and opening of the dura mater.

11.7.3 Opening of Cisterns and Drainage of Cerebrospinal Fluid

After opening the dura mater, the cisterns are opened to drain cerebrospinal fluid and reduce the pressure in the posterior fossa. Depending on the growth of the tumor occupying one or another portion of the cerebellopontine angle, the most accessible cisterns must be opened and drained.

11.7.4 Tumor Identification

The arachnoid plane of cleavage between the tumor and the nervous tissue is identified by exposing the maximal surface of the tumor. The tumor displaces the cranial nerves, but they are not as slender and flattened as they are in vestibular schwannoma. The artery adventitia is typically not invaded, and the arteries are typically displaced and free. Large-caliber arteries, such as the basilar artery or vertebral arteries, may be embedded in the tumor; however, an arachnoid plane of separation is consistently maintained between the tumor and the artery trunk. The veins may appear collapsed on the tumor's surface; however, they regain their original size upon their release.

11.7.5 Devascularization of the Tumor

Devascularization involves the search, identification, coagulation, and sectioning of the afferent arteries that are specific to each type of meningioma or those that have been detected in DSA. Nevertheless, this is not feasible in all cerebellopontine angle meningiomas, as they lack conspicuous arterial pedicles, except in cerebellar convexity meningiomas. This is a challenge in certain instances, as they are located at the posterior aspect of the tumor, which impedes tumor resection.

11.7.6 Internal Decompression

An aperture is created with a bipolar coagulator after the surface of the tumor has been coagulated, and the intracapsular emptying of the tumor is performed with an ultrasonic aspirator. The ultrasound aspiration must be comparatively low-powered. The resection is customarily performed to achieve hemostasis of any irregular intratumoral vessels that may appear. The resection is directed in all directions to hollow out the tumor in a regular manner, with a particular emphasis on the implantation base, as this is the source of the vascularization to the tumor that must be coagulated carefully. The wall aspirator can be used to press the tumor wall from outside, which can aid in the resection. It is crucial to refrain from perforating the capsule at any point in order to prevent the loss of the dissection plane and the injury of hidden structures.

11.7.7 Piecemeal Extirpation of the Tumor

As the tumor is emptied, the capsule is retracted with bipolar coagulation; it is separated from the vascular and nervous structures and progressively resected piecemeal into small fragments.

11.7.8 Tumor Implantation Management

It has been demonstrated that the Simpson grade of resection is correlated with the likelihood of recurrence of meningiomas in any location following microneurosurgical treatment. In meningiomas of the base of the skull, it is more challenging to achieve satisfactory grades of resection than in meningiomas of the convexity. However, in all cases, complete resection of the tumor should be pursued, as should the optimization of resection and intense coagulation of the dura mater if it cannot be removed. Resection of the dura mater surrounding the tumor implant to the greatest extent possible, as well as drilling of the underlying bone, are mandatory.

11.7.9 Anatomical Windows for Tumor Resection

The cerebellopontine angle nerves are anatomically organized in a highly stable and rigid manner, and, in contrast to arteries, they are not readily redeployed by the growth of tumors and have no anatomical variations. We can imagine that the cisternal course of the cranial nerves from the trigeminal to the vagal nerve runs on a plane that divides the cerebellopontine angle into two compartments. The deep compartment is located behind the nerves in the standard retrosigmoid approach and extends from this plane to the petroclival junction. Meningiomas of the tentorial notch, petroclival, and lateral meningiomas of the foramen magnum develop behind this plane. This implies that the neurosurgeon must operate between nerves to remove them. In this regard, there are several anatomical windows that, in a craniocaudal direction, are as follows: the space between the tentorium and the trigeminal nerve, the space between the trigeminal nerve and the facial–vestibulocochlear complex, the space between the facial-vestibulocochlear complex and the lower cranial nerves, and the space caudal to the lower nerves up to the first spinal nerve root. The sixth and hypoglossal nerves are located in the deeper compartment of the retrosigmoid approach. On the other hand, meningiomas of the convexity of the cerebellum, lateral and paramedian tentorial, premeatal and retromeatal petrosal are present in the most superficial compartment of the retrosigmoid approach before reaching the trigeminal-vagal plane. These meningiomas have the cranial nerves running in a deeper plane and are only discovered after the tumor has been partially decompressed and resected.

The systematic resection of the tumor is facilitated by the ability to work between the cranial nerves through these anatomical apertures, but the nerves' functionality is jeopardized. The nerves can be readily identified using anatomical references; however, intraoperative electrical stimulation may be beneficial in certain instances.

11.7.10 Transmeatal Access

Rand and Kurze proposed this access in 1964, which enables the resection of intracanalicular meningiomas or prolongations of petrosal meningiomas into the internal auditory canal. In essence, it involves the use of the Tübingen line as an anatomical reference to pierce the posterior wall of the internal auditory meatus. This access is primarily employed for the resection of the intracanalicular portion of vestibular schwannomas, as previously mentioned.

11.7.11 Suprameatal Access

In 1983, Samii introduced the suprameatal approach, which enables the resection of premeatal and petroclival petrosal meningiomas. The procedure primarily involves piercing the suprameatal tubercle, which is the portion of the petrosal bone located above and in front of the internal auditory meatus. This allows for the visualization and mobilization of the trigeminal nerve until it enters the Meckel's cave, thereby facilitating the resection of tumors that are medial to the nerve. After a meticulous dissection of the tumor from the fascicles of the trigeminal nerve, meningiomas that penetrate Meckel's cave are resected [18].

11.7.12 Transtentorial Access

The transtentorial approach can be used to accomplish the communication of the infratentorial space with the supratentorial space at the level of the middle fossa, which is necessary for the complete excision of certain cerebellopontine angle meningiomas that extend into the supratentorial space. In the transtentorial approach, a section of the tentorium is cut along the posterior border of the tumor from the junction between the tentorium and the petrosal bone at the level of the superior petrosal sinus and directed toward the tentorial notch. Subsequently, a second incision is made from the posterior edge of the tumor in an anterior direction, parallel to the edge of the petrosal bone, and approximately 2 mm away from it to prevent injury to the superior petrosal sinus. Thus, the tumor can be decompressed and mobilized until its upper limit is reached. The initial tentorial incision has been finished up to the incisura, and the second one is being worked on. This second incision crosses the trigeminal nerve as it enters Meckel's cave. The trochlear nerve may be injured at the anterior site of the tentorial incision, where it integrates into the tentorium. The ambiens cistern and its contents can be exposed and controlled by resecting the upper pole of the tumor in this manner.

11.7.13 Final Inspection

In the same manner as described in the chapter on the retrosigmoid approach to the cerebellopontine angle for vestibular schwannoma, the dura mater, craniotomy, and soft tissues are closed following meticulous hemostasis, the final inspection of the surgical field, and the final direct stimulation of the monitored cranial nerves.

11.8 Meningiomas that Require Specific Treatment

11.8.1 Cerebellar Convexity Meningioma

A suboccipital approach of appropriate size and location is employed to directly remove meningiomas of the cerebellar convexity in a similar way that with supratentorial convexity meningiomas. Resection of meningiomas of the cranial convexity is a technique that offers the additional benefit of a reduced eloquence of the underlying cerebellum in comparison to the cerebral hemispheres' cortex. The tumor's size increases the obligation of internal decompression. In the event of sinus wall invasion, the bone resection is prolonged by skeletonizing the dural sinus to assure tumor resection and sinus wall repair, if required. In the majority of patients, it is possible to ligate and divide both the transverse and sigmoid sinuses without repercussions in order to accomplish a complete resection of the tumor.

11.8.2 Petrosal Meningioma Located Posterior to the Internal Auditory Meatus

Small posterior petrosal meningiomas are removed straight away, as are those of the convexity of the cerebellum. However, bigger meningiomas are removed by separating their deeper portion from the cranial nerves at the conclusion of the tumor removal (Fig. 11.14). In order to accomplish complete tumor removal, the internal auditory canal must be resected using a transmeatal approach if the tumor extends into it. The posterior wall of the canal must be resected to the extent necessary to reach the tumor's end. An additional unique circumstance is the potential invasion of the sigmoid sinus wall. The tumor can be excised until the sinus wall is entirely free, as the sigmoid sinus restoration is a challenging endeavor. If a nondominant sinus or a sinus that has been completely or substantially obstructed by the tumor is involved, complete tumor resection entails the proximal and distal occlusion of the sinus. It may be necessary to extend the retrosigmoid approach with a presigmoid extension to sufficiently expose the sigmoid sinus for secure ligation.

11.8.3 Petrosal Meningioma Located Anterior to the Internal Auditory Meatus

Premeatal meningiomas are approached through the windows described according to the size of the lesion. The cranial window is located between the tentorium and the trigeminal nerve; the second window is between the trigeminal nerve and the facial-vestibulocochlear complex; the third window is between the facial-vestibulocochlear complex and the lower cranial nerves; and the most caudal window is located below the lower cranial nerves and extends to the foramen magnum (Fig. 11.15). The largest window is initially selected to execute internal decompression of the tumor. It is challenging to resect extensions to the internal auditory canal and jugular foramen due to the interposition of the cranial nerves, as well as the removal of the dura mater and underlying bone.

11.8.4 Petrosal Meningioma of the Internal Auditory Canal

The general technique for resection of these rare intracanalicular meningiomas is the same as for intracanalicular vestibular schwannomas, meaning a retrosigmoid approach with transmeatal access, despite the fact that presumptive preoperative accurate diagnosis from clinical data or imaging studies is very difficult. The facial and vestibulocochlear nerves can be preserved, as neither is the origin of the tumor, and nerve relationships are contingent upon the tumor growth

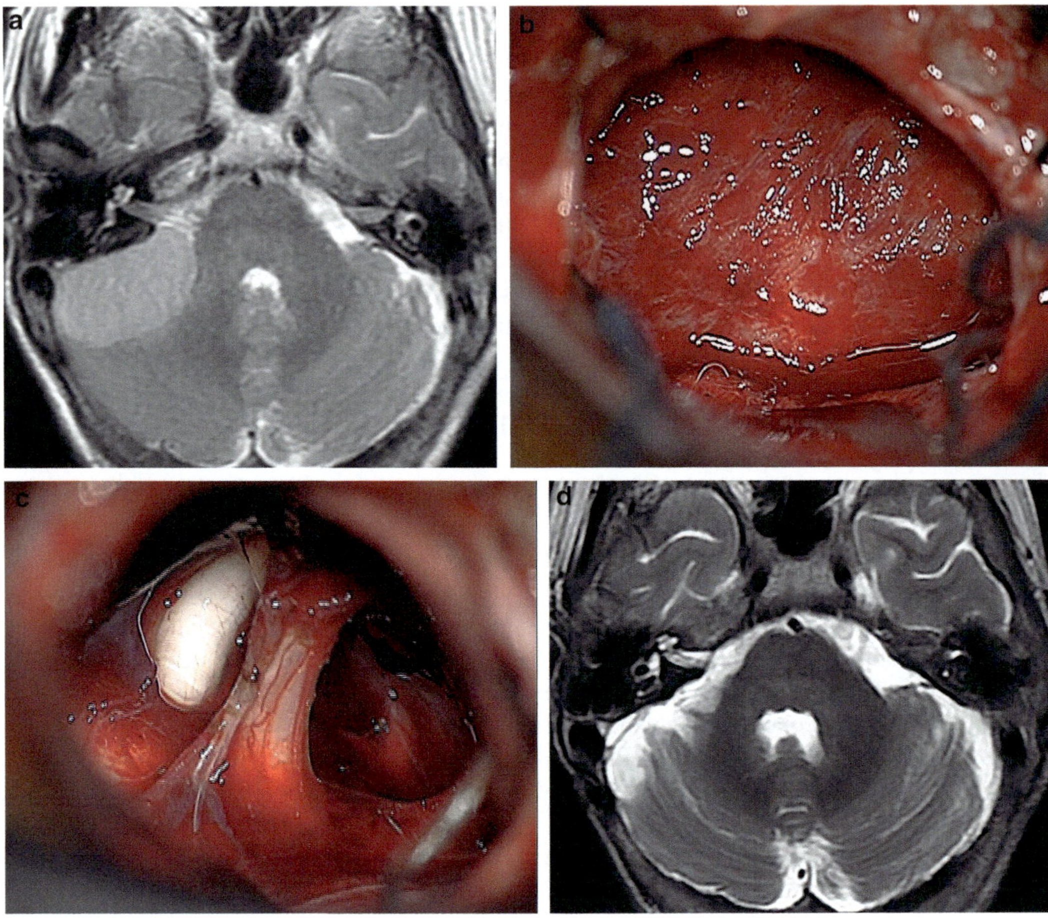

Fig. 11.14 Right retromeatal meningioma. (**a**) Axial T2-weighted MRI section. (**b**) Intraoperative picture displaying the tumor via a retrosigmoid approach. (**c**) Intraoperative picture after tumor resection, which now allows the visualization of the petrosal vein complex, the trigeminal nerve, and the facial-vestibulocochlear complex. (**d**) Postoperative axial T2-weighted MRI section, displaying the complete resection of the tumor

site. Nevertheless, the anatomic preservation of nerves that are embedded in the tumor may be challenging due to the restricted space in which they are located.

11.8.5 Jugular Foramen Meningioma

In a manner comparable to that of lower cranial nerve schwannoma, the microneurosurgical treatment of jugular foramen meningioma is dependent upon its degree of extension. The retrosigmoid approach is exclusively beneficial for the resection of the cisternal portion of these tumors, specifically type 2 and type 4. In any case, the retrosigmoid approach is not appropriate for the purpose of exploring the contents of the jugular foramen, resecting the tumor, and preserving the cranial nerves. In order to ensure safe access, a craniofacial approach is required, which involves the cervical dissection of the jugular vein and cranial nerves, the resection of presigmoid and retrosigmoid bone, and the ligation of the sigmoid sinus and jugular vein. This approach enables access to the jugular foramen and its contents for all types of tumors, as well as the intracranial portions of type 1 and 4 meningiomas and the extracranial portions of type 3

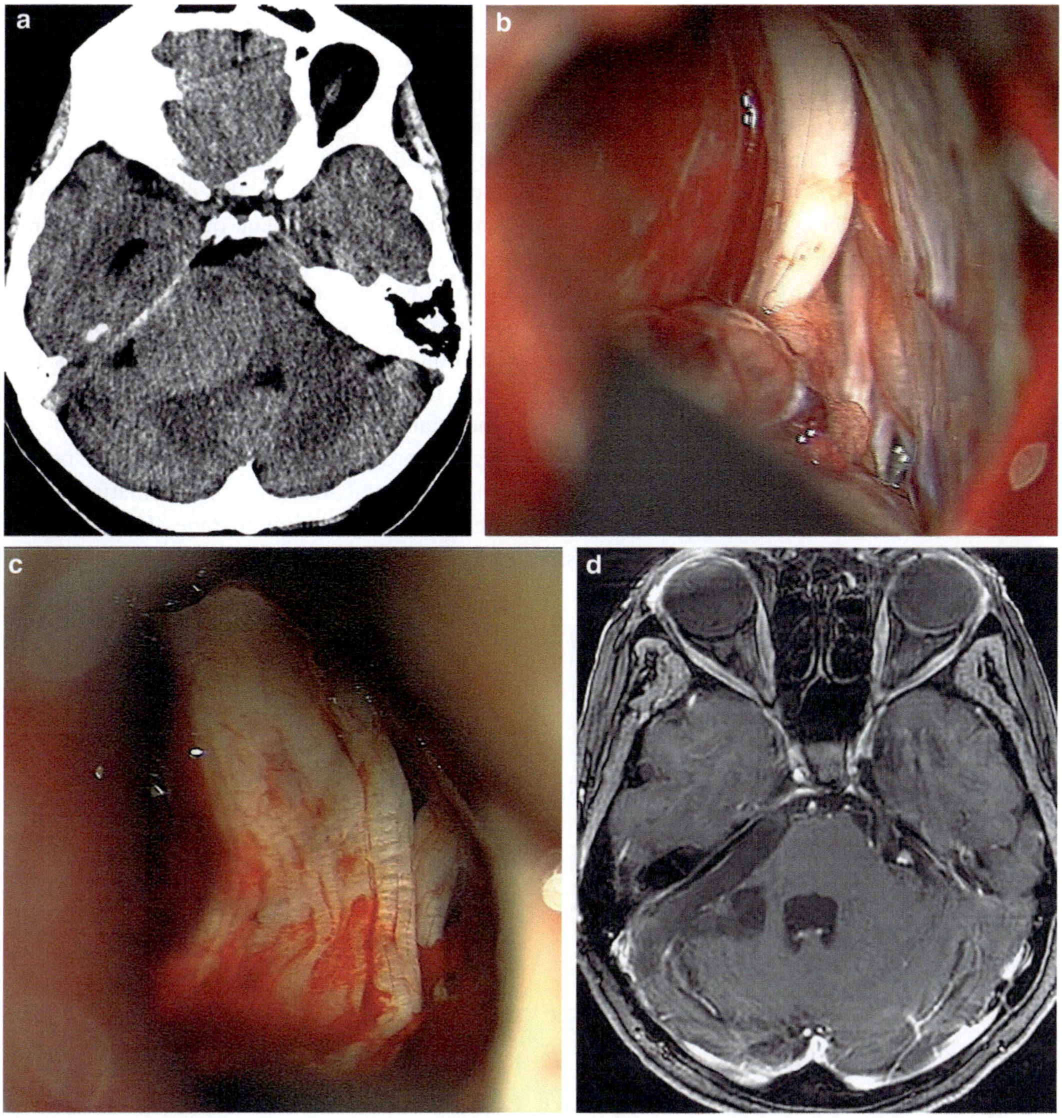

Fig. 11.15 Right premeatal meningioma. (**a**) Axial CT section of the lesion. (**b**) Intraoperative picture displaying the tumor via a retrosigmoid approach, which is located deeper than the facial–vestibulocochlear complex. (**c**) Intraoperative picture after tumor resection, which now allows the trigeminal nerve to be visualized and, in a more superficial and unfocused plane, the facial-vestibulocochlear complex. (**d**) Postoperative axial T1-weighted MRI section with gadolinium, displaying the complete resection of the tumor

and 4 meningiomas. A petrosectomy may be necessary if the tumor infiltrates the temporal bone into the middle ear and hearing is not functional. Conversely, an infralabyrinthine approach should be implemented if hearing is functional. Dissection, release, and mobilization of the facial nerve may be necessary for these petrosal approaches.

11.8.6 Petroclival Meningioma

Petroclival meningiomas necessitate highly intricate microneurosurgical treatment due to their size and profound location. The selection of an approach is contingent upon the surgeon's experience, the objectives of the surgery, and the extent of the lesion. The retrosigmoid approach allows the tumor's access and excision throughout its craniocaudal extension through the windows between the nerves. It is the most effective approach for tiny and small tumors (Fig. 11.16). In the case of large tumors, the retrosigmoid approach necessitates a sustained retraction of the cerebellum throughout the surgery. The surgical field is extremely deep, and the handling of the basilar artery is hazardous. Lastly, a radical resection of the lesion is challenging due to the extensions and the difficulty of accessing the tumor implantation in the dura mater for resection. In some cases, only profuse coagulation of the tumor implant is applicable. The transtentorial access that was previously described can be utilized to optimize resection. This is the reason why a supra-infratentorial posterior petrosal approach or an anterior petrosal middle fossa approach is recommended for large tumors, particularly those that extend to the cavernous sinus or middle fossa. This is significantly more technically challenging and intricate; however, it reduces the distance to the tumor and enables more effective treatment of the meningioma's implantation. Sometimes, these are laborious approaches that are scheduled in two operative sessions: one for the approach and another for the resection, which is scheduled a few days later. There is an alternative approach that is highly beneficial in certain circumstances: the two-stage surgical procedure. The infratentorial portion, which is typically the symptomatic one, is resected during the initial stage. The supratentorial portion of the cavernous sinus, or Meckel's

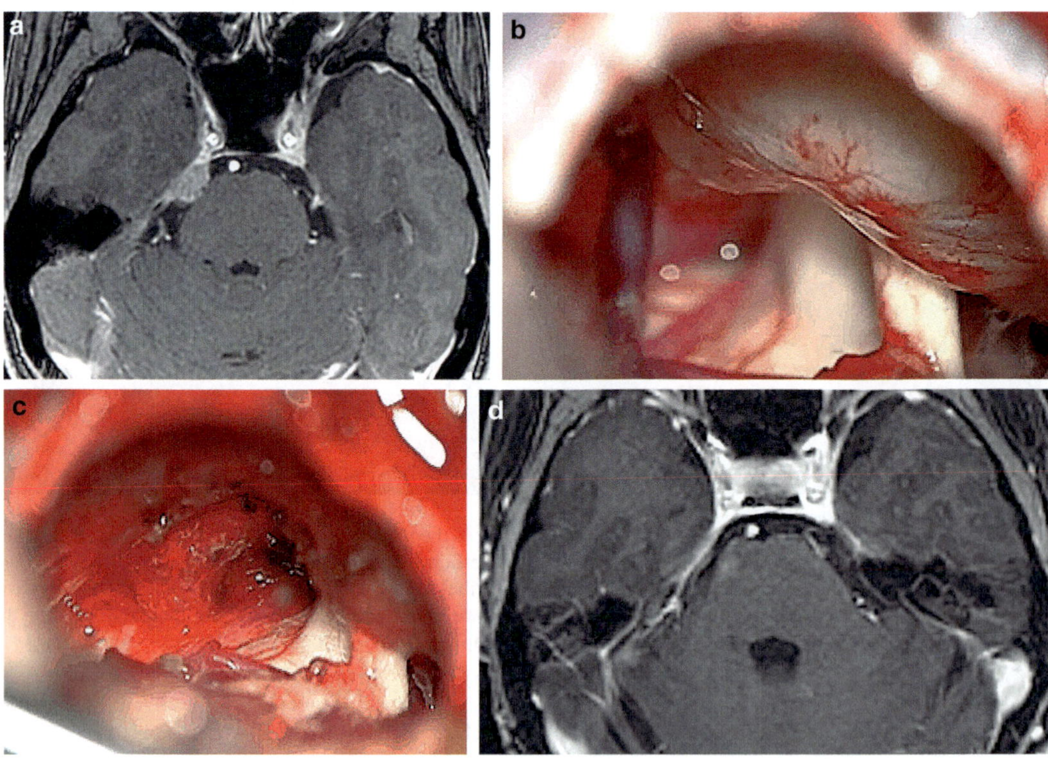

Fig. 11.16 Right small petroclival meningioma. (**a**) Axial T1-weighted MRI section after administration of gadolinium, displaying the tumor. (**b**) Intraoperative picture illustrating the retrosigmoid approach. A massive suprameatal eminence is visible, which obstructs the tumor's visualization. Visible are the trigeminal nerve, the superior petrosal vein complex, and the facial–vestibulocochlear complex, which is more superficial and focal. (**c**) Intraoperative picture following the completion of the suprameatal eminence drilling, which now enables the visualization of the tumor. (**d**) Postoperative axial T1-weighted MRI section obtained with gadolinium, demonstrating the complete resection of the tumor

cave, is the subject of a second stage. Alternatively, these parts of the tumor can be treated by stereotactic radiosurgery or, in cases of asymptomatic patients, imaging observation (Fig. 11.17). Although deep lesions or clival meningiomas are extremely profound lesions that frequently embed the basilar artery or its perforators, it is feasible to perform a complete resection using a retrosigmoid approach (Fig. 11.18). Furthermore, the anatomical and functional integrity of the cranial nerves is jeopardized by the necessity of microsurgical resection through the windows described, as these meningiomas are situated deeper than all of the cranial nerves. A transclival endonasal resection is an alternative technique that enables the early devascularization of the tumor and effective and regulated decompression of the brainstem and neurovascular structures. However, there is a significant risk of postoperative cerebrospinal fluid leak.

11.8.7 Foramen Magnum Meningioma

Posterolateral or anterolateral meningiomas of the foramen magnum are the preferred indication for the far-lateral approach, which is extended caudally with osteoplastic hemilaminectomy of the first cervical levels in accordance with the individual requirements of each patient. In this instance, the fundamental principles of the far-lateral approach and the resection of meningiomas of the cerebellopontine angle, as previously described (Fig. 11.19), are implemented. It is advisable to isolate and manage the vertebral in

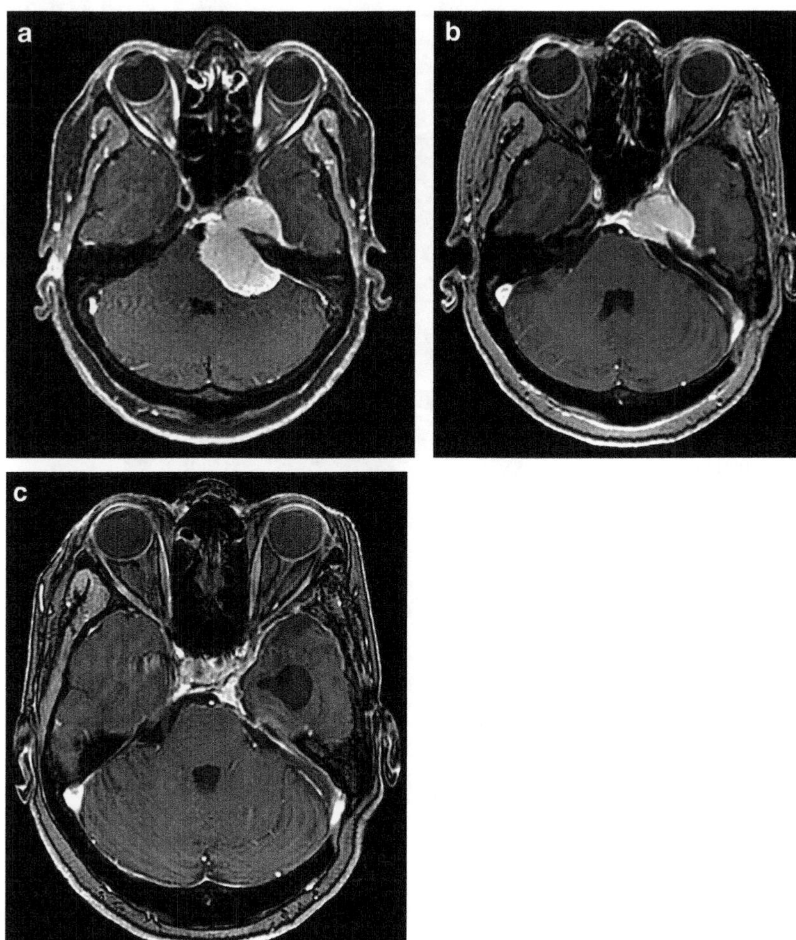

Fig. 11.17 Left petroclinoid meningioma with supratentorial extension. (**a**) An axial T1-weighted MRI section demonstrating a meningioma into the Meckel's cave and middle fossa and a component in the posterior fossa following gadolinium administration. (**b**) Postoperative axial T1-weighted MRI section with gadolinium following the resection of the infratentorial portion via a retrosigmoid approach. (**c**) Postoperative axial T1-weighted MRI section with gadolinium following the resection of the supratentorial portion through an extradural approach of the middle fossa with anterior petrosectomy

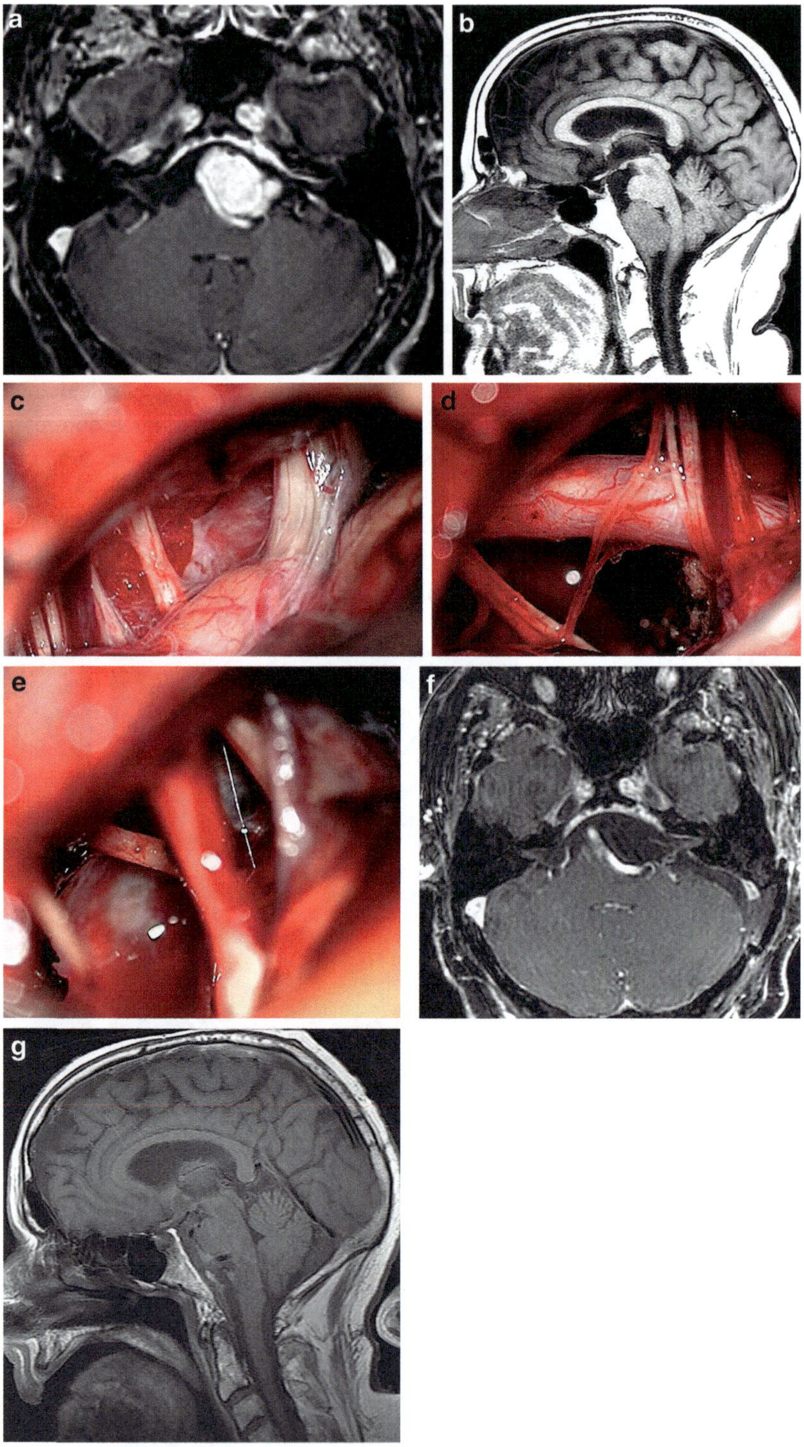

Fig. 11.18 Meningioma of the left clivus. (**a**) Axial T1-weighted MRI section following gadolinium administration, demonstrating the tumor's location, displacing the basilar artery medially. (**b**) Sagittal T1-weighted MRI section. (**c**) Intraoperative picture illustrating the facial–vestibul o–cochlear complex and the lower cranial nerves emerging from the brainstem, as well as the tumor in a deeper plane. (**d**) Intraoperative imaging after basilar artery release. (**e**) The anatomical integrity of all cranial nerves is demonstrated in this intraoperative picture following the entire resection of the tumor. (**f**) Postoperative axial T1-weighted MRI section with gadolinium, demonstrating the complete resection of the tumor and the enhancement of the basilar artery over the pons. (**g**) Postoperative axial T1-weighted MRI section demonstrating the complete resection of the tumor

its extradural V3 segment, as it may be surrounded by the tumor or have infiltrated the adventitia around its entry through the dura mater, despite the fact that it does not directly contribute to the vascularization of the tumor. This extradural vascular dissection enables the identification of a potential extracranial origin of the posterior inferior cerebellar artery and the

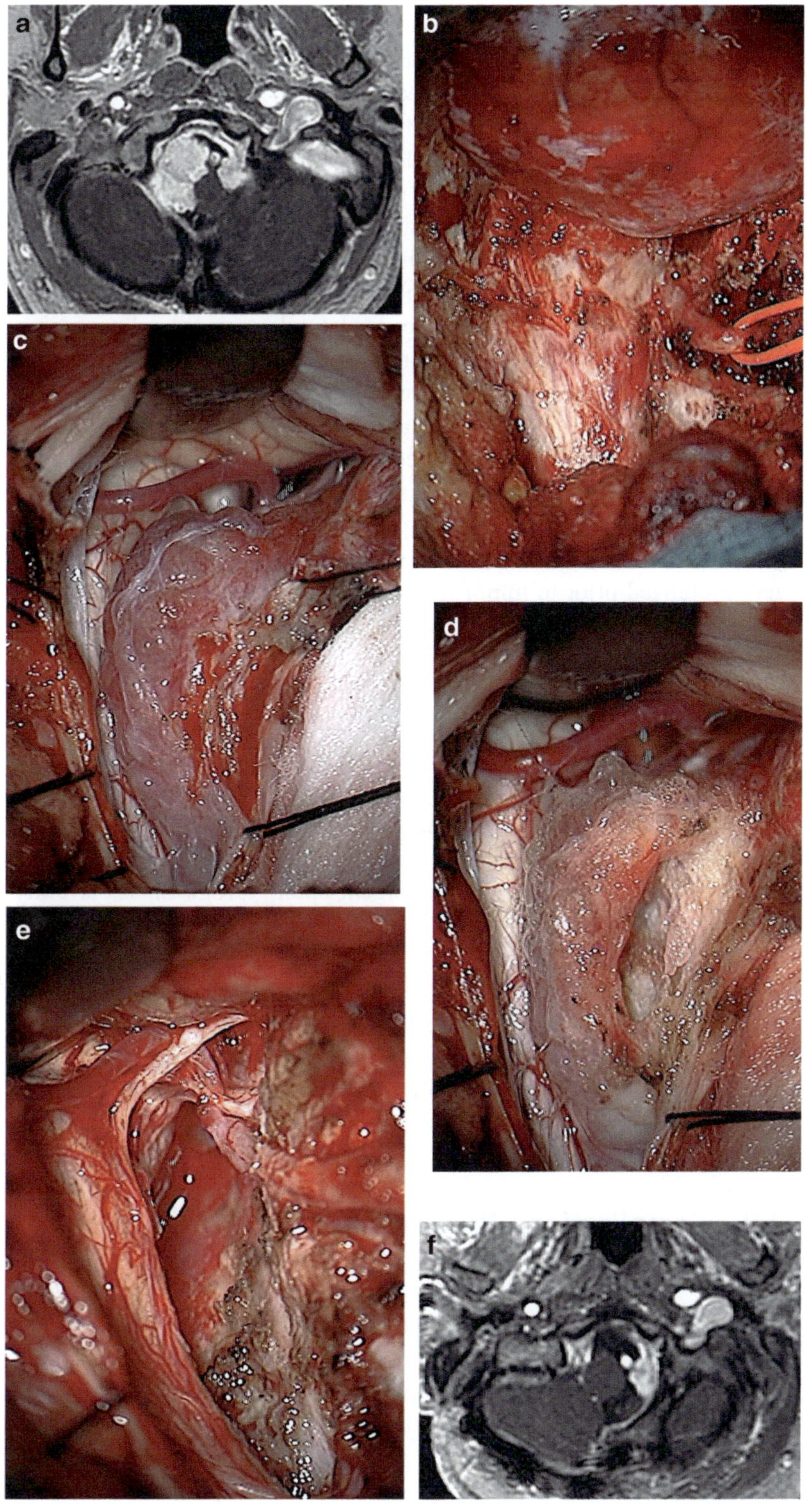

Fig. 11.19 Meningioma of the right foramen magnum. (**a**) Axial section of T1-weighted MRI after gadolinium administration, illustrating the tumor situated in the anterolateral region of the foramen magnum. A second, lesser tumor is present on the contralateral side. (**b**) Intraoperative picture illustrating the far-lateral craniotomy. For proximal control, the vertebral artery has been isolated extradurally. (**c**) Intraoperative picture followed by the release of the tumor following the opening of the dura mater. (**d**) Intraoperative picture following internal decompression. (**e**) Intraoperative picture following the complete resection of the tumor, illustrating the trajectory of the accessory nerve and the vertebral artery. (**f**) Postoperative axial T1-weighted MRI section demonstrating the complete resection of the tumor

coagulation of muscular and dural branches that contribute to the vascularization of the meningioma. The tumor is identified and decompressed with an ultrasonic aspirator after the dura mater is opened. The first insertion of the dentate ligament must be identified, and the relationship between the tumor and the second spinal nerve, the accessory nerve, and the remainder of the lower cranial nerves must be established. The dentate ligament is deeper in the far-lateral approach in posterolateral meningioma, and the vertebral artery is even deeper. Conversely, the dentate ligament and the vertebral artery at its entrance through the dura mater occupy a more superficial position in the far-lateral approach in anterolateral meningiomas. Consequently, the ligament must be sectioned and the vertebral artery mobilized prior to tumor manipulation. A small medial suboccipital approach associated with osteoplastic laminectomy of the first neural arch is the only secure method for resecting meningiomas that are posteriorly located.

11.8.8 Tentorial Meningioma

The selection of an approach is contingent upon the location and extent of each specific tumor. The retrosigmoid approach would be reserved for group 1, or incisural meningiomas, which exhibit caudal growth toward the posterior fossa (Fig. 11.20), and for group 5, or lateral tentorial meningiomas, which exhibit predominant growth toward the posterior fossa.

11.9 Complications, Prevention, and Management

The complications of microneurosurgery for meningiomas of the cerebellopontine angle can be categorized into two major categories: those that arise from the approach and those that arise from the treatment of the tumor. Meningitis, cerebrospinal fluid escape, headache, and venous sinus thrombosis are among the complications that may occur from the retrosigmoid approach. These complications have been previously examined in the retrosigmoid approach chapter. Vascular complications and cranial nerve dysfunction are among the complications that may arise as a consequence of tumor removal. Complications in the context of meningiomas are defined as the deterioration or loss of function of any cranial nerve in patients who are in a state of normal function at the time of surgery. In contrast to schwannoma, the anatomical relationships between the nerves and the tumor are more apparent, enabling the tumor to be more easily identified, individualized, and mobilized from the neurovascular structures. This is due to the presence of an arachnoid layer that separates the tumor from the nerve. Consequently, the prognosis is highly auspicious in the event of neurological dysfunction. Nevertheless, the prognosis is extremely cautious when the cochlear nerve is anatomically preserved and there is a postoperative hearing loss. The opening of the mastoid cells during the craniotomy may result in a sensation of ear fullness, which is frequently accompanied by a hearing loss. Fortunately, the prognosis is currently favorable. A cophosis may result from an injury to the internal auditory artery or the mechanical effect of the vibration caused by the high-speed motor, and the prognosis is extremely poor. Cerebellar function and the long sensory-motor pathways may also deteriorate, although this is typically transient or temporary. The arachnoid layer, which is aforementioned, ensures that the arteries are well separated from the tumor. However, in certain instances, the artery remains embedded within the tumor and must be extracted, with the perforating branches preserved. Removal is also facilitated by the presence of a clear plane of demarcation between the tumor and the nervous tissue. The cleavage plane is only lost in tumors that are extremely large or aggressive. In the chapter that is dedicated to the retrosigmoid approach and general aspects of vestibular

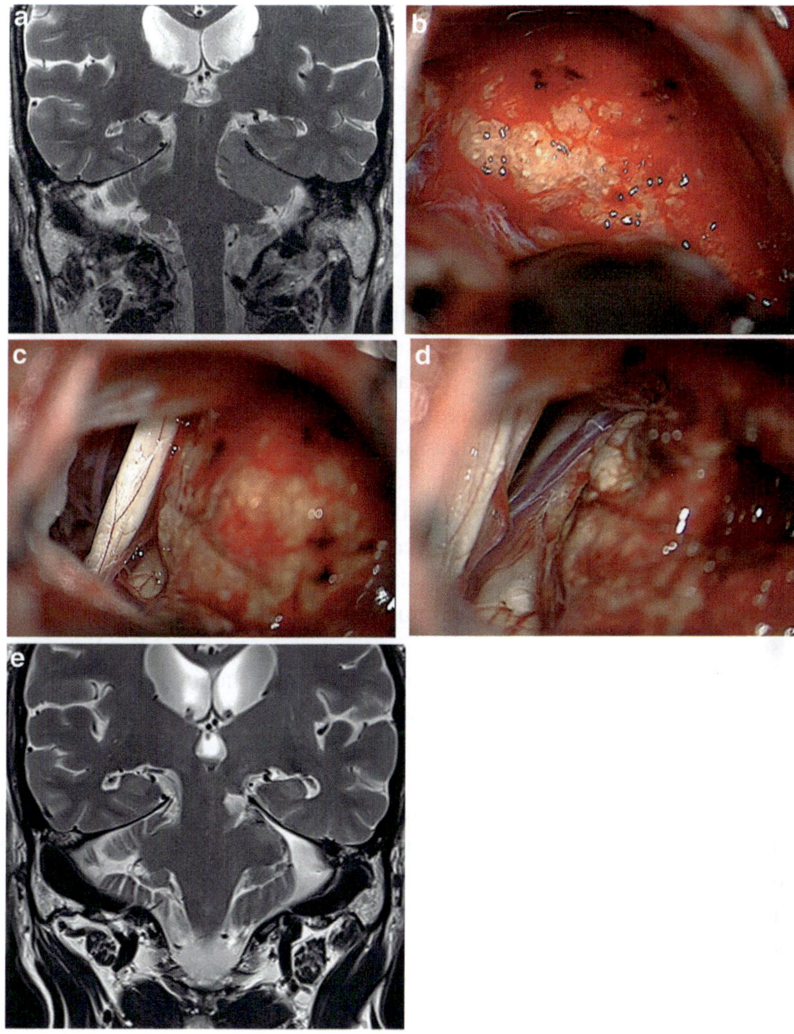

Fig. 11.20 Meningioma of the left tentorial incisure. (**a**) Coronal T2-enhanced MRI section. (**b**) Intraoperative picture illustrating the tumor via a retrosigmoid approach. (**c**) Intraoperative picture obtained following cranial mobilization of the capsule and internal decompression, which enables the visualization of the facial–vestibulocochlear complex. (**d**) Intraoperative picture illustrating the trigeminal nerve. (**e**) A postoperative coronal T2-weighted MRI section that demonstrates the complete resection of the tumor

schwannoma, the general principles of prevention and management of these complications have been reviewed.

11.10 Results, Prognosis, and Follow-Up

In this section, we will provide a comprehensive overview of the prognosis of cerebellopontine angle meningiomas, with a few observations regarding petroclival meningiomas, which are distinguished from other locations by their challenges in responding to microneurosurgical treatment.

In general, the rate of *gross total resection* (GTR) varies from 60% to 95% of cases, and perioperative mortality is less than 10%. Recurrence rates fall within the range of 0–30% of cases. Anatomical preservation of the cranial nerves is feasible in nearly all instances, in contrast to schwannomas, and the facial or vestibulocochlear nerve is functionally preserved in over 80% of cases. The deficitary clinical symptoms typically improve, and any deterioration is usually temporary. Nevertheless, the prognosis of patients with cerebellopontine angle meningiomas that are treated with microneurosurgery is influenced by a variety of factors. The initial factor is the meningioma's volume and location.

These outcome data are significantly worse as the depth of the meningioma in the cerebellopontine angle and the size of the tumor increase. In this regard, the meningioma's position in relation to the plane of the cranial nerves that we have delineated is crucial, as tumors that are situated at a greater depth are at a higher risk. Petroclival meningiomas are significantly more common than those in any other location in the cerebellopontine angle, as well as in any of the surgical series consulted, regardless of the surgeon's or center's experience. Subtotal or partial resection, morbidity, and mortality are significantly more common in petroclival meningiomas. This is likely to be followed by a meningioma of the foramen magnum. In the presence of these formidable lesions, meningiomas of the convexity of the cerebellum are the most suitable for the patient's radical and secure microsurgical resection.

The degree of resection is a second factor in the prognosis of meningioma of the cerebellopontine angle and the incidence of recurrence. The grades of resection of meningiomas were defined by Simpson in 1957 and are still valid: grade 1, with macroscopically complete resection of the tumor, including the tumor and the dura mater on which it grows and removing all the underlying abnormal bone, leading to a 10% recurrence rate at 5 years; grade 2, with macroscopic resection of the tumor and profuse coagulation of the underlying dura mater, with a 20% recurrence rate at 5 years; grade 3, with macroscopic resection of the tumor but without any action on the underlying dura mater, with a 30% recurrence rate at 5 years; grade 4, with subtotal resection of the tumor; and, finally, grade 5, with simple decompression of the tumor, which have high rates of progression and regrowth similar to the natural history of meningioma. Subsequently, a grade 0 resection was proposed, which involved the macroscopically complete resection of the tumor, the dura mater, and the underlying anomalous bone in addition to the resection of 4 cm of dura mater around the tumor implant or the resection of 2 cm of dura mater around the tumor implant with en bloc resection of the underlying hyperostotic bone. This radicality in the resection was derived from the observation that macronodules of meningothelial cells, which are typically 1–8 mm in diameter, or microscopic islands of meningothelial cells, are frequently present around meningiomas. These nodules are interspersed in the fibrous sheets of the dura mater or the fibrous tissue surrounding the dura mater, making it possible for the tumor to recur. Regrettably, grade 1 resection is exceedingly challenging to execute in cerebellopontine angle meningioma, and grade 0 resection is entirely unattainable. In contrast to 40% of skull base tumors, convexity meningioma patients achieve complete or grade 1 resection in 80% of cases. Consequently, the prognosis regarding survival and the absence of recurrence is considerably worse.

The WHO grade is another critical factor in the prognosis of cerebellopontine angle meningioma. After Simpson grade 1 resection, grade 1 meningiomas, which comprise approximately 90% of the total, have a five-year recurrence rate of 10–15% and a survival rate that is nearly 100%. Grade 2 meningiomas, which comprise approximately 6% of the total, have a recurrence rate of 40% after grade 1 resection and a survival rate of 80%. Grade 3 meningiomas, which comprise the remaining 4%, have a recurrence rate of over 70% after grade 1 resection and a survival rate of less than 10%. WHO grades 2–3 account for approximately 12% of cerebral convexity meningiomas, whereas this percentage is considerably lower in the case of skull base meningiomas, at approximately 3%. This most favorable prognosis is explicated by certain genetic and cell proliferation markers. This results in a more favorable overall prognosis for meningiomas of the cerebellopontine angle and the skull base [19].

The neurosurgeon can only positively influence the prognosis by accomplishing complete resection of the tumor and its dural implantation, thereby maximizing the degree of resection, as recurrence occurs from the same cell lines as those of the original tumor. Therefore, in 75% of recurrences, the same cell clones as in the original tumor are observed, whereas in the remaining recurrences, the same cell lines are discovered with the addition of some chromosomal mutations.

11.11 Management Modalities

Meningiomas are tumors that develop and typically necessitate treatment during the patient's lifetime. After the diagnosis of a cerebellopontine angle meningioma, there are three management options: clinical and imaging observation, stereotactic radiosurgery, and microneurosurgical treatment. Other pharmacological interventions are of marginal utility; however, they will also be examined.

11.11.1 Complete Microneurosurgical Resection

In general, the most effective treatment for meningioma is GTR, which has the lowest recurrence rate. Harvey Cushing defended and proposed this view in 1922 when he stated, in reference to spinal meningioma, that "There is today nothing in the whole realm of surgery more gratifying than the successful removal of a meningioma with subsequent perfect functional recovery, especially should a correct pathological diagnosis have been previously made."

In numerous cerebellopontine angle meningiomas, this approach is feasible; however, it is cumbersome in petroclival meningiomas of intermediate (2–4 cm) or large (>4 cm) dimensions. It has been demonstrated that 75% of asymptomatic petroclival meningiomas grow, and 60% of patients deteriorate over an average of 7 years. So the recommendation for small asymptomatic tumors is clinical and imaging observation and early microneurosurgical treatment in case of symptoms or relevant growth. The most effective treatment for small (<2 cm) symptomatic or paucisymptomatic petroclival meningiomas is radical microneurosurgical treatment, which is achieved in nearly all cases with a morbidity of less than 10% and without severe complications. This is attributable, in part, to the straightforward and straightforward nature of microneurosurgical treatment, which is conducted using a standard retrosigmoid approach.

In larger petroclival meningiomas, in a significant number of cases, the surgical approach itself is the cause of the elevated morbidity and mortality rates that follow gross total resection. Al-Mefty has defended this aggressive strategy for these tumors in recent decades. The rationale for this stance is that the tumor remains' behavior is unpredictable in terms of the speed of growth and prognostic grade of recurrence, that stereotactic is not always effective in controlling the growth of the tumor remains, that ionizing radiation of any type only delays the inevitable recurrence and could also induce a change in the grade of the tumor when it recurs, that the quality of life of the patient is improved in the medium or long term by the removal of the entire tumor, and, finally, that the surgical field is significantly altered by the previous surgery and/or stereotactic radiosurgery if a reintervention is necessary, and morbidity increases significantly.

11.11.2 Subtotal Microneurosurgical Resection

Although the aim of microneurosurgical treatment of meningiomas should be GTR with Simpson grade 1, this is not always feasible or desirable in all cases. We have already mentioned the difficulties in radical and extensive treatment of the dural implantation base and the underlying bone in tumors of different topographies, in addition to cases of invasion of the dural sinuses, lack of cleavage plane with the brain stem, invasion of the skull base foramina for cranial nerves, or extra-compartmental extension of the tumor. These factors render Simpson grade 1 resection impossible. To address this issue, an alternative strategy is NTR (*Near Total Resection*) or STR (*Subtotal Resection*) of the tumor, deliberately leaving tumor remains in compromised sites with a double justification. The initial objective is to prevent the exacerbation of neurological morbidity, particularly in the cranial nerves. This has resulted in the notion that it is preferable to maintain a tumor remnant rather than introduce a transient or permanent neurological deficit. This would be further supported by the demonstrated lower risk of recurrence of meningiomas of the skull base in comparison to those outside the skull base with the same histological type and degree of Simpson resection. The second justification is predicated on the potential for stereotactic radiosurgery treatment to be administered to the tumor remnants that are intentionally left after microneurosurgery.

11.11.3 Adaptive Resection

In complex and large meningiomas, an eclectic approach is to adjust the resection to the intraoperative difficulties and findings, excluding the portions of the tumor that are likely to compromise the neurovascular structures and brainstem, either anatomically or functionally, during the resection. This adaptive strategy reduces the percentage of GTR in exchange for a 50% reduction in added morbidity, despite the fact that it triples the recurrence rate. However, adaptive resection cannot be anarchic; it must adhere to a strict strategy.

Consequently, in the event of tumors that exceed the cerebellopontine angle, an effort must be made to complete the infratentorial resection. If infratentorial resection cannot be completed or the lesion is only infratentorial, resection of the cranial and/or caudal portions of the lesion is completed through the appropriate windows, then decompression of the tumor is performed as radically as possible through the other available windows, leaving behind the truly unresectable portion of the tumor, which is either observed or treated with stereotactic radiosurgery postoperatively. If the infratentorial resection is successful and the supratentorial tumor remains inaccessible due to extension to the cavernous sinus, as is frequently the case, the same approach is implemented. The residual tumor is either monitored through imaging or treated with stereotactic radiosurgery if it develops symptoms or expands. If the remaining supratentorial tumor is inaccessible following a complete infratentorial resection, despite transtentorial access, and has an extensive growth into the middle fossa, a second surgical procedure can be contemplated using the most appropriate supratentorial approach.

11.11.4 Staged Resection

Another surgical approach for large and complex cerebellopontine angle meningiomas is to plan their microneurosurgical resection in two or more stages. This involves beginning with a retrosigmoid approach to decompress the brainstem and cranial nerves, which alleviates the patient's symptoms and achieves the maximum possible tumor resection. Subsequently, a second and, eventually, a third approach are implemented to complete the resection of the remaining tumor (refer to case 14 in Chap. 21). This may be of interest in petroclival meningiomas, sphenopetroclival meningiomas, or tentorial meningiomas with a significant supratentorial component. The second approach should once again aim to achieve the maximal resection of the meningioma in that compartment and to connect this resection with that achieved by the retrosigmoid approach. Consequently, the upper limit of tumor resection that can be obtained with the retrosigmoid approach should be determined and acknowledged upon the implementation of the second supratentorial approach. The supratentorial approach is performed either days or weeks following the initial retrosigmoid approach, after the patient has recovered from the initial surgery or has made progress in addressing their clinical symptoms or additional neurological deficits. If the tumor remnant is asymptomatic, it can be subjected to imaging observation until it becomes symptomatic or an unmistakable growth is observed.

11.11.5 Stereotactic Radiosurgery

When microneurosurgical treatment is not feasible, when a portion of the tumor persists after microneurosurgical NTR or STR, or when the patient declines microneurosurgical treatment, stereotactic radiosurgery is a viable alternative for the treatment of cerebellopontine angle meningioma. If safe microneurosurgical gross total resection of the tumor is feasible, stereotactic radiosurgery should never be implemented as the initial treatment option. However, stereotactic radiosurgery has been employed primarily in a series of patients with petroclival meningiomas that are smaller than 30 mm. In 90% of cases, it has demonstrated tumor growth control. However, 5% of patients have new neurological deficits, some of which are severe due to brainstem injury. The average follow-up period is only 3 years. In any event, tumors exhibit a reduction in size in a relatively small number of instances. The treatment of tumor remnants with stereotactic results in the control of tumor growth in approximately 90% of patients, with a 10% rate of persistent complications. One of the major criticisms of stereotactic radiosurgery treatment of skull base meningiomas, whether as a first-line treatment or on tumor remains, is that studies have short follow-ups and that late recurrence is relatively frequent, even several years after treatment. Recurrence can have a higher grade and growth rate than the tumor initially treated. Nevertheless, stereotactic radiosurgery would be effective in tumors that are less than 25–30 mm in maximal diameter and 8–10 cc in volume. The high rate of complications associated with the use of ionizing radiation as a first-line treatment for large tumors, particularly in the form of cranial nerve dysfunction and brain stem edema, raises concerns about its efficacy in treating these types of large lesions [20].

11.11.6 Pharmacological Treatment

Historically, the predominance of women in the incidence of meningiomas and the presence of progesterone receptors in 70% and estrogen receptors in 30% of them were regarded as significant. Progesterone and estrogen antagonists were employed in instances of intractable recurrences or high-grade tumors because of this, but the results were generally unsatisfactory. The same has occurred with a series of chemotherapeutic agents, which have occasionally yielded promising results in in vitro studies but have demonstrated minimal efficacy in clinical practice. In the clinic, the most recent attempts at treatment with antiangiogenic agents, genetic therapies, or immunotherapy have not yielded beneficial results.

11.12 Key Messages

- *Meningioma is the second most prevalent tumor variety that develops in the cerebellopontine angle. The clinical appearance of the tumor is subject to significant variation due to the fact that it is contingent upon its location and size.*
- *Since the cerebellopontine angle is surrounded by meningeal and arachnoid layers with leptomeningeal cells, meningioma can develop at any point along the cerebellopontine angle. Cerebellopontine angle meningioma is classified in a variety of ways as a result.*
- *Meningiomas are typically benign WHO grade I lesions that can be effectively treated through aggressive resection. The cerebellopontine angle's restricted volume presents a challenge for Simpson grade 1 resection.*
- *A retrosigmoid technique can be used to remove the majority of cerebellopontine angle meningiomas. The microneurosurgical excision is systematic as it is conducted through the windows that compromise the cranial nerve roots of the cerebellopontine angle.*
- *Unless it is caused by ischemia, meningioma has a fair outcome, a very low recurrence rate, low mortality, and a favorable morbidity prognosis.*

References

1. Samii M, Tatagiba M, Carvalho GA. Retrosigmoid intradural suprameatal approach to Meckel's cave and the middle fossa: surgical technique and outcome. J Neurosurg. 2000;92:235–41. https://doi.org/10.3171/jns.2000.92.2.0235.
2. Chae R, Rodriguez RR. Anatomy of petrosal face. Handb Clin Neurol. 2020;170:143–56. https://doi.org/10.1016/B978-0-12-822198-3.00036-7.
3. Gonzalez-Darder JM, Quilis-Quesada V, Capilla-Guasch P, de Oliveira E. Abordajes neuroquirúrgicos

de la patología craneal y cerebral. 2nd ed. Barcelona: Elsevier España; 2020.

4. Rhoton AL Jr. The posterior fossa: microsurgical anatomy & surgical approaches. Neurosurgery. 2000;47(Suppl 3):S1–S279. https://doi.org/10.1097/00006123-200009001-00013.
5. Kerr K, Qualmann K, Esquenazi Y, et al. Familial syndromes involving meningiomas provide mechanistic insight into sporadic disease. Neurosurgery. 2018;83:1107–18. https://doi.org/10.1093/neuros/nyy121.
6. Yamanaka R, Hayano A, Kanayama T. Radiation-induced meningiomas: an exhaustive review of the literature. World Neurosurg. 2027;97:635–644.e8. https://doi.org/10.1016/j.wneu.2016.09.094.
7. Bakar B. Jugular foramen meningiomas: review of the major surgical series. Neurol Med Chir (Tokyo). 2010;50:89–96. https://doi.org/10.2176/nmc.50.89.
8. Macdonald AJ, Salzman KL, Harnsberger HR, et al. Primary jugular foramen meningioma: imaging appearance and differentiating features. AJR Am J Roentgenol. 2004;182:373–7. https://doi.org/10.2214/ajr.182.2.1820373.
9. Sanna M, Bacciu A, Falcioni M, et al. Surgical management of jugular foramen meningiomas: a series of 13 cases and review of the literature. Laryngoscope. 2007;117:1710–9. https://doi.org/10.1097/MLG.0b013e3180cc20a3.
10. Almefty R, Dunn IF, Pravdenkova S, et al. True petroclival meningiomas: results of surgical management. J Neurosurg. 2024;120:40–51. https://doi.org/10.3171/2013.8.JNS13535.
11. Giammattei L, di Russo P, Starnoni D, et al. Petroclival meningiomas: update of current treatment and consensus by the EANS skull base section. Acta Neurochir. 2021;163:1639–63. https://doi.org/10.1007/s00701-021-04798-z.
12. Van Havenbergh T, Carvalho G, Tatagiba M, et al. Natural history of petroclival meningiomas. Neurosurgery. 2003;52:55–62. https://doi.org/10.1097/00006123-200301000-00006.
13. Leon-Ariza DS, Campero A, Romero Chaparro RJ, et al. Key aspects in foramen magnum meningiomas: from old neuroanatomical conceptions to current far lateral neurosurgical intervention. World Neurosurg. 2017;106:477–83. https://doi.org/10.1016/j.wneu.2017.07.029.
14. Bir SC, Tanmoy K, et al. Foramen magnum meningiomas. Handb Clin Neurol. 2020;170:167–74. https://doi.org/10.1016/B978-0-12-822198-3.00038-0.
15. Nanda A, Patra DP, Savardekar A, et al. Tentorial meningiomas: reappraisal of surgical approaches and their outcomes. World Neurosurg. 2018;110:e177–96. https://doi.org/10.1016/j.wneu.2017.10.115.
16. Nakamura M, Roser F, Mirzai S, et al. Meningiomas of the internal auditory canal. Neurosurgery. 2004;55:119–27. https://doi.org/10.1227/01.neu.000012688.
17. Samii M, Gerganov V. Surgery of cerebellopontine angle lesions. Berlin-Heidelberg: Springer; 2013.
18. Seoane E, Rhoton AL Jr. Suprameatal extension of the retrosigmoid approach: microsurgical anatomy. Neurosurgery. 1999;44:553–60. https://doi.org/10.1097/00006123-199903000-00065.
19. McGovern SL, Aldape KD, Munsell MF, et al. A comparison of World Health Organization tumour grades at recurrence in patients with non-skull base and skull base meningiomas. J Neurosurg. 2010;112:925–33. https://doi.org/10.3171/2009.9.JNS09617.
20. Couldwell WT, Cole CD, Al-Mefty O. Patterns of skull base meningioma progression after failed radiosurgery. J Neurosurg. 2007;106:30–5. https://doi.org/10.3171/jns.2007.106.1.30.

Other Tumors of the Cerebellopontine Angle

12

12.1 Introduction

Schwannomas of the vestibular nerve are the most common tumors of the cerebellopontine angle, followed by meningiomas and epidermoid cysts. Vestibular schwannoma, meningioma, and epidermoid cyst account for over 90% of the cerebellopontine angle tumors, with the remaining 10% of cases containing other tumoral lesions. These tumors can present challenges in terms of differential diagnosis with the most common tumors, as well as in the selection of the treatment modality, particularly microneurosurgical treatment. In a separate chapter, we have addressed schwannomas of cranial nerves that are not the vestibular schwannoma. Additionally, we will later review cystic tumors that are not the epidermoid cyst. Other solid non-meningioma tumors that affect the cerebellopontine angle and others that are typically excised through the retrosigmoid approach will be examined in this chapter.

12.2 Classification

Given that this group of lesions is highly heterogeneous and has a relatively low incidence, there are numerous classifications [1–8]. In the book by Bambakidis, Megerian, and Spetzler, tumors of the cerebellopontine angle and petrosal bone are studied together and subdivided into tumors of the petrosal apex and petroclival region (petroclival meningioma, trigeminal schwannoma, cholesterol granuloma, among others), medial petrosal surface (vestibular and facial schwannoma, petrosal meningioma, and endolymphatic sac tumor), upper surface of the petrosal bone (middle fossa meningioma, schwannoma, and geniculate ganglion hemangioma), lateral area of the petrosal bone (tympanic paraganglioma, among others), and lower area of the petrosal bone (jugular paraganglioma, schwannomas of the lower cranial nerves and hypoglossal nerve, among others), leaving aside non-neoplastic lesions [1]. This classification fails to account for critical lesions such as meningiomas of the foramen magnum or intra-axial tumors of the brainstem. Conversely, it encompasses a substantial number of temporal bone tumors that are not amenable to resection through the cerebellopontine angle using a conventional retrosigmoid approach.

Several anatomical criteria will be employed in this section to classify the various tumor varieties in this chapter. The cerebellopontine angle can be characterized as a dihedral angle in a very general sense, with a medial plane formed by the brainstem, middle cerebellar peduncle, and petrosal surface of the cerebellum and a lateral plane formed by the posterior surface of the petrosal bone and occipital bone. These planes converge toward the petroclival junction, the deepest portion of the cerebellopontine angle.

J. M. González-Darder, *Microneurosurgery of Cerebellopontine Angle*,
https://doi.org/10.1007/978-3-032-03091-7_12

This concept enables the development of a topographic classification of tumors into three major categories: tumors that originate in the cisterns of the cerebellopontine angle, with the exception of schwannomas and cystic lesions; intra- or extra-axial tumors that originate in the medial surface of the cerebellopontine angle but occupy or invade this space; and, finally, tumors that originate in the lateral aspect of the cerebellopontine angle, with the exception of meningiomas, and that occupy or invade the cerebellopontine angle.

12.3 Tumors Originated Within the Cerebellopontine Angle

This category encompasses tumors that arise in the cerebellopontine angle's cisterns. The cisterns contain cranial nerves, arteries, and potentially embryonic remains, which are all embedded in the arachnoid membranes and cerebrospinal fluid (CSF). The majority of tumors that originate in the cerebellopontine angle structures are schwannomas that arise from the cranial nerves and various types of cystic lesions, which have been thoroughly examined in other chapters. Lipomas, paragangliomas, metastases, and a wide range of exceptional lesions are significantly less common.

12.3.1 Lipoma

The frequency of intracranial lipoma in autopsy or imaging investigations is established at 0.08% of intracranial tumors, with cerebellopontine angle lipoma accounting for 0.1% of tumors of this topography. There are 219 cases that have been described in a recent systematic review of the literature; however, a significant number of other observed cases have not been published. The pathogenesis of intracranial lipoma is not well understood. Lipomas are believed to be the result of the anomalous differentiation of specific cells in the primitive neural crest. The result is a very slow-growing lesion that envelops rather than displaces neurological structures. In reality, it is exceedingly uncommon to document the growth of an intracranial lipoma during the course of clinical or imaging examinations. Additionally, there are no documented instances of malignant transformation.

Clinically, they are diagnosed in the fourth decade of life, with an equal frequency in both sexes and on both sides. They may be bilateral in exceptional cases. In 70% of patients, hearing loss is the most common presenting symptom, followed by vertigo or instability in 50% and tinnitus in 50%. They may exhibit irritating symptoms, including hemifacial spasm or trigeminal neuralgia. Nevertheless, the number of asymptomatic lipomas is on the rise as a result of the increase in imaging studies. Both computed tomography (CT) and magnetic resonance imaging (MRI) are highly specific for imaging diagnosis, as they exhibit identical behavior to subcutaneous fat. In CT they are hypointense masses that are well-circumscribed and do not acquire contrast. They may exhibit some marginal calcification. In the T1-weighted sequence of the MRI, a hyperintense signal is observed. This signal is attenuated in fat suppression sequences and does not acquire contrast after the administration of gadolinium. In T2-weighted sequences, they exhibit the same intensity and signal characteristics as subcutaneous fat (Fig. 12.1).

The indication for microneurosurgical treatment is the most intriguing neurosurgical aspect of cerebellopontine angle lipomas, in addition to their rarity. In this context, resection is the sole appropriate course of action for patients who exhibit pertinent symptoms and are unresponsive to symptomatic medical treatment. Several cerebellopontine angle lipomas were investigated for biopsy and diagnostic confirmation prior to the development of imaging techniques. This was a common occurrence in the context of symptomatic lipomas. Of the symptomatic patients who underwent microneurosurgical resection, 20% of the symptomatic patients experienced some improvement in their symptoms, while 70% experienced new symptoms or a worsening of

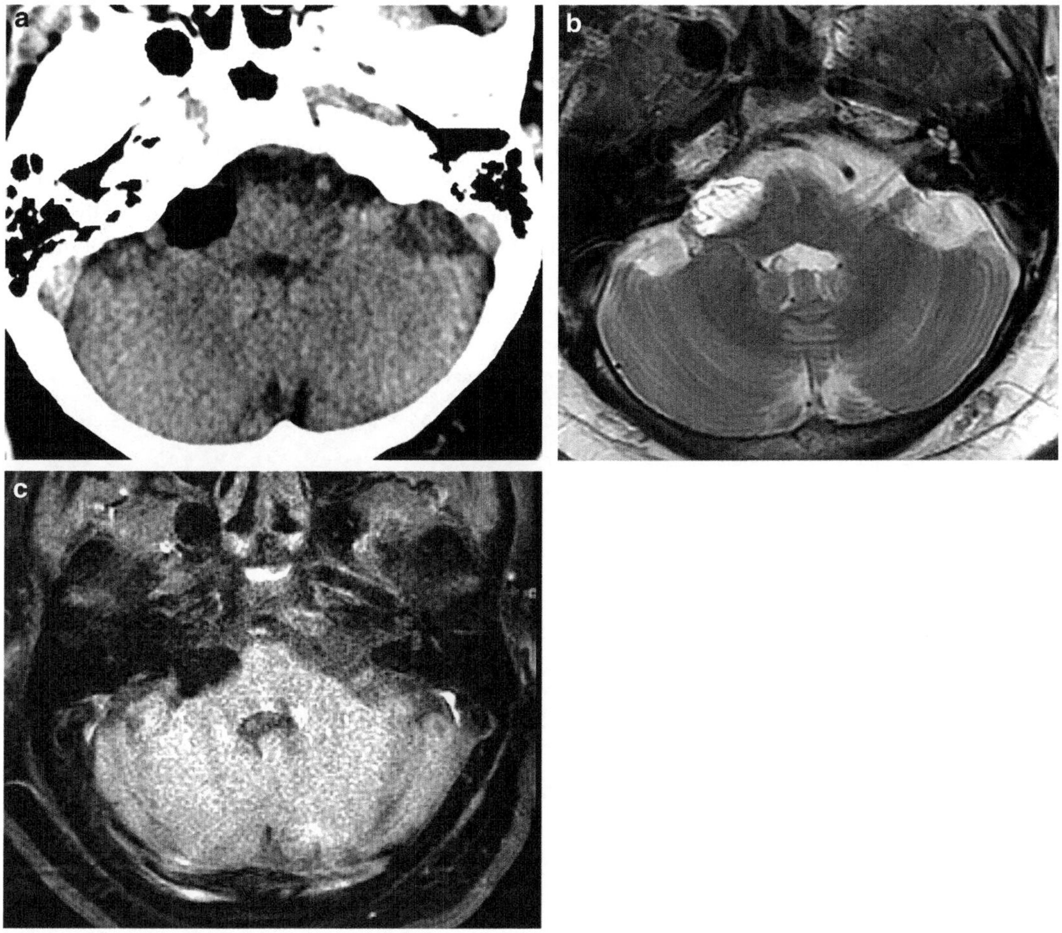

Fig. 12.1 Lipoma. A well-delimited lesion is seen in the right cerebellopontine angle, which has the same density as the subcutaneous fat. (**a**) Axial TC without contrast. (**b**) Axial T2-weighted MRI. (**c**) Axial fat suppression T1-weighted MRI

established ones. Fortunately, the nature and natural history of the lipoma have been better understood through the use of imaging techniques that enable the precise diagnosis and follow-up of the lesion. These tumors are usually quiescent, and there is no surgical indication to confirm the diagnosis or prevent potential growth or malignancy. Consequently, the sole indication would be in patients who experience symptoms such as intractable trigeminal neuralgia, hemifacial spasm, or severe vertigo. The emergence of new deficit symptoms is a possibility, and improvement is not guaranteed after surgery. The lipoma's growing pattern, which embeds the cranial nerves, renders the attempt at radical microneurosurgical resection, which involves the removal of all the fat tissue surrounding and adhering to the nerves, highly hazardous. It is advisable to implement internal decompression in a manner that is as generous as possible to alleviate tension and pressure on the nerves in the event of large lipomas. Even in small symptomatic lipomas, the recommendation is to reduce the volume of small lipomas and, if there are arteries that could cause symptomatic nerve compression symptoms, conduct an indirect microvascular decompression of the nerve by separating the arteries from the injured nerve root [9].

12.3.2 Paraganglioma

Paragangliomas are neuroendocrine tumors that arise from paraganglionic cells of the vessels and nervous system of the second branchial arch, which are derived embryonically from the neural crest. Consequently, paragangliomas are present in all regions of the adult body where this form of cell is present. In the head and neck, they form clusters in the middle ear in association with the Jacobson nerve, a branch of the glossopharyngeal nerve, and the Arnold nerve, a branch of the vagal nerve. Additionally, they are present in the jugular foramen in relation to the jugular vein and bulb and in the carotid body, which is situated at the bifurcation of the primitive carotid artery in the neck. Paragangliomas of the cerebellopontine angle may be the consequence of jugulotympanic tumor invasion (Fig. 12.2) or a metastasis of an uncommon malignant paraganglioma.

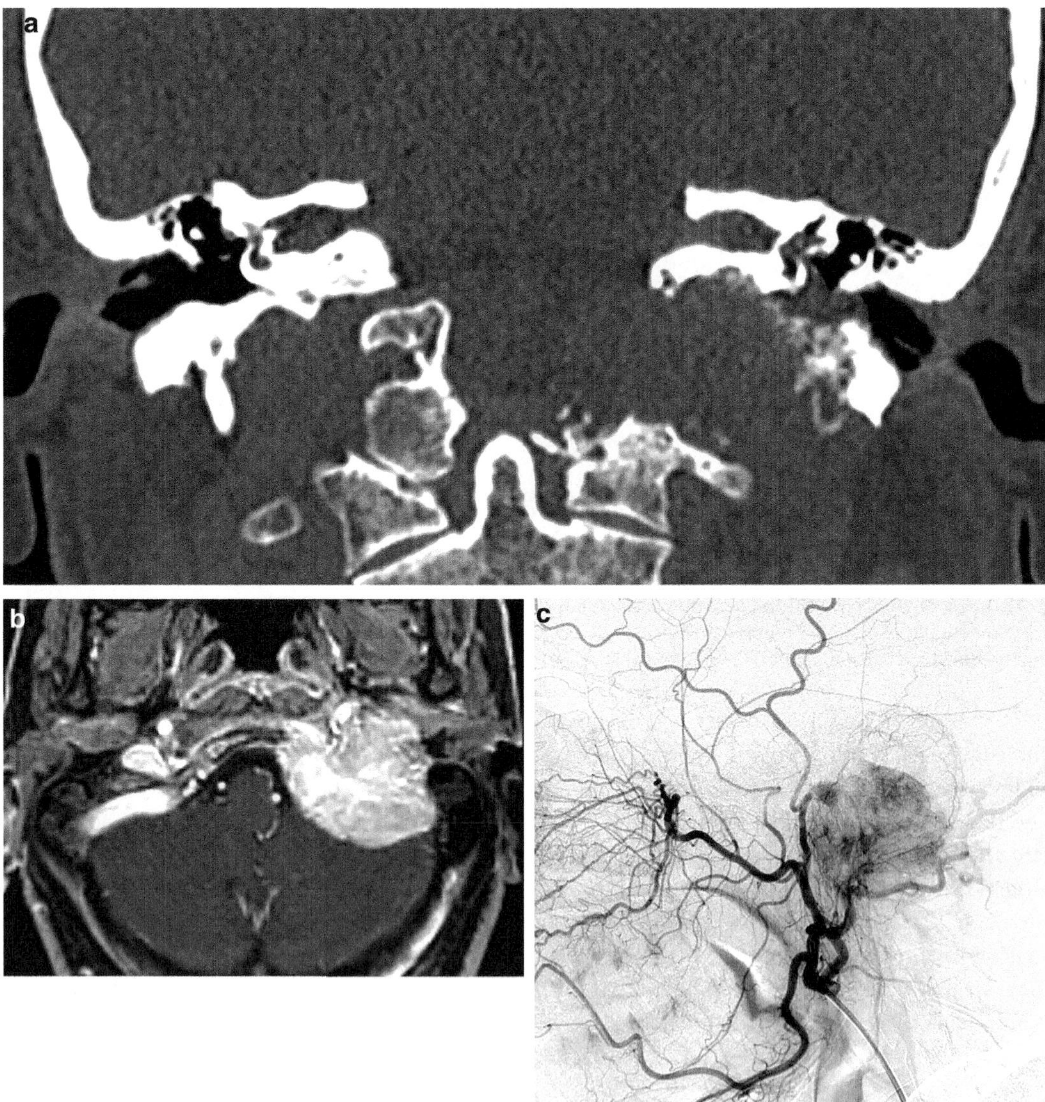

Fig. 12.2 Left jugular paraganglioma with invasion of the cerebellopontine angle. (**a**) Coronal CT scan with bony window displaying bone destruction of the infralabyrinthine portion of the petrosal bone, below the internal auditory canal and middle ear, as well as the occipital bone at the level of the jugular tubercle. (**b**) Axial section of T1-weighted MRI with gadolinium displaying the tumor's occupancy of the cerebellopontine angle. (**c**) DSA external carotid artery study, which exhibits hypervascularization of the tumor

Paragangliomas that originate predominantly in the cerebellopontine angle are exceptional, and only a handful of cases have been documented in the literature. In these instances, it is postulated that the tumor would arise from paraganglionic cells located in the cerebellopontine angle as a consequence of an abnormal migration of cells from the neural crest to their extracranial destinations or from the abnormal involution of fetal paraganglionic cells that, rather than dissipating, persist into adulthood.

Paragangliomas are hypervascular lesions that are benign and slow-growing. Catecholamines are present in all paragangliomas; however, only a small number of patients exhibit clinical symptoms as a consequence of the release of norepinephrine into the circulation or the detection of elevated levels of catecholamines in plasma or urine. Histopathologically, they are highly cellular tumors that form spheres or baskets (*zellballen*) and are bounded by a delicate fibrovascular stroma. The primary cells are cubic or polyhedral in shape, possess a prominent nucleus, and are devoid of pleomorphism, mitosis, or necrosis. Granules of catecholamine secretion are visible through electron microscopy in these cells. Supporting elements are other cells that surround the cellular globules and exhibit a more fusiform appearance. Ki67 and MIB-1 and other proliferative index indicators are not elevated. Immunohistochemical studies have demonstrated the presence of synaptophysin, chromogranin, and S-100 protein. The clinical symptoms of cerebellopontine angle paragangliomas are entirely nonspecific, and the exceptional amount of cases described renders it impossible to establish a pattern. The histopathological study is the determining factor in the definitive diagnosis, and it is the same with imaging studies or the surgical aspect. The imaging techniques demonstrate a well-defined lesion in the cerebellopontine angle that is challenging to distinguish from a meningioma due to its increased uptake of contrast. They do not exhibit bone erosion, as do tympanic or jugular paragangliomas. Diagnosis is exclusively achieved through cerebral digital subtraction angiography (DSA). The treatment involves the radical microneurosurgical resection of the tumor using a retrosigmoid approach. Devascularization of the tumor is the initial stage, which is followed by en bloc or piecemeal removal [10, 11].

12.3.3 Metastasis

Metastases in the cerebellopontine angle have been reported in the literature on unusual occasions. In certain instances, the metastasis may be solitary and nodular, resulting in a differential diagnosis of schwannoma or meningioma of the cerebellopontine angle. In other cases, bilateral and symmetrical lesions that occupy both internal auditory canals may lead to a differential diagnosis of neurofibromatosis type 2. Finally, there are cases of meningeal carcinomatosis with multiple nodular lesions or linear enhancement in the cerebellar folia. In general, the number of cerebellopontine angle tumors attributed to metastases varies between 0.2% and 2%, depending on the series.

The most significant neurosurgical challenge is the presence of single nodular lesions, which may demand microneurosurgical treatment in the event of a suspected schwannoma or meningioma in patients who have no known malignancy or in patients who have been diagnosed with cancer but have controlled or cured their disease. These patients might have another primitive tumor in the cerebellopontine angle. The clinical and imaging differential diagnosis between a benign cerebellopontine angle tumor and a metastasis can be challenging and is dependent on a set of criteria. Initially, benign tumors are significantly more prevalent than metastases, despite the fact that meningiomas are more prevalent in women with breast cancer. The exception in patients with metastasis is to present with subtle symptoms or be asymptomatic, and the usual presenting symptoms are unilateral involvement of one or more cranial nerves of the cerebellopontine angle. The clinical course of metastasis is more intense, progressive, and rapid than that of benign tumors. In general, the intensity of the clinical picture may be disproportionate to the size of the lesion. In imaging studies, the presence of perilesional edema and intensive tumor enhancement, often in a ring fashion, are the characteristic features of metastasis (Fig. 12.3). The presence of additional intra-axial or intracranial lesions or leptomeningeal enhancement that is indicative of carcinomatosis suggests metastasis. A rapid growth of the lesion is also an indirect indicator of malignancy. However, in the majority of the cases described, the diagnosis of metastasis is the result of the pathological analysis in patients whose lesion was initially diagnosed as a primary tumor of the cerebellopontine angle. Melanoma and lung and breast carcinomas are the most prevalent primary tumors. The mechanism of tumor emboli dissemination to the cerebellopontine angle is not yet fully understood; however, it appears that dissemination through the cerebrospinal fluid or leptomeningeal pathways is more probable than hematogenous dissemination. In patients with controlled or uncontrolled neoplastic disease, stereotactic radiosurgery may be indicated, and microneurosurgical indication for excision is exceptional [12, 13].

In the clinical setting, *meningeal carcinomatosis* may manifest with a meningeal syndrome and unilateral or bilateral involvement of multiple consecutive or nonconsecutive cranial nerves, as well as, in rare cases, with a syndrome of intracranial hypertension caused by hydrocephalus. Lung and breast tumors, melanoma, lymphoma, leukemia, hematopoietic tumors, and supratentorial malignant tumors with deposit metastases are the most frequent by origin. Multiple nodular lesions, typically of small size, are observed in the cerebellar folia, accompanied by unilateral or bilateral linear deposits, as demonstrated by imaging studies. A thickening of the meninges with a density comparable to that of the gray matter can be observed in T1- and T2-weighted pictures with MRI. An intense enhancement of the meningeal and leptomeningeal thickening is observed following the injection of gadolinium, particularly in the cerebellar sulci of the vermis, hemispheres, and flocculus. The pathognomonic feature of meningeal carcinomatosis is the thickening and enhancement of the cisternal and intracanalicular segments of the vestibulocochlear and facial nerves, as well as the trigeminal nerve root, regardless of whether it is unilateral or bilateral. There is no surgical indication for meningeal carcinomatosis.

12.3.4 Miscellaneous

There are other exceptional lesions of a different nature that grow in the cerebellopontine angle, forming masses, and that are not tumoral in nature but inflammatory, such as sarcoidosis;

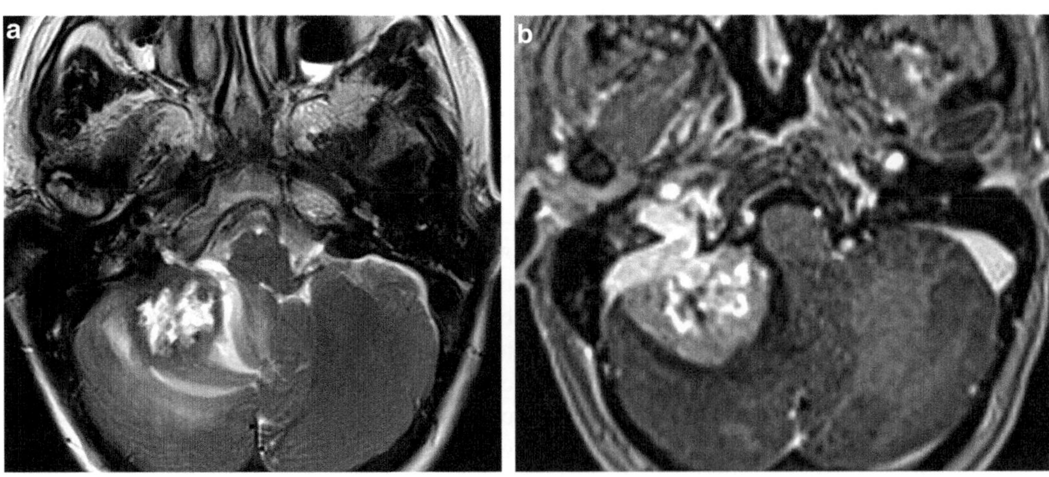

Fig. 12.3 Metastasis of breast carcinoma. (**a**) Axial T2-weighted MRI study displaying a nodular lesion in the right cerebellopontine angle with irregular signal intensity, perilesional edema, and mass effect. (**b**) An axial T1-weighted MRI analysis with contrast demonstrates the tumor's relationship with the sigmoid sinus and irregular contrast enhancement

infectious, such as tuberculosis; lesions of embryonic or malformative origin, such as hamartomas; or vascular lesions, such as large aneurysms.

12.4 Tumors Originating in the Brainstem and Cerebellum

The retrosigmoid approach is used to resect a significant number of brainstem and cerebellar tumors. However, in this section, we will focus on lesions that originate in these structures but that bulge, develop, or occupy the cerebellopontine angle.

12.4.1 Choroid Plexus Papilloma

Choroid plexus papillomas are uncommon tumors, comprising approximately 0.5% of intracranial tumors. The lateral ventricles (40%) and fourth ventricle (40%) are the typical sites of their growth. They are less common in the third ventricle (10%) and other extraventricular locations. The cerebellopontine angle is the most common extraventricular location of choroid plexus papilloma. The pineal, parasellar, intraparenchymal, or spinal regions are additional extraventricular locations. The origin of papillomas in the choroid plexus of the cerebellopontine angle can vary. Some are the consequence of the extension of an intraventricular papilloma of the fourth ventricle to the cerebellopontine angle via the foramen of Luschka. Others would result from the dissemination and deposit of an implant from a supratentorial intraventricular papilloma in the cerebellopontine angle. These are secondary papillomas in both instances and are the most common scenario. In an exceptional case, the cerebellopontine angle is the site of a choroid plexus papilloma that is devoid of any intraventricular papilloma, thereby defining the cerebellopontine angle as a genuine choroid plexus papilloma. It has been hypothesized that these extraventricular papillomas would arise from ectopic choroid plexus tissue or embryonic choroid cell remains (*Bockdalek flower baskets*). The pathology of choroid plexus papilloma is classified into three WHO prognostic grades: grade 1 or typical papilloma, grade 2 or atypical papilloma, with two or more mitoses per 10 high-power fields, and grade 3 or choroid plexus carcinoma. The majority of the cerebellopontine angle papillomas that have been described are classified as grade 1. The structure of these lesions is straightforward, with fibrovascular axes covered by a single layer of cells, devoid of mitoses or atypia, and exhibiting a high level of immunoreactivity against the S100 protein. However, they may also be positive for vimentin, synaptophysin, cytokeratins, EMA (*Epithelial Antigen Membrane*), or GFAP (*Glial Fibrillary Acid Protein*). Despite their benign nature, these tumors have the potential to grow to a significant size and exhibit a propensity for recurrences with an increase in grade, as well as the development of metastases through the spinal canal.

Cerebellopontine angle papilloma is almost exclusively found in adults and is equally prevalent in both sexes, whereas intraventricular papilloma is significantly more prevalent in minors than in adults. Headache and changes in the fifth to ninth cranial nerves are the most frequently observed symptoms at the time of diagnosis. The cranial nerves' involvement is contingent upon the papilloma's growth site. The fifth to eighth cranial nerves are affected by tumors that grow above the medullary-pontine sulcus; the lower cranial nerves are affected by tumors that grow below this level, and all cranial nerves are affected by tumors that grow at both levels. It is not uncommon for these slow-growing tumors to be large at the time of diagnosis and to be accompanied by symptoms of intracranial hypertension. In imaging studies, they are associated with hydrocephalus in over 50% of cases. This may be a result of the tumor's purported hyperproduction of cerebrospinal fluid or the compression or obstruction of the fourth ventricle's outflows.

Imaging reveals highly characteristic data, despite their rarity. On CT, they are depicted as well-defined structures that may be hypo- or hyperdense, occasionally containing calcifications of a wide range of patterns and distribution, and that exhibit a high degree of contrast uptake. On MRI, they are also depicted as circumscribed masses with a well-defined but irregular surface reminiscent of cauliflower. They are hypointense or isointense on T1-weighted sequences and hyperintense or isointense on T2-weighted sequences, with a homogeneous or heterogeneous appearance that is subject to the calcium and vessel content. After gadolinium administration, they enhance significantly. They are frequently linked to hydrocephalus, albeit at a significantly lower frequency than intraventricular papilloma. This has been attributed to the fact that they have a lower capacity for producing cerebrospinal fluid due to the fact that they have less vascularization than the intraventricular papilloma. However, it could also be argued that their extraventricular location does not increase the pulsatility of the intraventricular cerebrospinal fluid. Cysts may occasionally be observed, which are believed to be the result of the tumor's entrapment of the cerebrospinal fluid. By definition, true papillomas of the cerebellopontine angle lack an intraventricular component; however, they can be visually identified as plugging or obstructing the corresponding foramen of Luschka in coronal sections. The invasion of the petrosal bone or mastoid by the tumor and the presence of peritumoral edema are significantly more exceptional. The diagnosis is established by the following criteria: a well-defined, multilobed, or cauliflower-like mass in the cerebellopontine angle; compression or plugging of the foramen of Luschka in coronal sections; iso- or hyperdense mass, frequently with calcifications on CT; iso- or hyposignal on T1 sequences, with variable density on T2 due to calcifications or empty signal due to vascular flow; intense homogeneous or heterogeneous contrast enhancement on both CT and MRI; and occasional hydrocephalus. Digital DSA may demonstrate a staining pattern (blush), rapid flow with early discharging veins, or pictures of arteriovenous microfistulas within the tumor, which are indicative of a hemangioblastoma. These tumors receive arterial supply from branches of the anterior inferior cerebellar artery. Preoperative embolization is not beneficial, nor is DSA required for diagnosis.

The preferred treatment for these tumors is radical microneurosurgical resection using a standard retrosigmoid or far-lateral approach. The resection strategy should commence with the devascularization of the arterial afferents to the tumor, followed by internal decompression and complete segmental resection of the tumor. If it is impossible to remove fragments that are tightly affixed to the cranial nerve roots, they should be intensively coagulated. It is advisable to conduct an intraoperative biopsy to confirm the histopathology of the tumor, as its pathological diagnosis is highly direct. This will reduce the risk of metastasis by deposit by meticulously protecting and thoroughly cleansing the surgical field with saline solution. The prognosis is favorable following complete resection, with a recurrence rate of less than 10%. Occasionally, the recurrence is of a greater grade than the initial tumor being treated. In any event, postoperative radiotherapy or stereotactic radiosurgery is not advised, even for tumor remnants that may persist following subtotal resection. In these instances, it is advised to conduct follow-up imaging and contemplate reintervention in the event of recurrence. Radiotherapy should be administered if the degree of recurrence increases [14–16].

12.4.2 Intra-Axial Tumors Growing into the Cerebellopontine Angle

Brainstem gliomas are tumors that manifest distinct growth patterns and develop during infancy. The *H3-K27M* gene mutation is associated with a specific group of diffuse brainstem gliomas, which have a very poor prognosis and do not require microneurosurgical treatment. In contrast, gliomas of the midbrain tectum are typically pilocytic and have a favorable prognosis; however, they are not situated in the cerebellopontine angle and do not require microneurosurgical treatment as a rule. Other brain stem gliomas may exhibit asymmetric or exophytic growth below the pia mater, without invading the brainstem and may progress toward the cerebellopontine angle (Fig. 12.4).

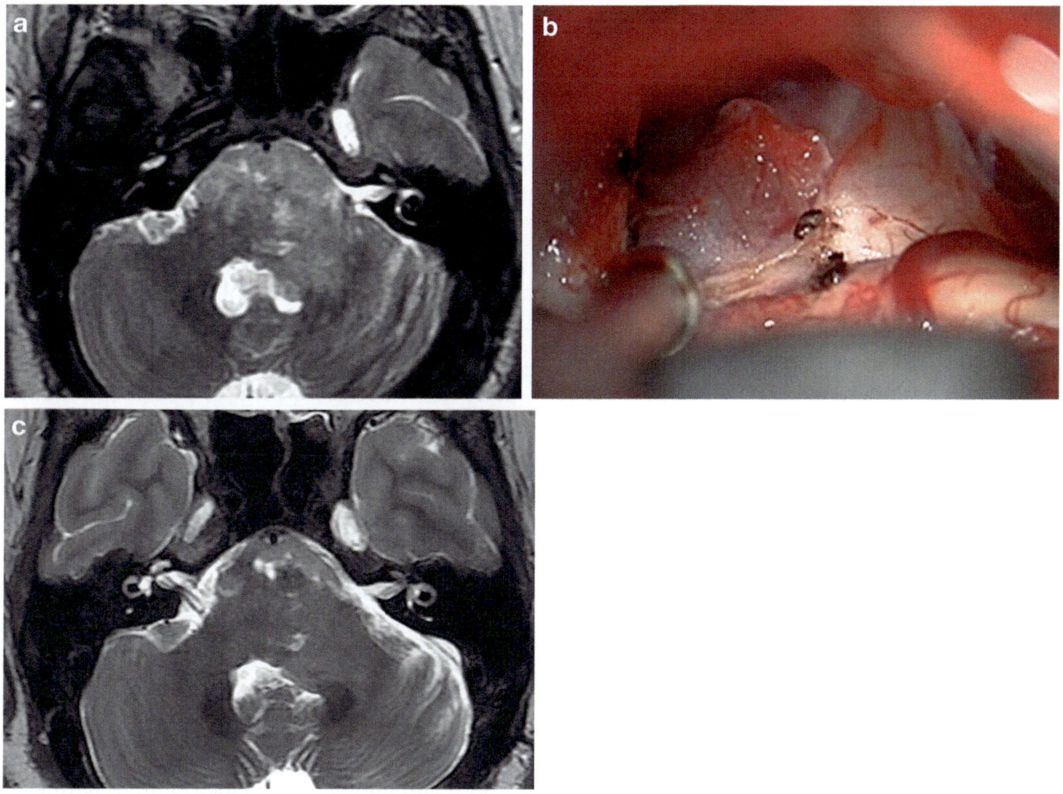

Fig. 12.4 Exophytic brainstem glioma. (**a**) An infiltrating and exophytic tumor is observed on the anterior aspect of the pons in an axial examination of T2-enhanced MRI. (**b**) Intraoperative imaging for the investigation of the left cerebellopontine angle via a retrosigmoid approach for biopsy. The tumor is observed to be expanding between the trigeminal nerve and the facial nerve. (**c**) Axial investigation of T2-weighted MRI 3 years after biopsy, demonstrating a decrease in the size of the lesion following treatment with immunotherapy and chemotherapy

Anaplastic ependymoma of the cerebellopontine angle has been documented in certain instances. It is relatively common for fourth ventricle ependymomas to extend into the cerebellopontine angle, exiting through one or both foramina of Luschka. Conversely, primary ependymomas of the cerebellopontine angle may arise from heterotopic arachnoid glial nests in exceptionally rare instances. The cranial nerves are typically embedded in the cerebellopontine angle cisterns by these tumors, which pose significant challenges for radical resection.

The cerebellopontine angle has also been the site of some cases of glioblastoma multiforme, which can develop exophytically and originate in the cerebellum. In other instances, glioblastoma develops directly in the cerebellopontine angle, in relation to the cranial nerves. This is feasible due to the fact that oligodendrocytes and astrocytes are present in the proximal regions of the cranial nerves, up to the Obersteiner–Redlich transitional zone, and they have the potential to form gliomas. Gliomas may also develop from heterotopic neuroglial cell clusters that are present in the arachnoid.

Lastly, medulloblastoma with predominant proliferation in the cerebellopontine angle has been described. Medulloblastoma is a neuroepithelial tumor that typically develops from the roof of the fourth ventricle and may manifest in the cerebellopontine angle through one or both of the foramina of Luschka's. The primitive cerebellopontine angle medulloblastoma is an exceptional condition that is believed to arise from the most lateral portion of the tela choroidea, which is also in close proximity to the cerebellopontine angle, or from remnants of the external granular layer of the cerebellar cortex in the flocculus, which is situated in the cerebellopontine angle.

Due to their extraordinary rarity, none of these tumors exhibits a clinical pattern that would permit diagnostic suspicion. Imaging studies replicate the tumor's characteristics in its most prevalent location; however, its extraordinary rarity renders diagnostic presumption exceedingly challenging prior to surgery. This enables intraoperative or postoperative diagnosis based on the pathological study. Gliomas are typically hypointense in T1, hyperintense in T2, and gain contrast in a variable manner. They originate in the brain stem. Ependymoma, medulloblastoma, and neuroepithelial dysembryoplastic tumor are hypointense in T1, hyperintense in T2, and gain contrast. The first of these tumors emerges from the fourth ventricle in an irregular and heterogeneous manner, the second from the cerebellum, and the third develops cysts.

Surgical exploration of the tumor in gliomas with an exophytic pattern of growth confirms its origin in the brain stem or cerebellum. Microsurgical resection of the tumor is continued in depth until a resection cavity is obtained that is consistent with the tumor's size. The limits of the resection are also marked by the navigation of the long pathways obtained through the tractography and intraoperative electrophysiological study. The resection is tailored to the histopathology and intraoperative electrophysiological monitoring in cases where tumors are amassing in the cranial nerves or within the cerebellopontine angle cisterns. Microneurosurgical resection adheres to the standard treatment protocol for each tumor type in its typical location of growth. The surgery is conducted in accordance with the accepted treatment guidelines for each tumor, which are determined by the pathology, grade, molecular biology, grade of resection, and other prognostic factors. The same is true for the postoperative oncological treatment.

12.4.3 Lymphoma

At present, the literature contains only approximately 20 cases of primitive lymphomas that affect the cerebellopontine angle. Around 10% of intracranial tumors are primitive lymphomas of the central nervous system, although the incidence appears to be on the rise in patients over the age of 65. Of these, only 10% are situated in the posterior fossa. There are two distinct clinical scenarios: lymphomas in immunocompetent patients, which are typical of patients in the fifth and sixth decades of life and do not exhibit any gender differences, and lymphomas in immunosuppressed patients, which are typical of younger patients in the third decade of life and are predominantly male. In CT studies, they are depicted as isodense or hyperdense lesions with poorly defined borders and minimal mass effect. These lesions uptake contrast in a uniform and intense manner. In MRI studies, they are depicted as cotton-like lesions that are iso- or hypointense on the T1-weighted sequence and that enhance avidly and intensely with gadolinium, with minimal perilesional edema. They are hypointense or isointense on the T2-weighted sequence. They exhibit a significant diffusion restriction on the DWI (*Diffusion Weighted Imaging*) sequence due to their high cell density. The picture is characterized by a minimal mass effect in relation to its apparent volume, perilesional edema, and the ability of the lesion to change in size spontaneously or following steroid treatment. This is pertinent because stereotactic biopsy should be conducted outside the cytotoxic effect of steroids when necessary to affirm the diagnosis in order to prevent a biopsy that lacks diagnostic value. The lesion's location may be intra-axial, extra-axial, or leptomeningeal. The treatment of primary central nervous system lymphoma is not universally accepted, but it is generally acknowledged that microneurosurgical treatment is not indicated and that the treatment is founded on the combination of radiotherapy and chemotherapy [17].

12.4.4 Hemangioblastoma

Cerebellar hemangioblastoma, which is frequently linked to von Hippel–Lindau disease, can be characterized by a large volume and the development of rapidly growing cysts with a highly vascularized tumor nodule. However, they are less frequently associated with a solid appearance without a cystic component. In either scenario, they may develop from the cerebellum, occupying the cerebellopontine angle. They are not problematic in the differential diagnosis or the selection of the microneurosurgical approach, as their aspect is so distinctive. The solid portion exhibits hypointense in the T1 sequence of the MRI and hyperintense in the T2 sequence, and it gains contrast rapidly following the administration of gadolinium. In sporadic cases, von Hippel–Lindau disease should be ruled out due to its prognostic implications and for family genetic counseling, and they should be studied with DSA. The primary objective of microneurosurgical treatment is to completely remove the tumor nodule in order to prevent its recurrence, as well as to empty the cyst.

12.4.5 Metastasis

Exophytic growth toward the cerebellopontine angle may also be observed in intra-axial metastases in the brain stem and cerebellum, with the most common sources being melanoma, breast, and lung [12, 13].

12.5 Tumors of the Cerebellopontine Angle that Originate at the Skull Base

Tumors that originate in the bony walls of the cerebellopontine angle and its dural membrane are included in this section. This category encompasses a substantial number of tumors that impact the petrosal bone, regardless of whether they are primitive, metastatic, or originate from regions near the base of the skull. This invasion may occur directly through bone growth or indirectly through the jugular foramen and other holes in the base of the cranium. The nature of the majority of these tumors may present diagnostic challenges; however, they do not present differential diagnosis issues with lesions of the cerebellopontine angle. Exceptionally, they are resected through a retrosigmoid approach. Consequently, we will be extremely selective in our description of them, concentrating on the most representative ones, such as the endolymphatic sac tumor and meningeal melanocytoma.

12.5.1 Tumor of the Endolymphatic Sac

The endolymphatic duct and sac are a portion of the membranous labyrinth of the inner ear, filled with endolymphatic fluid, and which in turn has two parts. A first portion, proximal and intraosseous, is a duct formed by the union of two channels arising from the utricle and the saccule, with a dilation called the sinus of the endolymphatic duct. The endolymphatic duct measures about 2 mm and is between 0.2 and 0.4 mm in diameter. More distally, the endolymphatic duct opens, forming the so-called endolymphatic sac. It is a flattened structure that expands in a fan-shaped contour, adopting a triangular configuration. The initial portion of the sac, approximately one-third, remains covered by a thin layer of compact bone on the posterior surface of the petrosal bone called the operculum. The wall of the initial portion of the sac, located under the bony operculum, has a structure forming roughness (*pars rugosa*), which gives it a pseudotubular appearance. The sac then becomes extraosseous through a bony cleft of widely varying size below the bony operculum. The endolymphatic sac now expands within the layers of the dura mater but marks a bony depression caudal to the operculum. The extraosseous portion of the endolymphatic sac measures 5–7 mm wide and 10–15 mm long, reaching and covering the dural wall of the sigmoid sinus in 40% of cases. The thickness of the sac depends on the endolymph content and is poorly evident on anatomical and imaging studies. The lumen of the endolymphatic duct and sac is lined by a monostratified, in some areas pseudostratified, epithelium of cuboidal or prismatic cells with villi.

Endolymphatic sac tumors are low-grade adenocarcinomas that are present in a small number of patients with von Hippel–Lindau disease. Von Hippel–Lindau disease is a syndrome that is associated with the inactivation of the tumor suppressor gene *VHL*, which is situated on the short arm of chromosome 3 (3p25–26). This gene is inherited in an autosomal dominant pattern and predisposes patients to the development of cystic tumors in the central nervous system and other organs, with a particular emphasis on single or multiple hemangioblastomas and endolymphatic sac tumors. The tumor of the endolymphatic sac is a rare tumor, with fewer than 300 occurrences documented in the medical literature. In the context of von Hippel–Lindau disease, half of the cases are diagnosed in adolescent patients with a female predominance, affecting one or both sides. In the remaining half of patients, who would be considered sporadic cases, the *VHL* gene mutation is present in nearly half of them. Sporadic varieties are unilateral and predominantly occur in adult male patients. It is crucial to identify a potential genetic mutation, as the endolymphatic sac tumor may be the initial symptom of von Hippel–Lindau disease. Conversely, any patient with von Hippel–Lindau disease may develop an endolymphatic sac tumor at any point in their life. 10% of patients with von Hippel–Lindau disease develop endolymphatic sac tumors, with an average age of 20 years at the time of diagnosis. In order to identify spinal or cerebral hemangioblastomas and endolymphatic sac tumors, it is advised that patients with von Hippel–Lindau disease undergo an annual MRI examination of the neuroaxis for the duration of their lives.

Although the endolymphatic sac tumor is a low-grade adenocarcinoma from a pathological perspective, it exhibits invasive local growth, extending into the petrosal bone and the cerebellopontine angle. The papillary pattern is the most common cytoarchitectonic pattern, in which the tumor cells develop on more or less florid fibrovascular axes, reminiscent of choroid plexus papilloma or thyroid carcinoma, despite the fact that the tumor can have other cytoarchitectonic structures. Nevertheless, the diagnosis of papilloma is prohibited by the immunohistochemical markers that are negative for GFAP (*Glial Acid Fibrillary Protein*) and transthyretin. The absence of atypia and pleomorphism, as well as other immunohistochemical data, excludes the diagnosis of thyroid carcinoma metastasis. The cells are PAS (*Periodic Acid Schiff*) positive, and immunohistochemical techniques have been employed to detect cytokeratins and specific neuronal enolase. A modest level of proliferation markers, including Ki67, is observed. The tumor exhibits a local growth pattern that is more or less aggressive; however, it does not metastasize and can only occasionally form intraspinal metastases as a result of deposits.

Numerous classifications have been devised to determine the tumor's extent. Bambakidis' proposed classification comprises four grades: grade 1, which denotes a tumor that is restricted to the temporal bone and middle ear; grade 2, which encompasses a tumor that extends to the posterior fossa; grade 3, which encompasses a tumor that extends to the middle fossa; and grade 4, which encompasses a tumor that extends to the clivus or sphenoidal wing bone. Schipper's classification employs significantly different criteria and differentiates three stages: grade 1, which is characterized by a tumor that is confined and does not cause bone erosion or infiltration of the dura mater; grade 2, which is characterized by the invasion of the bony labyrinth and neurosensory deafness; and grade 3, which is characterized by the invasion of the sigmoid sinus and jugular vein. Almost all patients manifest with hearing loss of varying severity at the time of diagnosis. Tinnitus or vertigo is experienced by half of the patients, and the facial nerve or other cranial nerves are involved less frequently. Occasionally, it may manifest as otalgia and otorrhea, which are indicative of a chronic middle ear infection. Given the clinical relationship between Ménière's syndrome and the endolymphatic sac, it is recommended that patients with a suspected diagnosis who exhibit atypical clinical characteristics undertake an imaging study to exclude an endolymphatic sac tumor. Hearing loss or impairment can be caused by endolymphatic sac tumors through various mechanisms. The first possibility is the direct invasion of the tumor into the anatomical structures of the inner ear, which would result in progressive hearing loss. The second possibility is the production of acute hemorrhage in the endolymphatic sac that extends to the inner ear, which would explain a complete and sudden loss of hearing in some patients. The final possibility is that the tumor blocks the drainage of endolymph and produces an increase in pressure or hydrops, which could explain progressive hypoacusis with a fluctuating course. The bone deterioration of the posterior part of the petrosal bone between the internal auditory canal, the bony labyrinth, and the sigmoid sinus is revealed by the thin-section CT imaging study. A heterogeneous appearance is observed in T1- and T2-weighted sequences with MRI due to hypervascularization, areas of bleeding, blood degradation products, cholesterol, residues of bone spicules, microcalcifications, and cysts. In an inhomogeneous manner, the lesion excitedly acquires contrast (Fig. 12.5). In the case of large and invasive tumors, DSA may be of interest; however, it is not recommended for minor tumors. Hypervascularization is identified in cases of significant extension from direct branches of the internal carotid artery or the vertebral artery, as well as from branches of the external carotid artery.

Radical microneurosurgical resection of the lesion is the preferred therapy for endolymphatic

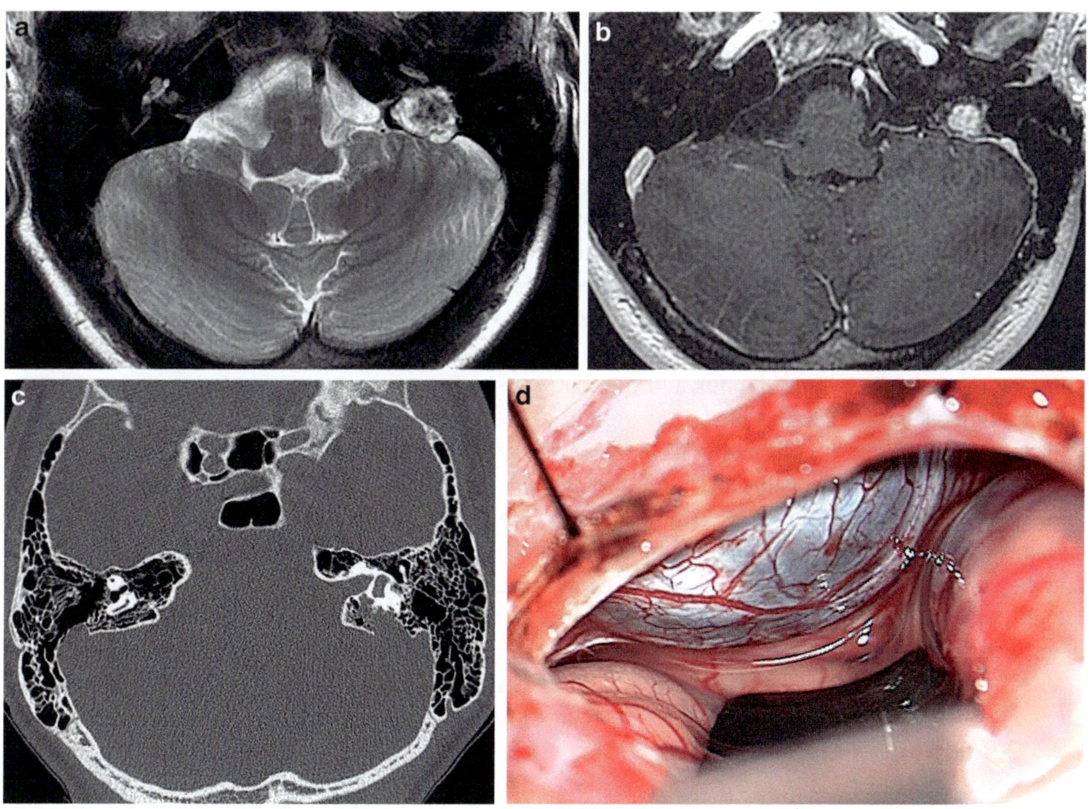

Fig. 12.5 Tumor of the endolymphatic sac. (**a**) Axial examination of T2-weighted MRI with a petrosal lesion of heterogeneous appearance that expands the cortical occupying the cerebellopontine angle. (**b**) Axial T1-weighted MRI study with contrast demonstrating nodular contrast enhancement. (**c**) Axial section of fine-cut CT with a bone window, demonstrating the disintegration of the infralabyrinthine bone and the fluid occupation of neighboring mastoid cells. (**d**) Intraoperative picture of the lesion obtained through a left retrosigmoid approach, demonstrating an extradural lesion with a cystic appearance and bluish content that suggests intratumoral hemorrhage

sac tumors. The method is contingent upon the tumor's size. Consequently, Schipper grade 1 tumors are removed using a standard retrosigmoid or transmastoid-retrolabyrinthine approach, which enables the patient to retain residual hearing. Grade 2 tumors are removed using a retrosigmoid-translabyrinthine approach, as the patients have deafness or no useful hearing. Grade 3 tumors necessitate an infratemporal approach, which enables the control and ligation of the sigmoid sinus and the internal jugular vein, if necessary. There are two varieties of tumors in surgical practice, which are distinguished by the extent of bleeding that occurs during resection. The majority of tumors that infiltrate the bone and adjacent structures are composed of fibrous tissue and exhibit minimal bleeding. Conversely, tumors that exhibit a cystic appearance and minimal infiltration exhibit a significant amount of bleeding during resection. DSA should be employed to investigate large and cystic tumors. If they exhibit substantial hypervascularization, preoperative embolization may be advantageous. Curettage of the lesion, piercing of the bone cavity until healthy-looking bone is achieved, and resection of the dura mater affected by the tumor are all components of microneurosurgical resection. Resection is performed segmentally using a retro-presigmoid approach when the sigmoid sinus is invaded. The sigmoid sinus and jugular vein are ligated and resected en bloc if the jugular vein is invaded. The rarity of the disease makes it challenging to assess the value of radiotherapy and stereotactic radiosurgery. Consequently, the series is exceedingly brief and diverse in nature, and they are exclusively reserved for instances in which complete resection of the lesion has not been accomplished [18–21].

12.5.2 Meningeal Melanocytoma

Meningeal melanocytomas are uncommon tumors; approximately 100 have been documented in the literature with respect to the intracranial region (refer to case 15 in Chap. 21). They are most frequently observed in the cerebellopontine angle (20%), followed by the sellar and parasellar regions, Meckel's cave, and the foramen magnum. In 15% of cases, they are linked to cutaneous lesions, such as the nevus of Ota, as the latter is derived from the same melanic cells in the neural crest. These symptoms are associated with the site of growth in adults of both sexes. However, the symptomatology has a long duration owing to the relatively slow growth pace. Melanocytoma is a neuroectodermal tumor that is derived from neural crest melanocytes. It is a member of a heterogeneous group of tumors that share the same origin, including meningeal melanocytoma, meningeal melanoma, melanocytosis, and meningeal melanomatosis. Meningeal melanocytoma of the cerebellopontine angle is characterized by a soft, well-circumscribed mass that is dark brown or black in color and is implanted in the dura mater. The mass does not infiltrate the underlying bone. The pathological examination reveals a tumor composed of spindle cells with a conspicuous nucleolus and an oval nucleus, without atypia, and a very low proliferative index. Melanocytes and melanophages are present in these extremely pigmented tumors. In immunohistochemical investigations, they may exhibit positivity for the S-100 protein, HMB-45, vimentin, and Melan-A, while they are consistently negative for GFAP, cytokeratins, and EMA. Intracellular melanosomes and promelanosomes are identified through electron microscopy. Except in rare instances, mutations in the *BRAF* gene, which are indicative of malignant melanoma, are not detected in molecular biology investigations [22]. Despite their histological benignity, these tumors exhibit a propensity for local recurrence and the development of leptomeningeal implants in the cistern where they are initially located or in neighboring cisterns. Additionally, they may induce metastasis by depositing in the spinal space. The histopathological aggressiveness of these recurrences or regional implants is not significantly increased. Differential diagnosis of meningioma is problematic with diagnostic imaging. They are implanted in the dura mater and appear as well-circumscribed extra-axial lesions on CT. The borders are well defined. They are hyperdense lesions that exhibit uniform contrast enhancement. In contrast to meningiomas, there is no dural tail, hyperostosis, calcifications, or bone invasion. On T1-weighted sequences, they are hyperintense on MRI, whereas they are iso- or hypointense on T2-weighted sequences. This behavior is a result of the high concentration of melanin pigment, which possesses paramagnetic properties. Following the administration of contrast, the signal intensity experiences a substantial increase, which may be homogeneous or heterogeneous, contingent upon the quantity of melanin present or the presence of intratumoral hemorrhages. The treatment for meningeal melanocytoma involves microneurosurgical excision, which involves the complete resection of the lesion, the dural implant, and the adjacent dura mater. The tumor resembles a meningioma during the microneurosurgical procedure when a precise preoperative diagnosis has not been established. Nevertheless, the absence of dural and bone invasion, the dark color, the weaker and pasty consistency, and occasionally a tar-like appearance are typical findings of meningeal melanocytoma. The recurrence rate after complete resection reaches 20% at 5 years, with a mean of 4.5 years until recurrence. Given the rarity of malignant transformation, the preferred treatment for recurrences is microneurosurgical resection, if feasible. Recurrence may manifest as multiple deposits of varying sizes in the vicinity or in the initially resected tumor bed, which presents a challenge for surgical treatment options. Consequently, radiotherapy has been advocated for the treatment of meningeal melanocytoma following subtotal resection or even total resection. Nevertheless, there has been no evidence to suggest that radiotherapy or stereotactic radiosurgery has any effect on disease control or survival. Additionally, chemotherapy does not influence the progression of tumors. Immunotherapy, which is advantageous in the treatment of malignant melanoma, is not applicable to melanocytoma unless there are *BRAF* gene mutations [23].

12.5.3 Miscellaneous

The cerebellopontine angle can be secondarily invaded by a skull base tumor, such as a paraganglioma, due to its unique development pattern. The two most common types of paraganglioma, tympanic paraganglioma and jugular paraganglioma, are resected through intricate skull base approaches and never with a retrosigmoid approach or its variants. The same is true for bone metastases in the petrosal bone or cranium base, bone tumors such as chondroma, chondrosarcoma, chordoma, or carcinoma, soft tissue sarcomas, and hematological lesions such as myeloma (Fig. 12.6). Pachymeningitis is a rare complication of inflammatory lesions; however, the cra-

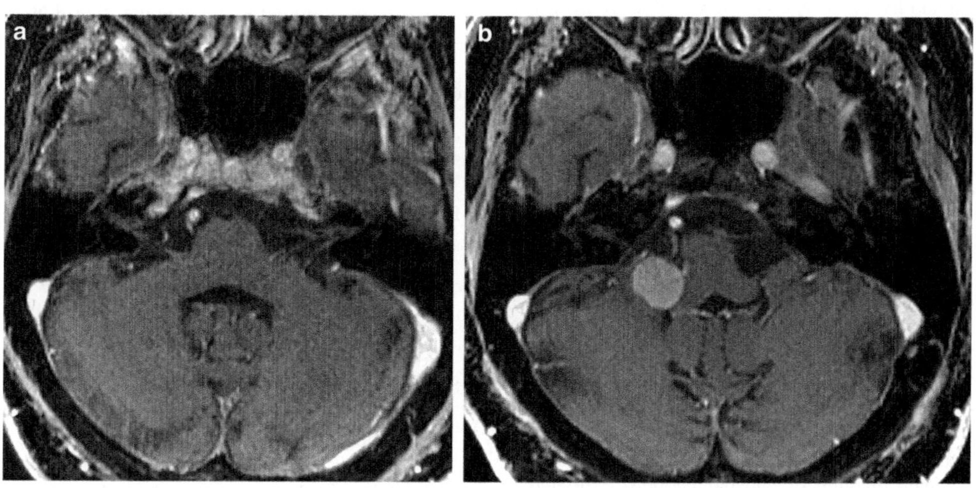

Fig. 12.6 Multiple myeloma. (**a**) Axial study of T1-weighted MRI with gadolinium in a patient with multiple myeloma in long-term remission, displaying the absence of lesions. (**b**) 9 months later, a new study shows an enhanced nodular tumor in the right cerebellopontine angle. The pathology showed that it was a focus of multiple myeloma

nial nerves may be affected, resulting in progressive neurological symptoms. The group also encompasses a variety of diseases, including idiopathic hypertrophic pachymeningitis and autoimmune pachymeningitis. The dura mater of the cerebellopontine angle exhibits a more or less conspicuous hypertrophy in imaging studies, which is exacerbated by the administration of contrast. The diagnosis is serological, and treatment is typically based on steroids. An open biopsy may be necessary.

12.6 Key Messages

- *The cerebellopontine angle is a place for a diverse array of tumors, in addition to vestibular schwannoma, meningioma, and epidermoid cyst.*
- *In general, tumors exhibit the same characteristics as those observed in imaging investigations of their most prevalent sites. The general treatment guidelines are also consistent.*
- *The endolymphatic sac tumor is a rare tumor that is exclusive to the cerebellopontine angle.*

References

1. Bambakidis N, Megerian CA, Spetzler RF, editors. Surgery of the cerebellopontine angle. Cham: Springer Nature; 2018.
2. Bonneville F, Sarrazin JL, Marsot-Dupuch K, et al. Unusual lesions of the cerebellopontine angle: a segmental approach. Radiographics. 2001;21:419–38. https://doi.org/10.1148/radiographics.
3. Bonneville F, Savatovsky J, Chiras J. Imaging of cerebellopontine angle lesions: an update. Part 1: enhancing extra-axial lesions. Eur Radiol. 2007;17:2472–82. https://doi.org/10.1007/s00330-007-0679.
4. Bonneville F, Savatovsky J, Chiras J. Imaging of cerebellopontine angle lesions: an update. Part 2: intra-axial lesions, skull base lesions that may invade the cerebellopontine angle region, and non-enhancing extra-axial lesions. Eur Radiol. 2007;17:2908–20. https://doi.org/10.1007/s00330-007-0680.
5. Demir MK, Özdamarlar U, Yılmaz B, et al. Magnetic resonance imaging of unusual neoplasms related to foramen of Luschka: a review for differential diagnosis. Indian J Radiol Imaging. 2022;32:71–80. https://doi.org/10.1055/s-0042-1743113.
6. Friedmann DR, Grobelny B, Golfinos JG, et al. Non-schwannoma tumors of the cerebellopontine angle. Otolaryngol Clin N Am. 2015;48:461–75. https://doi.org/10.1016/j.otc.2015.02.006.
7. Samii M, Gerganov V. Surgery of cerebellopontine angle lesions. Berlin-Heidelberg: Springer; 2013.
8. Springborg JB, Poulsgaard L, Thomsen J. Non-vestibular schwannoma tumors in the cerebellopontine angle: a structured approach and management guidelines. Skull Base. 2008;18:217–27. https://doi.org/10.1055/s-2007-1016959.
9. Totten DJ, Manzoor NF, Perkins EL, et al. Cerebellopontine angle and internal auditory canal lipomas: case series and systematic review. Laryngoscope. 2021;131:2081–7. https://doi.org/10.1002/lary.29434.
10. Deb P, Sharma MC, Gaikwad S, et al. Cerebellopontine angle paraganglioma—report of a case and review of literature. J Neuro-Oncol. 2005;74:65–9. https://doi.org/10.1007/s11060-004-5952-0.
11. Guevara N, Chays A, Bruzzo M, et al. Cerebellopontine angle paraganglioma. Otol Neurotol. 2003;24:469–72. https://doi.org/10.1097/00129492-200305000.
12. Buis DR, Peerdeman SM, Vandertop WP. Metastatic adenocarcinoma in the cerebellopontine angle, presenting as a meningioma: a case report of rare occurrence. Acta Neurochir. 2004;146:1369–72. https://doi.org/10.1007/s00701-004-0338-9.
13. Yuh WT, Mayr-Yuh NA, Koci TM, et al. Metastatic lesions involving the cerebellopontine angle. AJNR Am J Neuroradiol. 1993;14:99–106. PMID: 8427116
14. Adib SD, Hempel JM, Kandilaris K, et al. Surgical management of choroid plexus papilloma of the cerebellopontine and cerebellomedullary angle: classification and strategy. Neurosurg Rev. 2021;44:3387–97. https://doi.org/10.1007/s10143-021-015.
15. Luo W, Liu H, Li J, et al. Choroid plexus papillomas of the cerebellopontine angle. World Neurosurg. 2016;95:117–25. https://doi.org/10.1016/j.wneu.2016.07.094.
16. Shi YZ, Wang ZQ, Xu YM, et al. MR findings of primary choroid plexus papilloma of the cerebellopontine angle: report of three cases and literature reviews. Clin Neuroradiol. 2014;24:263–7. https://doi.org/10.1007/s00062-013-022.
17. Seevaratnam V, Li Y, Lee SLK, Olsson G. Primary central nervous system lymphoma at the cerebellopontine angle mimicking a trigeminal schwannoma: a unique case report and literature review. J Clin Neurosci. 2018;52:115–9. https://doi.org/10.1016/j.jocn.2018.01.016.
18. Gioacchini FM, Kaleci S, Chiarella G, et al. Symptoms and clinical features in patients affected by endolymphatic sac tumor: a systematic review and meta-analysis. Eur Arch Otorrinolaringol. 2022;279:5081–8. https://doi.org/10.1007/s00405-022-07469-6.

19. Lo WWM, Daniels DL, Chakeres DW, et al. The endolymphatic duct and sac. AJNR Am J Neuroradiol. 1997;18:881–7. 0195-6108/97/1805–0881.
20. Mendenhall WM, Suárez C, Skálová A, et al. Current treatment of endolymphatic sac tumor of the temporal bone. Adv Ther. 2028;35:887–98. https://doi.org/10.1007/s12325-018-0730-0.
21. Zechner G, Altman F. Histological studies of the human endolymphatic duct and tract. Pract Otorhinolaryngol (Basel). 1969;31(2):65–83. https://doi.org/10.1159/000274880.
22. Muñoz-Hidalgo L, Lopez-Gines C, Navarro L, et al. *BRAF* V600E mutation in two distinct meningeal melanocytomas associated with a nevus of Ota. J Clin Oncol. 2014;32:e72–5. https://doi.org/10.1200/JCO.2013.48.8718.
23. Prasad GL, Divya S. Intracranial meningeal melanocytomas: clinicoradiologic characteristics and outcomes. World Neurosurg. 2022;168:298–308.e8. https://doi.org/10.1016/j.wneu.2022.08.

13 Epidermoid Cyst

13.1 Introduction

In adults, the epidermoid cyst is the third most prevalent form of tumor in the cerebellopontine angle. It is responsible for approximately 1% of intracranial tumors and 10% of cerebellopontine angle tumors. The epidermoid cyst may be situated in various regions of the intracranial space and in the cranial bones. The cerebellopontine angle is the most common intracranial location, with an estimated 40% of intracranial epidermoid cysts located there. The parasellar area, middle cranial fossa, and various midline structures are also frequent locations. The pericallosal cistern, pineal region, fourth ventricle, and brainstem have all been described as locations of epidermoid cysts [1, 12].

The epidermoid cyst is immediately identifiable to the neurosurgeon due to its distinctive and unambiguous macroscopic appearance. The lesion is characterized by a pearly white appearance with iridescence and tiny concretions or bumps that, when observed under the surgical microscope, are reminiscent of the natural pearls that form in oyster shells. This particular aspect explains why they have been described in necropsy studies for centuries and referred to as a *pearl tumor* since 1829 by the French surgeon Jean Cruveilhier. Walter Dandy is purported to have stated that this tumor was the most exquisite lesion that could be discovered in the human body. Nevertheless, it is important to acknowledge that the pearly appearance is indicative of the contents of the cyst rather than the tumor itself. The tumor is a thin layer that creates a cyst that encases and envelops the beautiful pearly contents (Fig. 13.1).

The lesion and its significance must also be defined through a series of semantic and conceptual considerations [11]. In the neurosurgical environment, these tumors of embryonic origin are incorrectly referred to as cholesteatomas, a term that is both classical and vernacular. This terminology can lead to confusion with otologic lesions of the middle ear, which have a similar histopathological appearance but a distinct etiopathogenesis (true cholesteatoma), and there may be congenital cholesteatomas (true epidermoid cysts) in the middle ear. The confusion is exacerbated by the fact that otologists treat diseases of the middle ear and neurosurgeons treat lesions of the cerebellopontine angle. Consequently, the term *epidermoid cyst* should be reserved for congenital lesions, while *cholesteatoma* should be used to describe otologic lesions that are not congenital. The clinical, diagnostic, and management aspects of the congenital epidermoid cyst of the cerebellopontine angle will be examined in this chapter. The next chapter will focus on other cystic lesions of the cerebellopontine angle.

J. M. González-Darder, *Microneurosurgery of Cerebellopontine Angle*,
https://doi.org/10.1007/978-3-032-03091-7_13

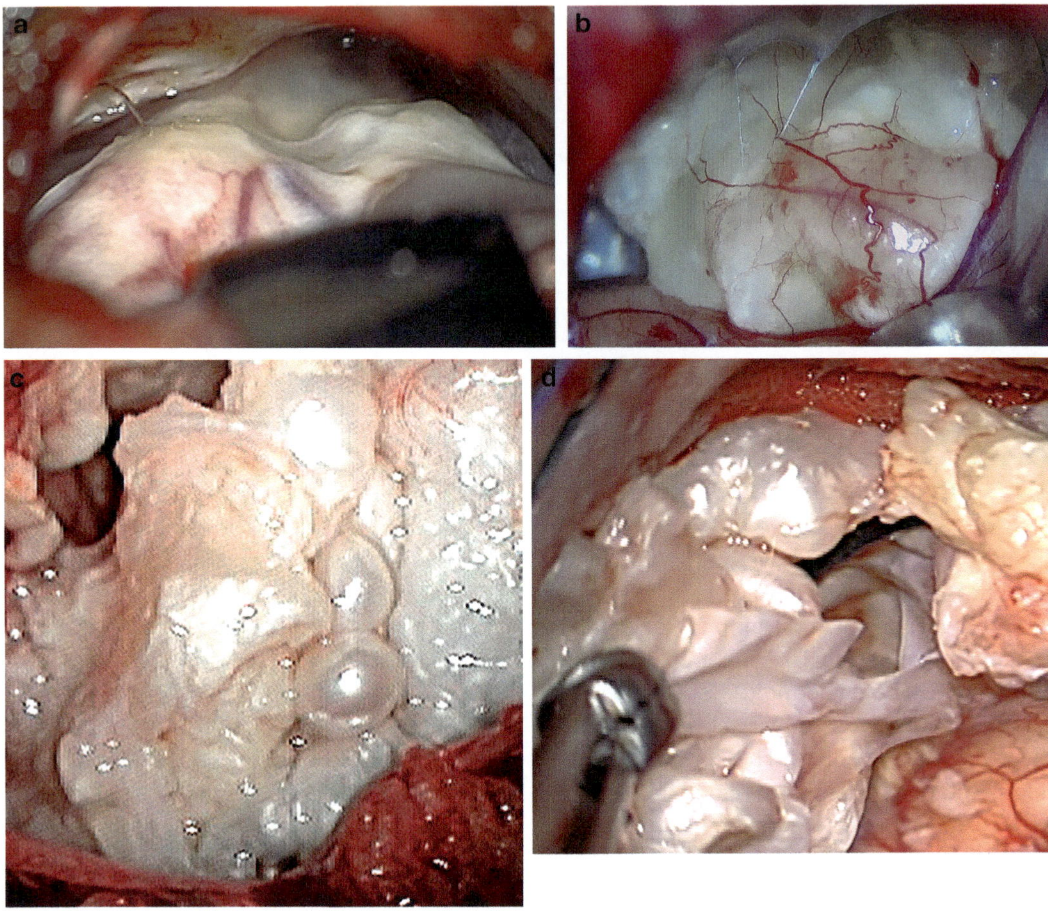

Fig. 13.1 Intraoperative pictures of epidermoid cysts in the cerebellopontine angle. (**a**) The tumor's surgical appearance, characterized by the distended arachnoid adhering to the cyst membrane. (**b**) An image of the tumor after the arachnoid has been removed, revealing the presence of some delicate vessels that travel along the membrane of the cyst. (**c**) Image of pearls after the cyst wall has been removed and the content is visible. (**d**) A portion of the cyst's membrane is removed with forceps, as it is nearly empty

13.2 Anatomical Considerations

13.2.1 Cerebellopontine Angle Cisterns

The cisterns of the posterior fossa, through which the lesion expands during its growth, must be reviewed due to the subarachnoid topography of the epidermoid cyst. The cisternal compartments can be categorized as follows at the infratentorial level: anterior midline cisterns (interpeduncular, prepontine, and premedullary), paramedial cisterns (cerebellar-medullary and cerebellopontine), and posterior midline cisterns (quadrigeminal, supracerebellar, and cisterna magna).

The *cerebellopontine cistern* is situated on the anterolateral aspect of the pons and cerebellum, and it is constructed from the external arachnoid membrane that is adjacent to the posterior surface of the petrosal bone. The lateral pontine-mesencephalic membrane facilitates superior communication with the ambiens cistern. The cistern communicates with the cerebellar-medullary cistern on its lower aspect. Finally, the cistern communicates with the prepontine cistern in the medial direction. The cisternal segment of the fifth to eighth cranial nerves, which extends from the apparent exit from the brainstem bony to their holes of the skull base, is located within the cistern. The cerebellopontine cistern is also the site of circulation and division for the superior cerebellar artery (SCA) and the anteroinferior cerebellar artery (AICA). The superior petrosal venous complex, a confluence of various veins, is the primary venous channel and discharges into the superior petrosal sinus.

The *cerebellar-medullary cistern* is situated caudally and laterally to the pontine-medullary junction, separated from the cerebellopontine cistern by the pontine-medullary membrane. It is bordered by the premedullary cistern medially. It encircles the lateral and dorsal surfaces of the medulla oblongata until it reaches the cerebellar biventral lobe. The lower cranial nerves are situated within the cistern, traveling in the direction of the jugular foramen. Additionally, the posteroinferior cerebellar artery (PICA) is located within the cistern, running dorsally toward the cisterna magna. The cistern extends caudally into the spinal subarachnoid space and communicates with the IV ventricle through the lateral Luschka recesses.

The *prepontine cistern* is a solitary midline cistern that is situated between the anterior surface of the pons and the lateral arachnoid membranes adjacent to the clivus. The cistern is separated from the interpeduncular cistern cranially by the mesencephalic membrane of Liliequist, and it is separated from the premedullary cistern caudally by the poorly defined medial pontine-medullary membrane at the pontine-medullary junction. The basilar artery is frequently formed by the confluence of both vertebral arteries at this level. The cistern is the location of the sixth cranial nerve and the basilar artery with its perforating branches, as well as the origin of the anteroinferior cerebellar arteries. The cerebellopontine cistern is connected to the cistern lateral to it by the anterior pontine membrane.

The *premedullary cistern*, which is also solitary and midline, is situated between the anterior surface of the brain stem and the lateral arachnoid membrane, which is adjacent to the most basal portion of the clivus. The medial pontine-medullary membrane borders it cranially, the cerebellopontine cistern and the dorsal portion of the medullary olive, and the premedullary cistern communicates freely with the anterior spinal cistern caudally. The cistern is the site of the circulation of both vertebral arteries, which results in the formation of anterior spinal arteries that will eventually coalesce into a single vessel at the anterior medial sulcus of the spinal cord. The roots that will form the hypoglossal nerve are directed in a lateral trajectory to locate the hypoglossal canal at the occipital condyle.

The anatomical structures that correspond to the pineal region are located in the *quadrigeminal cistern*, which is dorsal to the tectum of the midbrain and laterally connected to both ambiens cisterns. It establishes superior communication with the velum interpositum and the posterior pericallosal cistern. The trochlear nerve is situated on each side, and a multitude of arterial elements (calcarine and parieto-occipital arteries, terminal branches of the superior cerebellar artery, vermian and hemispherical artery branches of the superior cerebellar artery, posteromedial and lateral choroidal arteries, perforating arteries) and venous channels (internal cerebral veins, Rosenthal's basal vein, internal occipital veins, and the confluence of all of these venous structures and others to form the great vein of Galen) are present. The *posterior supracerebellar cistern* is situated between the lower surface of the tentorium and the upper surface of the cerebellar vermis. It communicates with the quadrigeminal cistern in the cranial direction and with the cisterna magna in the caudal direction. It communicates with the infratentorial subarachnoid space by extending over the cerebellar hemispheres laterally. It encompasses the superior vermian veins and cerebellar bridging veins, as well as the vermian and paravermian arteries, the most distal branches of the superior cerebellar artery.

Lastly, the *cisterna magna* is situated in the midline, dorsal to the vermis of the cerebellum and brainstem, and below the external arachnoid membrane that underlies the occipital bone. It communicates with the IV ventricle via the foramen of Magendie and continues caudally with the posterior spinal cistern. The posteroinferior cerebellar artery enters the cisterna magna and distributes throughout the cerebellum.

It is important to remember the ambiens and interpeduncular cisterns, as the epidermoid cyst frequently extends to these areas, occupying a topography between the supratentorial and infratentorial spaces. The *ambiens cistern* is situated between the midbasal region of the temporal lobe and the lateral aspect of the midbrain. The posterior border of the uncus and the crural cistern define its anterior boundary. It communicates with the quadrigeminal cistern in the posterior direction. The lateral geniculate body, the optic tract, and the pulvinar nucleus of the thalamus make up the roof of the ambiens cistern, arranged from front to back. It communicates with the cerebellopontine cistern on its caudal aspect. The ambiens cistern is home to the P2p segment of the posterior cerebral artery (PCA), as well as the posterolateral, posteromedial, short and long circumflex, thalamus-geniculate, perforating, inferior temporal, and parieto-occipital choroidal arteries. Additionally, the calcarine artery, the trochlear nerve, and segments of Rosenthal's basal vein are occasionally present.

Lastly, the singular, midline *interpeduncular cistern* is situated between the diencephalic and mesencephalic layers of the Liliequist membrane and the cerebral peduncles. The distal third of the basilar artery is the primary arterial element that runs within the cistern. It enters the cistern through the mesencephalic membrane and is the site of the origin of the superior cerebellar arteries; the basilar artery subsequently divides into both posterior cerebral arteries. The posterior perforated substance is the primary target of multiple perforating arteries that originate from the P1 segment of the posterior cerebral artery between its origin and the posterior communicating artery. The third cranial nerve, which travels between the superior cerebellar artery caudally and the posterior cerebral artery cranially, traverses this cistern [3, 10].

13.2.2 Neurovascular Content of the Cerebellopontine Angle

The neurovascular content of the cerebellopontine angle has been divided into three groups by Rhoton. The *superior neurovascular complex* includes the trochlear nerve and the trigeminal nerve, along with the superior cerebellar artery and its branches. The trochlear nerve originates at the back of the midbrain in the tectum and runs around the posterolateral border of the midbrain, leading to the free border of the tentorium between the posterior cerebral artery cranially and the superior cerebellar artery caudally, embedded in the arachnoid of the tentorial incisure. On the other hand, the apparent origin of the trigeminal nerve is in the center of the anterolateral aspect of the pons, just medial to the middle cerebellar peduncle, heading in an anterior-superior-lateral direction to enter Meckel's cave. The superior cerebellar artery arises near the division of the basilar artery and divides into a cranial branch and a caudal branch, which are distributed along the surface of the vermis and cerebellar hemisphere. The superior cerebellar artery relates anatomically to the trochlear nerve on the side of the tentorial incision and then to the upper aspect of the trigeminal nerve. These anatomical relationships will be deeply reviewed in the chapter devoted to the trigeminal neuralgia. The most important venous canal at the top of the cerebellopontine angle is the superior petrosal venous complex that drains into the superior petrosal sinus.

The *middle neurovascular complex* includes the abducens cranial nerve, facial nerve, and cochleovestibular nerve, along with the antero-inferior cerebellar artery. The abducens nerve has its apparent origin in the pontomedullary sulcus, just above the pyramid, and circulates in a superolateral direction to Dorello's canal. The facial and vestibulocochlear nerves originate more laterally, in the pontomedullary sulcus, just above the supra-olivary fossa. The facial-vestibulocochlear complex is directed in a superior-lateral direction to the internal auditory meatus. The anteroinferior cerebellar artery originates in the trunk of the basilar artery. The lateral pontine segment of the artery corresponds to the segment running along the cerebellopontine angle, where it is variably related to the facial–cochleo–vestibular complex. Venous drainage of this portion of the cerebellopontine angle is mainly done by the vein of the cerebellopontine angle fissure, formed by the confluence of several minor veins and running cranially towards the superior petrosal venous complex. Another venous channel is the vein of the middle cerebellar peduncle, originating in the pontomedullary sulcus and also running cranially to the superior petrosal complex.

Finally, the *inferior neurovascular complex* includes the glossopharyngeal, vagal, spinal or accessory nerve of Willis, and the hypoglossal nerves, along with the posteroinferior cerebellar artery. The lower cranial nerve is the hypoglossal nerve, which is formed by several branches originating in the anterolateral or pre-olivary sulcus of the medulla oblongata located between the pyramid and the olive. The other nerves are formed from a variable number of branches that emerge from the lateral aspect of the medulla oblongata in the posterolateral or retro-olivary sulcus, located between the lateral limit of the olive and the cuneiform fasciculus. All these rootlets run laterally below the choroid plexus that protrudes from the fourth ventricle through the foramen of Luschka in search of the jugular foramen. The cervical portion of the accessory nerve is formed by the union of a variable number of rootlets originating in the cervical spinal cord and climbs cranially through the foramen magnum. The nerve is applied to the inner surface of the jugular tuberculum and reaches the jugular foramen. The posteroinferior cerebellar artery has a very variable and complex origin, trajectory, and relationships from its origin in the vertebral artery. The anterior bulbar segment is related to the roots of the hypoglossal nerve, and the lateral bulbar segment is variably related to the rootlets of the rest of the lower cranial nerves. Venous drainage from the inferior compartment of the cerebellopontine angle is done through small veins that converge into the inferior petrosal sinus [3, 10].

13.3 Pathology

13.3.1 Epidermoid Cyst

The epidermoid cyst is a very simple lesion from the point of view of its histopathology, and the wall of the cyst and its contents can be considered separately. The wall is made up of a layered and well-differentiated squamous tissue, which is externally covered by a layer of connective tissue that, in turn, can adhere more or less indistinguishably to the pia mater or the arachnoid membranes. The contents of the cyst are made up of the products of the epithelial membrane. Tumoral growth results primarily from the desquamation of epithelial cells within the cyst, forming pearly, shiny debris, and also from the secretion of cholesterol and keratin within the cyst. These products are what determine the volumetric growth of the lesion and consequently the broadening of the surface of the epithelium producing these elements. The cyst is situated in the subarachnoid space; however, its precise origin is impossible to ascertain, with the exception of extremely small lesions. As they grow, they fill the cisterns of the cerebellopontine angle, forming fingers growing between and enveloping the nerves and vessels. The volume of the cyst can become complex as a result of the adhesion of these various digits of the cyst that are growing around the neurovascular structures, resulting in the appearance of anarchic septa or expansions. When the cyst reaches a large volume and occupies the cisterns, it may enter the fourth ventricle through the foramen of Luschka, extend to the contralateral side in front of the brainstem, or ascend into the supratentorial space into the ambiens or interpeduncular cisterns. Conversely, epidermoid cysts of the fourth ventricle or cisterna magna may grow toward the cerebellopontine angle. Although the soft contents and elastic wall of the lesion cause it to grow and adapt to neurovascular structures, when they reach large volumes, they will displace the brainstem. Exceptionally, cyst can rupture. The rupture of the arachnoid cyst allows the exit of its contents, resulting in an arachnoid and/or pial inflammatory reaction, which can be granulomatous and occasionally produce a general meningeal reaction with more or less acute and intense clinical symptoms. In 10% of instances, the cyst wall undergoes calcification.

The entrapment of ectoderm remnants during the closure of the neural tube of the embryo between the third and fifth weeks of gestation is the prevailing theory regarding the origin of these tumors. Classically, embryonal central nervous system tumors are considered to be midline, because the neural tube runs through the entire embryo from the anterior to the posterior neuropore along the midline of its dorsal aspect. It is hypothesized that the ectodermal remnants would be confined outside the midline by being swept away by the formation and migration of the otic and optic vesicles that develop later to explain the paramedial topography of cerebellopontine angle epidermoid cysts. Cysts located at the intraventricular or intracerebral level would result from entrapments that occurred before the third week, as this is the time at which cerebral vesicles are formed. Both of these mechanisms account for the topographic distribution of epidermoid cysts in the intracranial space and the cranium. Cysts of the fourth ventricle (10%) and intraparenchymal in skull bones (10%) are frequent locations, followed by the cerebellopontine angle (40%) and parasellar area (30%). The remaining locations are less frequent and are located in the brainstem, pineal region, or intraparenchymal in the brain or cerebellum.

The epidermoid cyst's slow growth rate is attributed to its benign congenital nature, which is characterized by a linear and constant cell growth that is comparable to that of the normal cutaneous epithelium. This growth is a result of the epithelial remains being trapped in embryonic development, as opposed to a more rapid, exponential, or irregular linear growth that would be found in an acquired tumor. This growth model posits that tumor growth is consistent with Collins's law, which was proposed in 1955 to account for the recurrence of childhood tumors. The Collins law defines the risk period for the recurrence of a tumor as the child's age at the time of diagnosis plus 9 months. In the same manner, the recurrence of a small tumor remnant of an epidermoid cyst would result in a recurrence of the same volume as the initial tumor after a period of time equal to the patient's age at the time of the intervention plus 9 months, assuming a linear and constant growth pattern. Nevertheless, certain cysts may experience sudden and rapid growth in the event of malignant transformation or hemorrhage.

13.3.2 Squamous Cell Carcinoma

Fortunately, the malignant transformation of the epidermoid cyst into squamous cell carcinoma has been described exceptionally [4]. The following criteria are used to determine the presence of a malignant transformation: the presence of benign squamous cells within the malignant tumor, the absence of metastatic carcinoma, the intradural nature of the tumor, and the exclusion of a nasopharyngeal tumor. The third cause of intracranial squamous cell carcinoma, following metastases and invasion by nasopharyngeal tumors, is malignant transformation of an epidermoid cyst, although only fifty cases have been documented in the literature so far. The mechanisms by which an epidermoid cyst transforms into squamous cell carcinoma remain unclear. The most common explanations are chronic inflammation as a result of recurrent cyst ruptures, previous incomplete surgeries, or the presence of islets of carcinoma in situ that have been present from the beginning and have grown unexpectedly. In the squamous cell carcinoma tumor cells are organized into well-defined cords and nests and exhibit a high level of mitotic activity. Interspersed are frequently regions of benign squamous epithelial tissue and those that exhibit indications of malignancy. Fingerings or invasion of the perivascular spaces of Virchow–Robin are the most common forms of infiltration of the nervous tissue. Occasionally, lesions that are circumscribed, only adhere to neighboring structures, or do not exhibit infiltration can be observed. Tumor cells can react with antibodies against cytokeratin and EMA (*Epithelial Membrane Antigen*) in an immunohistochemical test.

13.3.3 Cholesteatoma

The term cholesteatoma means fat-filled cyst and, in medical terminology, keratin-filled cyst. Otologists are responsible for the management of cholesteatomas in the middle ear, where they differentiate between congenital and acquired cholesteatomas.

The *congenital or embryonal cholesteatoma* is comparable to cranial and intracranial epidermoid cysts; however, it is situated in the middle ear, immediately behind the tympanic membrane, which is typically intact. Diagnostic criteria include the presence on otoscopy of a whitish mass behind a normal-appearing tympanic membrane and the absence of a history of otorrhea, tympanic perforation, or otologic surgery.

Acquired cholesteatomas, which are significantly more prevalent, have been attributed to a variety of primary etiological mechanisms. These mechanisms include metaplasia of the mucosa of the middle ear as a result of repeated or chronic inflammatory processes, migration of the epithelium from the outer aspect of the eardrum to the middle ear through a tympanic perforation, hyperplasia and migration of cells from the basal layer of the eardrum to the middle ear, and, finally, retraction of the eardrum to isolate a pocket of epithelial cells. Nevertheless, a significant number of middle ear cholesteatomas would be secondary to the implantation of epithelial tissue from the external ear canal through an eardrum defect as a consequence of trauma, surgical manipulations, or chronic infections of the external acoustic canal. The histopathology of acquired cholesteatomas reveals a content of keratin layers that are encircled by a wall of epidermal tissue or matrix, which is in turn surrounded by a connective stroma that is more or less dense, known as the perimatrix. The final layer typically exhibits angiogenesis and inflammatory changes, which facilitate bone resorption and the expansion of the lesion within the middle ear. This process results in the destruction of the eardrum and petrosal bone, as well as the erosion of the tegmen tympani.

13.4 Clinical Considerations

Clinical signs and symptoms vary greatly depending on whether the epidermoid cyst is located in the cerebellopontine cisterns, fourth ventricle, brainstem, or bone. There is undoubtedly a specific clinical condition associated with squamous cell carcinoma.

13.4.1 Epidermoid Cyst

From an epidemiological point of view, the *epidermoid cyst of the cerebellopontine angle* presents between the third and fifth decades of life, with a peak around the age of 40. The clinical course is indolent, and the diagnosis typically takes several years due to the low growth rate. The incidence is comparable between the sexes. Clinical symptoms are related to cranial nerve involvement or compression of the cerebellum or brainstem, while hydrocephalus or meningitis are significantly less common [2, 8]. The clinical symptomatology at onset and diagnosis is highly variable when the various series are analyzed. This is a result of the fact that the surgical series are not particularly large, have a highly heterogeneous composition in terms of the size and expansion of the lesions, and originate from geographical regions with varying levels of access to diagnostic resources and surgical treatment. Headaches are a prevalent symptom, with the suboccipital or nuchal region being the primary focus. Trigeminal neuralgia, hearing loss with or without tinnitus, vertigo, headache, diplopia, and facial paresis or hemifacial spasm are the most prevalent neurological symptoms. Some aspects of cranial nerve dysfunction are of interest. The trigeminal nerve is affected in 60% of patients, the cochleovestibular nerve in 70%, the facial nerve in 25%, and diplopia is present in 15% of patients, according to literature reviews. It is striking that the cranial nerves are highly affected in relation to, for example, schwannomas and meningiomas of similar size and topography and, thus, trigeminal neuralgia or hemifacial spasm occur more frequently in the case of epidermoid cysts. The cause of the high incidence of cranial nerve dysfunction is the result of the cyst's prolongations and evaginations, which can cause traction, compression, or angulation of the cranial nerve roots or displace the arteries that subsequently compress the nerve roots. Additionally, a mechanism of strangulation of the vascularization of the nerve between them may be present, which results in focal demyelination. The clinical manifestation would be more conspicuous, and functional recovery after resection of the cyst would not be very dazzling in some cases, as this focal lesion would lead to retrograde Wallerian degeneration of neurons in the nuclei of the brain stem, regardless of the mechanism. Although trigeminal neuralgia and hemifacial spasm are more common in the event of epidermoid cysts than in other cerebellopontine angle tumors, the relative frequency of trigeminal neuralgia is higher than that of hemifacial spasm in patients with epidermoid cysts [6]. This has been explained by the shorter length of the root entry zone of the facial nerve compared to that of the trigeminal nerve, since it is in this area that the pathophysiological changes that lead to the clinical manifestation would occur. It has also been argued that the root entry zone of the trigeminal nerve, in addition to being longer, is more exposed to compression in the cisterns than that of the facial nerve, which is more protected in the pontine-medullary sulcus and by the cochleovestibular nerve. Aseptic meningitis may result from the spontaneous rupture of the cyst, and if it is recurrent, hydrocephalus may develop. The sluggish growth of the lesion typically does not produce symptoms of intracranial hypertension, even in large lesions. If it does, it is through hydrocephalus, but acute hydrocephalus due to obstruction of the CSF circulation pathways is an exceptional occurrence.

The *epidermoid cyst of the fourth ventricle* is much less prevalent than the epidermoid cyst located in the cerebellopontine angle [7]. The age of presentation is the same and occurs more often in women. Clinical symptoms are also long-term until diagnosis, with an average of 4 years from the onset of symptoms. The clinical symptomatology has some particularities, since in almost all patients, there are symptoms and signs of cerebellar involvement, followed by cranial nerve involvement. Nevertheless, the nerves are injured in these lesions as a result of the compression of their nuclei on the floor of the fourth ventricle. Consequently, the trigeminal cranial nerve exhibits significantly less frequent dysfunction, while the cranial abducens, facial, and vestibulocochlear nerves are frequently implicated. Hemiparesis is present in 15% of patients who have experienced long-term motor tract involvement. In a third of cases, symptoms of intracranial hypertension and hydrocephalus are evident due to growth in the ventricle.

Much more exceptional is the *epidermoid cyst of the brainstem*, which presents clinically as a brainstem glioma, characterized by hemiparesis and predominance involvement of the sixth and seventh cranial nerves. The lack of clinical expressivity of these tumors is striking, as they often reach large size, some of which are completely intrinsic and others have exophytic growth [9].

Intraosseous epidermoid cysts can be located in the temporal bone or the occipital bone. Those in the petrosal bone produce otological symptoms, and the diagnosis is made with otoscopy, visualizing a white and shiny mass in the middle ear with the tympanic membrane intact. The diagnosis of the occipital bone is made based on the clinical symptoms of an indolent or painful local tumor, which can grow to a significant size due to the concealment of hair. The intratrophic occipital bone epidermoid cyst is an uncommon tumor that occasionally attains a substantial size. Although traumatic cases have been documented, the skin is trapped in the bone as a consequence of a wound, despite the fact that its origin is embryonic. Dermoid cysts, hemangiomas, arachnoid cysts, cholesterol granulomas, and/or bone tumors such as aneurysmal bone cysts, fibrous dysplasia, and eosinophilic granuloma are used to make a differential diagnosis. Dermoid cysts are frequently diagnosed in childhood and are typically situated along the midline. Hemangiomas are characterized by a honeycomb pattern. The DWI sequence on magnetic resonance imaging (MRI) can be used to differentiate arachnoid cysts from epidermoid cysts, which are very infrequently localized to the skull bone. Eosinophilic granulomas typically affect adolescents and young adults and exhibit contrast enhancement on MRI.

13.4.2 Squamous Cell Carcinoma

The duration from the onset of symptoms to the diagnosis of squamous cell carcinoma is exceedingly brief, lasting only a few weeks or months. The malignant transformation of a recurrence of an epidermoid cyst may occur during the first recurrence or after multiple recurrences and reoperations (refer to case 18 in Chap. 21). A malignant recurrence of the cyst can result from malignant transformation that can occur many years after the cyst was resected. In some cases, the malignant transformation occurs only a few months after the cyst is removed. This is more common in patients who have had imaging studies that revealed suspicious findings, such as compact nodules or contrast enhancement. In this instance, it is necessary to acknowledge that the carcinoma was already present in the operated epidermoid cyst and that the diagnosis was not detected during surgery or after histopathological examination due to the fact that malignant tissue was not sent to pathology or all of the submitted material was not examined. The basis for clinical suspicion is a rapid clinical deterioration, a sluggish and indolent recovery after surgery, or the imaging of an early recurrence. An additional risk factor is the presence of leptomeningeal enhancement nodules in imaging studies that are associated with a lesion that exhibits the typical characteristics of an epidermoid cyst. In all cases where imaging studies reveal this pattern, the patients have squamous cell carcinoma or a malignant transformation of the epidermoid cyst, as it is actually a meningeal carcinomatosis. In certain instances, it is feasible to diagnose carcinomatosis through the cerebrospinal fluid study or to exhibit cytological, biochemical, or markers that imply it [4].

13.5 Diagnostic Considerations

The MRI scan provides a highly accurate diagnosis of the epidermoid cyst [8]. The computed tomography (CT) data are less conclusive due to the cyst's lack of contrast enhancement and the confusion of its density with that of the cerebrospinal fluid (CSF). Calcifications or dense cysts, which are the result of alterations in their contents, are exceedingly uncommon. The study indicates the existence of a mass in the subarachnoid space that can displace the brainstem and cerebellum but does not infiltrate them. This mass has a well-defined and irregular limit. Alternatively, the mass may enter the fourth ventricle, expand into the supratentorial, contralateral, or spinal compartments, or occupy only the cerebellopontine angle.

The cyst may be slightly hyperintense in the T1-weighted sequence with respect to the cerebrospinal fluid on MRI. In the T2-weighted sequence, it is isointense or very slightly hyperintense with respect to the cerebrospinal fluid. The wall is not or very faintly enhanced in the T1 sequence with gadolinium. There are certain abnormal presentations, such as hyperintense cysts in T1 with respect to the parenchyma (white epidermoid) due to a high content of triglycerides or unsaturated fatty acids, hypointense cysts in T1 with respect to CSF (black epidermoid) due to the presence of solid keratin or cholesterol crystals, or the absence of triglycerides or unsaturated fatty acids, or hypointense cysts in T2 due to calcifications or the presence of iron pigments. They may exhibit a signal alteration in the FLAIR (*Fluid Attenuated Inversion Recovery*) sequence, typically a mixed alteration with isointense or hyperintense zones. The lesion appears highly bright in relation to cerebrospinal fluid and nervous tissue, as the contents of the cyst exhibit a high signal in the DWI (*Diffusion Restriction Study*) sequence, which is the most sensitive and specific discovery (Fig. 13.2). The FIESTA (*Fast Imaging Employing Steady-State Acquisition*) study, which employs highly T2-weighted sequences in all three planes, enables the precise delineation of the cyst's location and extensions,

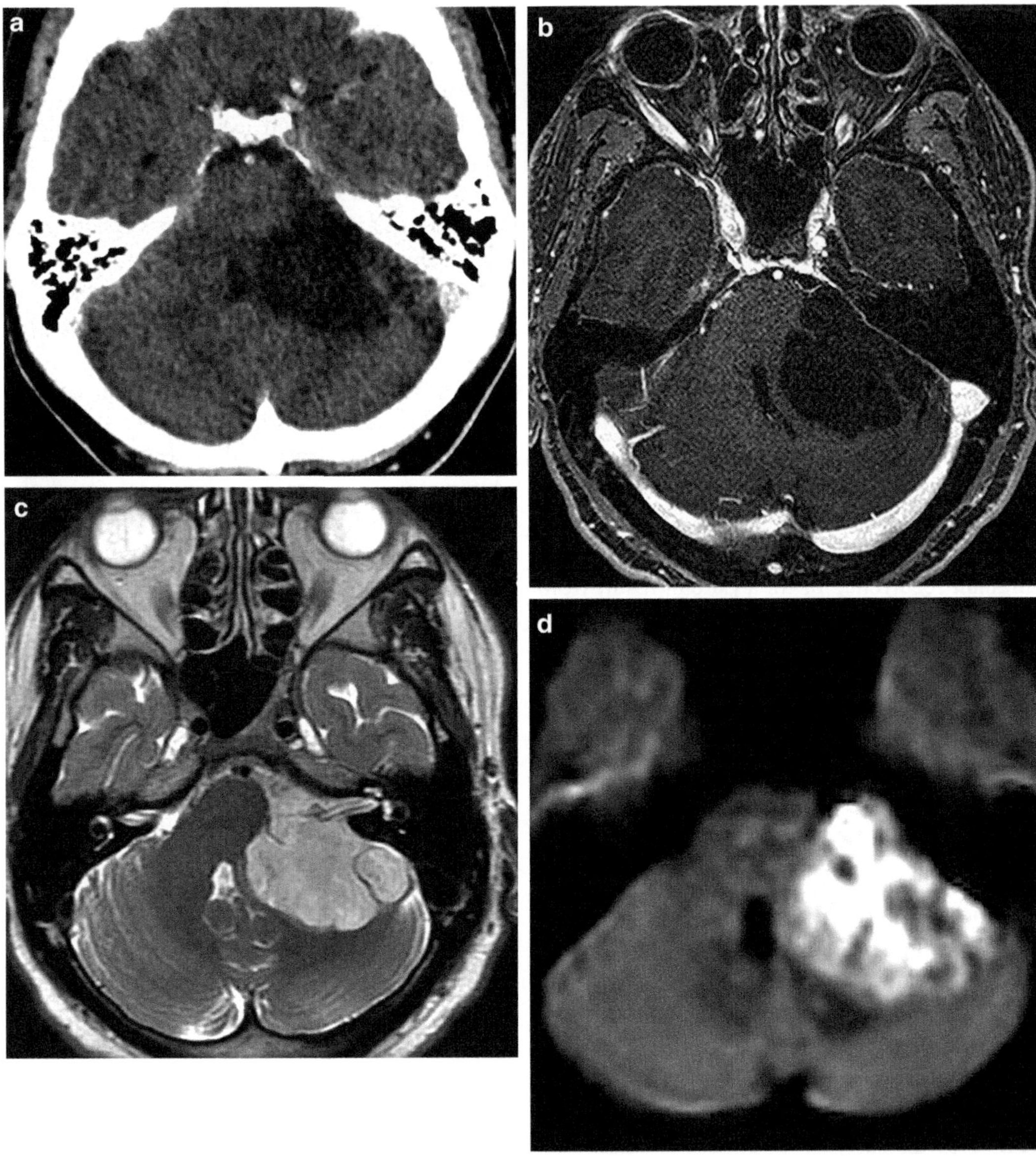

Fig. 13.2 Diagnostic pictures of the epidermoid cyst in the left cerebellopontine angle cisterns. (**a**) An axial CT slice without contrast and irregular hypointense lesions. (**b**) Axial slice of the T1-weighted MRI sequence, demonstrating a dark and irregular lesion that is isointense with the ventricular cerebrospinal fluid. (**c**) Axial section of the T2-weighted sequence of MRI demonstrating a faintly grayish lesion. (**d**) A vivid signal is visible in the axial section of the DWI sequence of an MRI

as well as its relationships with the cranial nerves, which are typically readily identifiable in these sequences. The differential diagnosis includes neurocysticercosis, hydatid cyst, dermoid cyst, and arachnoid cyst, which will be discussed in the subsequent chapter. Digitized subtraction angiography (DSA) reveals only artery displacement, without any aberrant vascularization.

The images of squamous cell carcinoma are entirely distinct. A lesion with a high focal or total enhancement is identified by the CT scan following contrast administration. MRI can reveal a variety of patterns; however, gadolinium is consistently uptaken enthusiastically, either in a focal or whole manner. Additionally, the adjacent nervous tissue undergoes modifications, including infiltration, edema, and mass effect. In some instances, it is possible to detect signs of meningeal carcinomatosis, such as multiple nodular or linear enhancements in the cerebral sulci or between the cerebellar folia.

13.6 Surgical Categories

The epidermoid cyst of the cerebellopontine cistern is distinguished by its variable size; however, at the time of diagnosis, they are typically large and exhibit expansions beyond the cerebellopontine angle. Consequently, it is crucial to establish the extent of the surgical procedure to determine the most suitable surgical approach. This criterion is employed by the majority of classifications. Type 1 lesions are limited to the cerebellopontine angle (40% of cases) (refer to case 16 in Chap. 21). Type 2 lesions have a cranial growth extension (25%) that extends to the supratentorial compartment and ultimately reaches the parasellar region or grows in the middle cranial fossa (refer to case 17 in Chap. 21). Type 3 lesions have a caudal growth extension (20%) through the foramen magnum. Type 4 lesions combine cranial and caudal growth (15%). Finally, the remaining lesions have a contralateral growth to the other cerebellopontine angle or enter the fourth ventricle through the lateral Luschka recesses.

13.7 Microneurosurgical Management

The retrosigmoid approach is employed to perform the radical resection of the epidermoid cyst of the cerebellopontine cistern type 1 in accordance with the subsequent steps and strategies [1, 3, 12, 13].

13.7.1 Position and Craniotomy

The retrosigmoid approach chapter does not contain any specificity with respect to the position, anatomical references, incision, craniotomy, and dural opening procedure. The craniotomy and dural opening must be positioned at the lower border of the transverse sinus and the posterior edge of the sigmoid sinus, with the cranial opening size being adjusted to the cyst's size.

13.7.2 Opening and Dissection of Cisterns

The lesion is immediately accessible after the opening of the dura mater, retraction of the cerebellum, and eradication of the arachnoid. The cyst is identifiable by its shiny and pearly appearance, well-delimited from the cerebellum, and a small venous vessel running along its surface. An initial attempt is made to expose the utmost surface area of the lesion while maintaining the cyst wall intact, always keeping in mind that the objective of the intervention is the removal of the cyst membrane. Even in tiny lesions, it is impossible to completely encircle the cyst due to its adhesion to the arachnoid, nerve tissue, nerve roots, and vessels.

13.7.3 Staged Resection of the Cyst

The membrane is opened in the widest and most accessible area when no additional surface area can be securely exposed. The contents of the cyst are meticulously evacuated to prevent the cyst wall from being inadvertently violated. This is accomplished by employing traditional wall aspiration, ultrasonic surgical aspirators with a very low power output, and large utensils or dissectors with blunt edges. The tumor is entirely avascular, which precludes any hemorrhaging. Additionally, the absence of pressure ensures that a broader dead space remains available as the emptying process advances. In order to reduce the likelihood of post-surgical aseptic meningitis, it is crucial to prevent the loss of fragments of the contents in the cisterns. Sequentially, these general maneuvers should be executed in accordance with the anatomical levels that the cyst occupies.

Begin at the caudal pole of the cyst if it is feasible to do so. It is typically challenging to isolate the cranial pole at the outset. If it is impossible to isolate the poles, begin with the central region. The neurovascular groups described by Rhoton and reviewed above are approximately equivalent to these three components. The cranial nerves (Fig. 13.3a) are surrounded and adhered to by the epidermoid cyst, which generally maintains their anatomical position. Consequently, it is imperative to identify any of the nerves, either anatomically or through direct nerve stimulation, to definitively determine the anatomical level at which we are located.

13.7.3.1 The Caudal Portion of the Cyst

The cyst should be resected after a thorough examination of the various cisterns in which the tumor is located. Nevertheless, the membranes that limit the cisterns are not identifiable due to their embedding and adhesion to the outer surface of the cyst membrane. Consequently, it is more advantageous to adhere to the neurovascular groups, using the cranial nerves as a guide, and to follow a strict order during the resection, ensuring that each compartment is entirely emptied before proceeding to the next. Typically, the rootlets of the hypoglossal nerve can be easily separated from the capsule in the caudal pole of the cyst. However, the vertebral artery and its branches may remain at the bottom of the surgical field, with the adventitia affixed to the capsule by some arachnoid fibrosis (Fig. 13.4). Easily detached from the cyst wall is the lateral aspect of the medulla oblongata. The lower cranial nerves that terminate at the jugular foramen run cranially. The accessory nerve is capable of evading adhesions and cyst expansions by running isolated over the dura mater that envelops the jugular tubercle. In contrast, the glossopharyngeal and vagal nerve rootlets are typically embedded in the cyst wall, with small cyst extensions insinuating among themselves. This renders the dissection and separation of the nerves from the cyst membrane challenging and perilous. This is particularly pertinent due to the fact that the nerves are highly expressive and have the potential to cause severe morbidity in the immediate postoperative period. At times, the cyst displaces and collects all of the rootlets, which simplifies the process of dissecting and cleansing these nerve roots (Fig. 13.5). The lateral Luschka recess can

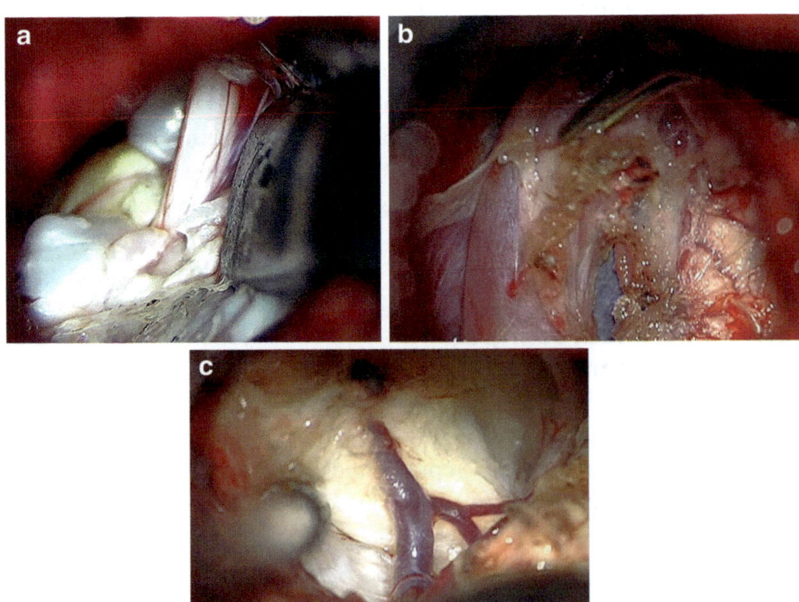

Fig. 13.3 Intraoperative pictures of the relationships of the epidermoid cyst of the cerebellopontine angle with the neurovascular structures. (**a**) Facial–cochleovestibular nerve complex. (**b**) Vertebral artery. (**c**) Superior petrosal vein complex

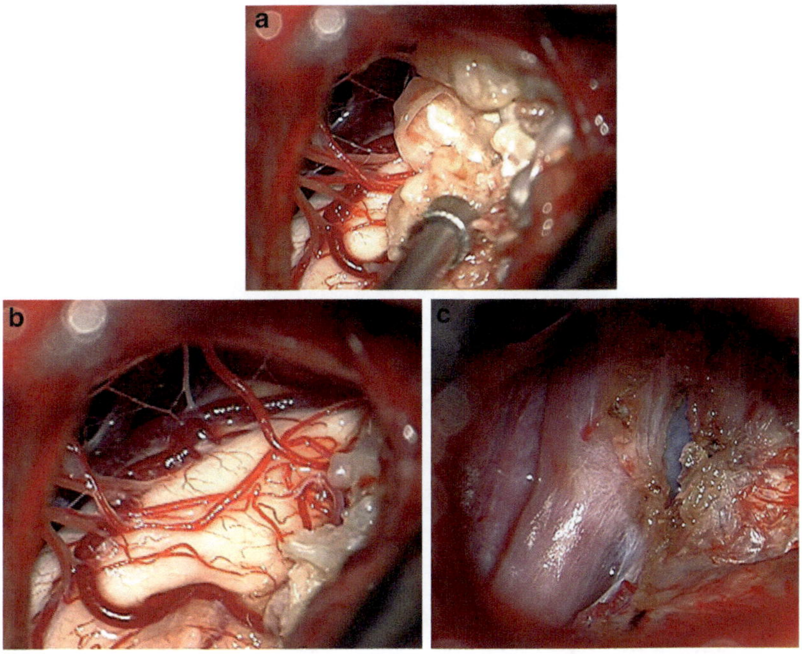

Fig. 13.4 Intraoperative pictures of the resection of a left epidermoid cyst of the cerebellopontine angle. (**a**, **b**) The lateral aspect of the medulla oblongata and the rootlets of the hypoglossal nerve are exposed following the excision of the lower pole of the cyst. (**c**) Both vertebral arteries are visible just prior to their union to form the basilar artery, with some adhesions still present between the adventitia, arachnoid membranes, and cyst membrane debris

be used to trace the cyst's expansion to the fourth ventricle and remove it completely. The choroid plexus, which is always located cranially, is used as a reference point, as it is dependent on the tela choroidea of the fourth ventricle. In the event of a cyst that has grown into the fourth ventricle, the far-lateral approach is recommended, as the standard retrosigmoid approach may be insufficient for this purpose.

13.7.3.2 The Central Portion of the Cyst

The facial-cochleovestibular complex is the next nerve that is almost always implicated in the cyst. The nerve complex can be identified as it progresses from the cyst to the internal acoustic meatus, and it can be verified through direct electrical stimulation of the facial trunk (Fig. 13.6). The cyst grows exceptionally into the internal auditory canal. Resection of the cyst and membrane contents can be continued until the abducens nerve and the basilar artery trunk are identified and released near midline, after the facial-cochleovestibular nerve complex is isolated and stripped from the cyst membranes until the inferior anterolateral aspect of the pons is exposed (Fig. 13.7a).

13.7.3.3 The Cranial Portion of the Cyst

The trigeminal nerve is situated further cranially and is typically displaced medially and encircled by the cyst. Consequently, the search and identification of the nerve are particularly challenging. The nerve's frequent dysfunction and fragility upon release are typically caused by its flattening and stretching (Fig. 13.7b). The cyst may occupy a lateral position in the lateral incisural space of the ambiens cistern or a medial position in the interpeduncular cistern during the transition between the infratentorial and supratentorial spaces at the midbrain level. The superior cerebellar artery and the trochlear nerve are typically both affected by the cyst in the initial scenario, which typically affects the midbrain. The nerve is situated just below the tentorium, more cranially, in the surgical access, while the artery is located first. The cyst can be removed by opening a window of sufficient size in the tentorium if it extends to the supratentorial level in a minor extension. It is advisable to maintain the tentorium in its current state and implement a subtemporal approach in a subsequent stage if the extension is extensive. When the extension is made in the direction of the interpeduncular cistern, it can be safely removed until the anatomical level of the

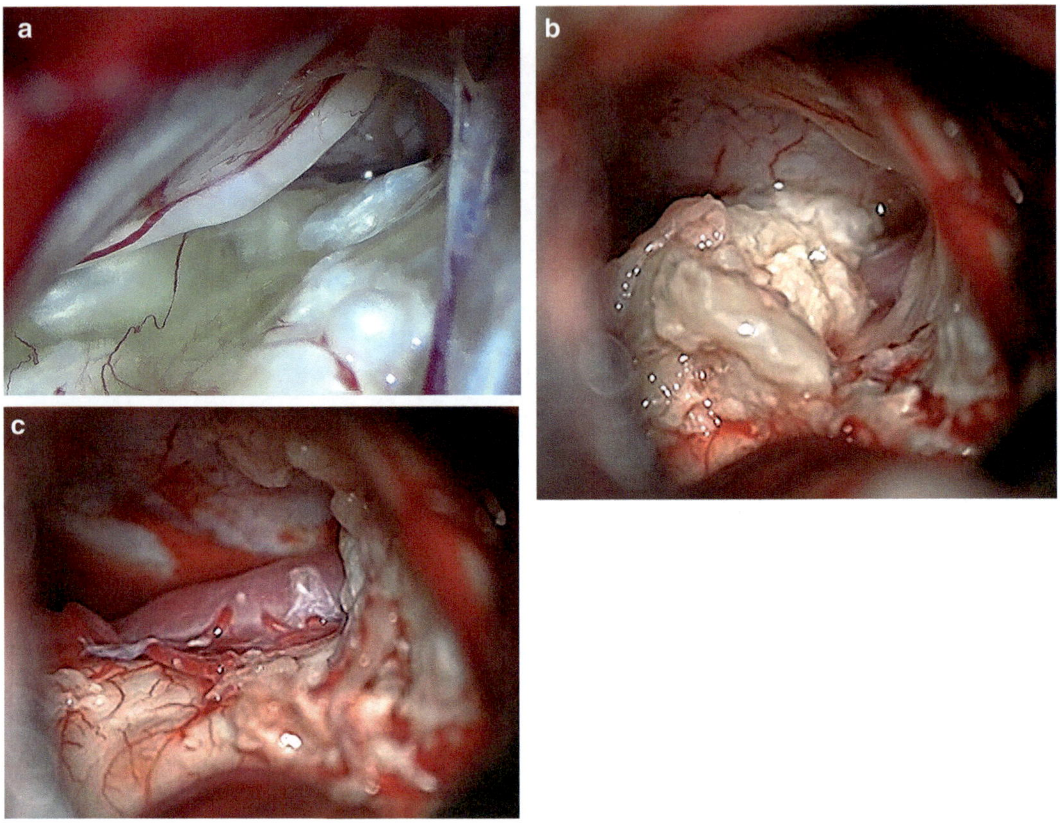

Fig. 13.5 Intraoperative pictures of the resection of a left epidermoid cyst of the cerebellopontine angle. (**a**) The accessory nerve is observed to be running outside the cyst, over the dura mater that envelops the jugular tuberculum. (**b**) The facial–cochleovestibular complex is exposed, and the fascicles of the vagal and glossopharyngeal cranial nerves are displaced cranially in a deeper plane after the tumor has been debulked. (**c**) Additional debulking enables the vertebral artery to be exposed, along with a few perforate arteries that extend to the anterior aspect of the medulla oblongata

oculomotor nerve is reached, which will expose the upper portion of the basilar artery, its branches, and bifurcation medially (Fig. 13.8).

13.7.4 Resection of the Cyst Wall

The radical cleaning of the nerve roots is only possible through numerous delicate manipulations, and the resection of the membrane affixed to the nerve roots is cumbersome and occasionally unproductive. The same principle applies to the separation of the membrane from the brainstem's surface, although the removal of pial adhesions is less challenging. Debris that is highly adherent or situated in blind areas may be left in place, although some authors suggest coagulating it. However, bipolar coagulation can also result in neurological damage as a result of the heating process. Consequently, it is imperative to conduct intraoperative neurophysiological monitoring of all cranial nerves in the posterior fossa, auditory evoked potentials of the brainstem (BEAPs), ascending pathway somatosensory evoked potentials (SSEPs), and descending motor electromyographic recording by transcranial cortical magnetic motor stimulation (TcMMEPs) in these patients. Arterial vessels are frequently grossly displaced by the cyst or implicated in the cyst membranes, and they exhibit a significant degree of individual variability. It is not feasible to indirectly identify

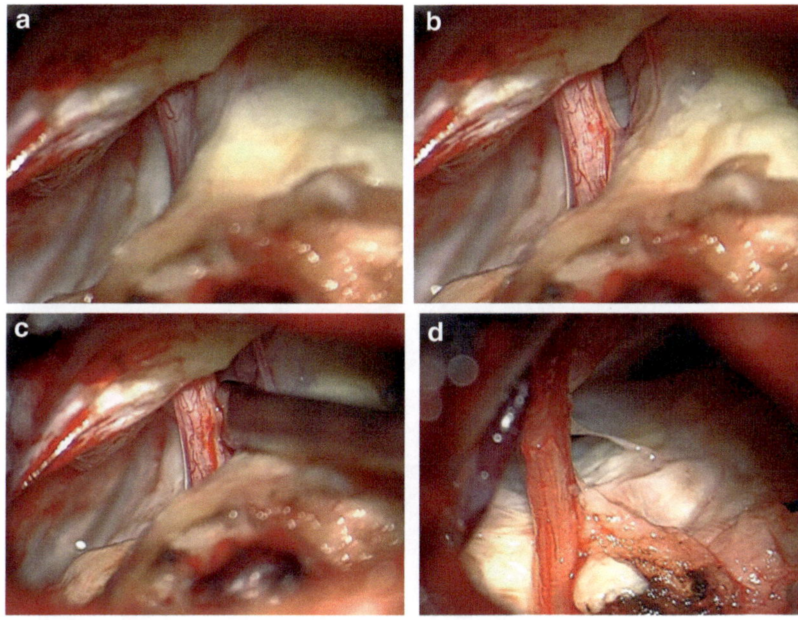

Fig. 13.6 Intraoperative pictures of the resection of a left epidermoid cyst of the cerebellopontine angle. (**a**, **b**) The facial nerve and cochleovestibular nerve are observed to emerge from the cyst and extend to the internal auditory meatus. (**c**) Direct electric stimulation of the facial nerve. (**d**) The nerves are in the advanced stage of dissection

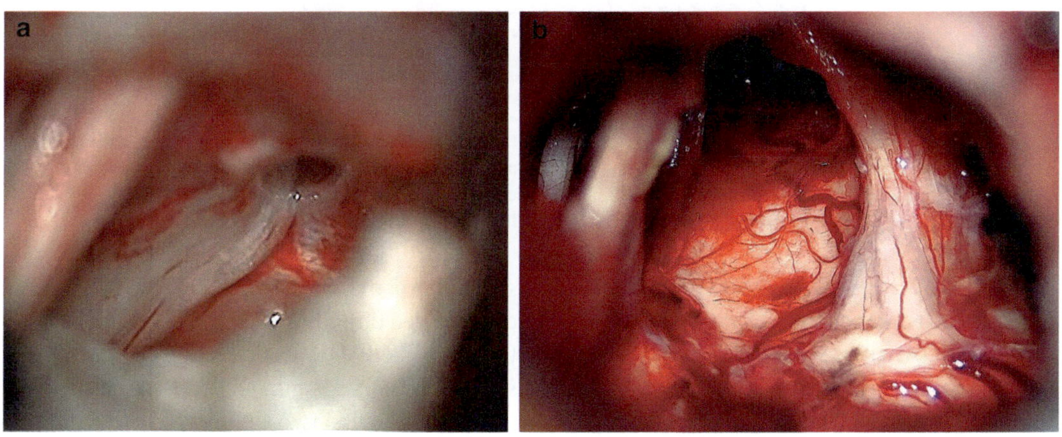

Fig. 13.7 Intraoperative pictures of the resection of a left epidermoid cyst of the cerebellopontine angle. (**a**) Image illustrating the sixth cranial nerve's entry into the Dorello's canal. (**b**) The trigeminal nerve is flattened and stretched following decompression

them with intraoperative aids. The adventitia of large vessels, such as the vertebral artery or basilar artery, may be affixed to the cyst membrane, which complicates any attempt at radical excision (Fig. 13.3b). In the first instance, the veins are either displaced or submerged in the cyst's membrane, as is frequently the case with those of the superior petrosal venous complex (Fig. 13.3c).

Complete communication with the neighboring compartment is guaranteed upon the completion of each compartment's resection. The whole surgical field is then extensively washed with warm saline to remove any undetected debris and to inspect for blind spots. Intraoperative endoscopy may prove advantageous in this endeavor. The placement of a barrier is guaranteed in the event of unresected expansions, which enables the limit of the resection to be identified in postoperative imaging studies and in an eventual access by a subsequent surgical approach.

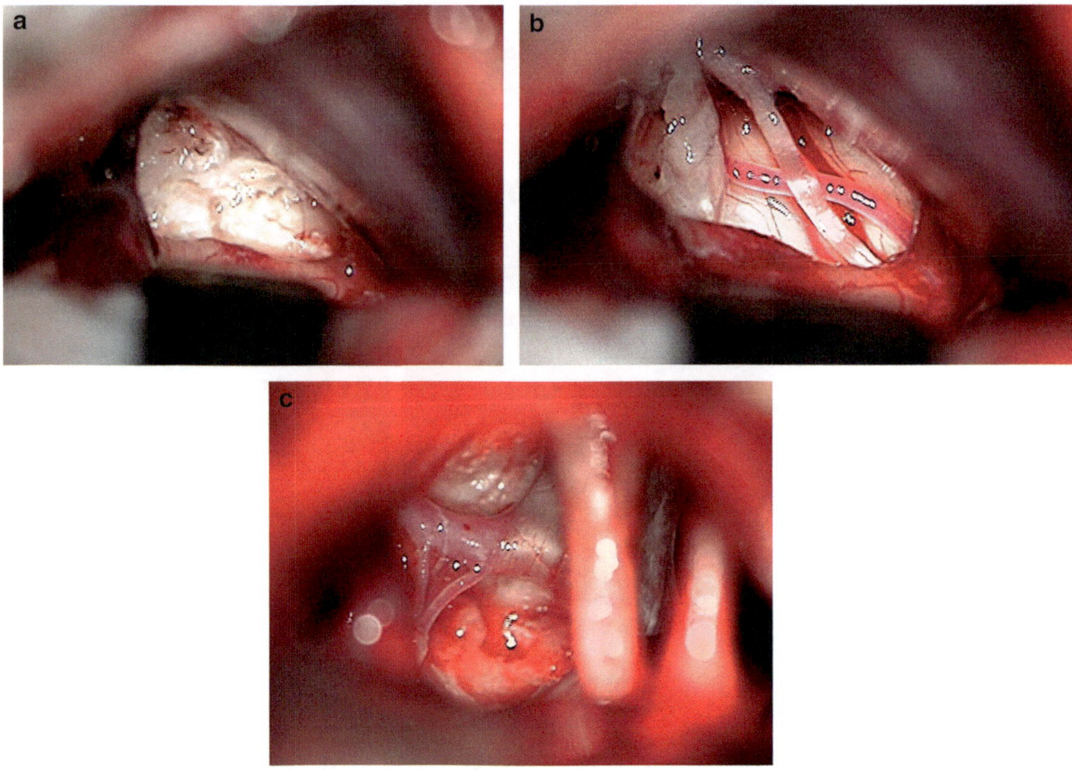

Fig. 13.8 Intraoperative pictures of the resection of a left epidermoid cyst of the cerebellopontine angle. (**a**) Image illustrating the epidermoid cyst, which is situated beneath the tentorium, filling the supracerebellar cistern. (**b**) The trochlear nerve and a branch of the superior cerebellar artery are exposed following the partial excision of the cyst. (**c**) Image of the interpeduncular cistern illustrating the bifurcation of the basilar artery

13.7.5 Neurovascular Decompression

The resolution of symptoms, particularly trigeminal neuralgia and hemifacial spasm, is a top priority of surgery when the most pertinent symptom for the patient is the dysfunction of one of the cranial nerves [6]. To this end, there are specific strategies that are complementary to those that have been previously described. In this regard, the relationships between the cyst and the neurovascular elements have been categorized into four types based on the pattern of relationship between the root entry zone of the trigeminal nerve and the root entry zone of the facial nerve: the nerve is completely buried by the tumor, but without displacement; the nerve is compressed and distorted by the tumor; the nerve is displaced in a cranial or caudal direction by the tumor and is compressed directly by an artery on the opposite side of the nerve; and, finally, the nerve is compressed directly by an artery displaced by the tumor located on the same side. The decompression of the nerve is guaranteed by the removal of the cyst in the first two situations. In the other two situations, the decompression of the nerve must be accompanied by the mobilization of the artery and, ultimately, the microvascular decompression by the placement of an interposed material to maintain the separation of the neurovascular elements. This process will be detailed in the chapters dedicated to cranial nerve rhizopathies.

13.8 Epidermoid Cysts that Require Specific Treatment

The fourth ventricle, the brainstem, the intradiploic occipital bone, and the petrosal bone epidermoid are the other topographies of posterior fossa epidermoid cysts.

13.8.1 Epidermoid Cyst of the Fourth Ventricle

The standard medial suboccipital approach is employed to treat cysts of the fourth ventricle (Fig. 13.9). They are typically visible through the arachnoid of the cisterna magna, as they expand into the cisterna that separates the cerebellar tonsils. The vallecula and the tela choroidea's section can be entirely exposed due to their opening. The general principles outlined for the cerebellopontine angle epidermoid cyst are applied to the removal of the fourth ventricle epidermoid cyst. Special attention is given to the separation of the deepest membranes of the cyst from the fourth ventricle floor to prevent morbidity. This maneuver is facilitated by the removal of the cyst's contents, provided that the membrane remains intact. The lateral recesses of the fourth ventricle are exposed to one or both sides to resolve the eventual uni- or bilateral expansion of the cyst to the cerebellopontine angle. In order to resolve or prevent the development of hydrocephalus, the permeability of the sylvian aqueduct must be verified and guaranteed [7].

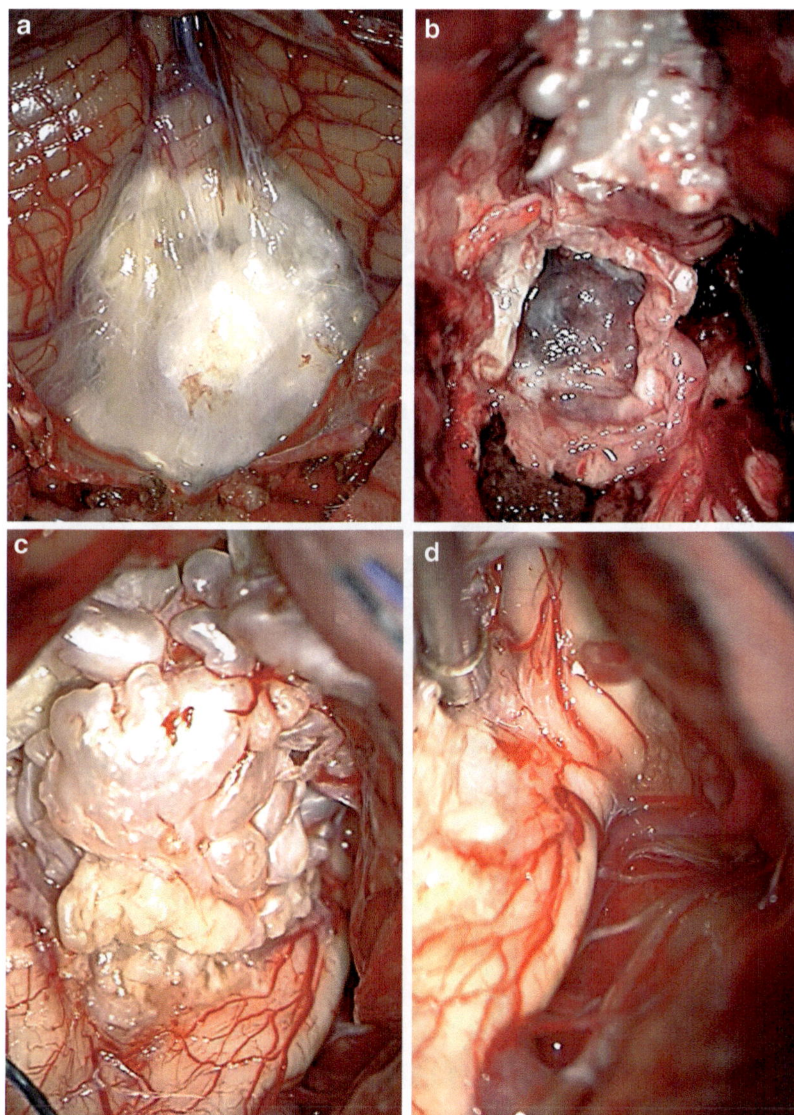

Fig. 13.9 Intraoperative pictures of the resection of an epidermoid cyst of the fourth ventricle. (**a**) Image showing the tumor occupying the cisterna magna before opening the arachnoid. (**b**) After emptying the contents, the capsule can be seen. (**c**, **d**) Images of the right lateral recess through which there was an extension of the cyst into the cerebellopontine angle, before and after its removal

13.8.2 Epidermoid Cyst of the Brainstem

The only treatment available for brainstem epidermoid cysts is palliative. A retrosigmoid approach is employed to access the most superficial point of the cyst near the pia mater or the area of exophytic growth. In the latter instance, the lesion is accessed through a cortectomy performed in one of the safe areas of entry to the brainstem. This access, which is typically extremely restricted, is used to evacuate the contents of the cyst and remove the membrane, which is almost always done in an incomplete manner [9].

13.8.3 Epidermoid Cyst of the Occipital Bone

Resection of the cyst is the standard treatment, which typically results in bone insufflation, deformation, and thinning. The dura mater is generally held in high regard. To guarantee the radical resection of the cyst and to perform a sufficient cranium repair using cranioplasty techniques (Fig. 13.10), it is recommended that a complete bone resection be performed. The functional and aesthetic prognosis is exceptional.

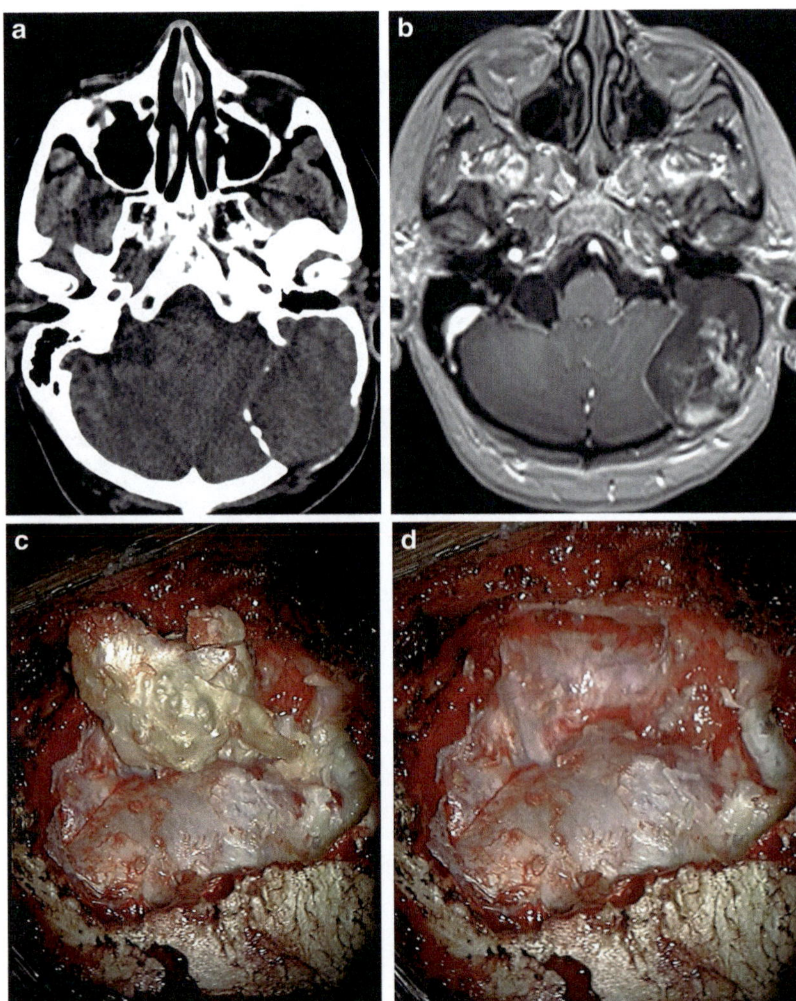

Fig. 13.10 Intradiploic epidermoid cyst of the occipital bone. (**a**) Axial CT section showing the lesion, insufflating and thinning the outer table and the inner table of the occipital bone. (**b**) Axial section in T1 sequence with gadolinium, showing an irregular enhancement. (**c**) Intraoperative image displaying the cyst and its contents over the dura mater following bone resection. (**d**) Image after total removal of the cyst, with the dura mater exposed

13.8.4 Epidermoid Cyst of the Petrosal Bone

Otologists are usually responsible for the management of congenital epidermoid cysts of the petrosal bone, which are exceedingly uncommon and only occasionally treated with microneurosurgical procedures. The cyst is operated on through a neurosurgical approach, typically a petrosectomy, in cases where there is an intracranial extension. This approach resolves the petrosal component of the cyst and, in conjunction with access to the intracranial component of the cyst through a presigmoid, retrosigmoid, or combined approach, resects the intracranial portion of the cyst (refer to case 19 in Chap. 21).

13.8.5 Primary Squamous Cell Carcinoma

The surgical treatment of primary squamous cell carcinoma of the cerebellopontine angle is conducted using the same strategies, approaches, and accesses as for the epidermoid cyst. However, the resection of the membrane must be much more aggressive and radical, which increases morbidity and mortality [4].

13.9 Results, Prognosis, and Follow-Up

The objective of surgical treatment for the epidermoid cyst is to decompress neurological structures by removing the cyst's contents and to prevent malignant transformation and recurrence by completely removing the cyst membrane. Nevertheless, the lesion's development pattern renders it impossible to guarantee that the cyst membrane has been completely resected. In certain instances, the membrane's complete removal is impossible due to adhesions to the neurovascular structures. Consequently, a *near-complete resection* (NTR) is attained in a subset of patients. It has been contended that incomplete resection may be adequate in elderly patients due to the delayed and slow rate of regrowth of the epidermoid cyst, which reduces morbidity and mortality with acceptable, very low recurrence rates. Nevertheless, the risk of malignant transformation and recurrence is a counterargument to incomplete resection. Additionally, neurovascular adhesions and fibrosis significantly increase morbidity and mortality in the event of a recurrence necessitating additional surgery, thereby making complete resection significantly more challenging. The rates of complete resection (GTR: *gross total resection*) in surgical series range from 50% to 80%.

The initial MRI imaging study should be conducted 6 months after surgery, with the DWI sequence being mandatory with respect to the lesion's follow-up. An imaging examination every 5 years may be sufficient for follow-up in the event of complete resection or minute residual tumors. An annual imaging investigation is advised if the residual is substantial. The literature reports a 20% recurrence rate, which does not necessarily indicate that the recurrences are symptomatic or necessitate additional microneurosurgical treatment. The aggressiveness of the resection is correlated with the recurrence rate. Consequently, the literature indicates that the recurrence rate may be nil after 5 years of subtotal resections, whereas in other series, recurrences are only identified in patients who underwent an incomplete resection. Nevertheless, it is exceedingly challenging to establish the extent of resection beyond the neurosurgeon's subjective assessment, which is invariably biased. It is important to keep in mind that the DWI sequence identifies the signal of the keratin content of the cyst but not of the membrane where the keratin-producing epithelium is located and necessitates a specific volume of keratin to be identified in the investigation. It is also possible for the cerebrospinal fluid to partially fill the cyst, which makes it more challenging to identify remnants or minor recurrences. The need for a novel microneurosurgical treatment is present when the recurrence or progression of a tumor remnant at the intervention site is accompanied by the emergence of new neurological symptoms or signs or the deterioration of residual clinical symptoms. In this regard, the simple remnant, recurrence, or regrowth of a tumor remnant does not, in and of itself, constitute a reason for a new surgical resection, unless there is a suspicion of the development of squamous cell carcinoma.

In fourth ventricle epidermoid cysts, literature references a complete resection in 50% of cases, frequent but transitory complications, and a favorable clinical evolution with improvement of preoperative symptoms in 75% of the patients who underwent surgery [7]. The postoperative morbidity and mortality rates of brainstem epidermoid cysts are extremely high, despite the fact that they have been significantly reduced in recent decades as a result of the refinement of the microneurosurgical technique and the knowledge and use of secure entry routes to the brainstem, neuronavigation, and intraoperative electrophysiological monitoring [9]. Overall, the prognosis of intraosseous epidermoid cysts is excellent.

Nevertheless, the prognosis of the squamous cell carcinoma is extremely bleak; the survival rate at 1 year is 80%, and at 5 years, it is a mere 20%. The benefits of complementary treatment with radiotherapy or stereotactic radiosurgery and chemotherapy are not well demonstrated due to the heterogeneity of cases and the limited number of patients [4].

13.10 Complications, Prevention, and Management

It is not uncommon for the cranial nerves that were subjected to manipulation during the surgical excision of the cyst to experience a temporary decline in function following the procedure. This phenomenon is observed in over 40% of patients. It is also common to develop new neurological deficits, such as facial paresis, hearing loss, or swallowing disorders. Nevertheless, these deficits are typically transient and resolve within a few weeks. Nevertheless, neurological morbidity may be more severe and persistent over time when there is ischemia of the cerebellar peduncle or brain stem.

To prevent postoperative aseptic meningitis caused by the leakage of material from the cyst into the subarachnoid space, which contaminates the cerebrospinal fluid, it has been suggested to wash the surgical field with a steroid solution (100 mg/l of hydrocortisone) or to administer high doses of steroids preemptively in the immediate postoperative period (dexamethasone 16–24 mg/day for 1 week) or for an extended period following the intervention in lower doses. Nevertheless, this complication is rare in the literature and has never occurred in our experience. Consequently, we only recommend the prevention of cyst material leakage during resection and the thorough washing of the surgical field with warm saline solution during the surgery and at the conclusion of the procedure. This method prevents potential complications associated with the use of steroids.

13.11 Management Modalities

13.11.1 Microneurosurgery

Microneurosurgical treatment is recommended for symptomatic patients and lesions that exhibit rapid growth or indications of malignant transformation on imaging studies. Microneurosurgery is advised for lesions that are substantial in size. Nevertheless, this does not substantiate the necessity of waiting for asymptomatic lesions to grow or reach a large size. The objective of surgery is to completely resect the cyst walls to prevent their recurrence and malignant transformation without introducing new neurological deficits. This has been demonstrated to be more straightforward and safer in smaller lesions.

A conventional retrosigmoid approach is employed to treat epidermoid lesions that are located in the cerebellopontine angle. The cranial extensions of the cyst, which occupy the interpeduncular and ambiens cisterns, can be reached up to the level of the third cranial nerve using this approach. Medial enlargement of the retrosigmoid craniotomy is necessary to facilitate lateral supracerebellar access for cranial extensions into the quadrigeminal cistern or supracerebellar space. A combined supra-infratentorial approach or a two-step approach is required when the supratentorial space is more cranial. We suggest a two-step approach: first, a retrosigmoid approach to access the symptomatic component of the cyst, which is typically the infratentorial one, and then a pterional or subtemporal approach to access the asymptomatic residual tumor. The interval between one intervention and the next may be extended until the residual tumor's growth is confirmed or symptoms manifest. This strategy necessitates the insertion of a sheet of non-absorbable material to indicate the upper limit of the resection and a radical resection of the infratentorial portion. A far-lateral approach is employed to remove the epidermoid cyst when it extends to the foramen magnum or the fourth ventricle. Contralateral extension in front of the brainstem can be pursued through the side of the initial approach, but the management of the vertebral arteries and basilar artery and their perforators is hazardous, so it can be completed with a second contralateral retrosigmoid approach.

13.11.2 Neuroendoscopy

Microneurosurgical resection is the preferred treatment for epidermoid cysts. Neuroendoscopy, which was initially employed to facilitate the visualization or resection of remains in blind spots or areas that are difficult to see under the surgical microscope, is now being used as a single method of treatment, despite the fact that resection is based on the microneurosurgical technique. The surgical approach for endoscopy is identical to that of microsurgery, namely the introduction of the neuroendoscope through a retrosigmoid craniotomy with a diameter of approximately 2 cm. An aperture is created in the cyst capsule after it has been identified, and the contents are aspirated to prevent the spread of the infection throughout the surgical field and postoperative aseptic meningitis. The capsule is subsequently resected in a sequential manner, running in conjunction with the nerves and arteries. The surgical field is thoroughly rinsed with saline or dexamethasone solution following the resection. Typically, the neurosurgeon employs one hand to hold the endoscope and the other for surgery. However, there are instances in which the assistant may be required to hold the endoscope to enable the surgeon to use both hands. The combination of a thorough understanding of the surgical anatomy of the cerebellopontine angle, systematic resection using the windows between nerves and arteries, reverence for nerve roots, arteries, and veins, and a significant amount of experience in the management of neuroendoscopy results in favorable outcomes. The degree of resection and clinical outcomes are comparable to those achieved through microsurgery in this scenario [5].

13.12 Key Messages

- *The epidermoid cyst is the most common embryonal tumor in the cerebellopontine angle cisterns and the third most common tumor in this topography. It is important to distinguish it from other cerebellopontine angle cysts, as well as from middle ear and petrosal bone cholesteatomas and epidermoid cysts.*
- *Other locations are the fourth ventricle, brainstem, petrosal, and occipital bone.*
- *Adults with epidermoid cysts may manifest a diverse array of symptoms, including cerebellar dysfunction, hydrocephalus, and headaches. Hemifacial spasm, trigeminal neuralgia, and hearing loss are among the most conspicuous indicators of cranial nerve involvement.*
- *The cyst membrane contains the tumoral epithelial layer that generates the cyst's contents and induces its expansion. This layer must be entirely removed and the contents evacuated during microneurosurgical removal.*
- *Regrowth is more probable when resection is subtotal and occurs over time. Furthermore, it increases the uncommon risk of malignant transformation. Nevertheless, the risk of neurologic morbidity is increased by complete resection, although this is typically temporary.*

References

1. Bambakidis N, Megerian CA, Spetzler RF, editors. Surgery of the cerebellopontine angle. Cham: Springer Nature; 2018.
2. Czernicki T, Kunert P, Nowak A, Wojciechowski J, Marchel A. Epidermoid cysts of the cerebellopontine angle: clinical features and treatment outcomes. Neurol Neurochir Pol. 2016;50:75–82. https://doi.org/10.1016/j.pjnns.2015.11.008.
3. Gonzalez-Darder JM, Quilis-Quesada V, Capilla-Guasch P, de Oliveira E. Abordajes neuroquirúrgicos de la patología craneal y cerebral. Barcelona: Elsevier España; 2020.
4. Hamlat A, Hua ZF, Saikali S, Laurent JF, Gedouin D, Ben-Hassel M, Guegan Y. Malignant transformation of intra-cranial epithelial cysts: systematic article review. J Neuro-Oncol. 2005;74:187–94. https://doi.org/10.1007/s11060-004-5175-4.
5. Hu Z, Guan F, Kang T, Huang H, Dai B, Zhu G, Mao B, Kang Z. Whole course neuroendoscopic resection of cerebellopontine angle epidermoid cysts. J Neurol Surg A Cent Eur Neurosurg. 2016;77:381–8. https://doi.org/10.1055/s-0035-1558818.
6. Kobata H, Kondo A, Iwasaki K. Cerebellopontine angle epidermoids presenting with cranial nerve hyperactive dysfunction: pathogenesis and long-term surgical results in 30 patients. Neurosurgery. 2002;50:276–85. https://doi.org/10.1097/00006123-200202000-00008.
7. Kumar S, Sahana D, Rathore L, Sahu RK, Jain A, Borde P, Tawari M, Madhariya SN. Fourth ventricular epidermoid cyst - case series, systematic review and analysis. Asian J Neurosurg. 2021;16:470–82. https://doi.org/10.4103/ajns.AJNS_539_20.
8. Nagasawa D, Yew A, Safaee M, Fong B, Gopen Q, Parsa AT, Yang I. Clinical characteristics and diagnostic imaging of epidermoid tumors. J Clin Neurosci. 2011;18(9):1158–62. https://doi.org/10.1016/j.jocn.2011.02.008.
9. Patibandla MR, Yerramneni VK, Mudumba VS, Manisha N, Addagada GC. Brainstem epidermoid cyst: an update. Asian J Neurosurg. 2016;11:194–200. https://doi.org/10.4103/1793-5482.145163.
10. Rhoton AL Jr. The posterior fossa: microsurgical anatomy & surgical approaches. Neurosurgery. 2000;47(3 Suppl):S1–S279. https://doi.org/10.1097/00006123-200009001-00013.
11. Rutkowska J, Özgirgin N, Olszewska E. Cholesteatoma definition and classification: a literature review. J Int Adv Otol. 2017;13:266–71. https://doi.org/10.5152/iao.2017.3411.
12. Samii M, Gerganov V. Surgery of cerebellopontine angle lesions. Berlin-Heildelberg: Springer; 2013.
13. Vernon V, Naik H, Guha A. Surgical management of cerebellopontine angle epidermoid cysts: an institutional experience of 10 years. Br J Neurosurg. 2022;36:203–12. https://doi.org/10.1080/02688697.2020.1867058.

Other Cystic Lesions of the Cerebellopontine Angle

14

14.1 Introduction

In this topography, the epidermoid cyst is the third most prevalent form of tumor and the most representative cystic lesion of the cerebellopontine angle. However, the cerebellopontine angle is home to a significant number of cystic lesions of varying types, each of which presents its own unique set of challenges. The arachnoid cyst is the classic differential diagnosis of the epidermoid cyst of the cerebellopontine angle. The dermoid cyst, neurenteric cyst, Rathke cyst, and craniopharyngioma are examples of true cysts that, like the epidermoid cyst, are characterized by a membrane or thin wall that is internally covered by an epithelium that generates the material that fills the cyst. The differential diagnosis by imaging with the epidermoid cyst, which was previously described in detail, will serve as a reference for the individual descriptions of these extremely uncommon lesions. Other lesions, such as cystic vestibular schwannoma and cystic cavernoma, are tumors or vascular lesions that may occasionally exhibit a more or less voluminous cystic component. However, this characteristic necessitates specific management strategies in comparison to the more prevalent solid forms. Additionally, there are infectious lesions, such as hydatidosis and cysticercosis, that present as cystic lesions in the cerebellopontine angle. Finally, it is necessary to evaluate effusions, apicitis, and cholesterol granulomas at the apex of the petrosal bone [2, 15].

14.2 Arachnoid Cyst

After the epidermoid cyst, the arachnoid cyst is the most prevalent cystic lesion in the cerebellopontine angle. It is, in turn, the second most common location of intracranial arachnoid cysts, following those located in the sylvian fissure, and accounts for approximately 10% of the total. While the cerebellopontine angle is the sole location of over half of them, a small number of them extend to the posterior aspect of the brainstem, either within the internal auditory canal or in the supracerebellar region. Arachnoid cysts that are exclusively confined to the internal auditory canal have been documented in exceptional cases.

The pathological structure and pathogenesis of these lesions are identical to those of any other topography. They are cerebrospinal fluid (CSF) collections that are situated between the arachnoid membranes. The cyst's wall is composed of a thin connective layer that is covered by meningothelial cells. The exact cause of this accumulation remains uncertain. The formation of an arachnoid diverticulum or a duplication of the arachnoid membranes, which is progressively filled with cerebrospinal fluid over time, is generally considered to be of congenital origin. This would be corroborated by the occasional association with other malformations and the presence of an increase in the size of the posterior fossa. Additional hypotheses include a traumatic etiology that is secondary to inflammation,

J. M. González-Darder, *Microneurosurgery of Cerebellopontine Angle*,
https://doi.org/10.1007/978-3-032-03091-7_14

infection, or hemorrhage in the arachnoid. The arachnoid cyst's growth rate is highly variable. Some remain asymptomatic for years or throughout one's life, while others increase in volume and develop symptoms. The growth mechanism is attributed to the progressive trapping of cerebrospinal fluid within the cyst through diffusion through the arachnoid or active secretion of the cyst wall. This process is induced by the osmolarity difference between the cyst fluid and the cerebrospinal fluid or by the production of small hemorrhages within the cyst. A valvular mechanism formed by the cyst membranes would be another factor that contributes to growth. This mechanism would permit the entry of cerebrospinal fluid from the cisterns rather than its departure, resulting in a net outcome that is advantageous to the cyst's growth. A few reports have also been made of the cyst's spontaneous reduction or disappearance.

Currently, the overwhelming majority of cerebellopontine angle arachnoid cysts are diagnosed incidentally in imaging studies due to trauma or in patients with nonspecific symptoms or symptoms unrelated to the injury. The symptoms in symptomatic cases are caused by hydrocephalus or compression of the cranial nerve roots, brainstem, or cerebellum. Consequently, the presenting symptoms include headache, dizziness or vertigo, hearing loss, tinnitus, gait disorders, and, in uncommon cases, dysfunction of the trigeminal nerve with secondary trigeminal neuralgia and of the facial nerve with hemifacial spasm. The symptoms are typically insidious and progressive, although sudden presentation is common in cases of spontaneous or traumatic hemorrhage within the cyst. They are typically diagnosed in young patients in the third decade of life, following a lengthy history of an average of five years of evolution. Computed tomography (CT) and magnetic resonance imaging (MRI) are both highly sensitive and specific methods of imaging diagnosis. In CT studies, the cerebellopontine angle is occupied by an isointense lesion that respects cerebrospinal fluid, is extra-axial, and displaces the nervous tissue. The lesion has rounded and clear borders, is generally devoid of septa or calcifications, and its thin wall does not acquire contrast (Fig. 14.1a). They may exhibit an increase in the size of the posterior fossa, which is highly characteristic and reflects the lengthy evolution of the cyst; even the bone adjacent to the lesion is thinning or bulging. This deformity may manifest in children prior to the closure of the cranium. The signal of arachnoid cysts is identical to that of cerebrospinal fluid in all MRI sequences. In MRI, the arachnoid cyst is hypointense in the T1 sequence and hyperintense in T2. Arachnoid cyst membranes do not enhance after contrast administration (Figs. 14.1b, c). The differential diagnosis of epidermoid cysts is based on the absence of hypersignal, which is a result of the absence of diffusion restriction in the DWI (*Diffusion Weighted Image*) sequence of MRI. Additionally, arachnoid cysts lack a specific signal in the FLAIR (*Fluid Attenuation Inversion Recovery*) sequence, and their limits are more rounded, lacking lobulations or finger-like extensions that are interspersed between the nerves and vessels, but rather displace them.

Arachnoid cysts that are asymptomatic should be monitored with clinical and imaging tests, but they do not necessitate treatment as they usually do not exhibit growth. The presence of hydrocephalus, neurological symptoms, and the demonstration of cyst growth are all indications for treatment. In this regard, there are several treatment options: microneurosurgical (Fig. 14.2) or endoscopic approaches (Fig. 14.3) which involve a retrosigmoid approach, fenestration of the cyst walls, marsupialization in the subarachnoid space, and/or resection of the wall; cystoperitoneal diversion of the trapped cerebrospinal fluid with an interposed programmable valve; and, finally, stereotactic puncture and evacuation. The most effective treatment appears to be microneurosurgical treatment, which involves the complete removal of the cyst walls. However, as with epidermoid cysts, subtotal resection is associated with lower morbidity and a higher incidence of recurrences, while radical resection is associated with a higher morbidity and a lower incidence of recurrences. In the majority of cases, patients have a favorable clinical prognosis, with subjective and objective neurological function recovery of the affected nerves. However, the relief of headache in patients who suffer from them chronically is more sporadic [3, 9].

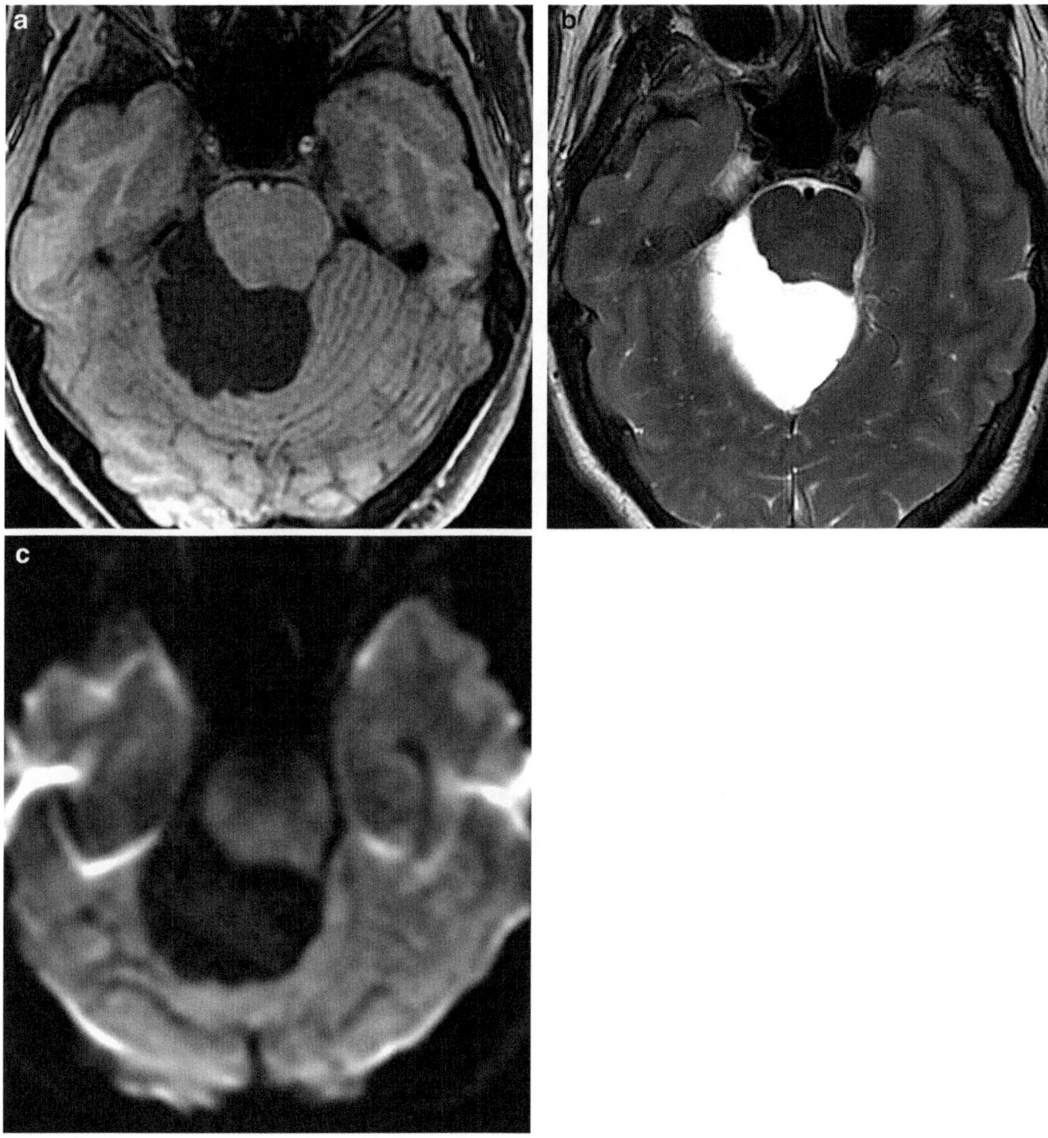

Fig. 14.1 Arachnoid cyst that extends into the quadrigeminal cistern from the cerebellopontine angle. (**a**) Axial T1-weighted MRI section, demonstrating a well-defined lesion with the same signal as the cerebrospinal fluid. (**b**) Axial T2-weighted MRI section, demonstrating a well-defined lesion with the same signal as the cerebrospinal fluid. (**c**) Axial MRI section in DWI sequence, demonstrating the absence of diffusion restriction, a characteristic of the cerebrospinal fluid that fills the arachnoid cyst

14.3 Dermoid Cyst

A dermoid cyst is a lesion that is the consequence of an embryonic development disorder. Dermoid cysts are most frequently observed in the parasellar region; however, they may occasionally be observed in the cerebellopontine angle as an isolated lesion or as a result of the caudal development of a parasellar cyst that is expanding toward the infratentorial space. Dermoid cysts are known to inhabit the midline in the nervous system, which is why their location in the cerebellopontine angle is so exceptional. The histopathology of the cyst must take into account the

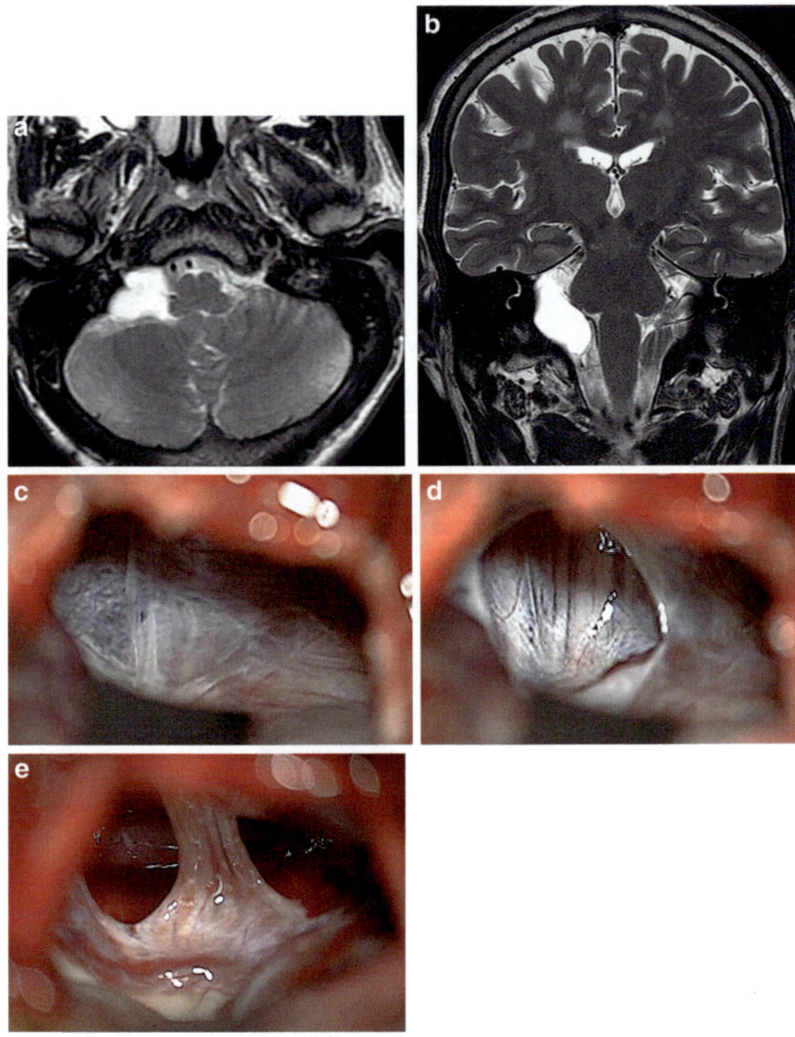

Fig. 14.2 Arachnoid cyst of the right cerebellopontine angle. (**a**, **b**). An arachnoid cyst occupying the cerebellopontine angle is demonstrated in axial and coronal T2-weighted MRI sections. (**c**–**e**) Intraoperative pictures of the lesion obtained through a microsurgical retrosigmoid approach, illustrating the most superficial wall of the cyst, the fenestration of this wall, the visualization of the deep wall that extends between the cranial nerves, and the fenestration of this wall through which the basilar artery is visualized in the prepontine cistern

cyst's wall and its contents, as is the case with other embryonic cysts. The dermoid cyst's wall is intricate, as it is composed of dermal elements, including fat, sweat glands, hair follicles, and sebaceous glands, in addition to epidermal epithelial elements. Consequently, the content is both highly variable in terms of its composition and appearance. In general, it is dense, pasty, and oily in appearance, and it contains epithelial and sebaceous desquamation material, as well as hairs and even dental structures. The cyst's growth is determined by this content, which is the outcome of cyst wall production. Midline dermoid cysts frequently exhibit a fistulous tract to the skin that is more or less conspicuous, with a depression or dermal sinus that is occasionally accompanied by cutaneous lesions [6]. This communication ascertains the potential for cystic infection, which may induce symptoms or exacerbate the lesion's size. Nevertheless, dermoid cysts of the cerebellopontine angle lack this external communication, resulting in a sluggish growth rate that is solely influenced by the secretion and production of material from the cyst wall. The symptoms are determined by the compression of the nerves, the brainstem, or the cerebellum, as well as hydrocephalus. The findings in imaging studies also demonstrate a very broad spectrum as a result of the variability of its structure and content. The wall of dermoid cysts

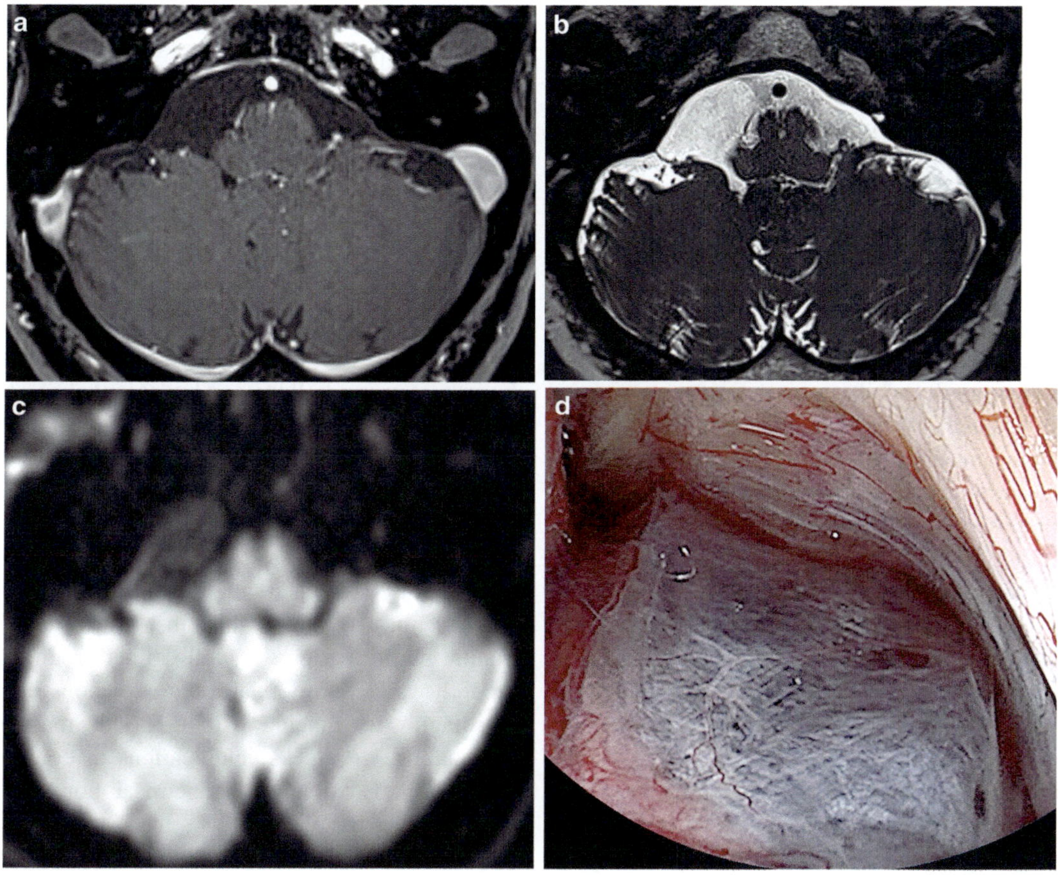

Fig. 14.3 Arachnoid cyst of the right cerebellopontine angle. (**a–c**). An arachnoid cyst occupying the cerebellopontine angle is demonstrated in axial T1-weighted with gadolinium, T2, and DWI MRI sequences. (**d**) Intraoperative picture of the lesion obtained through an endoscopic retrosigmoid approach, illustrating the most superficial wall of the cyst before fenestration

may spontaneously rupture, resulting in the discharge of small lumps of material and a meningeal reaction that is more or less significant, similar to epidermoid cysts. In CT, these lesions are well-defined and hypointense, with a solid wall and a rounded appearance. They may exhibit contrast uptake and calcifications. The adipose content is closely correlated with the lesion's appearance on MRI, resulting in a heterogeneous appearance with areas of hyperintensity on T1 and hypointensity on T2. Lastly, they exhibit diffusion restriction and are subsequently brilliant on diffusion-weighted DWI sequences. Growth and symptomatic cysts are the indications for treatment. The treatment is primarily microneurosurgical resection, which involves the tumor being accessed through a retrosigmoid approach. The treatment strategy involves the evacuation of the content and the complete resection of the wall. Nevertheless, the wall of a dermoid cyst is denser than that of an epidermoid cyst and may have significant and dense adhesions to arteries and nerve roots. Due to the minimal recurrence tendency of dermoid cysts, it is preferable to leave some remnants on the nerve structures rather than expose them to a significant risk of anatomical or functional damage. Nor does the risk of recurrence of the lesion appear to be elevated by the discharge and dissemination of the contents or remains of the cyst wall.

14.4 Neurenteric Cyst

The cerebellopontine angle neurenteric cyst is an exceedingly uncommon lesion, comprising approximately 0.1% of all lesions of this nature. It is typically situated in the midline, on the anterior surface of the cervical or thoracic spinal cord. However, some cases exhibit intracranial topography, with 90% of them located in the posterior fossa. Only 20% of the neurenteric cysts in the posterior fossa are situated in the cerebellopontine angle, while the remaining are situated on the anterior surface of the brainstem or in the fourth ventricle. This lesion is the consequence of an embryonic development disorder. Its wall is composed of an epithelium that secretes mucous and is likely of endodermal origin. As a result, the neurenteric cyst is a member of a group of cystic lesions that contain a variety of epithelia in their wall, including respiratory and pharyngeal epithelium. This group also includes the colloid cyst and the Rathke pouch cyst. This has resulted in the confusion of terminology and classifications. The neurenteric cyst would be the consequence of the entrapment of the embryonic neurenteric canal's remnants in its path through the notochord of the embryo, which would not vanish entirely, leaving a remnant trapped.

The histopathology of these lesions consists of a membrane with a pseudostratified cuboidal or columnar epithelium, secretory granules, and a well-defined basement membrane. This membrane is reminiscent of the mucosa of the intestinal or respiratory tract. Cases of squamous metaplasia have been documented. In other instances, benign mesenchymal content, such as adipocytes or muscle fibers, or neuroectodermal content, such as nerve filaments and ganglion cells, have been identified. The cells exhibit positivity in immunohistochemical assays for cytokeratins, EMA (*Epithelial Membrane Antigen*), and CEA (*Carcinoembryonic Antigen*), which are endodermal markers. By contrast, they do not exhibit a response to neuroectodermal immunohistochemical markers. The granules may be PAS (*Periodic Acid Schiff*) positive. The contents of the cyst are a milky-colored, mucinous secretion that is occasionally transparent or xanthochromic. The growth of the cyst is determined by this content, which is secreted by the membrane's epithelial cells.

The clinical symptoms are comparable to those of the other cystic lesions in this topography. The majority are incidental findings in imaging investigations that are the result of trauma or unrelated symptoms. The clinical manifestations are primarily characterized by disorders of the cochleovestibular nerves (dizziness or vertigo, hearing loss, tinnitus) and pain, which are the result of compression of the nervous structures, brainstem or cerebellum, and hydrocephalus. The fourth decade is the typical age of manifestation. In more than half of the cases, neurenteric cysts of the spinal cord are associated with other malformations or congenital anomalies of the vertebrae, neuraxis, and respiratory or digestive tract. However, cysts located intracranially are isolated and are not associated with other types of congenital malformations. A well-defined, rounded, smooth-walled extra-axial mass is demonstrated by diagnostic imaging with CT. This mass is hypointense and lacks calcifications or contrast absorption. Erosion of the petrosal bone may occasionally be observed. In the T1-weighted sequence, a well-defined mass of variable appearance is detected, which is hypointense and similar to the cerebrospinal fluid when the water and protein content of the cyst is low. However, it is isointense or hyperintense in relation to the parenchyma in T1 when the protein content is low. A dermoid cyst is typically hyperintense in T2-weighted and FLAIR sequences. The neurenteric cyst is dark in the DWI sequence because it does not exhibit diffusion restriction, in contrast to the epidermoid cyst, which exhibits hyperintensity in the DWI sequence due to its diffusion restriction.

Microneurosurgical treatment should be offered to patients with lesions that are symptomatic or exhibit growth on imaging studies. The objective of microneurosurgical treatment is the complete resection of the cyst wall and its contents using a retrosigmoid approach. Recurrences have been documented in the literature in one-third of cases, typically years following the initial intervention. The rule is that recurrences occur following incomplete resection of the cyst wall. Nevertheless, radicality is linked to a higher level of morbidity. In the event of severe adhesions between the cyst wall and nerves, it may be prudent to save a portion of the cyst wall and subject the patient to regular imaging follow-up [12, 16].

14.5 Rathke's Cyst and Craniopharyngioma

Some isolated cases of cystic lesions in the cerebellopontine angle have been described in the literature with the same histopathological appearance as that of Rathke's cysts and craniopharyngiomas. Both lesions have their usual topography in the midline, in the sella turcica or suprasellar space, and some, rarer, are located at the base of the skull or pharyngeal region. This characteristic topography is due to the fact that they are formed from remnants of Rathke's pouch in its course along the craniopharyngeal canal until forming the adenohypophysis. Two hypotheses have been described to explain why these lesions are also located in the cerebellopontine angle. The first is that they are expansions from suprasellar lesions located in the tuberal or infundibular portion of the hypophyseal stalk and that, as they grow, they access laterally to reach one of the cerebellopontine angles. The other would be the aberrant migration of the remains of Rathke's pouch towards the posterior fossa during embryonic development, becoming trapped in this location. The histopathology of Rathke's cysts and cystic craniopharyngiomas described in the cerebellopontine angle is similar to that of their usual location. However, the clinical and diagnostic imaging characteristics cannot be established, given the small number of cases described. In all patients, the diagnosis was made after pathological study [4, 13].

14.6 Cystic Cavernoma

In neurosurgical practice, cerebral cavernoma is a relatively common vascular lesion that is characterized by the compact accumulation of a network of multiple dilated vascular channels covered by a simple endothelial layer, embedded in hemosiderin deposits, and surrounded by gliosis. It is a dysplastic or hamartomatous lesion. Some cavernomas may be cystic, and 20% of them are situated in the cerebellopontine angle. The cyst wall is composed of fibrous tissue, inflammatory cells, neocapillaries, and hemosiderin deposits, while the nodule exhibits the pathological characteristics of a typical cavernoma. The exact mechanism by which solid cavernoma generates massive cysts remains unclear. It has been proposed that the condition may be the consequence of repeated hemorrhages that originate in the vascular channels of the cavernoma or in the neocapillaries of the periphery. This, in conjunction with the high osmolarity of the cyst contents, may result in the entry of fluid through the membrane. This mechanism is similar to that of chronic traumatic subdural hematoma of the convexity of the cerebral hemispheres. A number of patients have multiple lesions, and they are frequently familial cases.

CT imaging reveals a solid component within a spherical cystic mass. Contrast uptake may be observed in the solid component and cyst wall. In MRI, the cyst is iso or hyperintense in T1 and hyperintense in T2, while the nodule has a mixed signal in T1- and T2-weighted sequences in the MRI study. As with CT, gadolinium enhancement may be observed in both the nodule and the wall. The DWI MRI sequence reveals regions of hypointensity in the nodule or the vicinity of the cyst, which indicate the presence of hemosiderin or blood. Calcifications are occasionally observed. Cerebral digital subtraction angiography (DSA) demonstrates an avascular mass and enables the frequent association of a venous angioma, which is frequently already visible in the MRI study, to be ruled out.

Microneurosurgical treatment is advised for lesions that are symptomatic and exhibit growth or hemorrhage. Similar to other lesions described in this chapter, it is feasible to identify substantial adhesions between the cavernoma's wall and the cranial nerve roots, particularly the seventh and eighth. Consequently, if the process is non-tumorous, it may be permissible to retain a small amount of the capsule if it safeguards neurological function. The prognosis is favorable, and the likelihood of regrowth is nearly nonexistent [8, 11].

14.7 Hydatidic Cyst

Hydatidosis is a zoonosis that is caused by *Echinococcus granulosus*. The larvae of this parasite can inadvertently infest humans during their life cycle, resulting in the infection of various organs, including the liver and lungs. The subarachnoid space is an uncommon location for intracranial infestation, which occurs in only 2% of cases and is localized in the brain parenchyma. The cyst is typically solitary, although it may be multiloculated. The histopathology of the cyst demonstrates that the membrane is composed of three layers: an external layer, which is the inflammatory and fibrous response of the host, known as the pericyst, and a deeper layer that corresponds to the parasite and is divided into two layers: the intermediate laminar and acellular layer, the endocyst, and a deeper layer, the germinal epithelium, which forms a single vesicle. Occasionally, a single multiloculated cyst may contain multiple cysts or multiple vesicles. The larval forms of the parasite, known as scolex, are contained within the vesicles. The cyst's contents are liquid, pallid, or yellowish in color and consist of proteins, lipids, and polysaccharides, as well as the scolex of the ruptured vesicles. The clinical symptoms are non-specific, and the incidence is extremely low in developed countries, even in endemic areas. The lesion's appearance in imaging investigations is highly distinctive. CT imaging reveals a hypointense lesion that is rounded, well-defined, and has a density comparable to cerebrospinal fluid. It is devoid of calcifications and contrast uptake. The MRI scan reveals a single, well-defined lesion with a rounded limit and content that resembles cerebrospinal fluid. The lesion is hypointense in the T1-weighted sequence and hyperintense in the T2 sequence, with the exception of cases where the content has been altered due to infection or superimposed hemorrhage. In T2, the pericyst may be hyperintense. Serological investigations may verify the suspected diagnosis. The cyst is removed through a microneurosurgical retrosigmoid approach in the absence of a response to medical therapy. To prevent the subarachnoid space from becoming contaminated with scolices, it is recommended that the cyst be removed without rupturing the membrane, if feasible. Valsalva maneuvers, transient compression of the jugular veins, or injection of saline solution into the pericyst are employed to facilitate the expulsion of the cyst (*delivery of the cyst*) in larger surgical fields, such as brain lesions. Nevertheless, these maneuvers may be ineffectual or hazardous in cerebellopontine angle topography due to the limited available space or the presence of adhesions with the cranial nerves or vessels, which render the cyst mobilization impossible or risky. Consequently, it may be permissible to puncture the cyst with a very thin needle to aspirate and decompress the cyst, provided that the surrounding arachnoid has been removed and the cyst membrane has been exposed. This will prevent the release of the cyst's contents into the cisterns in any case. The walls of the cyst are microsurgically dissected from the neighboring structures after the cyst has been evacuated. In order to accomplish a cure for the disease, surgical treatment must be accompanied by pharmacological treatment [14].

14.8 Neurocysticercosis

Cysticercosis is a zoonosis caused by *Taenia solium*, which affects the central nervous system in more than half of patients. The parasite's life cycle is intricate and, intriguingly, differs when it infects the brain parenchyma versus the subarachnoid space. In the former scenario, it exhibits highly distinctive phases, including vesicular lesions, colloid type, granular nodules, and calcified nodules. In the subarachnoid space, numerous vesicles of varying sizes are capable of readily traversing the cisterns and occupying the entire cerebellopontine angle. The scolex is not present in all vesicles. The symptoms of these multicystic or racemose forms are the result of a non-specific inflammatory response, compression of the nervous structures, and obstruction of the cerebrospinal fluid circulation pathways. The obstruction is not typically a result of the mass effect; rather, it is the direct and abrupt obstruction of a vesicle in narrow points, which results in acute and frequently fatal hydrocephalus. The incidence in developed countries is exceptional and typically affects the immigrant population that has migrated from endemic regions. Vesicles are identified as polylobulated cystic lesions in CT imaging studies, without contrast uptake, calcifications, or bone erosion, and with a density comparable to cerebrospinal fluid. In the T1- and T2-weighted and DWI sequences of the MRI investigation, they are comparable to cerebrospinal fluid; however, they are hyperintense in the FLAIR sequence. The septa that distinguish cysts of varying diameters can be identified in the FIESTA (*Fast Imaging Employing Steady-State Acquisition*) sequence. The presence of a single cyst is exceptional. Gadolinium does not induce any enhancement. In consecutive investigations, the morphological change of the lesion is a pathognomonic sign, which is attributed to the mobility of the small cysts in the cisterns. The diagnosis of cysticercosis is verified by plasma and cerebrospinal fluid serology assays. To rule out any additional spinal lesions, an imaging examination of the entire neuraxis should be conducted. The microneurosurgical treatment uses a retrosigmoid approach. However, patients should also be treated pharmacologically with albendazole in conjunction with steroids and anticonvulsants. To prevent their fragmentation and loss in the surgical field, vesicles should be meticulously removed. Valsalva maneuvers can be executed intraoperatively in conjunction with transient compression of both jugular veins to expedite the search for vesicles [10].

14.9 Effusion and Apicitis of the Petrosal Apex

The tip, or apex, of the petrosal bone is the most medial portion of the bone, situated at the most cranial portion of the petroclival region, between the greater wing of the sphenoid and the clivus of the occipital bone. It has a pyramidal shape. The posterior surface of the apex is triangular in shape when viewed from the cerebellopontine angle. The upper border corresponds to the end of the petrosal crest and contains the groove through which the superior petrosal sinus runs. The inferomedial border corresponds to the petroclival suture and has a groove through which the inferior petrosal sinus runs. The base is a virtual line that runs in front of the internal acoustic meatus. The apex is cranially related to Meckel's cave and the middle cranial fossa, cranial to the inferior petrosal sinus and the jugular bulb, and anterior to the canal of the internal carotid artery in its petrosal segment and the bony labyrinth. Even though the sixth cranial nerve is not directly connected to the apex of the petrosal bone, it is a very intimate anatomical relationship and has implications for the clinical symptoms of petrosal apex pathology as it enters the cavernous sinus through the dural canal of Dorello. This is also the case for the trigeminal nerve, which enters Meckel's cave by resting on the bony fissure of the petrosal crest immediately behind the petrosal apex. The sympathetic plexus, which envelops the petrosal internal carotid artery, is the third neurological element that may have clinical implications. Petrosal apex internal structure is highly variable, as it may be aerated in one-third of cases, containing cells that communicate with the middle ear. These air-filled cells may become infected (*petrositis or apicitis*) or fill with liquid (*effusion*). In some cases, these cells may generate symptoms, which can be very severe and occasionally necessitate surgical treatment.

In 1904, the classic Gradenigo syndrome was described as the paradigmatic clinical presentation of apicitis. This syndrome is characterized by paresis of the sixth cranial nerve, facial pain that is distributed along the branches of the trigeminal nerve, and purulent otitis media. However, the diagnosis of the complete syndrome is now rare due to the early use of antibiotic therapy. Purulent otitis media symptoms and signs are observed in 60% of patients, retro-orbital pain in 50% of cases, and paresis of the sixth nerve in 15%. Ophthalmoplegia, trigeminal neuralgia, hypoesthesia, or facial paresis are uncommon combinations. The symptoms may be unilateral or bilateral, and in certain instances, thrombophlebitis of the cavernous sinus or orbit may follow a complete cavernous sinus syndrome. Apicitis is a condition that affects adult patients, with some individuals having immunodeficiencies that increase their susceptibility to infection. More than half of the cases are associated with *Pseudomona aeruginosa* when the causative germ is identified. The air cells are the primary pathway through which the infection enters this region; however, the hematogenous and lymphatic routes have also been proposed. The infection may be limited to the mucosa of the cells or influence the bone, in which case it is classified as a true osteomyelitis. The effusion's clinical presentation is also highly variable, with patients reporting a sense of ear oppression, hearing loss, vertigo, and facial spasms, as well as headaches. In imaging investigations, effusions are identified on MRI by their hypointense appearance on T1-weighted sequences and hyperintense appearance on T2-weighted sequences, without gadolinium enhancement. The bone trabeculae are preserved, and there is no contrast uptake on CT (Fig. 14.4). Additionally, there is no bone erosion. In juxtaposition, apicitis is also demonstrated on MRI as hypointense on T1-weighted sequences and hyperintense on T2-weighted sequences. However, there is ring-shaped gado-

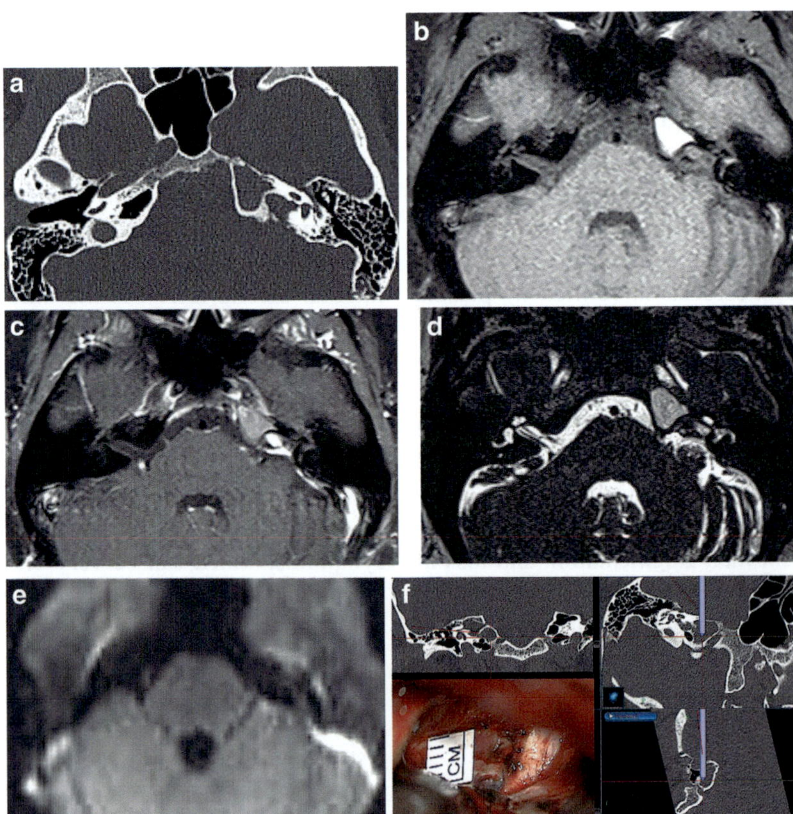

Fig. 14.4 Effusion within the left petrosal apex's cells. (**a**) Axial CT demonstrating the filling of a cell at the left petrosal apex. (**b, c**) Axial T1-weighted MRI study without and following gadolinium administration demonstrates a hypersignal in the apex, without gadolinium enhancement. (**d**) Axial T2-weighted MRI examination demonstrating hyperintensity at the apex of the petrosal bone. (**e**) MRI study demonstrating that the lesion does not exhibit any diffusion restriction on the DWI sequence, thereby ruling out the presence of infection. (**f**) The intraoperative picture and browser screenshots in the microneurosurgical extradural middle fossa approach to the cell through the Kawase triangle

linium enhancement and restriction in diffusion on DWI sequences, as well as bone erosion, bone trabeculae destruction, and contrast uptake on CT studies.

In cases of apicitis, the surgical indication is contingent upon the response to antibiotic treatment alone or in combination with otologic surgical treatment, which may involve minor procedures such as tympanostomy or the placement of ventilation tubes. At present, only approximately 10% of patients necessitate aggressive surgical intervention. Approximately 5% of instances result in mortality. Surgical indication is significantly more uncommon in the context of effusion. The treatment of asymptomatic cases is observation, while those that are secondary to a previous ear infection are treated with steroids and antibiotics. Direct drainage of the cells is only justified in cases that are refractory or have hearing loss or pain. The method of treatment for both apicitis and effusion is contingent upon the extent of the middle ear's structural involvement, auditory function, and the extent of the pathology. The sole direct approach to the apex of the petrosal bone is the extradural approach of the middle fossa through the Kawase triangle (Fig. 14.4f). From its exit from the geniculate ganglion through the fallopian hiatus until it passes under the V3 branch of the trigeminal nerve, the greater petrosal nerve forms one of the sides of the Kawase triangle, which is situated medially to it. From its departure from the gasserian ganglion to the petrosal nerve, the V3 branch establishes the second limit. Lastly, the third is defined by a line that extends from the fallopian hiatus to the dural foramen of Meckel's cavum. The anatomical relationships of the triangle are of great significance. The internal carotid artery, in its horizontal petrosal segment, passes through the anterior border of the triangle. The cochlea projects into the lateral angle of the triangle. The internal auditory canal is accessible by drilling the bone in its lateral portion. Finally, the lateral surface of the clivus and inferior petrosal sinus can be accessed by drilling the bony of the medial portion. The anterior petrosectomy, which involves the removal of the bony portion of Kawase's triangle, enables the entrance of the air cells at the apex and the resolution of both apicitis and effusion. Exceptionally, the petrosal apex can be reached using a retrosigmoid suprameatal approach [1, 5].

14.10 Cholesterol Granuloma of the Petrosal Apex

Cholesterol granuloma is a unilateral or bilateral expansive lesion of the apex of the petrosal bone that is distinguished by the presence of cholesterol crystals. The crystals are encircled by enormous foreign body cells, chronic granulomatous inflammation, and fibrous reaction. Only one of the pneumatized bone cells of the petrosal bone contains these elements. The lesion is believed to have originated from a hemorrhage within the air cell, which cannot be drained due to the obstruction of the ostium by the hemorrhage. This obstruction results in the accumulation of degradation products of hemosiderin and cholesterol, which in turn triggers an inflammatory response. Two potential explanations for the hemorrhage origin of cholesterol granulomas are described in the literature. In the past, it was believed that the reabsorption of air and inflammation of the mucosa would result in a negative pressure within the cell, which would be followed by hemorrhage. Currently, it is believed that the exuberant pneumatization of the cell would be the catalyst for the initiation of the process, which would erode the compact bone and expose the cancellous bone, which is loaded with bone marrow and has a propensity to hemorrhage. The chronicity of the process and the growth of the cell would be facilitated by the replication of hemorrhages, which could ultimately expand toward the cerebellopontine angle with the development of clinical symptoms. Despite the macroscopic appearance of the lesion, it is not a cyst, as there is no epithelium present nearby.

The prevalence and incidence are extremely low, 20 times lower than those of vestibular schwannoma. The symptoms are nonspecific and appear as headaches or unusual facial discomfort. Otological symptoms may result from obstruction of the Eustachian tube or serosal inflammation of the middle ear. Symptoms may manifest as a result of cranial nerve dysfunction when the cyst is sufficiently large. These symptoms include diplopia due to the involvement of the sixth pair, hearing loss, tinnitus, or vertigo due to the involvement of the eighth cranial nerve or destruction of the labyrinth or cochlea of the inner ear, and facial paresis due to the involvement of the facial nerve in its labyrinthine or tympanic segment, which is contingent upon the size of the lesion. The clinical evolution is inconsistent due to the presence of quiescent lesions and those that advance. The location in the apex of the petrosal bone is a critical element in the suspected diagnosis, as imaging modalities provide quite characteristic signs in CT and MRI. A cystic-looking lesion is observed in the CT scan, which erodes and expands the bone. The lesion is well-defined and does not exhibit contrast uptake. A lesion with identical morphological characteristics is observed in the MRI, exhibiting hypersignal in both T1- and T2-weighted sequences. Their appearance may be uneven as a result of hemosiderin or hemorrhage at varying stages of development. Similarly, while the general rule is that they do not enhance with gadolinium, sporadic enhancement is feasible in the presence of an abundance of granulation tissue. They are hyperintense on the FLAIR sequence and are typically hypointense on DWI diffusion. The differential diagnosis of epidermoid cyst and cholesteatoma is made in addition to their specific topography due to their low signal on T1 and DWI MRI sequences. Nevertheless, the clinical and imaging differential diagnosis of cholesterol granuloma is highly complex due to the extensive list of inflammatory lesions that can affect the apex of the petrosal bone. Mucoceles, encephaloceles, or apicitis comprise these lesions.

Surgical treatment is necessary for symptomatic or enlarging cholesterol cysts, contingent upon the patient's age and the size and extent of the lesion. The objective of surgery is to eliminate the lesion as completely as feasible without introducing any new neurological deficits. When planning and performing microsurgical resection, it is important to keep in mind that cholesterol granulomas are not cysts or tumors. Therefore, complete removal of the lesion is not necessary if this would compromise neurological function, particularly in geriatric patients. The lesion can be approached using a microneurosurgical or endoscopic transsphenoidal approach, an extradural subtemporal approach with access through the anterior petrosectomy described by Kawase, or an infralabyrinthine transpetrosal approach, depending on its extent. The standard retrosigmoid approach can be used to treat granulomas that expand caudally by piercing the bone directly over the lesion above the internal auditory and resecting the suprameatal tubercle. The contents of the lesion are evacuated as thoroughly as possible after it is opened, and the blind areas are inspected using an angled neuroendoscope. In order to prevent cerebrospinal fluid fistula and recurrence of the granuloma, the residual cavity is filled with an autologous adipose or muscle graft that is fixed with a biological sealing material. Other authors suggest that the cavity be drained simply by placing a drain tube to guarantee long-term emptying. The prognosis is favorable, as symptoms ameliorate, postoperative morbidity is minimal, and the recurrence rate is low, albeit transient. If a drainage conduit or sealing material is left in place, postoperative imaging monitoring of recurrence can be perplexing due to the supporting material implants left in place [7].

14.11 Key Messages

- *In addition to epidermoid cysts, there are numerous other forms of cystic lesions in the cerebellopontine angle, and these lesions are classified differently based on their pathophysiology.*
- *Cystic lesions typically replicate the characteristic features of their most prevalent sites in imaging investigations. The general treatment guidelines are also consistent.*
- *Apicitis, cholesterol granuloma, and petrosal apex effusion are a few uncommon lesions that are unique to the cerebellopontine angle.*

References

1. Arriaga MA. Petrosal apex effusion: a clinical disorder. Laryngoscope. 2006;116:1349–56. https://doi.org/10.1097/01.mlg.0000231301.79895.05.
2. Bonneville F, Savatovsky J, Chiras J. Imaging of cerebellopontine angle lesions: an update. Part 2: intra-axial lesions, skull base lesions that may invade the cerebellopontine angle region, and non-enhancing extra-axial lesions. Eur Radiol. 2007;17:2908–290. https://doi.org/10.1007/s00330-007-0680-4.
3. Caudron Y, Sterkers O, Bernardeschi D, et al. Objective improvement in adults with cerebellopontine angle arachnoid cysts after surgical treatment. Acta Neurochir. 2021;163:753–8. https://doi.org/10.1007/s00701-021-04721-6.
4. Fan J, Qi S, Peng Y, et al. An isolated primary Rathke's cleft cyst in the cerebellopontine angle. J Neurosurg. 2014;121:846–50. https://doi.org/10.3171/2014.3.JNS131837.
5. Gadre AK, Chole RA. The changing face of petrosal apicitis: a 40-year experience. Laryngoscope. 2018;128:195–201. https://doi.org/10.1002/lary.26571.
6. González-Darder JM, Feliu-Tatay R, Pesudo-Martínez JV, et al. Klippel-Feil syndrome associated with posterior fossa dermoid cyst. Case report Neurol Res. 2002;24:501–4. https://doi.org/10.1179/016164102101200258.
7. Hoa M, House JW, Linthicum FH, et al. Petrosal apex cholesterol granuloma: pictorial review of radiological considerations in diagnosis and surgical histopathology. J Laryngol Otol. 2013;127:339–48. https://doi.org/10.1017/S0022215113000091.
8. Huang H, Xu K, Qu L, et al. Cystic cavernous malformation of the cerebellopontine angle: case report and literature review. World J Surg Oncol. 2011;9:36. https://doi.org/10.1186/1477-7819-9-36.
9. Jallo GI, Woo HH, Meshki C, et al. Arachnoid cysts of the cerebellopontine angle: diagnosis and surgery. Neurosurgery. 1997;40:31–7. https://doi.org/10.1097/00006123-199701000.
10. Karegowda LH, Shenoy PM, Prakashini K, et al. A rare case of racemose neurocysticercosis of the posterior fossa. BMJ Case Rep. 2014;2014:bcr2014203955. https://doi.org/10.1136/bcr-2014-203955.
11. Ohba S, Shimizu K, Shibao S, et al. Cystic cavernous angiomas. Neurosurg Rev. 2010;33:395–400. https://doi.org/10.1007/s10143-010-0245-x.
12. Perrini P, Rutherford SA, King AT, et al. Enterogenous cysts of the cerebellopontine angle: short review illustrated by two new patients. Acta Neurochir. 2008;150:177–84. https://doi.org/10.1007/s00701-007-1483-8.
13. Powers CJ, New KC, McLendon RE, et al. Cerebellopontine angle craniopharyngioma: case report and literature review. Pediatr Neurosurg. 2007;43:158–63. https://doi.org/10.1159/000098394.
14. Rumboldt Z, Jednacak H, Talan-Hranilović J, et al. Unusual appearance of a cisternal hydatid cyst. AJNR Am J Neuroradiol. 2003;24:112–4.
15. Samii M, Gerganov V. Surgery of cerebellopontine angle lesions. Berlin-Heidelberg: Springer-Verlag; 2013.
16. Zarineh A, Leon ME, Saad RS, et al. Multiple neuroenteric cysts at cerebello-pontine angle and foramen magnum: a case report and review of the literature. Neurohistopathology. 2009;29:318–22. https://doi.org/10.1111/j.1440-1789.2008.00958.x.

Aneurysms 15

15.1 Introduction

Posterior circulation aneurysms represent about 15–20% of intracranial aneurysms, with only a subset found in the cerebellopontine angle (cerebellopontine angle). Posterior circulation aneurysms exhibit an elevated risk of hemorrhage and a poorer prognosis following subarachnoid hemorrhage (SAH) compared to anterior circulation aneurysms, as well as after endovascular or microneurosurgical treatment.

Posterior circulation aneurysms predominantly occur in the upper third of the basilar artery (BA), encompassing those at the BA bifurcation and the origin of the superior cerebellar artery (SCA). These aneurysms account for over 50% of posterior fossa aneurysms; however, they are situated outside the cerebellopontine angle and cannot be accessed via the retrosigmoid approach. Vertebral artery (VA) aneurysms and posterior inferior cerebellar artery (PICA) aneurysms that originate in the cerebellopontine angle are accessed through a retrosigmoid or far-lateral approach, representing the next most prevalent category of posterior fossa aneurysms. A small number of aneurysms also originate in the superior cerebellar artery (SCA) or anterior inferior cerebellar artery (AICA) as they traverse the cerebellopontine angle. The remaining posterior circulation aneurysms are anatomically situated outside the cerebellopontine angle, including BA and BA perforator aneurysms that develop in the prepontine cistern, which can be accessed through a retrosigmoid approach. Additionally, distal PICA aneurysms located in the cisterna magna can be approached via a medial suboccipital route. This chapter will concentrate on VA aneurysms and those at the origin of the PICA, as these are the most prevalent in the cerebellopontine angle, in addition to other less common aneurysms that may be addressed via a retrosigmoid approach.

15.2 Anatomical Considerations

The anatomical features of the arterial vessels in the posterior circulation and cerebellopontine angle have been extensively reviewed in the literature [1–5], as well as in the chapter dedicated to the anatomy of the cerebellopontine angle (Fig. 15.1).

15.2.1 Vertebral Artery

The vertebral artery (VA) has a long course from its origin to the vertebrobasilar junction to form the BA together with the contralateral VA. The intracranial course of the VA takes place within the cerebellopontine angle and corresponds to the anatomical segment V4. The VA passes through the dura mater in the lateral area of the occipitocervical junction through a dural ring that

J. M. González-Darder, *Microneurosurgery of Cerebellopontine Angle*,
https://doi.org/10.1007/978-3-032-03091-7_15

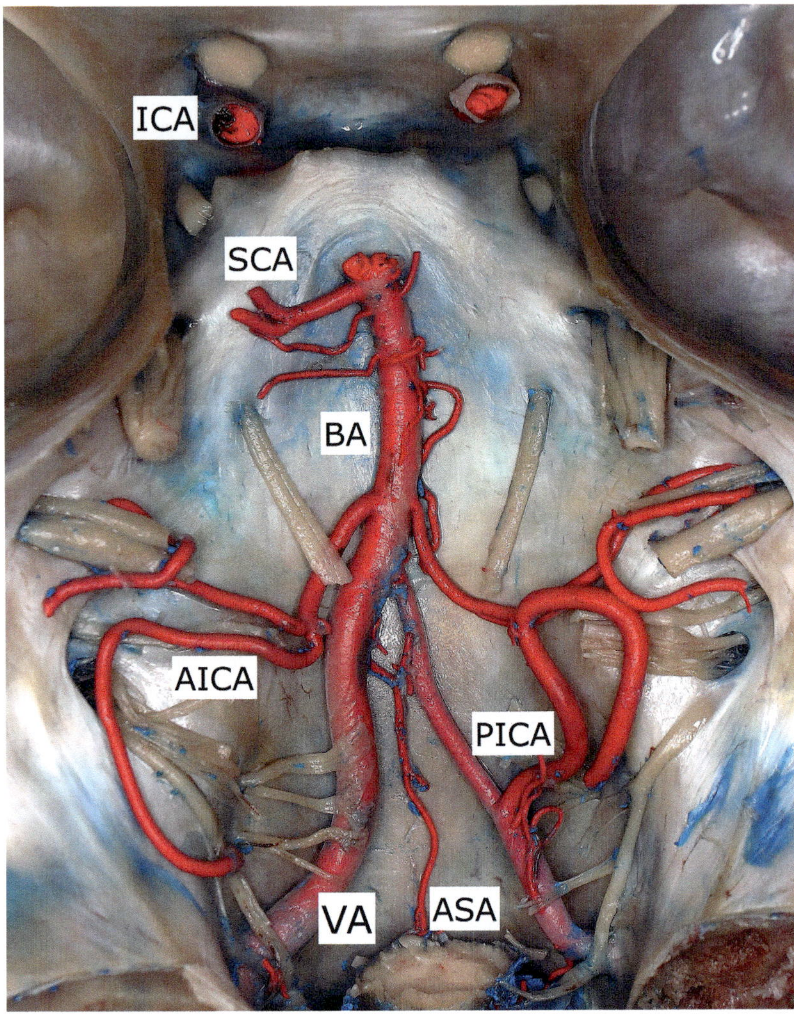

Fig. 15.1 Anatomical picture illustrating the intracisternal pathway of the posterior circulation arteries. An anatomical perspective of the posterior aspect of the clivus and petrosal bones following the resection of the cerebellum and brainstem. The cranial nerve roots have remained positioned appropriately. (ICA internal carotid artery, BA basilar artery, VA vertebral artery, SCA superior cerebellar artery, AICA anteroinferior cerebellar artery, PICA posterior inferior cerebellar artery, ASA anterior spinal artery)

surrounds the artery. At a distance of approximately 5 mm before its entry into the dura mater, the adventitia and the middle layer of the VA drastically reduce their thickness, and the same happens with the elastic fibers of the middle layer and the external elastic layer. The dura mater at this level is very thick and contains between its layers the continuation of the venous plexus of the VA that surrounds the artery in its extracranial portion. In this way, the wall of the intradural VA already has the structure of an intracranial artery, and it is free from the venous plexus.

As soon as the VA becomes intradural, it is wrapped in a fibrous sleeve that also binds the posterior spinal artery, the rootlets of the first spinal nerve, the spinal rootlets of the accessory nerve, and the first dentate ligament. The dentate ligament is formed by fibrous extensions of the arachnoid that surround the spinal cord and fix it laterally to the dura mater in its medial plane. The first anchorage of the dentate ligament is at the point where the VA becomes intradural. The accessory nerve passes behind the dentate ligament, which is related to the rootlets and spinal ganglion of the first spinal nerve in a variable manner. The accessory nerve is the only cranial nerve that runs through the foramen magnum and is formed by the confluence of ventral and dorsal rootlets from the first cervical spinal cord segments. The VA lies anterior to the plane of the dentate ligament and at this level gives off the posterior spinal artery, which is the first intradural branch of the VA, although it may occasionally have an extradural origin. The roots of the first spinal nerve are applied to the lower border of the VA and maintain this relationship in its course through the dural fibrous sleeve to the extradural region. Thus, the first spinal nerve always occupies a more superficial plane than the VA when the artery is visualized in its ascending course towards the posterior fossa in the retrosigmoid approach. In an even more superficial plane, the hypoglossal nerve is visualized, formed by several rootlets that emerge from the anterior surface of the medulla oblongata and run laterally towards the hypoglossal canal. The VA runs superiorly, anteriorly, and medially in a deeper plane, below the rootlets of the hypoglossal nerve, vagal nerve, and glossopharyngeal nerve, to surround the medulla oblongata until it fuses in the anterior median plane of the brain stem, at the level of the medullary-pontine sulcus, with the contralateral VA and forms the BA.

The first branch of the intradural VA is the posterior spinal artery, although it may originate in the extradural space or directly from the PICA. However, the most relevant branch is the PICA. Its point of origin in the VA, the level of origin in relation to the foramen magnum, the angle that marks the initial direction of the vessel with respect to the VA, the caliber, and the course of the PICA are highly variable. The next branch of the VA, already close to the BA, is the anterior spinal artery that joins with the contralateral one in the anterior medullary groove to distribute throughout the spinal cord.

15.2.2 Posterior Inferior Cerebellar Artery

The posterior inferior cerebellar artery (PICA) represents the primary division of the VA. The PICA typically originates from the intradural V4 segment of the VA; however, in approximately 10% of instances, it may have an extradural origin from the V3 segment. The PICA comprises five sections: anterior medullary segment, which extends from the origin of the PICA to the level of the anterior border of the olive (pre-olivary sulcus), is related to the roots of the hypoglossal nerve, usually passing deep to it, although the relationships are very variable; lateral medullary segment, which reaches the level of the posterior border of the olive (retro-olivary sulcus) where the rootlets of the cranial nerves emerge, the PICA is also variably related to the rootlets of the lower cranial nerves, always having a caudal course in relation to the facial- vestibulocochlear complex; tonsillar-medullary segment, describing a caudal loop that encircles the cerebellar amygdala caudally, its lowest point usually being above the level of the foramen magnum, and where in its ascending portion occupies a medial position and may be related to the contralateral artery; telovellotonsillar segment, that is a continuation of the previous segment, continuing up to the roof of the fourth ventricle, where it gives off branches to the tela choroidea and choroid plexuses, and drawing a second cranial loop, before the artery emerges above the cerebellar vermis, medially to the biventral lobe; finally, the artery continues with the last cortical segment, where bifurcates into two branches, one vermian and one hemispheric, which are distributed throughout the cerebellar cortex. PICA emits a series of perforating arteries to the medulla oblongata during its initial three segments, particularly from the first segment. The size of the PICA correlates with that of the AICA, as they compensate for the territories they serve; thus, a larger PICA corresponds to a smaller AICA, and vice versa. The point of origin in the VA and the connections of the PICA with the cranial nerves, medulla oblongata, and cerebellum are critical in the microneurosurgical management of aneurysms in this region.

15.2.3 Basilar Artery

The basilar artery (BA) is a singular trunk resulting from the fusion of both VAs at the medullary–pontine junction, extending to its bifurcation at the pontine-mesencephalic sulcus into the two posterior cerebral arteries (PCAs). The length of the BA varies, averaging between 30 and 35 mm. Despite the anatomical expectation that the BA follows a straight path along the midline within the prepontine cistern anterior to the brainstem, it is observed that over 50% of BAs exhibit a tortuous trajectory, deviating from the midline. The deviation occurs more frequently on the left side, attributed to the hemodynamic effects associated with the predominant influence of the left VA. The primary branches of the BA include the AICA and the SCA; however, it is essential to acknowledge the significant number of perforating arteries supplying the pons. The classification of these arteries is based on their course around the brainstem, distinguishing between direct and circumflex perforating arteries. The circumflex arteries exhibit a longer course and are further divided into short and long perforators.

15.2.4 Anterior Inferior Cerebellar Artery

In addition to the SCA, the primary trunk of the BA is the anterior inferior cerebellar artery (AICA). AICA originates from the BA, either as a single trunk or as multiple parallel branches of varying calibers, and extends towards the cerebellopontine angle. Initially, it is related to the abducens nerve, and more laterally, to the facial and vestibulocochlear nerves, the choroid plexus exiting through the foramen of Luschka, and the flocculus of the cerebellum. The relationships with the nerves are variable, potentially passing above, below, or between the facial nerve and the vestibulocochlear nerve. The arterial division pattern as a single trunk is variable, typically bifurcating into two trunks approximately 8 mm from its origin, either superior or inferior, before or after the level of the facial and vestibulocochlear nerves. The branches establish variable relationships with the nerves if the division occurs prior to their reach. The AICA is divided into four parts: anterior pontine segment, located between the clivus and the anterolateral region of the pons, related to the sixth cranial nerve; lateral pontine segment, which begins at the anterolateral margin of the pons and runs through the cerebellopontine angle above, below or between the facial and vestibulocochlear nerves, where the artery is closely related to the internal acoustic meatus, the lateral recess and the choroid plexus that protrudes from the foramen of Luschka, where arise the labyrinthine artery that gives blood supply to the facial nerve, the vestibulocochlear nerve and the vestibulocochlear labyrinth, some recurrent perforating arteries, which pass through the interior of the meatus but have a recurrent course to the brainstem, and, finally, the subarcuate artery, which enters the subarcuate fossa; flocculopeduncular segment, where the artery runs rostral or caudal to the flocculus until it reaches the middle cerebellar peduncle and the cerebellopontine fissure; and finally, the cortical segment, that corresponds to the distal branches that are responsible for supplying blood to the petrous surface of the cerebellum.

15.2.5 Superior Cerebellar Artery

From an anatomical perspective, the superior cerebellar artery (SCA) is the most consistent artery in the posterior fossa regarding its origin, course, and location. It typically originates caudal to the bifurcation of the BA and, in certain instances, may originate directly from the P1 segment of the PCA. SCA currently occupies the interpeduncular cistern and extends caudally to the oculomotor nerve. Following its origin, the artery courses caudally, encircling the brainstem, passing posterior to the trochlear nerve and anterior to the trigeminal nerve, ultimately reaching the cerebellar-mesencephalic fissure. The SCA divides into a rostral trunk and a caudal trunk along its course. The rostral trunk provides blood supply to the vermian and paravermian regions of the cerebellum, while the caudal trunk supplies the upper area of the suboccipital surface of the cerebellar hemisphere. It additionally releases distal perforating branches that extend to the brainstem and cerebellar peduncles. The SCA is categorized into four segments: anterior pontine-mesencephalic segment, which extends from its origin on the BA to the anterolateral region of the brain stem, running caudally to the oculomotor nerve; lateral pontine-mesencephalic segment, beginning at the anterolateral margin of the brain stem and projecting caudally to the lateral region of the upper half of the pons, terminating in the anterior region of the cerebellar-mesencephalic fissure, where it is closely associated with the trigeminal nerve; cerebellar-mesencephalic segment, traversing the cerebellar-mesencephalic fissure to reach the anterior region of the tentorial surface of the cerebellum; and the cortical segment, which encompasses the distal branches arranged around the tentorial surface of the cerebellum, divided into vermian and hemispheric groups. The SCA generates a variable number of perforating arteries throughout its course. The arteries are categorized into direct and circumflex perforating types according to their trajectory around the brainstem. The circumflex arteries exhibit an extended trajectory.

15.3 Pathology

15.3.1 Saccular Aneurysms

Saccular aneurysms represent the predominant type of aneurysms found in cerebral arteries. A typical saccular aneurysm comprises three main components: the neck, which connects the aneurysm lumen to the arterial lumen; the sac, characterized by the dilation of the arterial wall and containing blood and/or thrombi; and the dome or fundus, the distal portion of the sac where rupture most commonly occurs. The natural history of saccular cerebral aneurysms progresses through a sequence of distinct phases. The initial stage occurs before any observable morphological alterations in the artery and encompasses the factors that predispose, promote, or facilitate aneurysm formation. The second stage involves the formation of the initial aneurysm or microaneurysm, characterized by a weak area of the arterial wall that presents a slight bulge. The subsequent stage is the growth phase of the aneurysm, characterized by the lesion adopting a saccular shape, with the neck and sac becoming defined and the walls exhibiting notable pathological alterations. The aneurysm may proceed along two distinct trajectories from this stage. In certain aneurysms, the aneurysmal sac wall may fail under critical conditions, leading to rupture and subsequent hemorrhage. Following the rupture, a sequence of changes initiates that promotes the repair of the rupture and the reconstruction of the aneurysmal sac wall. This repair mechanism may be effective; however, it is typically temporary, leading to a subsequent rupture of the aneurysm wall and rebleeding. Complete ruptures of the sac wall can lead to bleeding, manifesting as subarachnoid, intracerebral, or intraventricular hemorrhage, which is frequently fatal. Incomplete ruptures can lead to intramural bleeding, which subsequently results in thrombus formation and initiates reparative processes. These processes may contribute to an increase in aneurysm size and are associated with thickening of the sac wall.

15.3.2 Dissecting Aneurysms

Dissecting aneurysms are typically located in the initial portion of the V4 segment of the VA. Dissecting aneurysms result from the rupture of the internal elastic lamina of the arterial wall, typically occurring just before the entry and within 10–20 mm following the passage of the VA through the dura mater, before the exit of the PICA. Histopathological examinations of normal VA reveal the common presence of focal defects in the internal elastic lamina prior to the VA passage through the dura mater and adjacent to the exit of the PICA, often correlated with intimal thinning. The interaction of these two factors establishes a region of reduced resistance advantageous to the formation of a dissecting aneurysm, frequently related with high- or low-energy traumatic incidents. Alongside the extension of the aneurysm along the VA, it is important to note that the dissection also results in an increase in volume and elongation of the artery [5–8].

15.3.3 Fusiform Aneurysms

At the level of the VA and the BA, fusiform aneurysms are identified, characterized by an extensive neck that aligns with the longitudinal axis of the artery, resulting in both arterial dilation and elongation. This pathophysiological category encompasses arteriosclerotic, dolichoectatic, dissecting, and serpentine aneurysms, as it is believed they share a common pathogenesis. From a morphological perspective, these lesions exhibit a fusiform shape, characterized by thickened, elongated, and occasionally tortuous vessels. They are usually large or giant lesions, possessing a notably thick arterial wall, with one or multiple vascular lumens that are irregularly covered by endothelium and demonstrate slow flow. Consequently, these exhibit significant differences from saccular aneurysms. Aneurysms are thought to arise from the rupture and fragmentation of the internal elastic lamina, facilitating vessel dilation and growth, resulting in increased length and caliber. The intima undergoes thickening and tearing, which promotes wall dissection, leading to the formation of hemorrhages and mural thrombosis, ultimately resulting in embolism or occlusion of branches and collaterals. Microhemorrhages occurring between the thickened and dissected intima and the adventitia may compromise the wall's integrity, potentially leading to rupture despite its thickness [9].

15.4 Clinical Considerations

Saccular aneurysms are more commonly associated with SAH, whereas fusiform aneurysms are more frequently linked to neurological symptoms due to compression or ischemia. Clinically, the most common aneurysms at the cerebellopontine angle, specifically VA aneurysms and those originating from the PICA at the VA junction, exhibit SAH in 70% of instances. In 15% of instances, they are findings in imaging studies, while in the remaining 5%, diagnoses are made based on neurological symptoms resulting from ischemia or neural compression. Certain cases are identified in imaging studies as a result of nonspecific symptoms such as headache, neck pain, or dizziness, or they occur as genuine serendipity.

Most saccular aneurysms are associated with SAH. Unruptured saccular or fusiform aneurysms are typically large and manifest compressive symptoms. Dissecting vertebral artery aneurysms are acute lesions that present with SAH in only 10% of cases, although they may bleed subsequently after a brief interval following diagnosis. The clinical grade of SAH and the bleeding intensity observed on computed tomography (CT) are greater than those associated with ruptured aneurysms in other locations.

15.4.1 Dissecting Aneurysms of the Vertebral Artery

Dissecting aneurysms of the VA exhibit a distinct clinical presentation that warrants individual consideration. The moment of dissection is clinically identified by the patient for the presence of acute suboccipital pain or headache and dizziness or vertigo, which may occur with or without neurological symptoms, and in cases of rupture, by the typical symptoms of SAH. The sudden onset of cranio-cervical pain accompanied by dizziness in a young patient, absent other suspected causes, strongly indicates a dissecting VA aneurysm. The neurological symptoms result from ischemia or compression. Ischemic symptoms can be transient, as seen in transient ischemic attacks, but they often persist or become permanent. Neurological symptoms resulting from compression of the medulla oblongata or cranial nerve roots due to the mass effect of the aneurysm exhibit rapid progression. SAH is an uncommon presentation of dissecting aneurysms, as it requires the dissection to be situated in the intradural segment of the VA, with a complete rupture of the arterial wall (refer to case 21 in Chap. 21). Dissecting aneurysms of the VA that present without SAH generally exhibit a favorable clinical prognosis in the majority of instances. Nonetheless, a specific percentage experiences unfavorable outcomes, characterized by bleeding occurring within the initial hours or 3–4 days following clinical presentation [6, 7].

15.5 Diagnostic Considerations

Today, the diagnosis of SAH is primarily conducted using CT, with lumbar puncture being required only in exceptional cases. Acute blood exhibits a high density in radiological studies, allowing for clear differentiation from brain tissue, which possesses a lower radiological density. The sensitivity of CT during the acute phase of SAH approaches 100%, enabling the identification of subarachnoid blood as well as intracerebral or intraventricular blood with equivalent sensitivity. After 6 hours, blood undergoes degradation and experiences a reduction in radiological density, eventually approaching the density of brain tissue over time. The sensitivity of CT for diagnosing SAH declines from nearly 100% within the first 2 to 3 days to approximately 30% by 2 weeks. This indicates that in instances of a negative CT study, yet with a strong clinical suspicion of a SAH occurring more than 2–3 days prior, a lumbar puncture should be conducted to investigate for xanthochromia or other analytical findings consistent with SAH, or preferably, a magnetic resonance imaging (MRI) should be utilized. The intensity of SAH on CT is assessed using the four-grade Fisher scale: grade 1 indicates no subarachnoid blood detected; grade 2 indicates diffuse hemorrhage in the basal cisterns or in the interhemispheric, insular, or ambiens cisterns with a thickness less than 1 mm; grade 3 indicates hemorrhage in the form of a clot located in the basal cisterns or in the interhemispheric, insular, or ambiens cisterns with a thickness greater than 1 mm; and grade 4 indicates an intracerebral or intraventricular clot associated with diffuse hemorrhage or without hemorrhage in the cisterns. MRI can diagnose SAH; however, due to the lengthy image acquisition time, higher costs, limited availability in emergency settings, and increased complexity of the examination in critical patients, its clinical application is significantly limited.

SAH resulting from basilar artery trunk aneurysms typically fills the cisterns around the brainstem in a diffuse and variable thickness, with intraventricular hemorrhage frequently occurring. *Perimesencephalic hemorrhage* represents a notable pattern of SAH, characterized by blood accumulation in the anterior cisterns of the midbrain, typically without the presence of an aneurysm. SAH resulting from the rupture of VA and PICA aneurysms is pronounced and localized within the cisterns of the posterior fossa on the side corresponding to the affected artery. Intraventricular hemorrhage and obstructive hydrocephalus are prevalent conditions. In cases of significant bleeding and large aneurysms, visualization of the aneurysm responsible for the bleeding may be achieved through negative imaging casts.

Three-dimensional CT angiography is a technique specifically developed for the diagnosis of aneurysms. High-quality studies demonstrate a sensitivity approaching 100% for aneurysms greater than 5 mm, whereas this sensitivity decreases to 80% for aneurysms smaller than 3 mm. MRI angiography is utilized for aneurysm diagnosis, employing T1-weighted sequences with contrast administration and TOF (*Time-On-Flight*) sequences that do not require contrast. The sensitivity of 3T machines exceeds that of 1.5T machines, approaching 95%. The sensitivity for detecting aneurysms smaller than 3 mm decreases to 85%, similar to CT findings. The specificity is 90%. Digital subtraction cerebral angiography (DSA) is considered the gold standard for diagnosing aneurysms. Despite being an invasive procedure with potential complications, it carries a very low risk of mortality (less than 0.05%) and low morbidity (less than 1%). DSA of all four cerebral vessels is essential, as the injection of contrast through both VAs is required to avoid missing lesions that may result from inadequate filling of the non-injected vertebral segment or its branches.

Cerebellopontine angle aneurysms can be identified on imaging studies as either saccular or elongated fusiform masses associated with one or both VAs or BA. Calcifications, intramural or intraluminal thrombi, and indications of ischemia are commonly observed. Fusiform aneurysms exhibit distinct features on DSA, CT, and MRI imaging studies, including focal or segmental stenosis and/or dilation of the artery, often referred to as string and pearl signs, or complete occlusion of the artery. Dissecting aneurysms exhibit pathognomonic signs, including the double-lumen image, pseudoaneurysm, and intimal flap. Furthermore, frequent observations of aneurysm changes occur in successive vascular studies, with documented instances of spontaneous improvement or healing, disappearance of the double lumen image, or even recanalization of the occluded artery (target sign). Large aneurysms exert a mass effect, leading to compression of the brainstem and potentially causing obstructive hydrocephalus (Figs. 15.2 and 15.3). Certain aneurysms, in non-contrast imaging studies, may mimic a cerebellopontine angle tumor. DSA may underestimate lesion size, as the vessel lumen can be narrow while the aneurysm volume may be significantly larger due to substantial wall thickening. CT and MRI studies are essential as they reveal the actual thickness of the vessel and the presence of intramural or intraluminal thrombosis.

15.6 Surgical Categories

Aneurysms located at the cerebellopontine angle encompass those of the VA trunk and those at the junction of the VA and PICA. Aneurysms at the VA–PICA junction, typically saccular, are of paramount importance in microneurosurgery. Aneurysms of the VA trunk typically present as dissecting or fusiform types. They may affect extensive lengths of the intradural segment of the VA, involve the exit of the PICA, and extend distally to the vertebrobasilar junction or the BA itself, as well as proximally to the extradural VA. Aneurysms of the BA and its branches can be accessed via a retrosigmoid approach and are thus included in this section. The classification of surgical types is derived from the intersection of the three fundamental aneurysm types (saccular, fusiform, and dissection) and the primary arterial vessels of the cerebellopontine angle (VA, VA–PICA junction, BA, main branches, and perforators).

15.6.1 Aneurysms of the Vertebral Artery and Posterior Inferior Cerebellar Artery Junction

Aneurysms at the VA–PICA junction represent a significant category in microneurosurgery (Fig. 15.4). Aneurysms in the territory of the VA and PICA comprise approximately 70% of cases of posterior fossa aneurysms in microneurosurgical series. Saccular aneurysms typically exhibit a neck positioned distally to the exit of the PICA; however, a large neck may encompass the exit of the PICA. The critical factor from a microneuro-

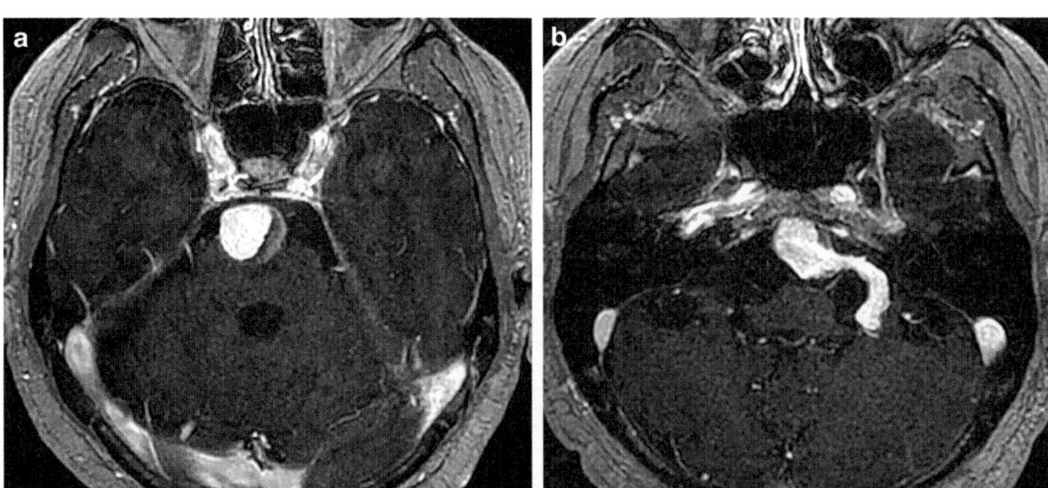

Fig. 15.2 Fusiform aneurysm of the basilar artery. (**a**, **b**) Axial T1-weighted MRI slices, displaying a vascular enhancement inside a large partially thrombosed aneurysm

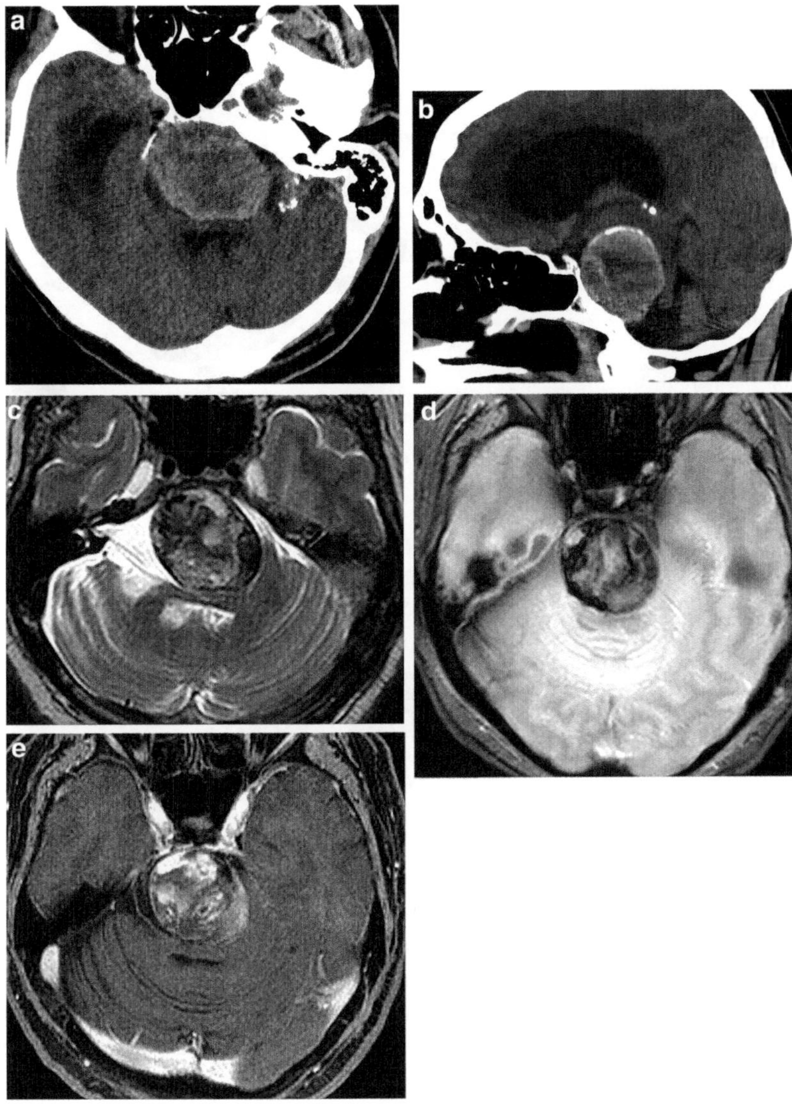

Fig. 15.3 Giant basilar artery aneurysm with a large intrasaccular thrombus. (**a**) Axial CT. (**b**) Sagittal CT. (**c**) Lateral projection. (**d**) Axial T2-weighted MRI. (**e**) Axial T2-weighted gradient MRI. Axial T1-weighted MRI after gadolinium administration

surgical perspective is the position of the exit of the PICA, and therefore of the aneurysms, along the VA, as the exit point of the PICA exhibits significant variability. Aneurysms linked to a very distal exit of the PICA are situated at the anterior medullary region, while more proximal aneurysms are found at the lateral medullary region. Aneurysms arising further proximally are in the tonsillar-medullary region. Lastly, aneurysms associated with a PICA emerging from the extradural V3 segment of the VA, occurring in 10% of cases, are located in the extradural space. The various topographies indicate distinct relationships with the cranial nerve roots and varying depths in the surgical field, resulting in unique characteristics for each group during microneurosurgical clipping [10–12].

15.6.2 Saccular Aneurysms of the Vertebral, Basilar, and Other Arteries

Typical saccular aneurysms not associated with the exit of the PICA may occur along the VA trunk, and they have the same considerations explained for VA–PICA junction aneurysms.

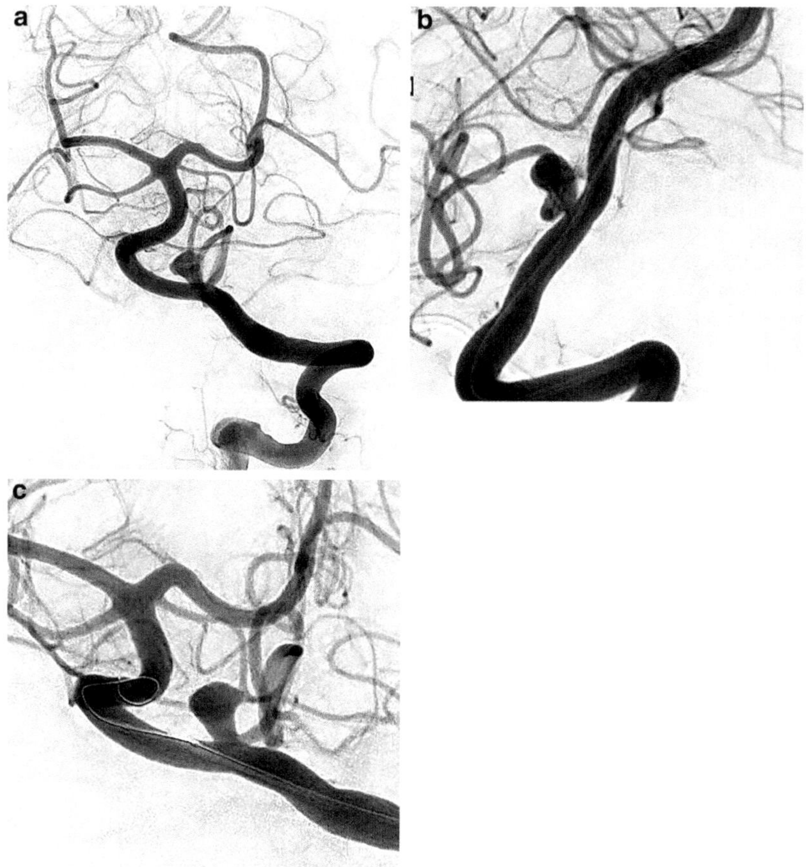

Fig. 15.4 Saccular aneurysm of the left vertebral artery and posterior cerebellar artery junction. (**a**) DSA of the vertebral artery in anteroposterior view. (**b**) Lateral projection. (**c**) Oblique projection

Saccular aneurysms of the BA trunk are infrequently observed [12]. Some originate directly from the BA trunk and may incorporate the BA in the neck without showing any apparent relation to its branches. Others are positioned concerning the emergence of the larger transverse branches, particularly the AICA. A notable proportion of cases is linked to the presence of persistent embryonic arteries that connect the posterior and anterior circulation. An extensively documented association exists with fenestration of the BA trunk. The low incidence of saccular aneurysms of the BA trunk, along with their frequent association with vascular abnormalities, indicates that these aneurysms likely develop in areas of weakness in the arterial wall rather than due to hemodynamic factors. Aneurysm size varies, typically being small, with the sac projecting laterally. The predominant clinical manifestation is SAH; however, large aneurysms may present symptoms resulting from compression of the pons, and some may be identified incidentally. Less than 200 cases have been recorded in the literature.

Saccular aneurysms of the perforating branches of the BA are characterized by a neck that is solely situated on the perforating artery, without any involvement of the BA trunk. This subtype of aneurysm is rare but holds significant clinical interest due to its association with perimesencephalic subarachnoid hemorrhage [13]. Fewer than one hundred cases have been recorded in the literature. The average size of these aneurysms at diagnosis is 3 mm, indicating they are relatively small. The clinical presentation consistently indicates SAH, usually localized to the prepontine and perimesencephalic regions, characterized by a low Fisher grade and similarly low scores on clinical assessment scales. Diagnosis using CT angiography is inconsistent due to its small size, and similarly, diagnosis with DSA is challenging, even with high-quality technical studies. Consequently, a notable proportion of patients receive a diagnosis of their aneurysm during the second vascular study. This phenomenon can be attributed to the possibility that the aneurysm or the artery was completely or partially thrombosed in the initial study. Conversely, their disappearance is noted in control studies on other occasions. This suggests that small aneurysms may account for angiographically negative perimesencephalic subarachnoid hemorrhage. Their true nature remains contentious, as they manifest in arteries characterized by low flow and minimal hemodynamic stress. Sequential imaging studies reveal changes, and spontaneous thrombosis is frequently observed, all of which are common in dissecting-type aneurysms.

Finally, AICA aneurysms are rare, with approximately 60 cases documented that have been treated using microneurosurgical or endovascular methods. These lesions are diminutive, typically situated at the arterial exit from the BA, and their common presentation is SAH, although symptoms related to cranial nerve dysfunction may also occur.

15.6.3 Dissecting Aneurysms of the Vertebral Artery

Aneurysms of the VA trunk are typically dissecting lesions, either spontaneous or associated with trauma. Aneurysms can exhibit a fusiform morphology characterized by arterial dilatation and elongation, which may involve the exit of the PICA and other branches of the VA. At this stage, the lesion may present neurological symptoms resulting from compression of the cranial nerves or the medulla oblongata or from ischemia secondary to occlusion of the arterial branches of the VA. Aneurysms can form intraluminal thrombi or thrombi within the arterial wall, leading to hemorrhage in the arterial wall, secondary dissection, and potential late rupture resulting in SAH. Aneurysms of this type progressively extend along the VA, resulting in gross deformation and thickening, ultimately affecting the BA and potentially the extradural V3 segment of the VA.

15.6.4 Fusiform Aneurysms of the Basilar Artery

Over 50% of aneurysms in the BA trunk are classified as fusiform aneurysms. The clinical symptoms indicative of the diagnosis include ischemia resulting from occlusion of perforating arteries, ischemia secondary to compression of the brain stem due to the increasing volume of the aneurysm, or SAH resulting from rupture. Headache can be associated with hydrocephalus.

15.7 Microneurosurgical Management

Aneurysms at the VA–PICA junction are particularly significant in microneurosurgery due to their higher prevalence and saccular nature, necessitating microneurosurgical treatment. Consequently, their treatment is extensively reviewed in the literature [10, 11, 14–16], and their microneurosurgical treatment will be described in detail in this section.

15.7.1 Preoperative Planification

Preoperative planning involves imaging studies to assess the aneurysm's size, neck dimensions, relationship to the PICA exit, position of the PICA exit from the VA, characteristics of the aneurysm, and evaluation of perforating arteries and collateral circulation (Fig. 15.5a). The feasibility of implementing a revascularization technique warrants consideration; thus, imaging studies should assess the occipital artery and the contralateral PICA for potential utilization in such procedures.

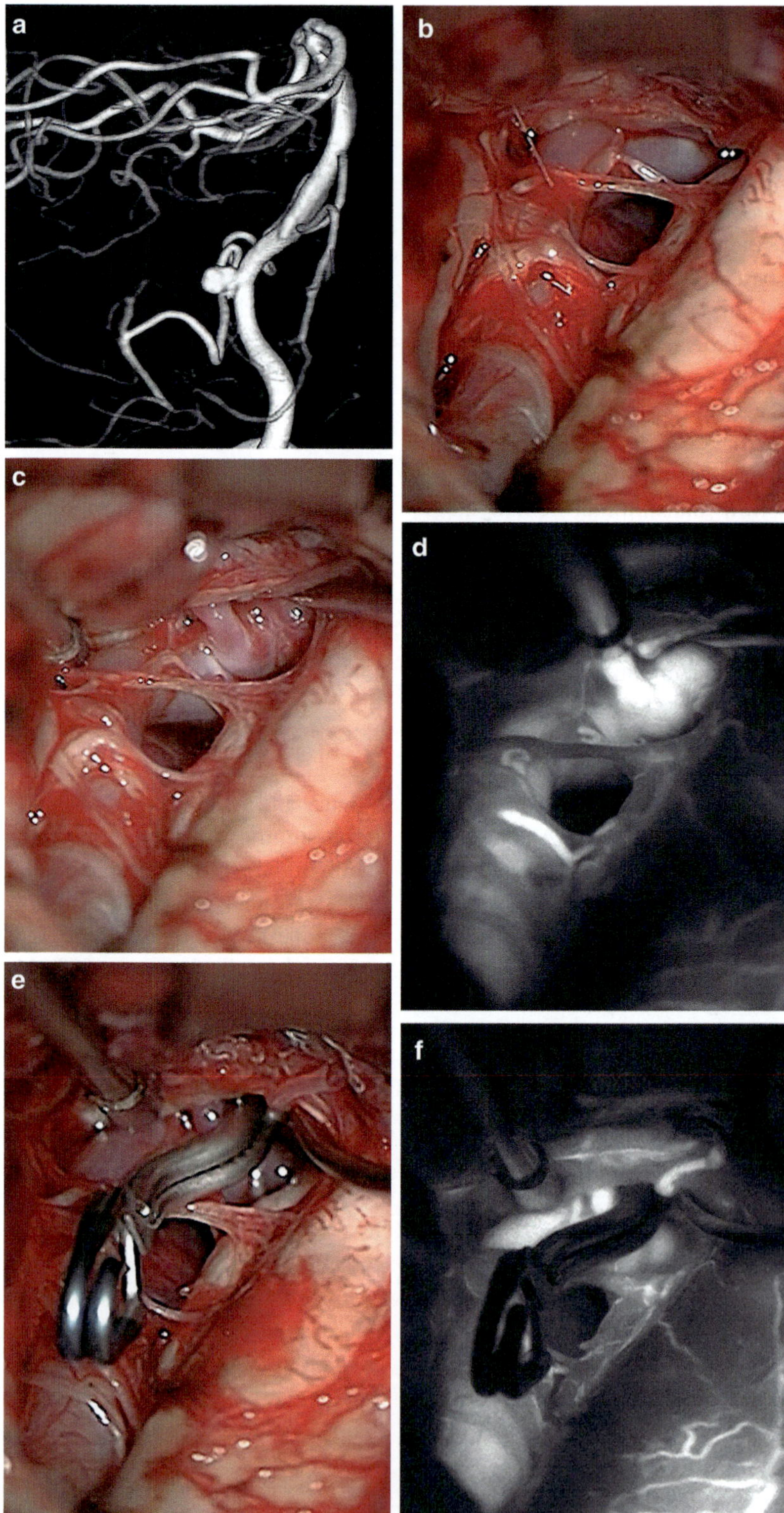

Fig. 15.5 Microneurosurgical clipping of a left vertebral artery and posterior inferior cerebellar artery junction ruptured aneurysm. (**a**) Three-dimensional DSA. (**b**) Intraoperative picture through a far-lateral approach, exposing the upper and lower triangles. (**c**). Dissection of the aneurysm, VA and PICA (**d**) ICG fluorescence. (**e**) Bayonet clipping. (**f**) Post-clipping ICG fluorescence

15.7.2 Surgical Approach

Accessing aneurysms at the VA–PICA junction universally requires a far-lateral suboccipital approach [17]. Certain aneurysms may be excluded through a standard suboccipital medial or lateral retrosigmoid approach; however, the far-lateral approach offers increased space, enhanced versatility for the neurosurgeon, and prompt and secure proximal control of the VA, even at an extradural level. The exposure and resection of the occipital bone may extend from the midline to the borders of the transverse and sigmoid sinuses. A critical component is that the lateral suboccipital craniectomy consistently involves extensive drilling of the foramen magnum rim. Resection of the posterior arch of the atlas is generally unnecessary; however, it is recommended to remove the periosteum to access the suboccipital space containing the suboccipital segment of the VA. The excision of fibroadipose tissue within the suboccipital triangle exposes the V3 segment of the VA, which is encircled by its venous plexus. The venous plexus, along with the muscular and dural branches of the VA, must be entirely or partially excised to facilitate the mobilization of the artery while ensuring that there is no extradural origin of the PICA. The aim of mobilizing the VA is to locate its entry into the dura mater to excise the indispensable bone, facilitating access to the dura mater just medial to the artery while also achieving proximal control. The VA can be further mobilized by releasing it from the transverse foramen of the axis to the dura mater. The VA is liberated from the osteofibrous canal of the posterior arch of the atlas through the sectioning and excision of the posterior occipitoatloid ligament. The posterior border of the transverse foramen of the atlas may be reamed or excised using a fine Kerrison punch to facilitate increased mobilization. The artery is traced medially to its entrance into the dura mater. The VA can be more effectively accessed at the transverse foramen of the axis by excising the abundant venous plexus in the region and dissecting and mobilizing the second spinal nerve. A rubber is positioned beneath the VA to facilitate cranial or caudal mobilization. The mobilization of the VA is significantly increased following total or partial resection of the ipsilateral half of the posterior arch of the atlas.

15.7.3 Position and Craniotomy

There is nothing special about the descriptions in the chapters to the far-lateral approach described above regarding position, anatomical references, incision, craniotomy, and opening of the dura mater.

15.7.4 Cistern Opening and Neurovascular Dissection

The treatment of intradural VA–PICA junction aneurysms involves a vertical incision of the dura mater, initiated in the suboccipital area posterior to the sigmoid sinus and extending to the cervical region, positioned just medial to the entry point of the VA. The dura mater may be circumferentially incised around the VA to facilitate further mobilization. Accessing the intradural space occurs through the opening of the dura mater at the lateral cerebellar-medullary cistern, allowing the VA to enter the premedullary cistern directly. The cisterna magna is located medially and can be accessed to evacuate cerebrospinal fluid (CSF). This procedure may also involve opening the vallecula to access the fourth ventricle, allowing for the removal of blood clots or aiding in the drainage of cerebrospinal fluid from the ventricular system, thereby alleviating pressure on the brain. Upon opening the dura mater, the roots of the first cervical nerve and the first dentate ligament may be safely divided, facilitating the release and further mobilization of the VA. The subsequent focus is on the identification and mobilization of the accessory nerve, followed by the dissection and mobilization of the hypoglossal nerve, located in a deeper plane anterior to the VA. The arterial branches of the VA are identified, specifically the posterior spinal artery and the PICA. The extradural origin of the PICA is common; therefore, this possibility should be examined in preoperative vascular imaging studies to avoid misidentifying and sectioning a PICA with an anomalous extradural origin rather than a large, irrelevant extradural muscular branch. The deep lateromedial plane is formed by the upper cervical spinal cord and the lower portion of the medulla oblongata, and the most anterior portion is formed by the clivus, foramen magnum, and odontoid process covered by ligaments and dura mater.

15.7.5 Vertebral Artery Dissection and Proximal Control

Comprehensive vascular management in the clipping of VA–PICA junction aneurysms necessitates dissection and control of the VA both proximally and distally to the aneurysm and the PICA. The initial point of control for the intradural VA occurs right after its passage through the dura mater, where it separates from the dentate ligament and prepares the initial segments of the artery for the application of a temporary clip. Extradural proximal control of the VA can be attained in the presence of a very proximal aneurysm. The PICA is readily identifiable in its tonsillar segment, located below the cerebellar tonsil, medially at the level of the caudal loop. The caliber, length, and relative position of the PICA in relation to the tonsil exhibit variability. At this stage, the control of the PICA is distal to the aneurysm; however, it is feasible to elevate the amygdala in a superior and medial direction to define an anatomical triangle encompassing the aneurysm. The triangle, as described by Lawton, is delineated medially by the lateral surface of the medulla oblongata and laterally by the trajectory of the accessory nerve, which adheres to the dura mater overlying the foramen magnum and the jugular tubercle, converging in a caudal direction. The upper boundary of the triangle is defined by the lower margin of the vagal nerve, with its rootlets extending from the retro-olivary sulcus of the medulla oblongata at the midline to the jugular foramen laterally, where they converge with the accessory nerve. In the microneurosurgical approach, the nerves are situated in a more superficial plane compared to the arteries, with the hypoglossal nerve traversing the triangle. Thus, the triangle is divided into two sections: one located below the hypoglossal nerve and another situated above it (Fig. 15.5b). The variability in vascular relationships indicates that access to the aneurysm should ideally be achieved through spaces defined by neurological structures, as the anatomical configuration of the brainstem and cranial nerves is significantly more stable than that of the arteries. Consequently, the clipping of the aneurysm neck may occur through either the upper or lower space, contingent upon the height of the PICA exit and the aneurysm's position. The aneurysm's size, along with the elongation or tortuosity of the VA, may alter the positioning of the aneurysm or the cranial nerves. Before dissecting the neck of the aneurysm, it is essential to secure distal control of the VA, as rupture may result in significant retrograde flow from the contralateral VA. The difficulty of this control increases as the PICA arises distally from the VA, given that the VA assumes a more anteromedial position with increasing distance from the aneurysm. After controlling the proximal and distal VA and the distal PICA, and identifying the cranial nerve roots, the proximal dissection of both arteries can be safely advanced to reach the neck of the aneurysm (Figs. 15.5c, d).

15.7.6 Clipping

The aneurysm is clipped with a straight or bayonet clip and temporary clipping of the proximal and, if possible, the distal VA. Fenestrated clips may be utilized to accommodate the nerves or the PICA within the clip window. Identifying and dissecting the perforating arteries is often unfeasible; therefore, precise clipping of the neck is essential to prevent compromising these small, irregularly distributed arteries. The exclusion of aneurysmal flow and preservation of flow through the VA and PICA arteries is confirmed using micro-Doppler and ICG (*Indocyanine Green*) fluorescence (Fig. 15.5e, f).

15.8 Aneurysms that Require Specific Treatment

15.8.1 Saccular Aneurysms of the Vertebral Artery, Basilar Artery, and Branches

The standard retrosigmoid approach to the cerebellopontine angle, involving a retrosigmoid craniotomy, may be useful for certain aneurysms located at the vertebrobasilar junction and the lower BA trunk [12]. This approach is well known among neurosurgeons, though it is constrained by the brainstem, lower cranial nerves, and the depth of the surgical field. The far-lateral approach represents a more extensive infratentorial technique. The two approaches can be linked to a presigmoid approach involving ligation and division of the sigmoid sinus. Saccular aneurysms may be managed through neck clipping and exclusion techniques. Surgical strategies for saccular aneurysms of the BA trunk are typically determined by their anatomical height. High-lying aneurysms may be accessed similarly to BA bifurcation aneurysms via a trans-sylvian pterional craniotomy, which can be extended using its variants (pretemporal, orbitozygomatic, transcavernous) or through the extended subtemporal approach (transtentorial, anterior petrosal). These approaches present challenges in achieving proximal vascular control. An extended retrosigmoid approach to the cerebellopontine angle is necessary for lower-lying aneurysms to adequately expose the BA trunk anterior to the brainstem. The extension is achieved through the implementation of a retrolabyrinthine presigmoid approach, a translabyrinthine approach, or a transcochlear petrosectomy. These approaches aim to secure extensive and parallel access to the prepontine space, facilitating proximal control of the BA and the aneurysm neck. Nevertheless, the outcome of these approaches consistently yields a confined and limited surgical field, presenting few alternatives for addressing unforeseen circumstances or intraoperative rupture. Many of these aneurysms are deemed unsuitable for clipping and are instead candidates for indirect treatment methods, including proximal occlusion or trapping, in conjunction with revascularization techniques or endovascular treatment.

Clipping saccular perforating artery aneurysms presents significant microsurgical challenges. Achieving proximal control is often difficult due to the aneurysms' proximity to the BA. Additionally, the neck of these aneurysms is poorly defined, complicating vessel reconstruction. The dissection of both the artery and the aneurysm is intricate and risks compromising the perforating artery and adjacent small perforating arteries. Similarly, achieving a complete exclusion of the aneurysm through endovascular treatment is noteworthy. An alternative involves sacrificing the perforating artery to achieve aneurysm exclusion. Traditionally, the occlusion of a perforating artery is regarded as high risk due to its role as a terminal circulation artery. Although significant collateral circulation exists among perforating arteries, this approach often results in ischemia, regardless of whether an endovascular or microsurgical technique is employed [16, 18–21].

15.8.2 Dissecting Aneurysms of the Vertebral Artery

Dissecting aneurysms of the VA cannot be addressed through clipping or clip reconstruction methods. The sole microneurosurgical treatment option involves the exclusion of the affected arterial segment through proximal and distal clipping (*trapping*) of the VA. The treatment options are contingent upon the arterial branches and the collateral circulation via the contralateral VA or the AICA. Aneurysms not involving the exit of the PICA may be addressed through endovascular or microneurosurgical methods, utilizing internal trapping or clipping of the aneurysmal segment of the artery. If the aneurysm occurs before the exit of the PICA, the flow is maintained in a countercurrent manner by the contralateral VA; conversely, if the aneurysm is located distal to the exit of the PICA, the flow is sustained by the VA itself. Aneurysms related to the exit of the PICA present a significant issue. Trapping is inadvisable in this scenario because of the significant risk of ischemia resulting from occlusion of the PICA and the perforating arteries that arise from the VA and PICA, even when a hypoplastic PICA is present. It is essential to conduct a balloon occlusion test to confirm effective collateral circulation or to devise a revascularization strategy in conjunction with the trapping of the VA [6–8, 16].

15.8.3 Fusiform Aneurysms of the Basilar Artery

The management of fusiform aneurysms primarily focuses on controlling lesion growth, alleviating its mass effect on the brainstem, and minimizing or eliminating vascular dilation to prevent rupture. Fusiform aneurysms, by definition, cannot be clipped, and their location complicates microneurosurgical exploration for evaluating potential microneurosurgical reconstruction of the artery. Aneurysmal dilatation can only be addressed effectively if it is characterized by eccentricity, brevity, or positioning in regions devoid of perforating arteries. Before the advent of endovascular treatment, fusiform aneurysms of the BA were managed by ligating one or both VAs or the trunk of the BA proximal to the aneurysm. This approach was contingent upon the presence of one or both fetal-type posterior communicating arteries, which maintained distal flow through the BA. This strategy has also been employed in endovascular techniques. Both approaches have not yielded satisfactory outcomes, and each treatment modality is linked to significant morbidity and mortality rates. Consequently, revascularization techniques represent a logical alternative approach [9].

15.9 Complications, Prevention, and Management

Complications associated with microneurosurgery for aneurysms can be categorized into two primary groups: those arising from the surgical approach and those resulting from the treatment of the aneurysm itself. The complications associated with the approach include cerebrospinal fluid leak, meningitis, venous sinus thrombosis, neck pain or headache, and occipito-cervical instability, which are discussed in the chapter on retrosigmoid and far-lateral approaches. Complications arising from aneurysm clipping encompass cranial nerve dysfunction and vascular issues.

The manipulation of aneurysms at the VA–PICA junction poses a risk of injuring the lower cranial nerve roots. The prevalence of this complication in the literature is contingent upon the interest in data collection, resulting in variability across different series, with some reporting occurrences in over one-third of cases. The clinical implications are significant in cases of severe combined injury to the glossopharyngeal and vagal nerves, potentially resulting in swallowing disorders and impaired vocal cord mobility, which may necessitate temporary or permanent tracheostomy or gastrotomy. Hearing loss may occur alongside a sensation of ear fullness, often resulting from the filling of mastoid cells that were accessed during craniotomy. The prognosis is currently favorable. Deafness has a poor prognosis and may result from injury to the internal auditory artery or from the mechanical effects of vibration caused by high-speed motor use. A temporary deterioration in cerebellar function and long sensory-motor pathways may occur. These disorders are challenging to identify and assess in patients with diminished consciousness requiring prolonged mechanical ventilation, a common scenario in individuals who have experienced a high-grade posterior fossa SAH. In these patients, the typical neurological presentation is not evident; however, they exhibit insufficient cough, increased secretions, blood gas abnormalities, and recurrent pneumonia due to repeated silent aspiration. This condition prolongs critical situations and elevates mortality risk. Most cranial nerve damage typically results from nerve manipulation during dissection and clipping, leading to low-intensity lesions (neuroapraxia). Consequently, spontaneous functional recovery is observed within several weeks to a few months.

The primary complication associated with microsurgical treatment of aneurysms is ischemia. Ischemic syndromes resulting from occlusion of the posterior circulation arteries exhibit significant syndromic complexity and typically progress at a slower rate. Initial symptoms are often nonspecific, including vertigo, nausea, headache, or neck pain. Prodromal symptoms may occur hours or days before a confirmed stroke. The clinical manifestation of VA occlusion is contingent upon the specific region affected by ischemia. The initial symptoms may be nonspecific, including vertigo or dizziness, nausea or vomiting, and headache or neck pain. Additional signs and symptoms encompass hemiparesis, ataxia, diplopia, pupillary abnormalities, dysarthria, and changes in the level of consciousness. Occlusion of the perforating arteries may lead to ischemia in the lateral region of the medulla oblongata, resulting in Wallenberg syndrome. This condition is characterized by reduced thermo-algesic sensitivity on the ipsilateral face and the contralateral side of the body, along with Horner syndrome, limb ataxia, dysphonia, and dysphagia. Bilateral pontine ischemia resulting from occlusion of the BA trunk is among the most severe syndromes. The final clinical presentation resembles a state of coma, which is, in fact, indicative of pentaplegia. In this condition, only conjugate vertical ocular movements and blinking are preserved, while the patient remains fully conscious yet entirely incapable of interacting with their surroundings. This condition is referred to as *locked-in syndrome*. The acute phase of this situation is associated with a significantly high mortality rate. Occlusion of the circumferential perforating arteries can lead to ischemia in the lateral region of the pons, typically resulting in contralateral motor deficits, potentially accompanied by cerebellar symptoms such as ataxic hemiparesis or Gasperini syndrome. This syndrome involves the damage of the trigeminal, abducens, and facial nerve nuclei, along with contralateral hemi-hypoesthesia and hypoacusis. Ischemia of the AICA results in symptoms associated with brainstem involvement, including hearing loss, facial paresis, ipsilateral facial hypoesthesia, contralateral body hypoesthesia, Horner syndrome, axial and limb ataxia, and vertigo.

15.10 Outcome, Prognosis, and Follow-Up

Definitive conclusions regarding the specific outcomes of cerebellopontine angle aneurysms are challenging to establish, as systematic reviews are lacking due to the rarity of these lesions. A meta-analysis of the literature on posterior circulation aneurysms indicates that there are no statistically significant differences in post-procedure and late mortality rates between endovascular and microneurosurgical treatments, applicable to both ruptured and unruptured aneurysms. Endovascular treatment yields superior outcomes concerning the incidence of permanent neurological deficits, while microneurosurgical clipping demonstrates advantages related to the necessity for retreatment (refer to case 20 in Chap. 21).

15.11 Management Modalities

The management of cerebral aneurysms typically involves the identification, prevention, and treatment of vascular risk factors; imaging surveillance; microneurosurgical intervention; and endovascular therapy [22–24].

Unruptured saccular aneurysms located in the posterior circulation exhibit a significant risk of rupture; therefore, endovascular or microneurosurgical intervention is advised. Ruptured saccular aneurysms in the posterior fossa represent a neurosurgical emergency, necessitating prompt endovascular or microneurosurgical intervention to avert early rebleeding, which can have severe consequences. Aneurysms diagnosed before rupture should be treated promptly due to their significant risk of growth or rupture, which remains largely unpredictable. Similar to saccular aneurysms, urgent treatment is required if they present with SAH. In the context of dissecting aneurysms, treatment options include both endovascular and microneurosurgical approaches. While endovascular treatments are more commonly employed, they often serve a palliative purpose. Conversely, microneurosurgical options are limited and primarily palliative as well. Treatment with anticoagulants or antiplatelet agents for dissecting aneurysms presenting with ischemia or mural or intraluminal thrombi is not advised. Treatment options for fusiform aneurysms are limited and generally ineffective. If microneurosurgical solutions are inadequate, endovascular solutions also prove ineffective, exhibiting a high incidence of complications and mortality. Furthermore, these approaches often result in incomplete treatments, recurrences, and the necessity for retreatments, which rarely alter the disease's natural progression, ultimately resulting in aneurysm growth, exacerbation of neurological symptoms, and rupture.

15.12 Key Messages

- *Cerebellopontine angle aneurysms represent a subtype of posterior circulation aneurysms, arising from the arteries of the posterior circulation as they traverse the cerebellopontine angle.*
- *Posterior circulation aneurysms may be addressed through either a standard retrosigmoid or far-lateral approach or by extended approaches.*
- *Saccular, fusiform, or dissecting aneurysms located at the cerebellopontine angle are different types of aneurysms. The VA and BA trunks, perforators, and the VA–PICA junction are common locations for the formation of saccular aneurysms. Dissection occurs frequently in both BA and VA. The VA and the BA are implicated in fusiform aneurysms.*
- *Cerebellopontine angle aneurysms may lead to bleeding as well as nonspecific symptoms or those related to compression of the brain stem, cranial nerves, or cerebellum.*
- *Microneurosurgical intervention is recommended for saccular aneurysms located at the VA–PICA junction. There are precise indications for other types and locations. Endovascular therapy represents an alternative approach.*
- *The prognosis for cerebellopontine angle aneurysms is generally unfavorable.*

References

1. De Oliveira E, Tedeschi H, Rhoton AL, et al. Microsurgical anatomy of the posterior circulation: vertebral and basilar arteries. In: Carter LP, Spetzler RF, editors. Neurovascular Surgery. New York: McGraw-Hill; 1995.
2. Djulejić V, Marinković S, Milić V, et al. Common features of the cerebral perforating arteries and their clinical significance. Acta Neurochir. 2015;157:743–54. https://doi.org/10.1007/s00701-015-2378-8.
3. Pai BS, Varma RG, Kulkarni RN, et al. Microsurgical anatomy of the posterior circulation. Neurol India. 2007;55:31–41. https://doi.org/10.4103/0028-3886.30424.
4. Rhoton AL Jr. The posterior fossa: microsurgical anatomy & surgical approaches. Neurosurgery. 2000;47(Suppl 3):S1–S279. https://doi.org/10.1097/00006123-200009001-00013.
5. Sedat J, Chau Y, Mahagne MH, et al. Dissection of the posteroinferior cerebellar artery: clinical characteristics and long-term follow-up in five cases. Cerebrovasc Dis. 2007;24:183–90. https://doi.org/10.1159/000104475.
6. Gottesman RF, Sharma P, Robinson KA, et al. Imaging characteristics of symptomatic vertebral artery dissection: a systematic review. Neurologist. 2012;18:255–60. https://doi.org/10.1097/NRL.0b013e3182675511.
7. Iihara K, Sakai N, Murao K, et al. Dissecting aneurysms of the vertebral artery: a management strategy. J Neurosurg. 2002;97:259–67. https://doi.org/10.3171/jns.2002.97.2.0259.
8. Kai Y, Nishi T, Watanabe M, et al. Strategy for treating unruptured vertebral artery dissecting aneurysms. Neurosurgery. 2011;269:1085–91. https://doi.org/10.1227/NEU.0b013e3182262adf.
9. Nussbaum ES, Mendez A, Camarata P, et al. Surgical management of fusiform aneurysms of the peripheral posteroinferior cerebellar artery. Neurosurgery. 2003;53:831–4. https://doi.org/10.1227/01.neu.0000084162.29616.43.
10. Al-khayat H, Al-Khayat H, Beshay J, et al. Vertebral artery-posteroinferior cerebellar artery aneurysms: clinical and lower cranial nerve outcomes in 52 patients. Neurosurgery. 2005;56:2–10. PMDI: 15617580.
11. Batjer HH, Kopitnik TA, Purdy PD, et al. Vertebral and posteroinferior cerebellar artery aneurysms. In: Carter LP, Spetzler RF, editors. Neurovascular surgery. New York: McGraw-Hill; 1995.
12. Higa H, Ujiie H, Kato K, et al. Basilar artery trunk saccular aneurysms: morphological characteristics and management. Neurosurg Rev. 2009;32:181–91. https://doi.org/10.1007/s10143-008-0163-3.
13. Kapadia A, Schweizer TA, Spears J, et al. Nonaneurysmal perimesencephalic subarachnoid hemorrhage: diagnosis, pathophysiology, clinical characteristics, and long-term outcome. World Neurosurg. 2014;82:1131–43. https://doi.org/10.1016/j.wneu.2014.07.006.

14. Gonzalez-Darder JM, Quilis-Quesada V, Capilla-Guasch P. Aneurismas cerebrales. Barcelona: Elsevier España; 2022.
15. Lawton MT. Seven aneurysms. Tenets and techniques for clipping. New York: Thieme; 2011.
16. Yasargil MG. Microneurosurgery. New York: Thieme; 1984.
17. González-Darder JM, Quilis-Quesada V, Capilla-Guasch P, de Oliveira E. Abordajes neuroquirúrgicos de la patología craneal y cerebral. 2nd ed. Barcelona: Elsevier España; 2020.
18. Chau Y, Sachet M, Sédat J. Should we treat aneurysms in perforator arteries from the basilar trunk? Review of 49 cases published in the literature and presentation of three personal cases. Interv Neuroradiol. 2018;24:22–8. https://doi.org/10.1177/1591019917734531.
19. Garcia-Gonzalez U, Cavalcanti DD, Agrawal A, et al. Anatomical study on the "perforator-free zone": reconsidering the proximal superior cerebellar artery and basilar artery perforators. Neurosurgery. 2012;70:764–73. https://doi.org/10.1227/NEU.0b013e3182351f8e.
20. Gross BA, Puri AS, Du R. Basilar trunk perforator artery aneurysms. Case report and literature review. Neurosurg Rev. 2013;36:163–8. https://doi.org/10.1007/s10143-012-0422-1.
21. Marinković SV, Gibo H. The surgical anatomy of the perforating branches of the basilar artery. Neurosurgery. 1993;33:80–7. https://doi.org/10.1227/00006123-199307000-00012.
22. Fountas K, Spyrou M, Konovalov N. Clipping versus coiling in posterior circulation intracranial aneurysms: a meta-analysis. Chin Neurosurg J. 2019;5:16. https://doi.org/10.1186/s41016-019-0163-x.
23. Lawton MT, Abla AA, Rutledge WC, et al. Bypass surgery for the treatment of dolichoectatic basilar trunk aneurysms: a work in progress. Neurosurgery. 2016;79:83–99. https://doi.org/10.1227/NEU.0000000000001175.
24. Lehto H, Niemelä M, Kivisaari R, et al. Intracranial vertebral artery aneurysms: clinical features and outcome of 190 patients. World Neurosurg. 2015;84:380–9. https://doi.org/10.1016/j.wneu.2015.03.034.

16 Arteriovenous Malformations

16.1 Introduction

Arteriovenous malformations (AVMs) located in the cerebellopontine angle (CPA-AVMs) represent a specific subtype of cerebral AVMs, characterized by distinct topographical features that influence their clinical presentation and treatment approaches [1, 5, 9, 10, 12]. CPA-AVMs are situated in the posterior fossa, a small intracranial region characterized by a high concentration of critical neurological structures that hold significant clinical and vital importance.

The basic structure of cerebral AVMs includes one or more arterial afferents, a nidus where arteriovenous shunts are situated, allowing arterial blood to flow directly into the venous segment, bypassing the capillary network, and one or more drainage veins that transport blood to the dural venous sinuses. The nidus of the cerebral AVMs is situated on the pial surface of the brain, cerebellum, and brainstem, with potential extension into deeper structures. Consequently, CPA-AVMs ought to be situated on the surface of the cerebellum and brainstem related to the cerebellopontine angle, as well as on the surface of the cranial nerve roots at their origin from the brainstem. CPA-AVMs are defined as rare lesions, typically small, that have a close connection with cranial nerve roots and extend minimally onto the pial surface of the brainstem. CPA-AVMs can be defined as those requiring microneurosurgical treatment accessed via a retrosigmoid approach or its variations.

The incidence of cerebral AVMs is approximately 1 to 1.5 cases per 100,000 individuals annually, with a prevalence of less than 1%. Posterior fossa AVMs represent 7–15% of the total incidence, with 70% situated in the cerebellum, 20% in the brainstem, and 10% partially or preferentially located in the cerebellopontine angle.

16.2 Anatomical Considerations

AVMs replicate the vascular structure of the anatomical region in which the nidus is situated. Consequently, CPA-AVMs receive afferent blood supply from the arteries of the posterior circulation and drain into the dural venous sinuses of the posterior fossa via the veins of the cerebellopontine angle [3, 13]. Various aspects of the vascular anatomy of the cerebellopontine angle have been reviewed in other chapters and therefore will be summarized in this section.

16.2.1 Cerebellopontine Angle Arteries

The vertebral artery (VA) follows an extensive course both extracranially and intracranially, extending from its origin to the vertebrobasilar

J. M. González-Darder, *Microneurosurgery of Cerebellopontine Angle*,
https://doi.org/10.1007/978-3-032-03091-7_16

junction. This course is divided into four segments, with segment V4 traversing the cerebellopontine angle after crossing the dura mater. The initial branch of the intradural VA is the posterior spinal artery, which may arise from the extradural space or directly from the posterior inferior cerebellar artery (PICA). Nonetheless, the principal branch of the VA is the PICA, which may also originate from an extradural source. The subsequent branch of the VA, adjacent to the basilar artery (BA) trunk, is the anterior spinal artery, which connects with the contralateral artery in the anterior medullary groove to supply the spinal cord. The PICA represents the primary branch of the VA. PICA is categorized into five segments: anterior medullary, lateral medullary, tonsillar-medullary, telovellotonsillar, and cortical segment, where it bifurcates into two branches, one vermian and one hemispheric, which are distributed across the cerebellar cortex. The BA is a singular vessel created by the convergence of both VAs at the medullary–pontine junction, extending to its bifurcation at the pontomesencephalic sulcus. The primary branches of the BA include the anterior inferior cerebellar artery (AICA) and the superior cerebellar artery (SCA), along with numerous smaller perforating arteries supplying the pons. The AICA originates from the BA in close proximity to its source. The AICA comprises four segments: anterior pontine, lateral pontine, flocculus-peduncular, and cortical. This cortical segment corresponds to the distal branches that supply blood to the petrosal surface of the cerebellum. The SCA arises a few millimeters from the bifurcation of the BA into the posterior cerebral arteries. The SCA typically divides into two branches, one superior and one inferior, before its relation with the trigeminal nerve. SCA is categorized into three segments: anterior pontine-mesencephalic, lateral pontine-mesencephalic, and cerebellar-mesencephalic, culminating in the terminal distribution by the cortex of the cerebellum.

16.2.2 Cerebellopontine Angle Veins

The venous architecture of the posterior fossa consists of a systematic arrangement of transverse and longitudinal venous channels at varying levels. These channels drain into bridging veins that connect to the superior and inferior petrosal sinuses, the vein of Galen, and the transverse and sigmoid dural venous sinuses.

The superficial venous group is responsible for draining the cortex of the cerebellum and is categorized based on the specific surface areas of the cerebellum they serve: tentorial, petrosal, or suboccipital. The tentorial surface is drained by the superior hemispheric and superior vermian veins; the suboccipital surface is drained by the inferior hemispheric and inferior vermian veins; and the petrosal surface is drained by the anterior hemispheric vein. The deep venous system is associated with three deep fissures situated between the brainstem and the cerebellum: the vein of the cerebellar-mesencephalic fissure, the vein of the cerebello-pontine fissure, and the vein of the cerebello-medullary fissure. The primary veins are interconnected by proximal collectors, including the vein of the superior cerebellar peduncle located in the cerebellar-mesencephalic fissure, the vein of the middle cerebellar peduncle situated in the cerebellopontine fissure, and the vein of the inferior cerebellar peduncle found in the cerebellar-medullary fissure. This venous group also encompasses the tonsillar veins.

The veins draining the brainstem are categorized based on the specific region they serve (midbrain, pons, or medulla oblongata), the surface area they drain (anterolateral, anteromedial, or lateral), and their projection direction (transverse or longitudinal). The primary longitudinal veins of the brainstem include the anteromedial pontomesencephalic vein, anteromedial medullary vein, anterolateral pontomesencephalic vein, anterolateral medullary (pre-olivary) vein, lateral mesencephalic vein, and lateral medullary (retro-olivary) vein. The primary transverse veins include the peduncular vein, posterior communicating vein, pontomesencephalic sulcus, transverse pontine vein, medullary-pontine sulcus, and transverse medullary veins.

The bridging veins result from the convergence of the distal branches of the aforementioned venous groups. The galenic group comprises veins that converge on the vein of Galen, including the superficial veins of the tentorial surface and the deep veins of the cerebellar-mesencephalic fissure. The tentorial group is responsible for draining the superficial veins located on the suboccipital surface and the posterior rami of the tentorial surface. The petrosal drainage group comprises all veins that drain into the superior and inferior petrosal sinuses. The superficial veins of the lateral cerebellum, deep veins of the cerebellopontine and cerebellar-medullary fissures, along with the majority of the brainstem drainage veins, will converge at this location.

The primary venous structure in the upper region of the cerebellopontine angle is the superior petrosal venous complex, which drains into the superior petrosal sinus. A single drainage channel, known as the Dandy vein, typically arises from the convergence of two or more veins originating from the surface of the cerebellum or brain stem. Occasionally, multiple individual trunks may drain into the superior petrosal sinus. The pontine-trigeminal vein terminates in the superior petrosal complex or directly in the sinus and may have a close relationship with the trigeminal root. The venous drainage of the middle level of the cerebellopontine angle primarily occurs via the vein of the cerebellopontine fissure, which is formed by the confluence of multiple smaller veins and ascends towards the superior petrosal venous complex. The vein of the middle cerebellar peduncle is another venous channel, originating in the medullary-pontine sulcus and extending cranially toward the superior petrosal complex. The venous drainage of the lower compartment of the cerebellopontine angle occurs via small veins that converge into the inferior petrosal sinus.

16.3 Pathology

AVMs have traditionally been classified as congenital lesions characterized by a complex angioarchitecture. Despite this complexity, a classic vascular pattern can be identified, comprising feeding afferent arteries, a nidus, and drainage veins, all of which exhibit a clear anatomical correspondence with the vascular anatomy of the area where they develop. Clinical observations and an increasing understanding of the biological mechanisms governing cerebral angiogenesis indicate that not all AVMs may have congenital origins. Furthermore, a dynamic behavior has been observed in certain AVMs, wherein the angioarchitecture of the traditional vascular network undergoes spontaneous changes over time. The outcome of this dynamic process typically reveals that most AVMs exhibit a complex angioarchitecture at the time of diagnosis. This architecture involves one or more of the three compartments and reflects the classic patterns associated with regular AVMs, including variations in the size of the nidus, the number of afferent arteries or drainage veins, and instances of spontaneous occlusion of the AVM. However, some AVMs exhibit a range of novel and atypical alterations in their angioarchitecture, including arterial flow aneurysms; transdural arterial supply; occlusion of afferent arteries leading to the formation of neovascularization resembling moyamoya disease; and signs of proliferative cerebral angiopathy. Spontaneous changes in the AVM may occur alongside alterations resulting from incomplete treatment via microneurosurgery, radiation, or endovascular techniques.

16.4 Clinical Considerations

16.4.1 Cerebellar Arteriovenous Malformations

Posterior fossa AVMs exhibit a significantly elevated risk of hemorrhage compared to the overall incidence associated with cerebral AVMs. The incidence of bleeding in posterior fossa AVMs exceeds that of supratentorial AVMs by more than twofold. The presence of an AVM in the posterior fossa constitutes a significant risk factor for spontaneous bleeding. In more than 80% of cases, the clinical presentation of posterior fossa AVM is characterized by spontaneous bleeding, which may manifest as subarachnoid hemorrhage, intraparenchymal hemorrhage, or a combination of both types. This results in a significant risk of direct mortality due to bleeding, impacting two-thirds of patients. Posterior fossa AVMs present a significant risk of rebleeding, with an annual rebleeding incidence of 17.8%. The risk of rebleeding is notably elevated during the first year following the initial hemorrhage. Various risk factors have been identified in relation to these observations, including a high incidence of associated flow aneurysms; the tendency for many AVMs to receive afferent supply from small-caliber perforating branches that exhibit limited resistance to hemodynamic stress; a high prevalence of deep venous drainage occurring in confined spaces, where vein angulations may lead to increased retrograde pressure; and, lastly, the small size of the nidus. Progressive neurological deficit due to mass effect, ischemia, or hydrocephalus is the second most prevalent presentation of posterior fossa AVMs. In some instances, cases are identified in patients exhibiting non-specific symptoms such as headache, dizziness, or vertigo. Alternatively, these may represent true serendipitous findings observed in imaging studies conducted for reasons unrelated to neurological issues. The incidence of AVMs diagnosed through this method is increasing and is likely to continue to rise in the future due to improved access to imaging studies for the general population. Due to their topography, posterior fossa AVMs typically do not manifest as epileptic seizures. However, in instances of hemorrhage, patients may experience seizures either acutely or subsequently, attributable to the irritative effect of subarachnoid blood on the cerebral cortex.

Cerebellar AVMs exhibit a clinical presentation similar to that of posterior fossa AVMs. Over 75% of patients experience bleeding, 12% present with headaches or neurological deficits, while the remaining cases are identified in asymptomatic individuals.

16.4.2 Brainstem Arteriovenous Malformations

AVMs of the brainstem, although infrequent, exhibit a significant incidence of hemorrhage (>75%) as the primary event prompting diagnosis. The annual bleeding incidence exceeds 15%, accompanied by a high mortality rate. Other cases are diagnosed through a diverse range of symptoms, including headache, dizziness, facial pain, paresis, or hydrocephalus.

16.4.3 Cranial Nerve Arteriovenous Malformations

Genuine CPA-AVMs, or intrinsic cranial nerve root arteriovenous malformations, occur alongside intraparenchymal and/or subarachnoid bleeding, manifesting as trigeminal neuralgia or hemifacial spasm. From an epidemiological perspective, the age of clinical presentation for this type of AVM is significantly higher, with an average of 55 years, compared to cerebral AVMs.

Particularly, since the beginning of the exploration of the trigeminal nerve root for the treatment of trigeminal neuralgia with microvascular decompression, cases began to be described in which small AVMs were unexpectedly found whose nidus or one of the afferent arteries or drainage veins exerted compression on the entry area of the trigeminal root. The initial descriptions pertained to small AVMs or microangiomas that were not detected in preoperative imaging studies, such as magnetic resonance imaging (MRI) angiography or digital subtraction angiography (DSA), and were consequently termed cryptic or angiographically occult angiomas or AVMs (refer to case 27 in Chap. 21). Additionally, cases of AVMs and dural arteriovenous fistulas were documented in patients with trigeminal neuralgia, where vascular tangles were noted in proximity to the trigeminal nerve root or associated dilated arterial or venous vessels. The nidus of the AVM is often situated on the petrosal surface of the cerebellum, where compression occurs due to a dilated afferent artery or drainage vein. This phenomenon is also observed in dural arteriovenous fistulas, where compression typically results from significantly dilated veins caused by elevated pressure in the dural sinus. Trigeminal neuralgia resulting from an AVM is observed in less than 2% of cases. However, approximately 10% of patients with a posterior fossa AVM exhibit clinical symptoms of trigeminal neuralgia, with a notably higher incidence in AVMs situated in the cerebellopontine angle or those intrinsic to the trigeminal nerve root.

In the early treatment series for hemifacial spasm via microvascular decompression of the facial nerve root, the occurrence of AVMs, including the nidus, arterial or venous vessels, or aneurysms associated with the facial nerve, was reported in a small percentage of cases (1–2%).

16.5 Diagnostic Considerations

The imaging diagnosis of uncomplicated AVMs is typically straightforward using computed tomography (CT) angiography and MRI angiography, ideally with three-dimensional reconstruction. This diagnosis relies on the identification of a cluster of vessels exerting minimal mass effect on adjacent nervous tissue, along with the observation of serpentine and dilated arterial and venous vessels. MRI T1- and T2-weighted sequences reveal a honeycomb appearance attributed to flow void signals. MRI enables accurate localization of the nidus within the cerebellum, brain stem, and cranial nerve roots. The adjacent nervous tissue and any residual tissue between the vessels exhibit hyperintensity on T2 and FLAIR (*Fluid Attenuation Inversion Recovery*) sequences, attributable to gliosis. Intraparenchymal hemorrhage can complicate the diagnosis of AVM during the acute phase. Cerebral DSA is the diagnostic gold standard, essential for confirming diagnoses, understanding angioarchitecture, and gathering necessary information for treatment selection and design.

In posterior fossa AVM, a complete DSA study of the following vessels is essential: both vertebral arteries, both internal carotid arteries, and both external carotid arteries, assessed in anteroposterior and lateral projections. Rotational angiography facilitates three-dimensional reconstructions. Microneurosurgical planning requires knowledge of the following: the number and origin of afferent arteries; the size and anatomical location of the nidus; the number, destination, and size of drainage veins; flow aneurysms associated with the AVM; occlusion of afferent arteries, particularly the VA and aberrant arterial circulation of the moyamoya type; the pattern of proliferative cerebral angiopathy, characterized by normal-sized arterial afferences with significant interposed brain tissue, normal flow velocity, and non-dilated draining veins; and, finally, VA dominance and collateral circulation from the internal carotid arteries via the posterior communicating arteries. Imaging studies provide data regarding the size of the nidus, the type of venous drainage, and the eloquence of the nidus location, which facilitate the assessment of surgical risk using the Spetzler-Martin and supplementary scales [5].

16.6 Surgical Categories

Accurate localization of the AVM nidus in a specific anatomical region is crucial for microneurosurgical planning, given its correlation with arterial afferents and venous drainage, which influences the choice of optimal access and surgical approach. Therefore, the topographic classifications of AVMs are highly pertinent (Fig. 16.1).

16.6.1 Cerebellar Arteriovenous Malformations of the Cerebellopontine Angle

Cerebellar AVMs are categorized based on the cortical surface of the cerebellum where the nidus arises into five types: suboccipital, tentorial, vermian, petrosal, and tonsillar. Notably, only petrosal and tonsillar AVMs are related to the cerebellopontine angle, comprising 20% of cerebellar AVMs. The nidus of petrosal AVMs is located on the petrosal surface of the cerebellum, constituting the medial wall of the cerebellopontine angle. This area extends laterally from the cerebellopontine fissure and is divided into two portions by the horizontal or petrosal fissure. The arterial supply is provided by the AICA and its branches, while venous drainage occurs toward the petrosal sinuses via the anterior hemispheric

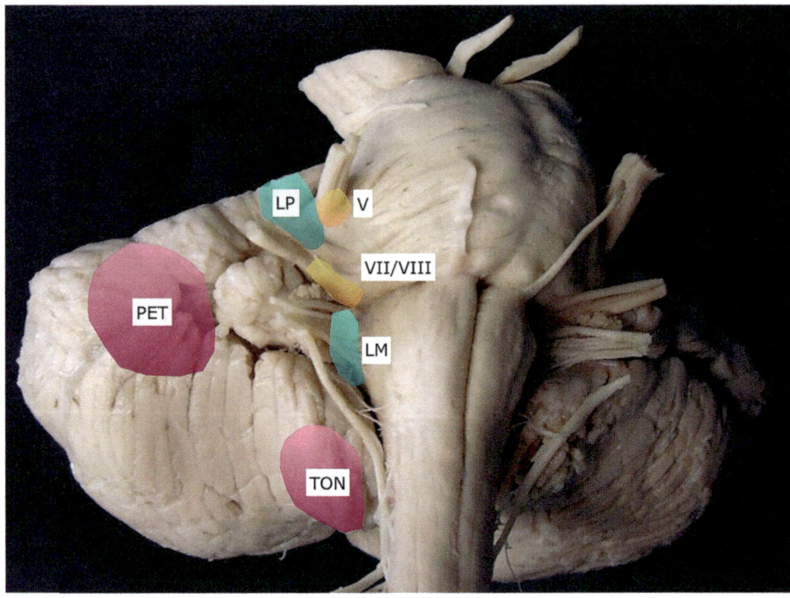

Fig. 16.1 An anatomical picture of the brainstem illustrates the right cerebellopontine angle, highlighting the topography of the AVMs situated in the cerebellar cortex, indicated in pink (PET: petrosal; TON: tonsillar), in blue those of the brainstem (LP: lateral pontine; LM: lateral medullary), and in yellow those intrinsic to the cranial nerves (V: trigeminal nerve; VII/VIII: facial-vestibulocochlear nerves)

vein and the vein of the cerebellopontine fissure. Tonsillar AVMs originate in the cerebellar tonsil, represent the least common type of cerebellar AVMs, receive blood supply from branches of the PICA, and exhibit superficial drainage via the tonsillar veins [5].

16.6.2 Brainstem Arteriovenous Malformations of the Cerebellopontine Angle

Brainstem AVMs are categorized into six types based on anatomical planes and levels: anterior and posterior mesencephalic, anterior and lateral pontine, and anterior and lateral medullary. Only pontine and medullary lateral AVMs are associated with the cerebellopontine angle. The nidus of lateral pontine AVMs is situated on the surface of the pons, positioned between the apparent origin of the trigeminal nerve and the cerebellopontine sulcus. It receives blood supply from branches of the AICA and, less frequently, from branches of the SCA. Venous drainage occurs towards the superior petrosal sinus via the superior petrosal venous complex. The nidus of lateral medullary AVMs is situated within a confined area, bordered cranially by the medullary-pontine sulcus and medially by the pre-olivary sulcus, posterior to the hypoglossal nerve rootlets. Afferent input originates from the VA and PICA, with drainage occurring through the lateral medullary veins [4, 5, 7].

16.6.3 Cranial Nerve Arteriovenous Malformations of the Cerebellopontine Angle

Cranial nerve-related AVMs are found in two distinct locations. The most common occurrences are associated with the trigeminal nerve root, supplied by branches of the SCA and perforating arterial branches of the BA, though they may also receive afferents from the AICA. The arterial supply consists of multiple small-caliber trigeminal arteries that typically create a network surrounding the root of the trigeminal nerve, originating from the SCA, AICA, and perforating branches of the BA. Venous drainage occurs cranially via the superior petrosal venous complex toward the superior petrosal sinus. AVMs associated with the facial–vestibulocochlear complex receive blood supply primarily from branches of the AICA, with contributions from the SCA occurring only in rare instances. Venous drainage exhibits considerable variability in both cranial and caudal courses [5, 8, 14].

16.7 Microneurosurgical Management

Microneurosurgical management of ACP-AVMs follows the established principles for cortical AVMs, which involve the progressive disconnection of arterial afferents, isolation of the nidus, and ultimately, disconnection of the venous drainage. Each deep cerebral AVM requires a specific treatment strategy, and the various types of CPA-AVMs will be detailed individually in the following section.

16.8 Arteriovenous Malformations That Require Specific Treatment

Next, we will describe the particularities for the microneurosurgical resection of each type of CPA-AVM, following our classification (Fig. 16.1) [3, 5].

16.8.1 Petrosal Arteriovenous Malformations

Resection is conducted through a broad retrosigmoid artery approach, revealing the inferior margin of the transverse sinus and the posterior margin of the sigmoid sinus. Following cerebrospinal fluid (CSF) drainage, the petrosal surface of the cerebellum is exposed and medially retracted using a spatula, directing attention to the origin of the facial–vestibulocochlear complex within the medullary-pontine sulcus. The flocculus is situated between the nidus and the facial–cochleovestibular complex, and more caudally it is positioned the choroid plexus between the nidus and the lower cranial nerve roots. The exposure of the nidus can be enhanced by incising the petrosal fissure of the cerebellum. The AICA is located caudally; however, the branches supplying the AVM are likely not observable due to the anterior position of the nidus. Arterialized venous drainage is routed cranially via the superior petrosal venous complex. The nidus is surrounded by cerebellar cortex, facilitating the resection and evacuation of the associated hematoma following prior bleeding. This facilitates the mobilization of the nidus to coagulate and sequentially section the arterial afferents from the AICA. The nidus is ultimately isolated from the blue drainage veins, which are subsequently coagulated and sectioned.

16.8.2 Tonsillar Arteriovenous Malformations

Small AVMs of the tonsil can be addressed using a lateral suboccipital approach; however, larger AVMs may require a far-lateral approach. The strategy involves a systematic exposure of the anatomical boundaries of the tonsil. Medially, the vallecula is incised, allowing for the separation of both tonsils. Cranially, the tonsillar-biventral sulcus is dissected to isolate the tonsil at the tonsillar peduncle. Laterally and anteriorly, the tonsil is detached from the posterior surface of the medulla oblongata up to the medullary-cerebellar fissure. Ultimately, the caudal pole of the tonsil is mobilized in a cranial direction. The initial segments of the PICA are identified by skeletonizing through the identification, coagulation, and sectioning of the branches leading to the nidus of the AVM (refer to case 22 in Chap. 21). The PICA typically terminates in the nidus, while its branches extend to the cerebellar vermis, with occlusion having minimal functional impact.

16.8.3 Brainstem Arteriovenous Malformations

Brainstem AVMs confined to the pial surface, lacking intraparenchymal extension, generally receive arterial supply from enlarged branches of the SCA or AICA and are amenable to complete resection. Brainstem AVMs with intraparenchymal extension generally receive arterial input from perforating branches and are often not amenable to complete resection due to the potential for neurological deterioration resulting from surgical manipulation, heat from bipolar coagulation, or ischemia (Fig. 16.2). In this context, in

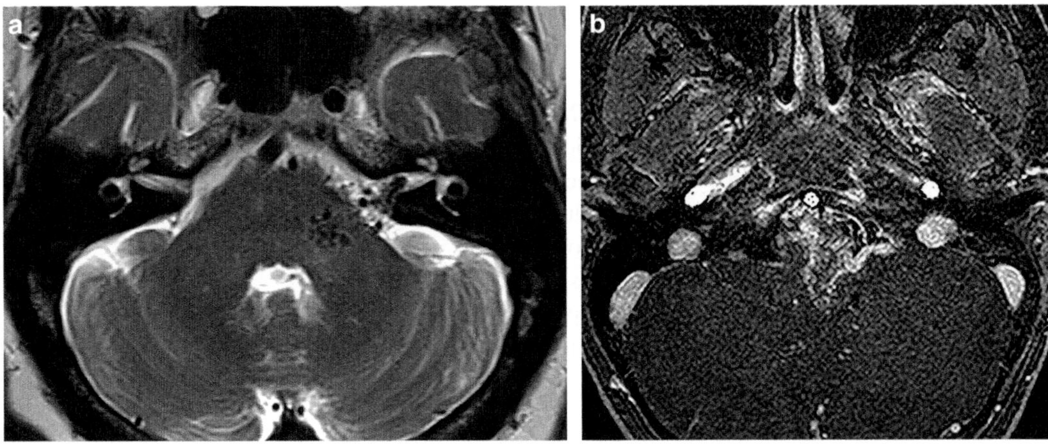

Fig. 16.2 Brainstem arteriovenous malformations with deep nidus. (**a**) Lateral pontine AVM with a pial component related to the facial–vestibulocochlear nerves and a deep component in the middle cerebellar peduncle. (**b**) Anterolateral medullary AVM with a huge nidus occupying the entire section of the medulla oblongata

situ coagulation represents a viable alternative, especially for lesions that have not experienced bleeding. In cases of AVMs that have experienced hemorrhage, the hematoma may facilitate dissection and mobilization of the nidus. The decision-making process in intrinsic AVMs of cranial nerves occurs during surgical exploration and involves either the removal of the nidus, in situ coagulation of the nidus or arterial afferents, or microvascular decompression in selected cases [4, 7].

16.8.3.1 Lateral Pontine Arteriovenous Malformations

The method and access to the AVM are consistent with the previously described approach (Fig. 16.3). The nidus is located in a deeper position within the petrosal sulcus corridor, situated above the flocculus and at the anatomical level of the facial–vestibulocochlear complex. The nidus is situated on the surface of the pons, rather than in the cerebellum, and may extend in depth into both the pons and the middle cerebellar peduncle. In cases of deep AVMs, it is essential to mobilize the nidus through parenchymal dissection conducted as near to the nidus as feasible, minimizing the risk of neurological deterioration (refer to case 24 in Chap. 21).

16.8.3.2 Lateral Medullary Arteriovenous Malformations

These AVMs are located anatomically beneath the medullary-pontine sulcus and receive afferent connections from both the VA and the PICA. Therefore, access requires a far-lateral approach, which facilitates the drainage of cerebrospinal fluid, elevation of the amygdala, proximal control of the V4 segment of the VA immediately after its entry through the dura mater, and opening of the cerebellar-medullary fissure. The arachnoid is subsequently dissected to reveal, in a superficial plane, the lower cranial nerves that traverse the field horizontally, as well as the accessory nerve that ascends longitudinally. A triangle in the midline is defined by the lateral surface of the medulla oblongata, laterally bordered by the course of the accessory nerve that converges caudally. The upper boundary of the triangle is indicated by the lower border of the vagal nerve, with its rootlets extending from the retro-olivary sulcus of the medulla oblongata in the midline to the jugular foramen, where they converge with the vagal nerve. The microneurosurgical approach reveals that cranial nerves are positioned in a more superficial plane compared

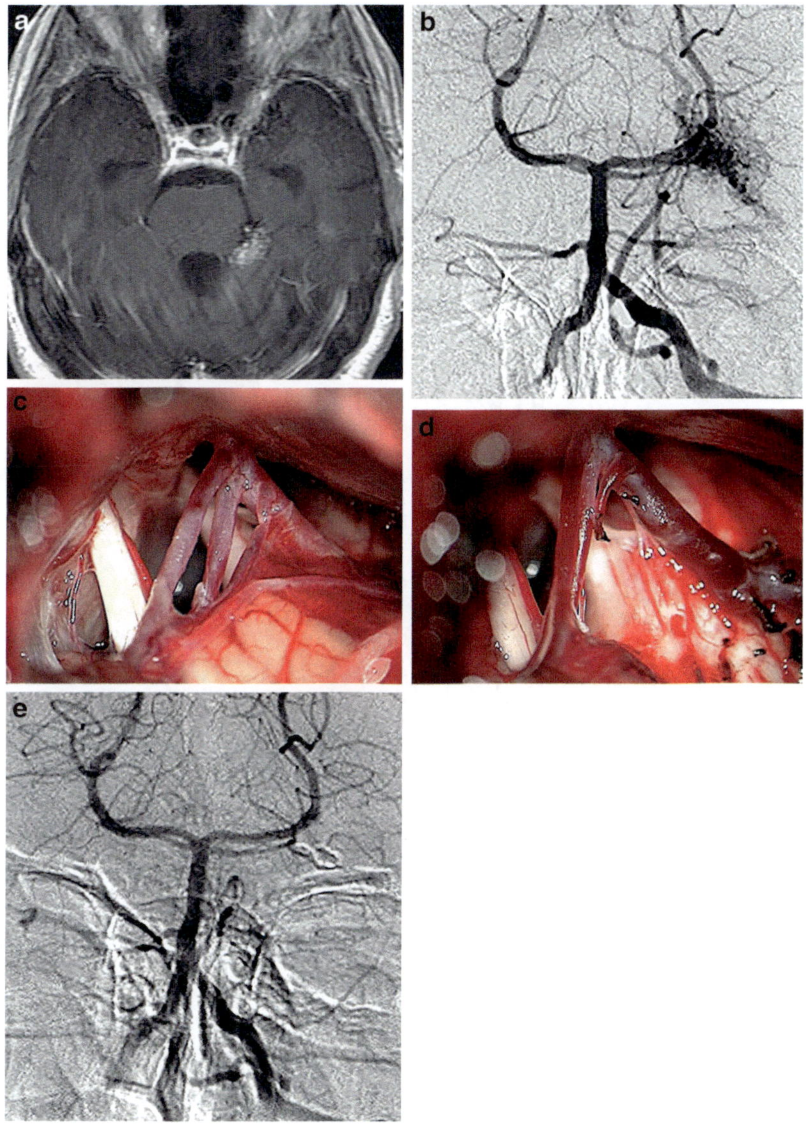

Fig. 16.3 Lateral pontine AVM. (**a**). Axial T1-weighted MRI with gadolinium demonstrates the location of the nidus on the lateral aspect of the pons and in relation to the left cerebellar peduncle. (**b**). Vertebral artery DSA demonstrating the AVM dependent on the superior cerebellar artery. (**c**, **d**) Intraoperative pictures depict the petrosal vein complex with arterialized blood before resection and with venous blood after resection. (**e**) Postoperative vertebral artery DSA

to the arteries, resulting in the nidus of the AVM being situated beneath them, along with the arterial input from the VA and PICA and the venous drainage. The hypoglossal nerve is located at a deeper level, traversing the trunk of the vertebral artery. The anterior and lateral arterial inputs to the nidus are dissected, coagulated, and sectioned until the VA and the origin of the PICA are skeletonized, facilitating the mobilization of the nidus. Nevertheless, controlling the medial inputs may pose challenges, and resecting the intraparenchymal portion of the nidus embedded in the medulla oblongata may be complicated until the blood flow through the draining veins ultimately appears blue (refer to case 23 in Chap. 21).

16.8.4 Intrinsic Arteriovenous Malformations of the Trigeminal Nerve

The approach and access adhere to the general microneurosurgical principles outlined above (Fig. 16.4). The lesion is confined to the root of the trigeminal nerve at its exit from the pons. Often, this consists of a network of small trigemi-

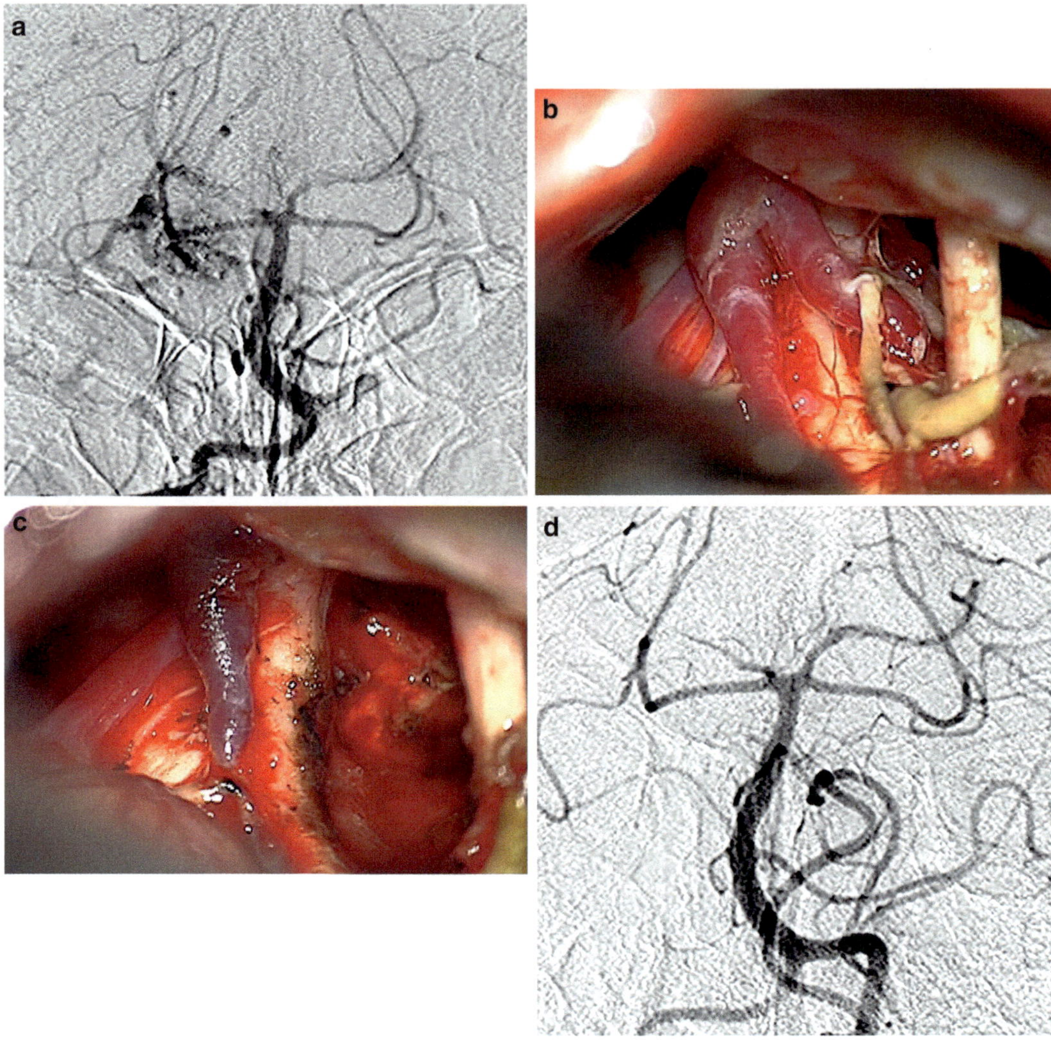

Fig. 16.4 Intrinsic AVM of the trigeminal nerve. (**a**) Vertebral DSA demonstrates the AVM nidus supplied by the superior cerebellar artery. (**b**, **c**) Intraoperative pictures illustrate the petrosal vein complex displaying arterialized blood before resection and venous blood after the resection of the nidus. (**d**) Postoperative vertebral artery DSA

nal arterial vessels that encircle or interweave with the root of the trigeminal nerve. In this scenario, the arterioles are coagulated and severed until the root is liberated and normal blue venous flow is restored, indicating in situ arterial occlusion. In cases where the SCA or a drainage vein is believed to significantly compress the root of the trigeminal nerve in patients with trigeminal neuralgia, microvascular decompression may be indicated (refer to case 27 in Chap. 21). In half of the cases involving patients with trigeminal neuralgia associated with AVM who undergo surgical exploration, it is found that the trigeminal neuralgia is attributable to the compression of arteries and/or veins. In patients without a history of bleeding, microvascular decompression may be adequate if the removal of the nidus is deemed risky; however, this approach does not completely mitigate the risk of bleeding [8, 14].

16.8.5 Intrinsic Arteriovenous Malformations of the Facial–Vestibulocochlear Nerve

The approach and microneurosurgical technique are consistent with the previously outlined description. Nevertheless, the nidus is situated deeper within the petrosal groove corridor, medial to the flocculus. Consequently, separation of the flocculus and choroid plexus is necessary to access the medullary-pontine groove and the origin of the facial–cochleovestibular complex, where the AVM is found.

16.8.6 Superior Petrosal Sinus Arteriovenous Fistula

These lesions do not represent true AVMs; however, they may be mistaken for other vascular lesions or tumors located in the cerebellopontine angle. The superior petrosal sinus arteriovenous fistula represents a subtype of tentorial arteriovenous fistulas characterized by direct communication between dural branches of the external carotid arteries (such as the middle meningeal artery) or the internal carotid artery (specifically the tentorial artery of Bernasconi–Casinari) and the superior petrosal sinus. This condition results in retrograde filling and dilation of veins in the posterior fossa and cerebellopontine angle, including the petrosal vein and the basal vein of Rosenthal. Large venous aneurysmatic dilatations may resemble cerebellopontine angle tumors until a suitable vascular study is conducted (Fig. 16.5). The management of these lesions is either endovascular or, preferably, microneurosurgical. The fistula is accessed via a standard retrosigmoid or infratentorial supracerebellar approach and is disconnected through direct and progressive bipolar coagulation of the venous channels. The outcome is favorable, despite the arterial supply remaining intact [6].

16.9 Complications, Prevention, and Management

Complications related to the approaches are common to all cerebellopontine angle pathologies and have been reviewed in the corresponding chapters. Microneurosurgical treatment of intrinsic AVMs of the cranial nerves faces the problem of leading to complete or incomplete, transient or permanent injury of the trigeminal nerve, facial nerve, or vestibulocochlear nerve, as a consequence of the manipulation of the nerves or the heat generated by bipolar coagulation of the arterial afferents that are related to the nerve root. The petrosal surface of the cerebellum is not considered an eloquent area, so a neurological deficit should not be expected due to the removal of the cerebellar tissue necessary for resection of the nidus. The middle cerebellar peduncle is a very inelastic structure, and the nidus of lateral pontine AVMs can be safely removed if it extends into the parenchyma, but the lateral aspect of the medulla oblongata is more eloquent in case removal of the nidus of a parenchyma-embedded lateral pontine AVM is required.

16.10 Outcome, Prognosis, and Follow-Up

Microneurosurgical intervention for CPA-AVMs typically results in the complete resection of the AVM and angiographic resolution in nearly all instances. In skilled hands, 60% of patients with tonsillar AVMs experience stability or improvement post-surgery, whereas the remaining 40% may deteriorate or succumb. Alongside vermian AVMs, they exhibit the poorest prognosis. Patients with petrosal AVMs exhibit the lowest grades on both the Spetzler–Martin scale and the supplementary scale. Pontine and lateral medullary AVMs exhibit the most favorable prognosis among brainstem AVMs when surgically treated by skilled professionals, achieving neurological stability or improvement in 100% and 75% of cases, respectively. Intrinsic AVMs of the cranial nerves are exceedingly rare, with only isolated cases documented, making it challenging to

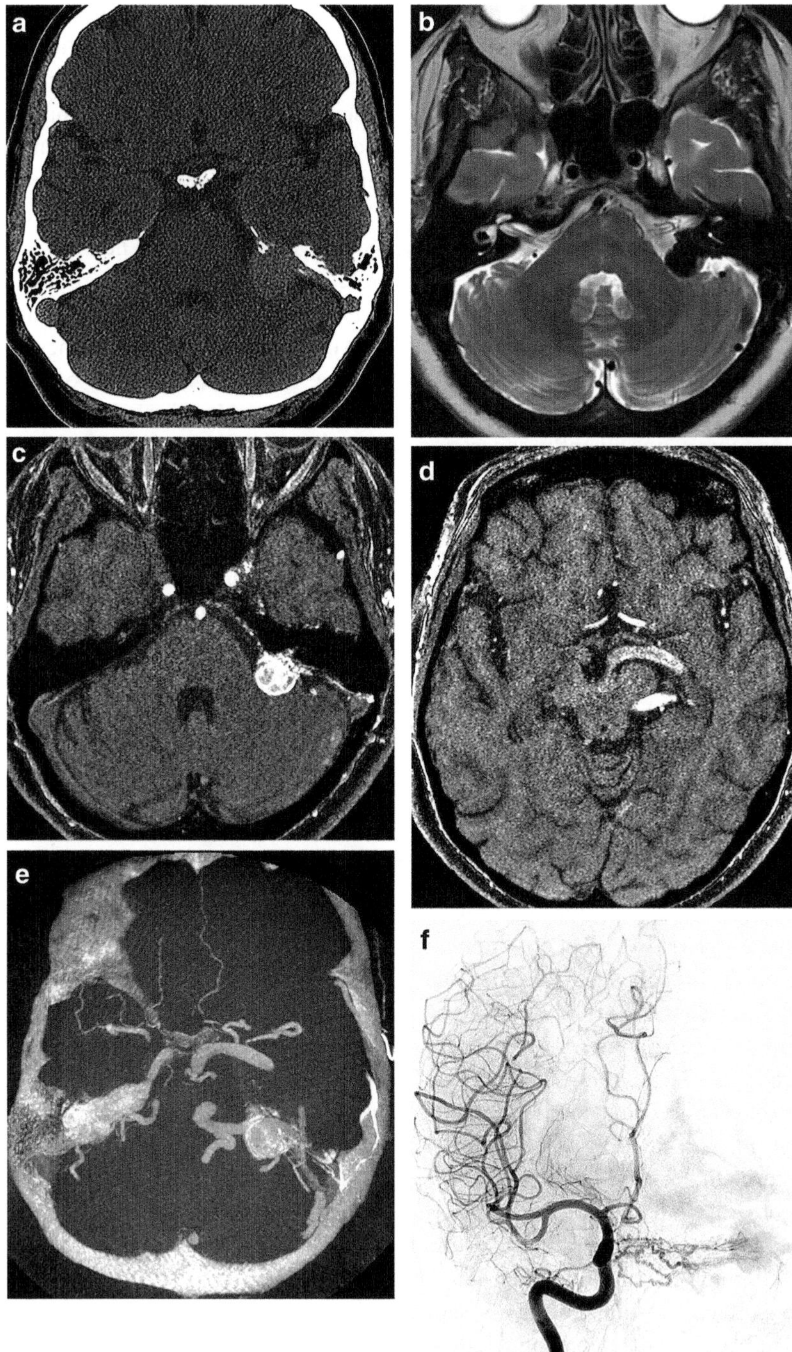

Fig. 16.5 Arteriovenous fistula of the superior petrosal sinus. (**a**) CT scan slice without contrast, demonstrating a rounded mass in the left cerebellopontine angle, slightly hyperintense relative to brain tissue. (**b**) Axial T2-weighted MRI demonstrates a hypointense, rounded lesion. (**c**, **d**) Axial T1-weighted MRI with gadolinium demonstrates significant enhancement of the lesion and dilation of the basal vein of Rosenthal. (**e**) CT angiography reveals a dilated basal vein of Rosenthal along with the presence of a venous aneurysm. (**f**) Right internal carotid artery DSA demonstrating dural vessels supplying the fistula. (**g**) Left internal carotid artery DSA. (**h**) Left external carotid artery DSA demonstrating the arteriovenous fistula

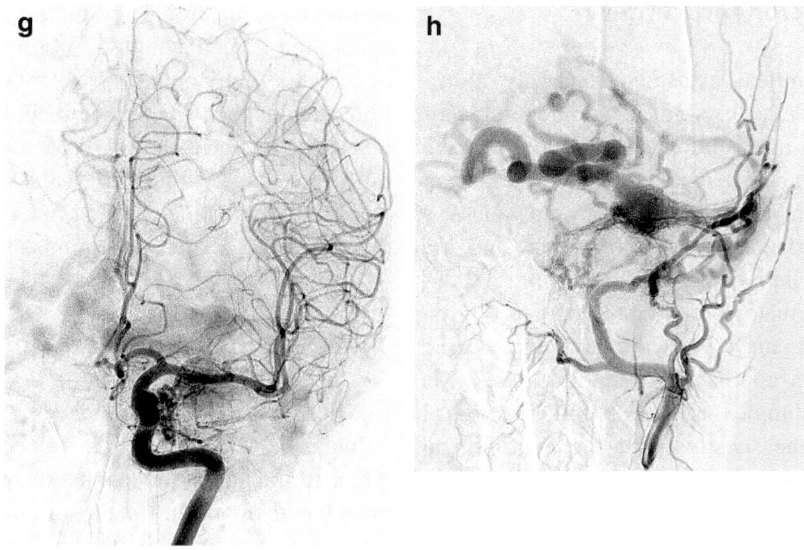

Fig. 16.5 (continued)

derive definitive conclusions in this area. Furthermore, variability exists in microneurosurgical treatments, which include nidus removal, in situ coagulation, and microvascular decompression. Conversely, numerous cases are addressed using stereotactic radiosurgery. The verification of the resolution of a treated AVM is achieved via cerebral DSA. In lesions managed through microneurosurgery, a vascular assessment is advised several months post-intervention, unless there are uncertainties regarding the completeness of removal, in which case DSA should be performed in the immediate postoperative period prior to hospital discharge. Following treatment of the lesion with stereotactic radiosurgery, it is advisable to conduct an annual MRI angiography study for follow-up. A DSA study is indicated if there are no signs of AVM closure after 3–4 years to confirm the persistence of the AVM and to evaluate the possibility of retreatment with stereotactic radiosurgery. Should closure of the malformation be suspected in the annual MRI angiography, confirmation via cerebral DSA is necessary to definitively verify the healing of the lesion.

16.11 Management Modalities

The management of cerebral AVMs is multifaceted, encompassing observation with symptomatic care, embolization and various endovascular approaches, stereotactic radiosurgery along with other radiation modalities, and ultimately microneurosurgical intervention. The selection of the most appropriate treatment involves numerous factors, including the surgical risk, the patient's symptoms, clinical status, expectations, and desires, as well as the specialist's experience and available technology. Treatment may involve a singular therapeutic option or a sequential combination of multiple approaches. The primary objective in designing treatment for AVMs is to achieve complete exclusion of the lesion while minimizing the risk of producing or exacerbating the patient's neurological sequelae. The management of AVMs involves the isolated or combined application of microsurgery, endovascular treatment, or stereotactic radiosurgery, in conjunction with symptomatic treatment or imaging monitoring tailored to the patient's specific needs [2, 5].

16.11.1 Microneurosurgery

Microneurosurgical excision effectively eliminates the immediate risk of bleeding or rebleeding. Surgical intervention for AVMs that have experienced hemorrhage should be done during the subacute phase, characterized by patient stability, reduced edema in nerve tissue, and the onset of clot liquefaction. While urgent evacuation of the hematoma and concurrent resolution of the AVM may be warranted in specific instances, this approach is rare in CPA-AVMs due to the complex anatomy, limited surgical access, and the sensitivity of the neurological structures involved. Microneurosurgical treatment offers the benefit of excising the AVM, thereby eliminating the significant risk of bleeding or rebleeding, particularly associated with posterior fossa AVMs. It can promptly address specific clinical symptoms, particularly those related to a potential intraparenchymal hematoma. The primary issue is the exacerbation or development of new neurological symptoms, especially pertinent in brainstem AVMs due to the density and significance of the neurological components involved. Stereotactic radiosurgery has emerged as a viable alternative for lesions of this topography.

16.11.2 Stereotactic Radiosurgery

Stereotactic radiosurgery, in contrast to microsurgery, results in delayed obliteration of the AVM, sustaining the risk of bleeding until the AVM is fully closed, with complications arising from radiation-related toxicity manifesting at a later stage. The surgical risk associated with resection of an AVM is influenced by the eloquence of the anatomical location, the size of the nidus, and the venous drainage. In contrast, stereotactic radiosurgery is not affected by the location or venous drainage; its primary determinant is the volume of the nidus receiving more than 12 Gy of irradiation. The obliteration rates for brainstem AVMs treated with stereotactic radiosurgery range from 50–60%. This obliteration typically occurs 3–5 years postirradiation, with an annual postoperative bleeding frequency of less than 5% and irradiation-related symptoms observed in 5–10% of patients. The brainstem's tolerance to irradiation remains inadequately defined; however, it is generally accepted that if AVM obliteration has not taken place within 3–5 years, retreatment is warranted due to the elevated risk of bleeding or rebleeding associated with brainstem AVMs.

16.11.3 Endovascular Treatment

Endovascular treatment achieves a curative outcome in 10–20% of patients with cerebral AVMs when administered independently, and it is associated with morbidity and mortality risks. This treatment is recommended as a palliative measure before microneurosurgery or stereotactic radiosurgery. It has been observed that embolization treatment for AVMs significantly diminishes the efficacy of stereotactic radiosurgery. Several arguments have been proposed to elucidate this paradoxical effect: recanalization of embolized vascular channels not targeted by radiation; the conversion of compact nidus into more diffuse forms with boundaries that are harder to delineate and irradiate; the attenuation of radiation effectiveness by embolic agents; the reactive angiogenic response to tissue hypoxia resulting from embolization; and, lastly, the tendency for larger or more complex AVMs to undergo embolization before stereotactic radiosurgery.

16.11.4 Medical Treatment

Recent investigations have explored pharmacological treatments for AVMs that are not amenable to other treatments. These medical treatments aim to block or modify specific biological mechanisms that regulate the life cycle of these lesions, especially those affecting growth and rupture. Bevacizumab, an anti-VEGF monoclonal antibody, has been studied due to the critical role of VEGF (*Vascular Endothelial Growth Factor*) in regulating and stimulating angiogenesis in the central nervous system. Elevated VEGF levels are observed in patients with AVMs, present in both plasma and pathological specimens. Thalidomide has been evaluated for its positive impact on pericytes and PDGF-beta (*Platelet-Derived Growth Factor*), a marker for pericytes. Pericytes play a crucial role in preserving the integrity of the blood-brain barrier by regulating the junctions between endothelial cells. In patients with AVMs who have experienced microhemorrhages or bleeding, there is a reduction in the number of pericytes. MMPs (*Matrix Metalloproteinases*) regulate the extracellular matrix through protein degradation. Their excessive activity is associated with vessel wall instability and hemorrhage in aneurysms and AVMs. Inhibition of MMPs using tetracyclines may offer protective benefits against rupture. Additional pharmacological agents associated with neuroprotection during ischemic events, as well as the management of inflammation through the use of aspirin or heparin coagulation factors, have been suggested. Numerous trials have been conducted on patients with hereditary hemorrhagic telangiectasia or Rendu–Osler syndrome. In many instances, the trials have either not progressed to the clinical phase or, if they have, they have yielded unsatisfactory results or a significant risk of complications [11].

16.12 Key Messages

- *AVMs may infrequently occur at the cerebellopontine angle, affecting the surface of the brainstem, cerebellum, and certain cranial nerves.*
- *A subarachnoid or intraparenchymal hemorrhage originating from the nidus is the prevalent manifestation of AVMs located at the cerebellopontine angle.*
- *The risk of rebleeding associated with cerebellopontine angle AVMs is significant.*
- *VMs located in the cerebellopontine angle require treatment following diagnosis due to their significant propensity for bleeding and rebleeding.*
- *Microneurosurgical intervention for AVMs effectively eliminates the risk of hemorrhage or rehemorrhage. Resection of brainstem lesions with parenchymal involvement carries a significant risk of morbidity; thus, stereotactic radiosurgery presents a valid alternative.*

References

1. Arnaout OM, Gross BA, Eddleman CS, et al. Posterior fossa arteriovenous malformations. Neurosurg Focus. 2009;26:E12. https://doi.org/10.3171/2009.2.FOCUS0914.
2. Cohen-Inbar O, Ding D, Chen CJ, et al. Stereotactic radiosurgery for deep intracranial arteriovenous malformations, part 1: brainstem arteriovenous malformations. J Clin Neurosci. 2016;24:30–6. https://doi.org/10.1016/j.jocn.2015.11.007.
3. González-Darder JM, Quilis-Quesada V, Capilla-Guasch P, de Oliveira E. Abordajes neuroquirúrgicos de la patología craneal y cerebral. 2nd ed. Barcelona: Elsevier España; 2020.
4. Han SJ, Englot DJ, Kim H, et al. Brainstem arteriovenous malformations: anatomical subtypes, assessment of "occlusion in situ" technique, and microsurgical results. J Neurosurg. 2015;122:107–17. https://doi.org/10.3171/2014.8.JNS1483.
5. Lawton MT. Seven AVMs. Thieme, New York: Tenets and techniques for resection; 2014.
6. Lawton MT, Sanchez-Mejia RO, Pham D, et al. Tentorial dural arteriovenous fistulae: operative strategies and microsurgical results for six types. Neurosurgery. 2008;62(Suppl 1):110–24. https://doi.org/10.1227/01.neu.0000317381.68561.b0.
7. Madhugiri VS, Teo MKC, Vavao J, et al. Brainstem arteriovenous malformations: lesion characteristics and treatment outcomes. J Neurosurg. 2018;128:126–36. https://doi.org/10.3171/2016.9.JNS16943.
8. Maher CO, Atkinson JL, Lane JI. Arteriovenous malformation in the trigeminal nerve. Case report J Neurosurg. 2003;98:908–12. https://doi.org/10.3171/jns.2003.98.4.0908.
9. Nishino K, Hasegawa H, Morita K, et al. Clinical characteristics of arteriovenous malformations in the cerebellopontine angle cistern. J Neurosurg. 2017;126:60–8. https://doi.org/10.3171/2015.12.JNS152190.
10. O'Shaughnessy BA, Getch CC, Bendok BR, et al. Microsurgical resection of infratentorial arteriovenous malformations. Neurosurg Focus. 2005;19:E5. https://doi.org/10.3171/foc.2005.19.2.6.
11. Raper DMS, Winkler EA, Rutledge WC, et al. An update on medications for brain arteriovenous malformations. Neurosurgery. 2020;87:871–8. https://doi.org/10.1093/neuros/nyaa192.
12. Rodríguez-Hernández A, Kim H, Pourmohamad T, et al. University of California, San Francisco Arteriovenous Malformation Study Project.

Cerebellar arteriovenous malformations: anatomic subtypes, surgical results, and increased predictive accuracy of the supplementary grading system. Neurosurgery. 2012;71:1111–24. https://doi.org/10.1227/NEU.0b013e318271c081.

13. Sumioka S, Kondo A, Tanabe H, et al. Intrinsic arteriovenous malformation embedded in the trigeminal nerve of a patient with trigeminal neuralgia. Neurol Med Chir (Tokyo). 2011;51:639–41. https://doi.org/10.2176/nmc.51.639.
14. Yuan Y, Zhang Y, Luo QI, et al. Trigeminal neuralgia caused by brain arteriovenous malformations: a case report and literature review. Exp Ther Med. 2016;12:69–80. https://doi.org/10.3892/etm.2016.3277.

17 Cerebellopontine Angle and Brainstem Cavernomas

17.1 Introduction

Cavernomas are vascular malformations located within the nervous tissue. Rarely, extra-axial cavernomas can be detected in the sellar and parasellar regions as well as in the cavernous sinus. Just 18 cases were reported in the cerebellopontine angle in a recent review of the literature, and a retrosigmoid technique was used for their microneurosurgical treatment [26]. On the other hand, brainstem cavernomas are prevalent and will be discussed collectively since, while not all of them are removed using a retrosigmoid technique, a considerable portion of them is [1, 4, 5, 9, 11, 12, 14].

17.1.1 History of Microneurosurgical Treatment of Cavernomas of the Brainstem

Cerebral cavernomas of any location were historically found at autopsy or in pathological studies of hemorrhagic materials in patients with spontaneous intracerebral bleeding. Their angioarchitecture characteristics make it impossible to diagnose them with cerebral digital subtraction angiography (DSA), which is why they were called *angiographically occult intracranial vascular malformations*. With the introduction of computed tomography (CT), they began to be diagnosed in patients without bleeding, and, later, their diagnosis was made extraordinarily easier after the introduction of magnetic resonance imaging (MRI), which allows for a quick and safe diagnosis. The massive diagnosis of patients with symptomatic and asymptomatic cavernomas has allowed us to understand in a fairly deep way the natural history of these lesions and consequently has allowed us to make recommendations and algorithms for their more effective and safe treatment.

This same line of reasoning can be applied to cavernomas of the brainstem. However, cavernomas of the brainstem have several peculiarities. The first is that cavernomas of the brainstem show a particularly aggressive clinical natural history and frequently require urgent microneurosurgical treatment. The second is that the brainstem is difficult to access, since it is located in a deep area of the posterior fossa, and its anterior surface is applied to the clivus. The third is that the brainstem is the area of the central nervous system with the highest density of neurological structures, both nuclei and ascending and descending pathways, many of them vital, so they are difficult to access without adding morbidity and mortality. All of this meant that, classically, access to brainstem lesions was exceptional in neurosurgical practice.

Despite these difficulties, the frequent diagnosis of brainstem cavernomas with or without symptoms or associated hemorrhage prompted an effort by some leading neurosurgeons to

J. M. González-Darder, *Microneurosurgery of Cerebellopontine Angle*,
https://doi.org/10.1007/978-3-032-03091-7_17

resolve these lesions safely, just as had been done with cavernomas in other locations. Initially, exophytic lesions, or those that could be safely recognized directly on the surface of the brainstem during microneurosurgical exploration, were preferably addressed, particularly those located in the rostral portion of the brainstem and accessible through midline approaches to the brainstem or the fourth ventricle. Later, different authors, such as Robert Spetzler, took advantage of the development of approaches to the skull base to establish a new strategy for accessing intrinsic lesions of the brainstem, based, whenever possible, on avoiding the approach through the fourth ventricle and choosing a more lateral entrance to the brainstem, particularly through the point where the lesion is located more superficially. With this strategy, once the lesion is identified in CT or MRI diagnostic studies, a line is drawn between the central point of the lesion and the closest point to the pia mater or to an accessible entry point in the brainstem, which serves as a guide to then select the most appropriate surgical approach following this line from the surface, with some independence from the complexity of the approach (*2-points approach*). This was the first holistic proposal for microneurosurgical access to brainstem cavernoma based on choosing the shortest route to the lesion from the pial surface, an access adjusted to the consideration of two aspects. The first was that a standardized cranial approach should be followed, more or less modified or expanded. The second was that, on the way to the lesion, crossing eloquent nuclei or pathways should be avoided [1, 2]. This approach led to the need to carry out complex approaches to the skull base to meet the requirements described, which led to complex, long-term surgeries that were a source of morbidity and mortality related to the approach itself, as these were infrequent approaches in the general neurosurgical practice that required a long learning curve.

A paradigm shift was subsequently introduced with the introduction of the concept of *safe entry zones*, where the priority is to select the safest access route to the lesion via a standard approach [6, 7, 10, 13–15, 21, 27]. This more simplistic approach gave a new impetus to surgery for brainstem cavernoma, placing the route through the brainstem to the lesion as the focus. The development of these safe entry zones was based on the study of microneurosurgical neuroanatomy. Safe entry zones can thus be defined as areas on the surface of the brainstem that are easily identifiable by means of unequivocal anatomical landmarks and where the underlying neurological structures are not, at least theoretically, clinically relevant for the patient and can be used as a corridor to reach the deeper located lesion. This concept of safe entry zones had already been developed in the 1990s for access to intrinsic lesions of the brainstem located in the floor of the fourth ventricle. In this case, reference structures were defined: the facial colliculus and the internal wing of the floor of the fourth ventricle, corresponding to the hypoglossal nucleus, which could be defined anatomically or with direct electrical stimulation. Using these references, two safe paramedian entry zones through the floor of the fourth ventricle, the *supracollicular zone* and the *infracollicular zone*, were proposed to resect rostral lesions [23]. With regard to anterolateral lesions of the brainstem, it was initially Evandro de Oliveira's group, in 2007, that described three safe entry zones to the brainstem, one for the midbrain (*lateral mesencephalic sulcus*), another for the pons (*peritrigeminal area*) and, finally, a third for the medulla oblongata (*inferior olivary nucleus*), all of them accessible through a retrosigmoid approach [21]. In response to this simplistic approach, there was an explosion of safe brainstem access routes and sites associated with safe approaches, again confusing the selection of the most appropriate route to the cavernoma. Our objective in this chapter is to present the safe brainstem access sites that are accessible through the retrosigmoid approach and are capable of resolving the vast majority of brainstem cavernomas and tumors (*refer to case 26 in* Chap. 21).

17.2 Anatomical Considerations

This section will outline the brainstem safe entry points that can be reached through the cerebellopontine angle with the retrosigmoid approach, which enables the excision of almost all brainstem cavernomas and other intra-axial lesions. The genuine cavernomas of the cerebellopontine angle are located on cranial nerve roots, and the microneurosurgical anatomy of the cisternal course of the cranial nerves in the cerebellopontine angle has been thoroughly detailed elsewhere.

17.2.1 Corticospinal Tract in the Brainstem

The brainstem has a high density of neurological structures, with nuclei and ascending, descending, and transverse fiber tracts. Access to intrinsic lesions in the brainstem can therefore only be made through a few safe routes based on anatomical references. It is currently possible to reconstruct the pyramidal tract with tractography and follow the tract along the brainstem from where it enters the midbrain, forming the cerebral peduncle, although anatomical references are essential, and neurophysiology can be helpful, so this will be the only anatomical structure of the brainstem that we will review. The pyramidal tract in the pons splits into many fascicles, which reassemble in the anterior region of the medulla oblongata. The cortical-medullary tracts for the medullary nuclei and the cortical-spinal tract can be projected on the surface of the pons, gathering between two imaginary lines, one medial, which goes from the most medial point of the pontine-mesencephalic sulcus to the point where the pyramid joins the medullary-pontine sulcus, and another lateral, which goes from the lateral portion of the peduncle and pontine-mesencephalic sulcus to the point where the pyramid joins the medullary-pontine sulcus. At the medullary-pontine level, a part of the fibers takes a posteromedial direction to form the pyramidal decussation. A second group of descending fibers forms the corticopontine tract that ends in the motor nuclei of the pons, from where prolongations emerge in a transverse direction that reach the contralateral cerebellum through the middle cerebellar peduncle.

17.2.2 Safe Entry Zones to the Brainstem

Safe entry zones in the brainstem are based exclusively on the anatomy of the area that allows access to deep areas without producing any foreseeable additional neurological deficit attributable to the access. As we have said, the initial proposal of Evandro de Oliveira's group included three zones, one for each segment of the brainstem in its anterolateral portion (Fig. 17.1) [21]. Subsequent anatomical work with white matter dissection substantially increased the number of safe zones. Different anatomical studies from Albert Rhoton's school in 2015 described 11 safe entry zones: anterior midbrain (perioculomotor area), middle (supracholicular and infracolicular) and paramedial (lateral mesencephalic sulcus); anterior pons (supratrigeminal area; peritrigeminal area) and posterior (suprafacial, interfacial, infrafacial); anterior medullary (transolivary) and posterior (midline) [28]. In a later anatomical study from 2017, the supratrigeminal area was not described, and, on the contrary, the transolivary access was duplicated in an anterior olivary access and a posterior olivary access [6]. Robert Spetzler's group, in 2016, described a total of 13 safe areas of entry to the brainstem: anterior midbrain (anterior mesencephalic area), lateral (lateral mesencephalic sulcus) and posterior (intercollicular region); anterior pons (peritrigeminal area; supratrigeminal area), lateral (lateral pontine area) and posterior (supracollacular and infracollacular areas; middle sulcus of the fourth ventricle); anterolateral medulla (anterolateral sulcus; olivary area); posterolateral (lateral bulbar area or inferior cerebellar peduncle) and posterior (posterior middle sulcus) [7].

17.2.2.1 Lateral Mesencephalic Sulcus

The safe entrance to the anterolateral midbrain is through the lateral mesencephalic sulcus (Fig. 17.1). From the medial geniculate body of the thalamus to the pontine-mesencephalic sulcus, the lateral mesencephalic sulcus divides the peduncular and tegmental regions of the midbrain. It has a supratentorial and an infratentorial

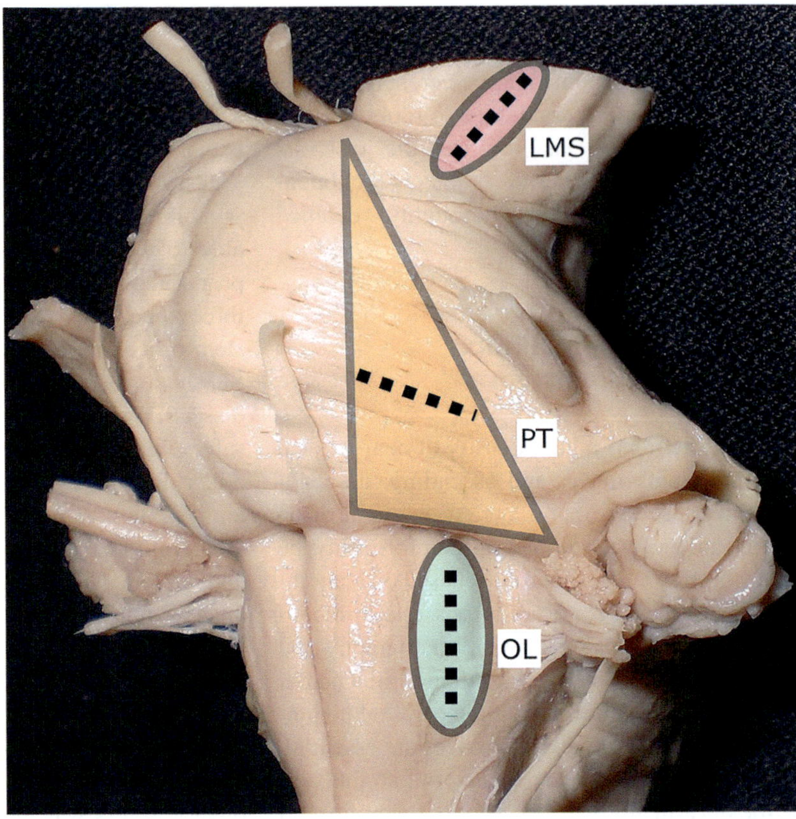

Fig. 17.1 The topographical safe entrance zones are depicted in this brainstem anatomy picture, which displays the left cerebellopontine angle. The olivary zone (OL) is green, the peritrigeminal zone (PT) is yellow, and the lateral mesencephalic sulcus (LMS) is pink

portion. The sulcus is followed by the lateral mesencephalic vein, crossed by the posterior cerebral artery in its cranial portion, and by the trochlear nerve and superior cerebellar artery in its caudal portion. A vertical incision that follows the sulcus in depth is used to make the entry. The working channel is around 8 mm in length, while the sulcus is around 10 mm. By entering perpendicular to the midbrain's surface, the red nucleus is accessed, which is situated at a depth of roughly 4.5 mm. Thus, the approach should be oriented approximately 45 degrees forward, leaving the lateral lemniscus rostrally and the substantia nigra ventrally. The distance between the lateral mesencephalic sulcus and the trochlear and oculomotor nuclei is approximately 9.5 mm.

17.2.2.2 Peritrigeminal Zone

The anterolateral pons can be safely accessed through the peritrigeminal zone (Fig. 17.1). The medullary-pontine sulcus forms its caudal border, a craniocaudal line that traces the inner edge of the trigeminal nerve's apparent exit from the pons to the pontine-mesencephalic sulcus forms its outer border, and a line that connects this intersection with the medullary-pontine sulcus on the outside of the sixth cranial nerve's exit traces the medial border of the triangle. Outside of the corticospinal tract, which extends medially towards its decussation, this entry zone is situated rostral to the trigeminal nucleus, which is about 11 mm deep from the surface of the pons. Here, a transverse incision is performed to follow the transverse pontocerebellar fibers of the pons, leaving about 8 mm of safety between the corticospinal tract and the trigeminal nerve's exit. The safety distance between the corticospinal tract and the facial nerve exit is 9.2 mm. If a longitudinal incision is performed, the height of the facial nerve's exit from the pons should not be surpassed caudally to prevent damage to the sixth nerve's pontine fibers. The nucleus of the sixth nerve, which is situated deeper, behind the trigeminal nucleus, close to the surface of the fourth ventricle, is surrounded by the facial nerve's anteroposterior fibers.

17.2.2.3 Olivary Zone

The olive is the safe entry zone to the anterolateral medulla oblongata (Fig. 17.1). The olive is a prominence on the anterolateral surface of the medulla oblongata, delimited medially by the anterolateral sulcus and the pyramid with the corticospinal tract and laterally by the posterolateral sulcus. The olive measures about 13.5 mm in length and extends 5–7 mm in depth. The approach through the anterolateral sulcus does not injure the olive but is very close to the pyramidal tract and the rootlets of the hypoglossal nerve. The approach through the posterolateral sulcus also does not injure the olive but is close to the inferior cerebellar peduncle and the rootlets of the glossopharyngeal and vagal nerves.

17.3 Pathology

Cavernoma is a type of vascular lesion of the central nervous system, along with arteriovenous malformations, venous angiomas, and telangiectasias. All of them were classically considered malformations and consequently stable once formed in the embryological development, beyond the changes imposed by complications or hemodynamic factors. However, it is now proved that cavernomas are lesions that change and evolve over time due to intrinsic factors. The mechanisms by which they form, grow, and break are also known. Finally, the genetic mechanisms that explain their sporadic or familial appearance are well elucidated. Cavernomas of the cerebellopontine angle and the brainstem follow, in this sense, the general patterns of cavernomas of the central nervous system.

17.3.1 Histopathology

Macroscopically, intra-axial cavernoma appears as well-defined, granular-looking masses of red, dark blue, or purple color. Size varies greatly, from a few millimeters to a few centimeters, which is unusual for a brainstem cavernoma. The lesion is compact and well-defined from the surrounding nervous tissue. The nervous tissue frequently has a brown or golden color stain as a result of microhemorrhages and subsequent hemosiderin deposition. When the cavernoma has bled beyond the limits of the lesion, it is surrounded by blood of different appearances depending on the volume of bleeding, the time since the bleeding, and whether there has been repeated bleeding. The cerebellopontine angle cavernoma may be predominantly solid or cystic and present as reddish or bluish lesions, well demarcated with cavities filled with blood or fluid with xanthochromia, growing from one of the cranial nerves and firmly adherent to the nerve and surface of the brainstem.

The histopathology of cavernomas is the same for any location, and they are characterized by being formed by vascular spaces filled with blood and surrounded by nervous tissue without a separating fibrous capsule. The nervous tissue may extend more or less deeply and irregularly into the lesion between the vascular spaces, but the center of the cavernoma lacks nervous tissue. The wall of the vascular spaces is formed by fibrous tissue, occasionally with calcifications or metaplasia in the form of bone tissue. The interior layer of the wall of the vascular spaces is lined by endothelial cells. These vascular spaces are agglutinated by acellular fibrous tissue with hemosiderin-filled macrophages. The lumen of vascular spaces contains blood, sometimes with thrombi at different stages of development and occasionally with neoangiogenesis [19].

17.3.2 Molecular Biology

Cavernomas may occur sporadically, which occurs in 80–90% of cases, or in a familial manner. *Sporadic cavernomas* are usually single, although in 20% of patients, they may be multiple (*cavernomatosis*). In contrast, *familial cavernoma* is usually multiple at the time of diagnosis; its number usually increases with follow-up time, and the hereditary pattern is autosomal dominant. Therefore, nonfamilial multiple cavernomas constitute a group of patients that are difficult to classify and provide advice on. Finally, there is a particular group of cavernomas that develop induced by the application of ionizing radiation to the brain.

Familial cavernomas are caused by loss of function due to mutation of any of the following genes: *KRIT1* (*Krev Interaction Trapped Protein*) at locus 7q21.2, *CCM2* (*Cerebral Cavernous Malformation 2 Protein*) at locus 7p13, or *PDCD10* (*Programmed Cell Death Protein 10*) at locus 3q26.1. The mutation of only one of these genes is sufficient to trigger the disease. The mutations occur in the endothelial cells of the vascular spaces, are variable and multiple, but determine a loss of function in the proteins encoded by the genes. This explains the different clinical expression of patients with familial cavernoma, although the predominant mutation of each of the genes may explain some differential characteristics in the intensity or clinical expression of the patients. On the other hand, there seems to be a somatic mutation that would favor the activation of the lesion, both in familial and sporadic forms. Thus, it is observed that the *PIK3CA* gene (*Phosphoinositide 3-Kinase*) located at locus 7q26.32, which controls cell development, and the *CCM* gene would be mutated in the cavernoma and also in somatic cells, and that the *MAP 3 K3* gene (*Mitogen-Activated Protein Kinase*) at locus 17q23.3 would be mutated in somatic cells, which explains the different clinical presentations through a double or triple impact mechanism.

Patients with familial cavernoma would have an inherited genetic alteration in their biallelic somatic endothelial cells in the *CCM* gene that would produce multiple quiescent cavernomas. Some of these lesions would develop mutations in the *PIK3CA* gene, which would favor their growth. In sporadic cavernomas, the chain of events would be different. At the somatic level, a double mutation in the *CCM* gene in the same cell or a mutation in the *MAP 3 K3* gene is required, which forms an initial quiescent lesion, followed or preceded by a somatic mutation of the *PIK3CA* gene, which would favor its growth. Most patients in familial cases of Hispanic-American ethnicity have a mutation in the *CCM1* gene (*Q455X* or common Hispanic mutation).

As regards cavernomas induced by ionizing radiation, the pathophysiological mechanism is different, although the histopathological structure of the lesion is the same. The patterns in induced cavernomas are the following: they usually present as multiple cavernomas, and they appear in patients irradiated in childhood or adolescence who received high doses of ionizing radiation. It is hypothesized that the development of cavernomas is due to the association of multiple mutations in the DNA of somatic cells induced by radiation [25].

17.3.3 Growth Patterns

The growth of the lesion is initially due to the division of endothelial cells that progressively form new vascular spaces. However, from a clinical point of view, the abrupt growth secondary to intra- or extralesional bleeding or thrombosis of vascular spaces is more relevant since these events are usually associated with a change in clinical symptoms. The most serious event in the evolution of cavernoma is rupture with the consequent bleeding of greater or lesser intensity, inside or outside the lesion. Electron microscopy studies show that there is a loss of intercellular junctions between endothelial cells in the vascular spaces of cavernoma, which could explain the tendency to bleed. The *KRIT1* gene is known to encode some proteins involved in dense intercellular junctions. In addition to this purely structural mechanism, there are other molecular mechanisms that explain the tendency of cavernoma to bleed. It has been discovered that cerebral vessels have low levels of thrombomodulin and *EPCR* (*Endothelial Protein C Receptor*) in relation to the vessels of the rest of the body, which confers a certain pro-hemostatic effect, while the endothelial cells of cavernoma have high levels of both, which would favor hemorrhagic diathesis. The high levels of thrombomodulin and EPCR receptors would be a consequence of the tendency of blood contained in vascular spaces, which are wide and have a very slow flow, to thrombose. The thrombolytic action would be, paradoxically, protective against the rupture of vascular spaces in the case of intraluminal thrombosis [16, 27].

17.4 Clinical Considerations

17.4.1 Cavernomas of the Cerebellopontine Angle

The few cases described of cavernoma of the cerebellopontine angle are located in the cranial nerve roots, so the predominant symptoms are related to their dysfunction. The vestibulocochlear nerve is affected in 90% of patients, followed by the trigeminal nerve in 54% of patients and the facial nerve in 30%, while some patients present involvement of the lower cranial nerves due to displacement by the cavernoma. One-third of patients present cerebellar or long pathway symptoms due to the mass effect of the cavernoma. No patient presented with extralesional bleeding in the form of subarachnoid hemorrhage or hematoma in the cerebellopontine angle [26].

17.4.2 Cavernomas of the Brainstem

The incidence of cavernoma of the brainstem in the general population is 0.5–1%, but they account for one-third of symptomatic intracerebral cavernomas. The most common age of presentation is between 20–50 years, with a mean of about 30 years. Although cavernomas occur in all races and ethnic groups, a higher incidence has been observed among Hispanic Americans in the southwestern United States and northern Mexico.

Overall, the most common presenting symptom is epileptic seizures (50%) followed by intraparenchymal bleeding (25%) and neurological deficits without signs of recent bleeding (25%), although an increasing number of asymptomatic patients are found at the time of diagnosis, reaching 25–50% depending on the series, due to the availability and widespread use of MRI as a means of diagnostic imaging test. Brainstem cavernomas cannot present with epilepsy. Therefore, the most common presentation of brainstem cavernoma is bleeding, although they also have a higher risk of bleeding than cerebral cavernoma. Bleeding from cavernoma in general, and from cavernoma of the brainstem in particular, may be intralesional or extralesional. In both cases, symptomatic bleeding must be distinguished from asymptomatic bleeding, which is detected in imaging studies. In symptomatic bleeding, the clinical impact and the volume of the hemorrhage are relevant. The bleeding rate from cavernomas of the brainstem is around 4% per patient per year, almost double that of cavernomas in other intracranial locations, and is lower in sporadic cavernomas than in familial ones. This means that, at diagnosis, 75% of patients with brainstem cavernoma had suffered a recent hemorrhage, and 85% of patients had some focal neurological deficit symptoms, including cranial nerve involvement in 66% of cases, long pathway involvement in 60%, and extrapyramidal involvement in 25%, although in 30% of cases they are associated with minor or nonspecific symptoms or are incidental.

In general, the risk of bleeding decreases over time from diagnosis, which implies that there are some years where the risk of bleeding accumulates and then, as the patient gets older, it is significantly reduced. The risk of bleeding is also related to the location in the brainstem or having previously bled and, to a lesser degree, to female sex, size of the lesion, and multiple cavernomas. Another worrying problem with brainstem cavernoma is that, if they have bled, the rate of rebleeding reaches 45% of cases in the following five years, which increases the risk of death. This rate of rebleeding is higher than that of cavernomas in other locations, which is less than 10%. In contrast, neurological symptoms tend to improve or stabilize in 80–90% of patients. The remaining patients worsen over time, especially patients with lesions that cross the midline, are associated with a venous angioma, or have rebleeding [13, 16, 27].

17.4.3 Familial Cavernoma

The risk of bleeding from a specific cavernoma is the same as for sporadic cavernoma, but the risk per patient is higher because patients often have multiple lesions. Approximately 20% of cavernoma cases are familial with autosomal dominant inheritance, although penetrance is incomplete in many cases and clinical presentation is variable. There is a clear relationship with the Hispanic population of the southwestern United States and northern Mexico, where a high prevalence of mutations related to the development of cavernoma has been demonstrated. Most patients with familial cavernoma have multiple lesions. Patients with familial cavernoma increase the number of lesions identified on MRI over time, with a variable increase of 0.5–2.5 new lesions per year depending on the series. This increase is noted in childhood and adolescence and then stabilizes. The disease is transmitted in an autosomal dominant pattern, such that 50% of the offspring of each affected parent will receive and transmit the mutation. To rule out a family origin in patients with multiple cavernomas and attribute it to a sporadic mutation, the family history must be determined with certainty up to the third generation. There are systemic genetic tests that confirm the mutation of the *CMM1–3* genes, and genetic counselling can be given to those affected, and a recommendation is made for a screening of family members. There are also some biological markers in blood that are related to the disease, such as calciferol levels, non-HDL cholesterol, and others.

17.5 Diagnostic Considerations

17.5.1 Cerebellopontine Angle Cavernoma

Cerebellopontine angle cavernomas present on imaging studies as solid or cystic lesions. Solid lesions are usually small, hyperintense on T1-weighted MRI sequences, and lack contrast enhancement. Given their anatomical relationship to the facial–vestibulocochlear complex and the possibility of being introduced into the internal auditory canal, they may be confused with vestibular schwannoma. Cystic lesions, on the other hand, are larger and multilobulated, with a heterogeneous signal resulting from the presence of blood in different stages of degradation and calcifications, together with contrast enhancement. Thus, they may be confused with atypical or cystic schwannomas or meningiomas.

17.5.2 Brainstem Cavernoma

CT imaging studies offer poor sensitivity and specificity for diagnosing brainstem cavernoma. The only finding on CT may be calcification or intraparenchymal bleeding. In contrast, MRI is the test of choice, as it offers virtually 100% sensitivity and the highest specificity. On T1-weighted sequences, a cavernoma has a variable appearance depending on the state of the blood and the time of evolution of bleeding. They usually have a granular appearance with a mixture of rounded hyperintense and hypointense spaces. There is usually no gadolinium enhancement. Vascular sequences may be useful to rule out an associated venous angioma. On T2-weighted sequences, cavernomas have a similar appearance but are typically surrounded by a dark hypointense ring due to the accumulation of hemosiderin. Large vascular spaces can be seen at that level. Highly enhanced T2 sequences, like FIESTA (*Fast Imaging Employing Steady-State Acquisition*) or SWAN (*Susceptibility-Weighted Angiography*), are particularly useful for diagnosing cavernomas, while gradient-echo T2 sequences are particularly sensitive for identifying small lesions in the case of multiple cavernomas, due to their high sensitivity in identifying hemosiderin and calcifications (Fig. 17.2). All these imaging findings are distorted in a very striking way when bleeding occurs that exceeds the limits of the cavernoma and forms an intraparenchymal hematoma. In this case, the time of evolution of the bleeding and the possibility of repeated bleedings cause large changes in the T1- and T2-weighted sequences that camouflage the cavernoma up to days or weeks after the first hemorrhage (Fig. 17.3). The differential diagno-

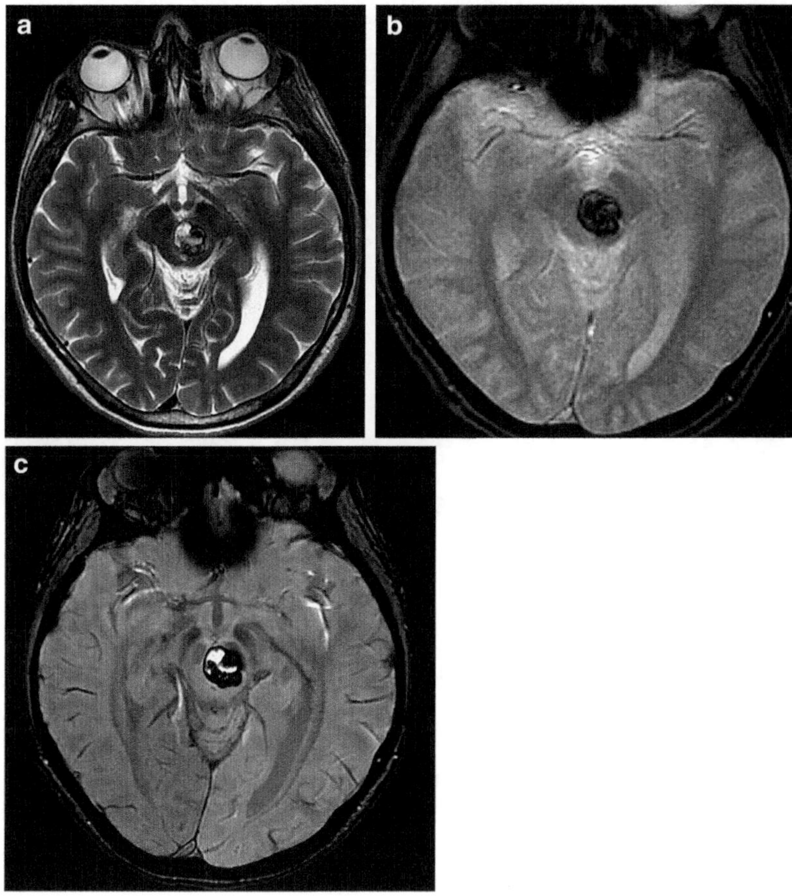

Fig. 17.2 Midbrain cavernoma. (**a**) Axial T2-weighted MRI slice. (**b**) Axial gradient T2-weighted MRI slice. (**c**) Axial T2-weighted SWAN MRI slice

sis is based on small hemorrhagic metastases or calcified tumors. Finally, the preoperative study can be completed with a DTI (*Diffusion Tensor Imaging*) MRI study and fiber tractography, especially the descending corticospinal and ascending lemniscus pathways (Fig. 17.4). The digital subtraction angiography (DSA) is almost always normal and only useful to exclude an arteriovenous malformation or for the identification of an associated venous angioma.

17.6 Surgical Categories

In this chapter, we review the cavernomas of the cerebellopontine angle and the cavernomas of the brainstem that are removed through a surgical approach through the cerebellopontine angle. The latter are classified topographically into cavernomas of the midbrain, pons, and medulla oblongata, and also medullary-pontine and pontine-mesencephalic junctions. In terms of frequency, the most frequent ones subjected to microneurosurgical treatment are the pontine cavernomas (45%), followed by the midbrain cavernomas (20%), with the rest of the topographies being equally distributed with 10–15% of the cases for each one of them. Within each brainstem segment, the lesions located in the anterior or ventral, posterior or rostral, and lateral portions are usually considered, subdivided by some authors into lesions of anterolateral and posterolateral location. We will now describe the general technique of microneurosurgical removal of cavernomas and then detail the particularities of each of the different topographies.

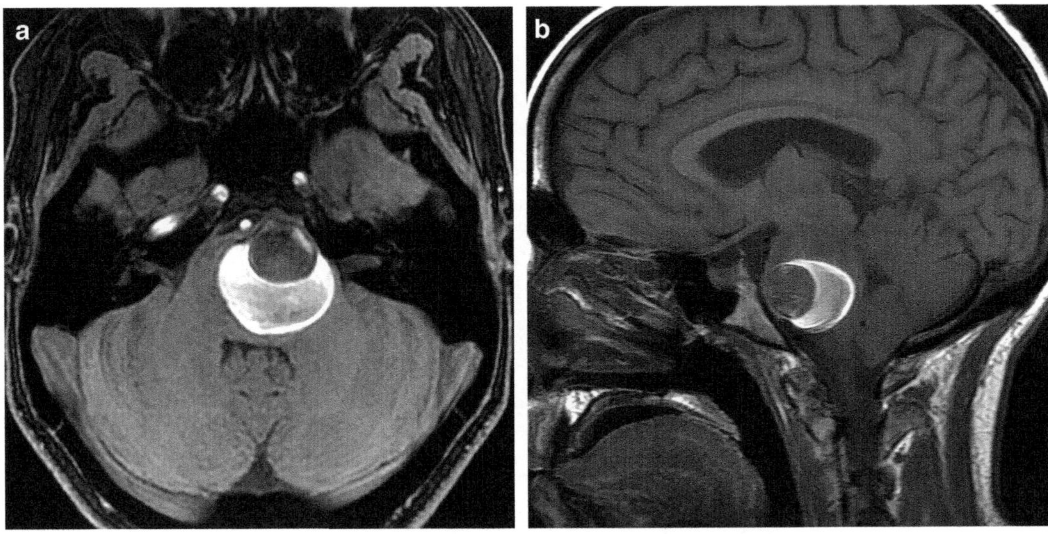

Fig. 17.3 Pontine cavernoma, with an acute and a subacute hemorrhage. (**a**) Axial T1-weighted MRI slice. (**b**) Sagital gradient T1-weighted MRI slice

17.7 Microneurosurgical Management

17.7.1 Cerebellopontine Angle Cavernoma

Cavernomas of the cerebellopontine angle develop in the cranial nerves in their cisternal segment. The approach is through a standard retrosigmoid craniotomy. Microneurosurgical treatment is based on internal decompression of the cysts or hemorrhagic areas and careful coagulation of the capsule to achieve retraction of the lesion and its separation from the nerve root, in which they grow, to achieve an *en bloc* resection of the lesion. Loss of the capsule plane, which can occur in large lesions, can lead to bleeding, leave a remnant, or injure the underlying nerve [26].

17.7.2 Brainstem Cavernoma

Microneurosurgical resection of brainstem cavernomas, in any location, is a highly complex procedure, requiring high technical requirements from the neurosurgeon and surgical team, and with a high risk of morbidity and mortality for the patient [4, 5, 14, 15, 18]. As a result, surgical planning needs to be done as thoroughly as feasible.

17.7.2.1 Preoperative Setup

Preoperative imaging studies should include high-resolution, multi-slice T2-weighted MRI sequences in all planes, with a sufficient number of slices for intraoperative navigation with these sequences. A DTI MRI is useful for pyramidal tractography. Once the location of the lesion has been defined, the safe entry zone in the brainstem is determined, and finally, the approach route. Intraoperative aids include anatomical, lesional, and pyramidal pathway neuronavigation; electrophysiology with monitoring of somatosensory evoked potentials (SSEP) and transcranial electric motor evoked potentials (TcMMEP) and brainstem auditory evoked potentials (BAEP); as well as continuous electromyographic recording and direct monopolar or bipolar electrical stimulation of the cranial nerves and pyramidal pathway [22].

The timing of surgery after bleeding is another element of consideration. Early surgery was initially advocated based on the emergent decompressive effect of surgery in evacuating the hematoma. Furthermore, it has been shown that

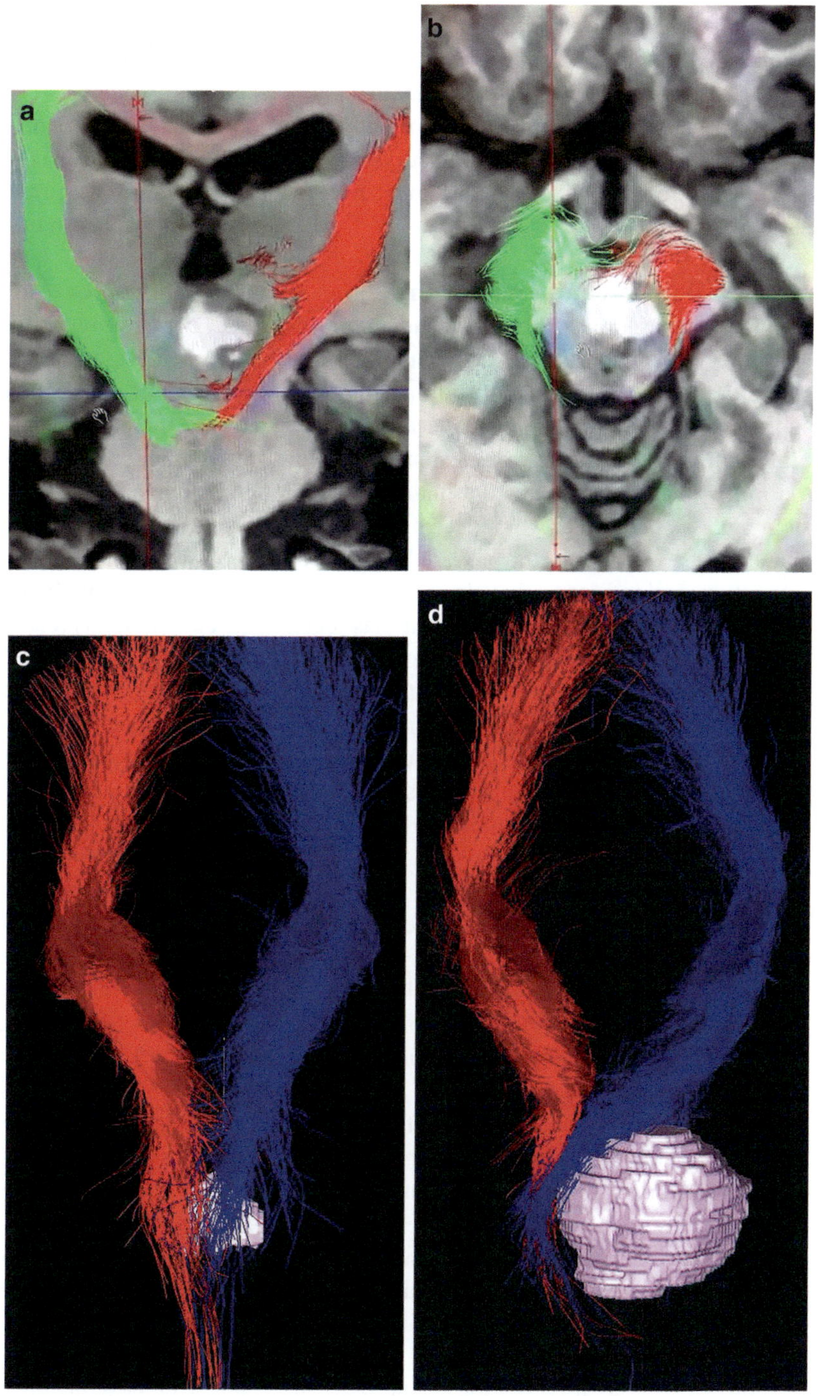

Fig. 17.4 Pyramidal tractography in brainstem cavernomas. (**a**, **b**) Axial and coronal cuts displaying both pyramidal tracts in a case of left paramedial midbrain cavernoma with acute hemorrhage. (**c**, **d**) Axial view of the distortion and displacement of the pyramidal tract in two examples of pontine cavernoma, one small and another larger

over time, hematomas are reabsorbed, organized, and form a scar that is continuous with the glial scar, which smudges the separation between the cavernoma and the nervous tissue. There is now a general agreement that the recommended time window for microneurosurgical treatment of cavernomas that have bled would be between 4–6 weeks after the hemorrhagic event, when the hematoma is still liquid, edema of the brain tissue has reduced, and there is no scarring. This period allows the patient to stabilize or improve their neurological deficit and allows time for the etiological study of the bleeding and confirmation that it is due to a cavernoma. On the other hand, as contrary to ruptured cerebral aneurysms, the risk of early rebleeding is very low (*refer to case 25 in* Chap. 21).

17.7.2.2 Position and Craniotomy

Brainstem cavernomas with lateral and anterolateral topography can be removed through a retrosigmoid or paramedial infratentorial supracerebellar approach. When accessing the brainstem in the area where the lesion is located, the limits of the safe entry zone into the brainstem must be delimited, which is achieved using anatomical references, data provided by neuronavigation, and intraoperative electrophysiology. There is no particularity in all that has been described in the chapter on the retrosigmoid approach regarding the position, anatomical references, incision, craniotomy, and dural opening. The access to the lateral aspect of the brainstem can be facilitated by opening the cistern of the petrosal fissure of the cerebellum [20].

17.7.2.3 Cisternal Dissection

The cisterns of the cerebellopontine angle are easily opened because there is no lesion in the cerebellopontine angle. Arachnoid adhesions are released to isolate, identify, and mobilize all cranial nerve roots and arteries in the surgical field, and the pial surface of the brainstem is exposed. Regarding the lesion, we can face different situations during microneurosurgical examination. In some cases, the lesion is exophytic and is clearly recognized by its appearance on the surface of the brainstem. In other cases, it is possible to recognize the presence of the intra-axial lesion by indirect signs, such as a bulge produced by the cavernoma or, more frequently, by the hematoma, or a brown or golden coloration of the pial surface of the brainstem that reflects the transudation of blood or the existence of an underlying hematoma. Finally, in other cases where the lesion is deeper or has not bled sufficiently, the surface of the brainstem does not show any signal about the location of the underlying cavernoma (Fig. 17.5a). The final decision on the location of the cortectomy, its size, and its direction depends on the surgeon's assessment, evaluating the data obtained from the preoperative studies, anatomy, neuronavigation, electrophysiology, and appearance of the pial surface of the brainstem in the microneurosurgical examination.

17.7.2.4 Cortectomy

The cortectomy should always be performed within the safe entry zones described above. In the event of exophytic lesions, the emerging portion of the cavernoma is surrounded, and in the remaining cases, the cortectomy is performed going deeper through the brainstem following the increasingly brown color of the white matter or until white matter with a brown color is found, and, in this way, the hematoma or the surface of the cavernoma is reached.

17.7.2.5 Cavernoma Excision

The presence of a hematoma helps dissect the cavernoma, while if the hematoma has been reabsorbed or the cavernoma has not bled, there is a more or less conspicuous plane of gliosis between the nervous tissue and the lesion. When the cavernoma is reached, it is not necessarily done at the ideal point, since the access direction, often oblique, does not necessarily lead to the center of the lesion. The cavernoma is then dissected with microdissectors, trying to systematically surround and separate it from its adhesions to achieve an en bloc resection when it has been completely released (Figs. 17.5b, c). Given the limited space available, the dissection by the surgeon is exclusively bimanual, with a microaspirator that serves to keep the cortectomy lips open and aspirate the blood, and with the microdissector of adequate size and shape, which is used to mobilize the cavernoma. Once the cavernoma is removed, the cavity is washed profusely and a hemostatic material is applied for a few minutes (Fig. 17.5d). Small arterial vessels related to the cavernoma can be identified, which can be coagulated, but if a relatively large vein is identified, visible or not in the imaging studies, it must be respected since it may be a venous angioma.

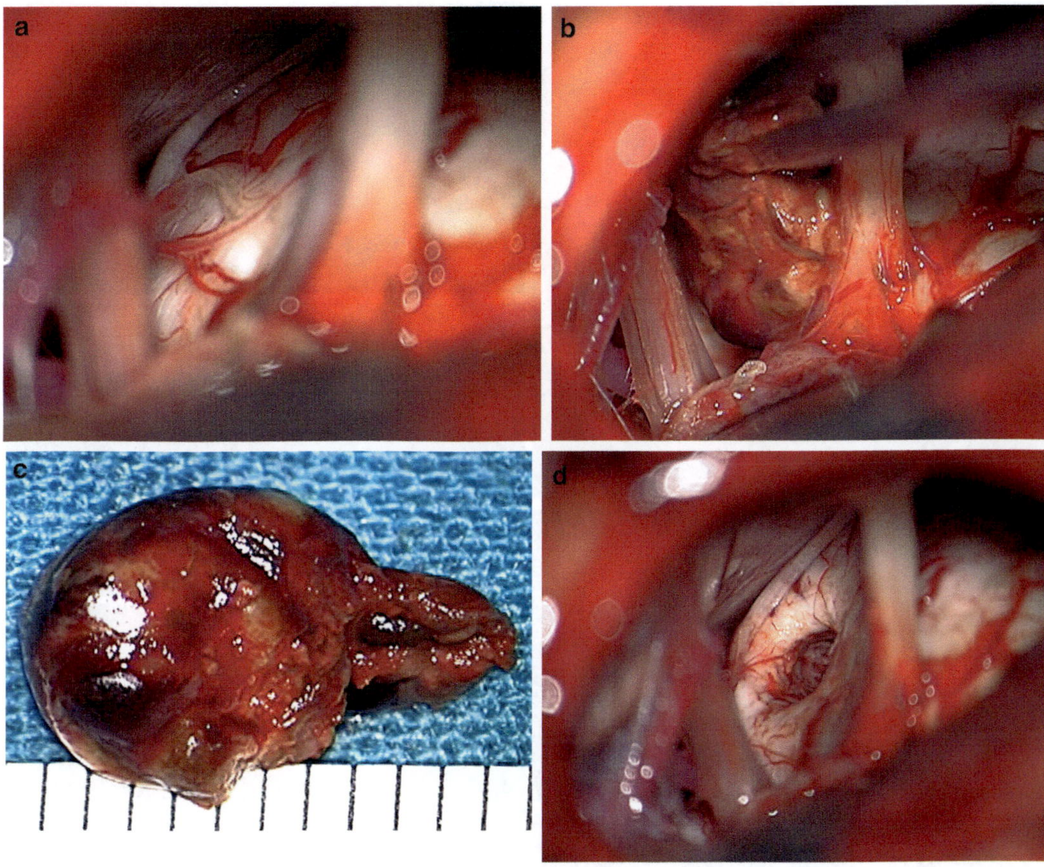

Fig. 17.5 Microneurosurgical excision of a pontine cavernoma through a left retrosigmoid approach. (**a**) Intraoperative picture of the anterolateral surface of the pons, bulging by the cavernoma. From left to right: glossopharyngeal and vagal nerves; flocculus, above the peritrigeminal safe entry zone of the pons, and above the abducens nerve and the dura mater of the clivus; and facial and vestibulocochlear nerves. (**b**) Image displaying the en bloc excision of the cavernoma. (**c**) Image of the cavernoma. (**d**) Image showing the cortectomy, cavity of resection, and collapse of the pons following the complete resection of the cavernoma

17.8 Cavernomas That Require Specific Treatment

17.8.1 Cavernomas of the Midbrain

Cavernomas of the midbrain located in the lateral or anterolateral portion are removed through a lateral mesencephalic sulcus approach, which can be accessed through a standard retrosigmoid or paramedian infratentorial supracerebellar approach, although they can also be accessed through a subtemporal approach. Strictly anterior cavernomas are removed through an approach through the peri-oculomotor area via an extended trans-sylvian pterional approach, such as an orbitozygomatic approach, but if they are large or with a large hematoma, they can be resected through the lateral mesencephalic sulcus access. Finally, cavernomas of the posterior portion of the midbrain located in the tectal region are removed by a medial infratentorial supracerebellar approach.

In the approach through the lateral mesencephalic sulcus, the anatomical key-point reference is the lateral mesencephalic vein that runs along the sulcus, although its caliber is variable, and sometimes it may not be recognized (Fig. 17.6). Navigation provides reliable data, and the neurophysiological study helps to locate the pyramidal pathway in the most ventral portion of the pedun-

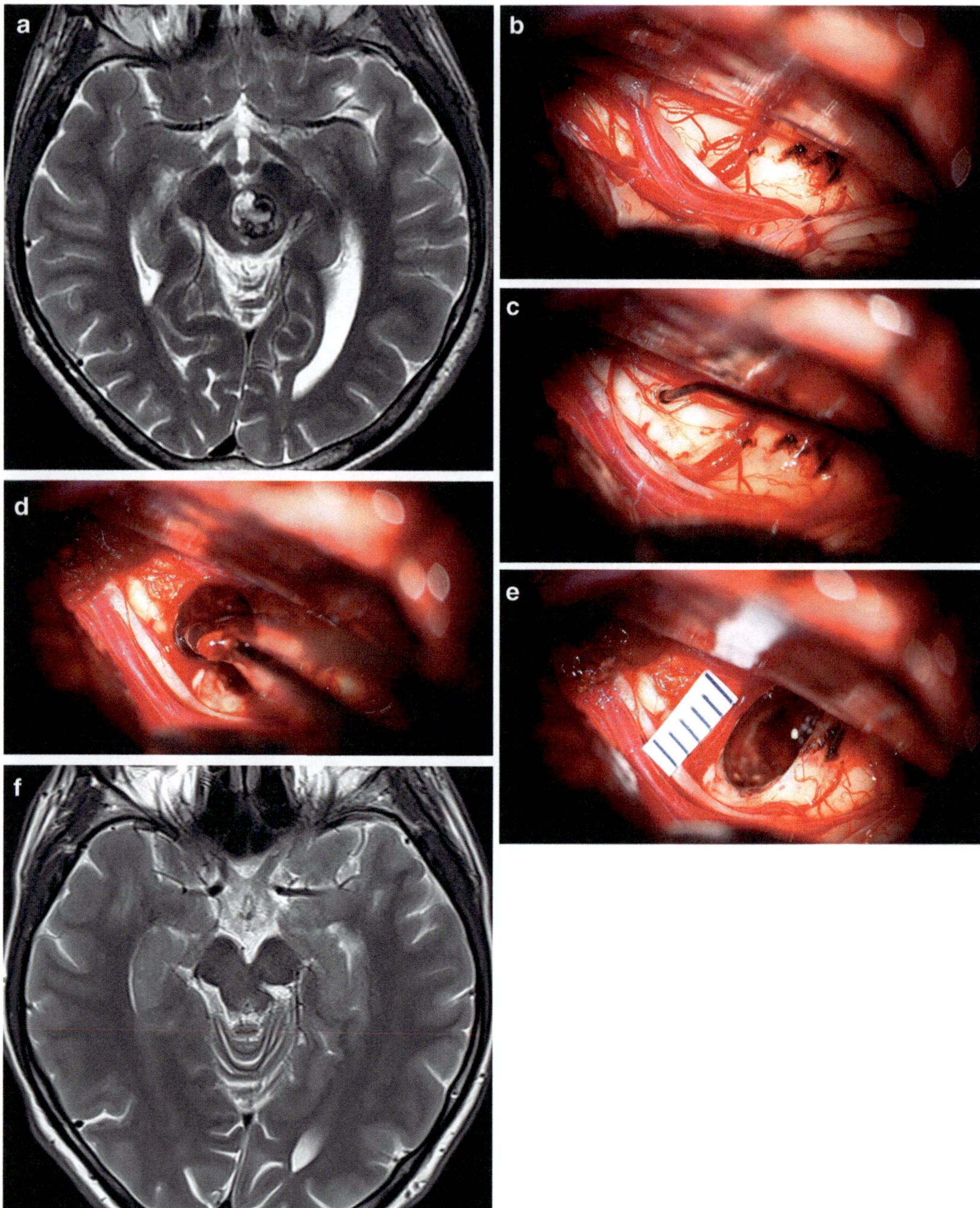

Fig. 17.6 Microneurosurgical excision of a midbrain cavernoma through a left retrosigmoid approach. (**a**) Axial T2-weighted MRI displaying the cavernoma, with an acute bleed. (**b**) Intraoperative picture of the lateral mesencephalic safe zone entry. From above to below: tentorium, lateral aspect of the midbrain with the lateral mesencephalic sulcus and vein; trochlear nerve; and superior cerebellar artery. (**c**) Direct monopolar electrical stimulation of the lateral peduncle. (**d**) Image showing the excision of the cavernoma. (**e**) Final result showing the cortectomy of around 5 mm, and the cavity of resection. (**f**) Postoperative axial T2-weighted MRI slice demonstrating the complete resection of the cavernoma

cle. The anatomical elements to be preserved are the superior cerebellar artery, the trochlear nerve, and, more cranially, the superior cerebral artery and its branches.

17.8.2 Cavernomas of the Pons

Cavernomas of the pons located in its lateral or anterolateral portion are removed through an access through the peritrigeminal area, which can be accessed through a standard retrosigmoid approach. Those strictly anterior can theoretically be removed better through a presigmoid approach, but the access is more restricted, and this approach does not help to access the cavernoma more perpendicularly. In any case, if the cavernoma is large or there is a hematoma, the retrosigmoid approach is adequate. Finally, cavernomas in the posterior portion of the pons should be removed through a midline approach through the fourth ventricle, which is reached by a medial suboccipital approach.

In the approach through the peritrigeminal area, the anatomical reference elements are the exit of the trigeminal nerve from the pons, the medullary-pontine sulcus, and the exit of the facial and abducens nerves (Fig. 17.7). There are usually no relevant arteries on the surface of the pons, and the small pial arterioles that are distributed irregularly can be coagulated, although any circumferential artery must be preserved at all costs. Navigation provides reliable data, and the neurophysiological study helps to locate the pyramidal pathway in the most medial portion of the pons. The anatomical elements to preserve are the cranial nerves and the pyramidal tract.

17.8.3 Cavernomas of the Medulla Oblongata

Cavernomas of the medulla oblongata located in its lateral or anterolateral portion are removed through access through the olivary zone, which is accessed through a standard retrosigmoid approach. Strictly anterior and caudal anterolateral locations can theoretically be removed better through a far-lateral approach, but if the cavernoma is large or there is a hematoma, the retrosigmoid approach is satisfactory. Finally, cavernomas of the posterior portion of the bulb should be removed through a midline posterior access to the medulla oblongata, which is reached through a medial suboccipital approach.

In the approach through the olivary zone, the anatomical reference elements are the medullary-pontine sulcus and the exit of the rootlets of the glossopharyngeal nerve from the retro-olivary sulcus in its cranial portion and of the rootlets of the hypoglossal nerve from the pre-olivary sulcus in its caudal portion (Fig. 17.8). The anterior inferior cerebellar artery, the posterior inferior cerebellar artery, or even the basilar artery trunk can establish very variable anatomical relationships and may require their mobilization for a safe identification of the olive. Navigation provides unreliable data given the small size and location of the olive, while the neurophysiological study helps to safely identify the nerves and locate the pyramidal pathway in the most medial portion of the medulla oblongata. The anatomical elements to preserve are the cranial nerves and arteries, while the lesion of the olive does not seem to provide any additional neurological symptoms or signs to the patient.

17.9 Complications, Prevention, and Management

The complications of surgery for cavernomas of the cerebellopontine angle and brainstem are the same as those for benign and well-defined tumor lesions of the cerebellopontine angle and brainstem, both those related to the approach and to the microneurosurgical resection itself. There is always the fear of bleeding when a cavernoma is inadvertently opened. The problem of cavernoma fragmentation does not lie in the hemorrhage itself, which is easily controlled, but in the fact that the limited space available and the eloquence of the neighboring neurological structures make the use of bipolar coagulation dangerous due to

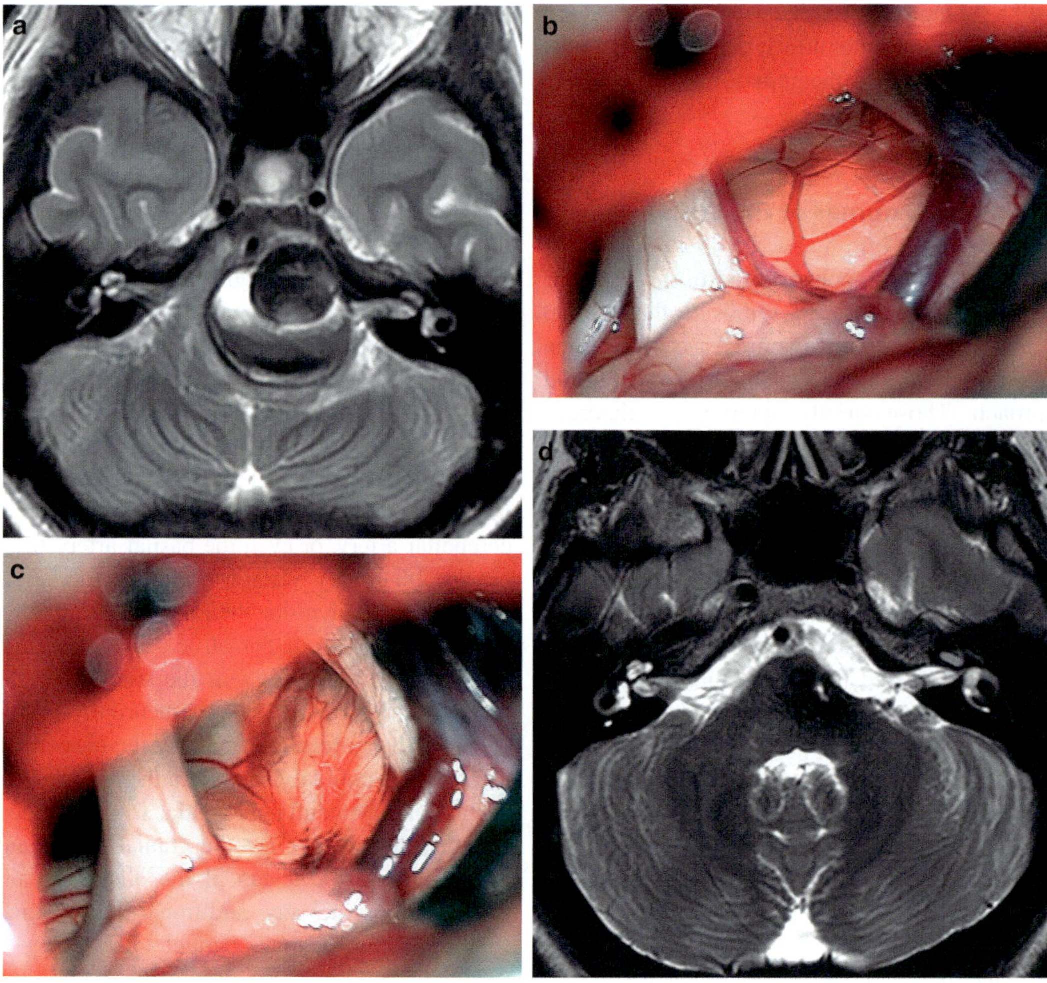

Fig. 17.7 Microneurosurgical excision of a pontine cavernoma through a left retrosigmoid approach. (**a**) Axial T2-weighted MRI slice displaying the cavernoma, with a large acute bleed. (**b**) Intraoperative picture of the peritrigeminal safe zone entry. From left to right: the trigeminal nerve, pons bulging due to the underlying hematoma, and ascending pontine vein. (**c**) Final result displaying the cortectomy and the collapse of the pons. (**d**) Postoperative axial T2-weighted MRI slice showing the total resection of the cavernoma

the heat dissipated. The same happens with the use of hemostatic materials due to the compression they exert. In addition, the fragmentation of the lesion and the bleeding may leave a small residual fragment unnoticed which allows growth or a late rebleeding. As with cavernomas of any location, no venous channel adjacent to the lesion should be coagulated, since venous angiomas carry blood from normal territories where, in this way, a symptomatic venous infarction can occur.

17.10 Outcome, Prognosis, and Follow-Up

17.10.1 Cerebellopontine Angle Cavernomas

The prognosis for resection of cerebellopontine angle cavernomas is good, with improvement of symptoms in 60% and stability of neurological deficits in 20%.

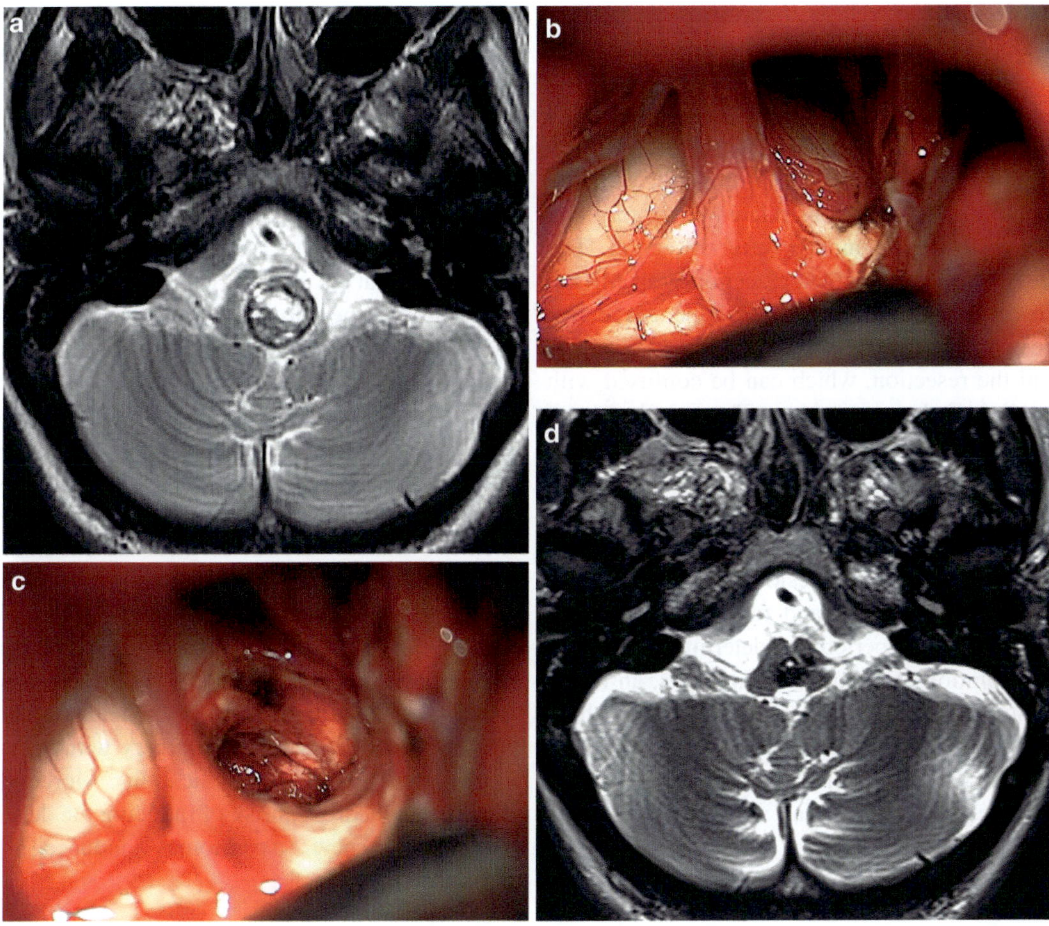

Fig. 17.8 Microneurosurgical excision of a medulla oblongata cavernoma through a left retrosigmoid approach. (**a**) Axial T2-weighted MRI slice displaying the cavernoma with an acute bleed. (**b**) Intraoperative picture of the olivary safe zone entry. From left to right: the inferior olive; glossopharyngeal and vagal nerves crossing the surgical field; the superior olive with a golden coloration and bulging due to the underlying hematoma; and the vestibulocochlear nerve. (**c**) Final result showing the cortectomy and the cavity of resection. (**d**) Postoperative axial T2-weighted MRI slice displaying the complete resection of the cavernoma

17.10.2 Brainstem Cavernomas

In the old microneurosurgical series, the results of the resection of these lesions were discouraging. However, since the safe entry zones to the brainstem have been described, the morbidity and mortality have been substantially reduced. However, published results are coming from relatively short series and in the hands of surgeons and centers with great experience who collect patients referred from other neurosurgical units. The results show that more than 75% of the patients improve, remain stable, or return to their condition before diagnosis after microneurosurgical resection. A large percentage of patients return to their usual preoperative activities. Mortality is anecdotal. Finally, the resection of the lesion eliminates the risk of rebleeding.

However, a percentage of patients worsen or develop new temporary neurological deficits, and around 10% worsen.

The follow-up of cavernomas is not well defined. Sporadic cavernoma is monitored with a CT study in the immediate postoperative period to rule out complications related to surgery and with an MRI six months after resection. The assessment of cavernoma resection with MRI is very problematic since MRI sequences detect traces of blood, gliosis, or hemosiderin resulting from the resection, which can be confused with remains of the cavernoma. The small size of brainstem cavernomas contributes to this confusing situation. Patients with multiple cavernomas require more careful monitoring. In the case of patients in childhood or adolescence, it is common for the number of lesions visible with MRI to increase over time and to stabilize later, so controls must be periodic to determine the extent and evolution of the disease. In adults, an imaging study should only be performed when there are symptoms that justify a new imaging study, although the anxiety and concern of patients justify repeated examinations with very low diagnostic yield [8, 24].

17.11 Management Modalities

The treatment of cavernomas of the cerebellopontine angle and brainstem is based on microneurosurgical resection [3]. In this topography, the general recommendations for the treatment of cerebral cavernomas must be followed, that is, microneurosurgical resection of symptomatic cavernomas that are surgically accessible and that have a risk of morbidity and mortality less than or equal to that of the natural history of the disease. Brainstem cavernomas that have bled should be treated with microneurosurgery, although some authors consider that this should be done after a second bleeding, given the risk of morbidity and mortality after resection. In our opinion, cavernomas should be resected when they have bled and produce symptoms as a result of this, particularly if they are relevant. On the contrary, there is no indication for microneurosurgical treatment of asymptomatic cavernomas or those with minimal intralesional bleeding that do not produce clinical symptoms. There is a series of surgical criteria that would favor the recommendation for microneurosurgical resection. The first is that the lesion should be raised or bulging on the pial surface of the brainstem, since this means that the neurosurgeon does not have to walk through the normal nervous tissue to reach the lesion. In general, the more superficial the lesion, the easier the resection will be. The second factor is an acute and large extralesional hemorrhage, which, in addition to producing neurological symptoms of greater intensity, favors the resection of the cavernoma. Other elements to consider for the surgical indication are the verification of repeated intralesional hemorrhages with progressive neurological deterioration or the presence of a large intralesional or extralesional hemorrhage with a significant mass effect. The alternative to microneurosurgical resection is stereotactic radiosurgery with highly controversial results and indications. Moreover, there is the theoretical risk of inducing the development of new cavernomas induced by radiation.

17.12 Key Messages

- *Cerebellopontine angle cavernomas are uncommon and found on the surface of the brain's nerves. Brainstem cavernomas are more common and might present sporadically or with a familiar pattern. They can be single or multiple.*
- *Brainstem cavernomas must be treated after diagnosis due to their high rate of bleeding and rebleeding.*
- *Brainstem cavernomas frequently manifest as bleeding and carry a high risk of rebleeding.*
- *Nowadays, microneurosurgical techniques that employ safe entry zones, a retrosigmoid approach, and a delicate microneurosurgical technique may safely treat the majority of brainstem cavernomas.*

References

1. Abla AA, Lekovic GP, Turner JD, et al. Advances in the treatment and outcome of brainstem cavernous malformation surgery: a single-center case series of 300 surgically treated patients. Neurosurgery. 2011;68:403–14. https://doi.org/10.1227/NEU.0b013e3181ff9cde.
2. Abla AA, Turner JD, Mitha AP, et al. Surgical approaches to brainstem cavernous malformations. Neurosurg Focus. 2010;29:E8. https://doi.org/10.3171/2010.6.FOCUS10128.
3. Akers A, Al-Shahi Salman R, Awad I A, et al. Synopsis of guidelines for the clinical management of cerebral cavernous malformations: consensus recommendations based on systematic literature review by the Angioma Alliance Scientific Advisory Board Clinical Experts Panel. Neurosurgery. 2017;80:665–80. https://doi.org/10.1093/neuros/nyx091.
4. Asaad WF, Walcott BP, Nahed BV, et al. Operative management of brainstem cavernous malformations. Neurosurg Focus. 2010;29(3):E10. https://doi.org/10.3171/2010.6.FOCUS10134. PMID: 20809751
5. Bradac O, Majovsky M, de Lacy P, et al. Surgery of brainstem cavernous malformations. Acta Neurochir. 2013;155:2079–83. https://doi.org/10.1007/s00701-013-1842-6.
6. Cavalcanti DD, Preul MC, Kalani MY, et al. Microsurgical anatomy of safe entry zones to the brainstem. J Neurosurg. 2015;9:1–18. https://doi.org/10.3171/2015.4.JNS141945.
7. Cavalheiro S, Yagmurlu K, da Costa MD, et al. Surgical approaches for brainstem tumors in pediatric patients. Childs Nerv Syst. 2015;31:1815–40. https://doi.org/10.1007/s00381-015-2799-y.
8. Dukatz T, Sarnthein J, Sitter H, et al. Quality of life after brainstem cavernoma surgery in 71 patients. Neurosurgery. 2011;69:689–95. https://doi.org/10.1227/NEU.0b013e31821d31b7.
9. Ferroli P, Schiariti M, Cordella, et al. The lateral infratrigeminal transpontine window to deep pontine lesions. J Neurosurg. 2015;123:699–710. https://doi.org/10.3171/2014.11.JNS141116.
10. Flores BC, Whittemore AR, Samson D, et al. The utility of preoperative diffusion tensor imaging in the surgical management of brainstem cavernous malformations. J Neurosurg. 2015;122:653–62. https://doi.org/10.3171/2014.11.JNS13680.
11. Garcia RM, Ivan ME, Lawton MT. Brainstem cavernous malformations: surgical results in 104 patients and a proposed grading system to predict neurological outcomes. Neurosurgery. 2015;76:265–77. https://doi.org/10.1227/NEU.0000000000000602.
12. Garrett M, Spetzler RF. Surgical treatment of brainstem cavernous malformations. Surg Neurol. 2009;72(Suppl 2):S3–9. https://doi.org/10.1016/j.surneu.2009.05.031.
13. Giliberto G, Lanzino DJ, Diehn FE, et al. Brainstem cavernous malformations: anatomical, clinical, and surgical considerations. Neurosurg Focus. 2010;29:E9. https://doi.org/10.3171/2010.6.FOCUS10133. PMID: 20809767
14. Gonzalez Darder JM, Capilla-Guasch P, Real-Peña L. Retrosigmoid approach: a simple and safe way to resect intrinsic pontomedullary lesions. JNSB. 2020;81:223–31. https://doi.org/10.1055/s-0039-1685536.
15. González-Darder JM, Quilis-Quesada V, Capilla-Guasch P, de Oliveira E. Abordajes neuroquirúrgicos de la patología craneal y cerebral. 2nd ed. Barcelona: Elsevier España; 2020.
16. Li D, Zheng JJ, Weng JC, et al. Neurological outcomes of untreated brainstem cavernous malformations in a prospective observational cohort and literature review. Stroke Vasc Neurol. 2020;6:501–10. https://doi.org/10.1136/svn-2020-000608.
17. Mai JC, Ramanathan D, Kim LJ, et al. Surgical resection of cavernous malformations of the brainstem: evolution of a minimally invasive technique. World Neurosurg. 2013;79:691–703. https://doi.org/10.1016/j.wneu.2012.04.030.
18. Marotta D, Hendricks BK, Zaher M, et al. Resection of brainstem cavernous malformations: pearls and pitfalls for minimizing complications. World Neurosurg. 2022;159:390–401. https://doi.org/10.1016/j.wneu.2021.08.072.
19. Mosnier JF, Brunon J, Nuti C. Anatomie pathologique des cavernomes du système nerveux central. Neurochirurgie. 2007;53(2–3 Pt 2):131–5. https://doi.org/10.1016/j.neuchi.2007.02.004.
20. Ohue S, Fukushima T, Friedman AH, et al. Retrosigmoid suprafloccular transhorizontal fissure approach for resection of brainstem cavernous malformation. Neurosurgery. 2010;66 Suppl Operative 6:306–12. https://doi.org/10.1227/01.NEU.0000369703.67562.BB.
21. Recalde RJ, Figueiredo EG, de Oliveira E. Microsurgical anatomy of the safe entry zones on the anterolateral brainstem related to surgical approaches to cavernous malformations. Neurosurgery. 2008;62(Suppl 1):9–15. https://doi.org/10.1227/01.neu.0000317368.69523.40.
22. Sarnthein J, Bozinov O, Melone AG, et al. Motor-evoked potentials (MEP) during brainstem surgery to preserve corticospinal function. Acta Neurochir. 2011;153:1753–9. https://doi.org/10.1007/s00701-011-1065-7.
23. Strauss C, Lütjen-Drecoll E, Fahlbusch R. Pericollicular surgical approaches to the rhomboid fossa. Part I Anatomical basis J Neurosurg. 1997;87:893–9. https://doi.org/10.3171/jns.1997.87.6.0893.
24. Schwartz C, Grillhösl A, Schichor C, et al. Symptomatic cavernous malformations of the brainstem: functional outcome after microsurgical

resection. J Neurol. 2013;260:2815–22. https://doi.org/10.1007/s00415-013-7071-3.
25. Snellings DA, Hong CC, Ren AA, et al. Cerebral cavernous malformation: from mechanism to therapy. Circ Res. 2021;129:195–215. https://doi.org/10.1161/CIRCRESAHA.121.318174.
26. Tarabay A, Rocca A, Maeder P, et al. Extra-axial cavernoma of the cerebellopontine angle: a case study and review of literature. World Neurosurg. 2019;128:415–21. https://doi.org/10.1016/j.wneu.2019.05.034.
27. Xie MG, Li D, Guo FZ, et al. Brainstem cavernous malformations: surgical indications based on natural history and surgical outcomes. World Neurosurg. 2018;110:55–63. https://doi.org/10.1016/j.wneu.2017.10.121.
28. Yagmurlu K, Rhoton AL Jr, Tanriover N, et al. Three-dimensional microsurgical anatomy and the safe entry zones of the brainstem. Neurosurgery. 2014;10(Suppl 4):602–19. https://doi.org/10.1227/NEU.0000000000000466.

18 Trigeminal Neuralgia

18.1 Introduction

Currently, three etiological types of trigeminal neuralgia (TN) are distinguished: classical, secondary, and idiopathic (Fig. 18.1). Classic TN is caused by vascular compression of the trigeminal root, and its microneurosurgical treatment is microvascular decompression (MVD) of the trigeminal nerve root. MVD is a pathophysiological and curative intervention. Secondary TN is due to a series of neurological diseases and neurosurgical disorders, including tumors and other structural lesions of the cerebellopontine angle and other regions of the head and face, that damage the trigeminal root, ganglion, or nerves. In this group of patients, treatment of TN involves microsurgical removal of the lesion. In idiopathic TN, there is no neurological disease or lesion that can explain the neuralgic pain. In TN secondary to neurological diseases and in idiopathic NT, there is no rationale for MVD, but there is occasionally room for some other types of symptomatic neurosurgical treatment.

Microneurosurgical treatment of TN with MVD of the trigeminal nerve root is a successful case in the neurosurgical treatment of neurological diseases. Currently, the therapeutic arsenal for the treatment of TN is very effective and reaches practically all patients and includes, in addition to pharmacological treatment, neurosurgical treatment options with MVD, minimally invasive percutaneous techniques, and stereotactic radiosurgery. MVD is a pathophysiological treatment technique, one of the few non-exeretic and non-lesive treatments available in the neurological surgery armamentarium. MVD has a short history, since it was introduced in the second half of the twentieth century, thanks to the work and drive of a group of pioneers in a history not free of rivalry and controversy between them until the recognition and widespread acceptance of the value of the technique.

18.1.1 History of the Microvascular Decompression

TN is a devastating condition for the patient, which currently has an excellent pharmacological and surgical solution. However, this has not always been the case, and, as far as the surgical solution is concerned, it has compelled the development of complex approaches and very specific craniotomies that the ongoing pathophysiological knowledge of the disease has led to their definitive abandonment. The objective of the surgical procedures developed at the end of the nineteenth century and the beginning of the twentieth century was oriented towards achieving the sectioning of all the sensory inputs coming from the cutaneous area of the trigeminal nerve (*neurectomy of the peripheral branches of the trigeminal nerve*). In the event of a poor outcome, the state-of-the-art method at the time was *retrogasserian*

J. M. González-Darder, *Microneurosurgery of Cerebellopontine Angle*,
https://doi.org/10.1007/978-3-032-03091-7_18

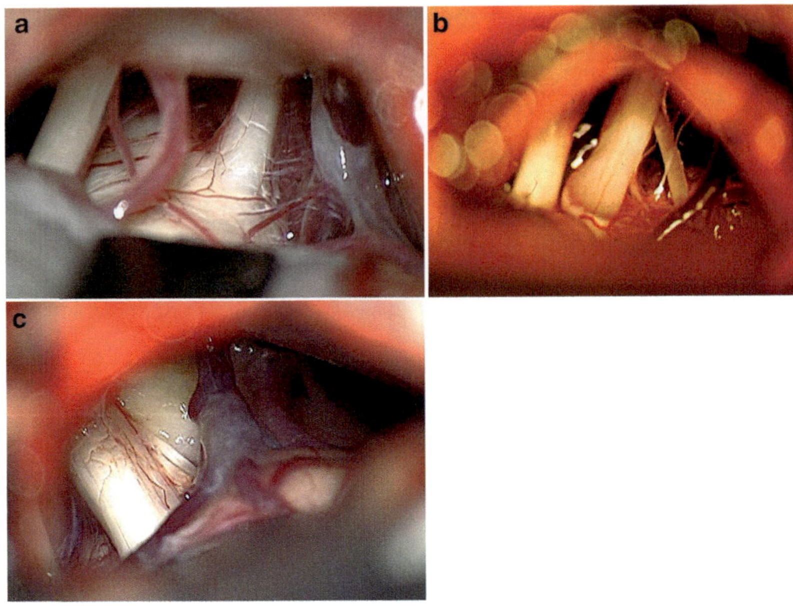

Fig. 18.1 Intraoperative pictures of the trigeminal root in the cerebellopontine angle. View through a left retrosigmoid approach (left to right: facial–cochleovestibular complex; trigeminal nerve; superior petrosal venous complex). (**a**) Normal appearance of the cerebellopontine angle. (**b**) Patient with classic trigeminal neuralgia, with root compression by a branch of the superior cerebellar artery. (**c**) Patient with secondary TN, with a root compression by a small epidermoid cyst

section of the root of the trigeminal nerve in Meckel's cave, *resection of the semilunar ganglion of Gasser*, or *section of the main branches of the trigeminal nerve*. For these procedures, several surgical approaches were developed independently but practically simultaneously by Victor Horsley (1857–1916) and Frank Hartley (1856–1913) in the United States, Eugène Louis Doyen (1859–1916) in France, and Fedor Krause (1857–1937) in Germany. Because of the hidden nature of the approach, bleeding, anatomical or terminological confusions, and a lack of in-depth anatomical knowledge of the area, these surgeons frequently struggled to identify the precise neurological structure they sectioned or removed. In any case, the approach was made always with a temporal craniotomy and extradural access to the trigeminal nerve root, ganglion, or nerve branches. Due to the severe atrophy of the temporal and masseteric muscles caused by the section of the motor root or the third branch, as well as the frequent loss of the eye due to keratitis secondary to the sensory denervation of the conjunctiva and cornea dependent on the first branch of the trigeminal nerve, these surgeries were especially mutilating for the patient. Hemorrhage from the cavernous sinus or the middle meningeal artery, an unintentional severing of the superior cerebellar artery in the rhizotomy, damage to the facial nerve at the level of the geniculate ganglion and other cranial nerves related to the cavernous sinus, cavernous sinus thrombosis, intraoperative or postoperative shock, or infection were among the common and devastating surgical complications. The most successful and recognized technique was the retrogasserian section of the trigeminal nerve root via a subtemporal approach, known as the Spiller–Frazier technique.

In the meantime, some authors advocate and try the trigeminal rhizotomy through the posterior fossa. Doyen documented in 1917 one such attempt using an endoscope with a 20 mm diameter that was placed through a cranial hole at the level of the asterion. However, Walter Dandy (1886–1946) is credited with creating the *retrogasserian trigeminal rhizotomy through a retrosigmoid approach*. The advantages attributed to this approach were ease and speed, selective section of sensory fibers without significant loss of sensitivity and therefore less risk of keratitis, preservation of motor fibers, and less injury to the facial nerve and other cranial nerve. In 1932, Dandy stated that, of approximately 500 cases he operated on, 10% had tumors or aneurysms compressing the trigeminal nerve root; nevertheless, "in almost every additional case, the nerve is grooved or bent by a loop of the anterior inferior cerebellar artery (sic). This, I believe, is the cause of tic douloureux." Despite this surgical observation made decades before the introduction of the surgical microscope, Dandy never considered this neurovascular relationship as a core cause of TN, and for a few decades, the Spiller–Frazier retrogasserian trigeminal rhizotomy with an extradural subtemporal approach or the Dandy retrogasserian trigeminal rhizotomy with a retrosigmoid approach were still carried out.

However, this shift in focus in the treatment of TN was continued with a number of new techniques aimed at decompressing the root of the trigeminal nerve root in order to cure TN without damaging the nerve. Palle Taarnhøj proposed in 1951 "to treat patients with trigeminal neuralgia by dividing the dural sheath enclosing the root and ganglion without dividing the root itself." For this author, "good decompression is secured by running a nerve hook along the posterior trigeminal root." Through a subtemporal approach, without the aid of a surgical microscope, he performed the opening of the proximal dura mater of the gasserian ganglion through the superior petrosal sinus and 1 cm above the tentorium to widen the foramen of the Meckel's cave and release the root of the trigeminal nerve. As a result, it was the first surgical method to cure TN without necessarily causing a sensory impairment. James Gardner (1898–1987) refined the method years later in 1959 when he noted that the neurolysis or manipulation of the trigeminal nerve's sensory root at the point where it crosses the apex of the petrosal bone of the temporal bone to enter the Meckel's cave appeared to be the crucial part of the procedure. Gardner suggested that the sensory root be released from its dural sheath, then gently manipulated with a cotton swab and cleaned with Ringer's solution. Sixty percent of positive outcomes were recorded using this *nontraumatic manipulation of the trigeminal nerve root*. When the subtemporal method failed, Gardner operated on his patients again, now using the retrosigmoid technique, which allowed him to once more see how arteries and veins compressed the trigeminal nerve root. Then, in addition to nontraumatic manipulation, he began to place a gelatin sponge pad (Gelfoam) between the nerve root and the vessels.

Peter Jannetta (1932–2016) was a resident at UCLA between 1963 and 1966, where Rand and Kurze introduced the surgical microscope, and Rand asked him to study the anatomy of the cranial nerves in the laboratory under the surgical microscope, and he again observed the relationship of vessels with the root of the trigeminal nerve. In 1965, together with Rand, Jannetta observed a patient with TN where a pulsating artery compressed the root of the trigeminal nerve and exclaimed, "That's the cause of the tic!" postulating in 1966 that hemifacial spasm would have the same pathophysiology as TN. Jannetta presented cases as a resident and later, together with Rand, proposed the "release of the artery without nerve section" or *microvascular decompression of the trigeminal nerve root*. As a senior working in New Orleans, he abandoned the subtemporal transtentorial approach, adopted the microsurgical retrosigmoid approach, and defined microvascular compression as the cause of TN, asserting that "trigeminal neuralgia is a symptom due to an abnormality at the root entry zone of the trigeminal nerve at the pons. It is due to vascular cross-compression in most cases" and unifies other neuropathies of the cranial nerves under the same physiopathology, defining the neurovascular compression syndromes. Jannetta received criticism for his youth, his use of the microscope, his defiance of accepted doctrines, his genuineness and candor, and his sincerity. Rand stated in 1981 that Gardner should be credited with the idea and creation of the MVD process, which is sometimes mistakenly referred to as the "Jannetta operation." These harsh accusations weighed heavily on Jannetta, as he was always very careful to refer to his predecessors and never claimed the invention of the MVD as his original idea. In any event, regardless of credit issues, what matters is that MVD continues to be the preferred microneurosurgical procedure for treating typical NT [4, 13].

18.2 Anatomical Considerations

In accordance with Albert Rhoton, the neurovascular composition of the cerebellopontine angle can be categorized into three groups. The trochlear nerve root, the trigeminal nerve root, the superior cerebellar artery and its branches, and the superior petrosal vein complex are all part of the superior neurovascular complex.

The trigeminal nerve appears to originate on the anterolateral side of the brainstem, midway between the upper and lower borders of the pons and just medial to the middle cerebellar peduncle. It then travels anteriorly, superiorly, and laterally to enter Meckel's cave. This apparent origin of the trigeminal nerve actually corresponds to its entry into the brainstem, since it is an eminently sensitive nerve. That is the reason that the nearest portion of the cranial nerve root to the pial surface of the brainstem is broadly known as the *root entry zone*. With a diameter of roughly 5 mm, the trigeminal nerve is the biggest cranial nerve in the posterior fossa. A big sensory root (*pars major*), a tiny motor root (pars minor), and a variable number of aberrant rootlets make up the internal structure of the trigeminal nerve. The classic somatotopic distribution of the sensory fibers of the trigeminal nerve is as follows: the fibers of the third branch are located in the caudolateral zone, those of the first branch in the rostro-medial zone, and those of the second branch between the two. The motor fibers are located rostrally, relating to the sensory fibers of the third branch. However, the trigeminal nerve is subject to a large number of anatomical variations and variability in the distribution of sensory and motor fibers. Although the results differ according to the studies, the total number of nerve fibers is around 25,000 in V1, 50,000 in V2, and 75,000 in V3, while the motor root would have about 7500 fibers. The root of the trigeminal nerve enters Meckel's cave, forming an angle of variable amplitude, where the most distal portion of the root, called retrogasserian, and the semilunar ganglion of Gasser are housed, with the pars minor occupying the deepest topography. As the root passes along the edge of the petrosal bone to enter the cave, the sensory fibers have a large number of anastomoses in the so-called triangular plexus. The Meckel's cave, with very variable dimensions, is filled with cerebrospinal fluid (CSF) dependent on an arachnoid expansion of the cisterns of the cerebellopontine angle.

The superior cerebellar artery arises near the division of the basilar artery and divides into four parts: the anterior pontine-mesencephalic segment, the lateral pontine-mesencephalic segment, the cerebellar-mesencephalic segment, and finally, the cortical segment. At widely varying distances from its origin, the superior cerebellar artery divides into a cranial and a caudal branch. The main trunk of the superior cerebellar artery is anatomically related to the trochlear nerve on the lateral part of the tentorial notch, where the artery runs caudally to the nerve and the two elements may have points of contact. The main superior cerebellar artery or its branches are related to the cranial surface of the trigeminal nerve. This relationship is a contact or loop of the superior cerebellar artery trunk, its cranial branch, its caudal branch, or both, which may contact, deform, or distort the trigeminal nerve root.

The most important venous channel in the upper part of the cerebellopontine angle is the superior petrosal venous complex, which drains into the superior petrosal sinus. This is a structure characterized by its great anatomical variability. There is usually a single drainage channel or Dandy vein formed by the union of two or more veins that come from the surface of the cerebellum, midbrain, and pons. These veins frequently join together in two channels, the ascending cerebellopontine trunk and the transverse pontine vein. Sometimes two or more individual trunks drain into the superior petrosal sinus. The pontine-trigeminal vein, which ends in the complex or in the superior petrosal sinus, may also have a close relationship with the trigeminal nerve root. These neurovascular relationships have been considered relevant in the etiopathogenesis of TN [3, 9]

18.3 Pathology

As we have reported, it was Walter Dandy who was the first to note the close anatomical relationship between the vessels and the trigeminal root in patients with TN who were operated on through a lateral suboccipital approach to perform a partial rhizotomy. This observation was validated microsurgically years later and led Jannetta to hypothesize the MVD of the trigeminal root as a pathophysiological treatment for TN. Different histological, anatomical, and neurophysiological research and clinical observations have shown that TN is due to the formation of anomalous connections between sensory nerve fibers in the so-called *Obersteiner–Redlich transitional zone* that generate aberrant nerve impulses that are interpreted by the patient as pain. The glioneural sheath, which is supplied by oligodendroglia and the outer support of astrocytes, still covers the nerve fibers of cranial nerve roots at their entry zone and up until this transitional zone. The myelin sheath, which is supplied by Schwann cells and supported by endoneurium connective elements like fibroblasts and extracellular matrix filaments like collagen, protects the nerve fibers distal to the transitional zone. The transition between the central and peripheral myelin sheath does not occur at the same level in all fibers, but over a few microns, adopting a conical morphology throughout the root, that is, more distally in the center of the nerve root. In the case of the trigeminal nerve, the average distance of the central myelin sheath is 4.2 mm, which represents approximately one-third of the intracranial length of the root, which measures between 8 and 15 mm [1, 14, 15].

18.3.1 Classic Trigeminal Neuralgia

In classic TN, the etiology of compression of the trigeminal root is of vascular origin and is carried out by anatomical arterial or venous vascular structures, but generally with an abnormal or elongated anatomical configuration or course. The nerve root exhibits compression-related alterations, including color and size changes in addition to contact or compression (Fig. 18.1b). In this regard, the elements of compression, the area of the compressed root, and the trigeminal branch where the pain is referred must be considered [1, 2].

18.3.1.1 Offending Vessels

The most common cause of compression is the superior cerebellar artery (SCA), which contacts the superolateral or superomedial portion of the nerve root, particularly in its bifurcation or by its caudal branch. On the lower portion of the nerve root, an upper loop of the anterior inferior cerebellar artery (AICA) more infrequently causes compression. 60% of microvascular decompression procedures for NT are found to be pure compression via the superior cerebellar artery or anteroinferior cerebellar artery. An extremely cranial path of the vertebral artery (VA), posterior inferior cerebellar artery (PICA), or its branches, or an elongated or fusiform basilar artery (BA) may be the cause of vascular compression. In these situations, it is not uncommon for additional cranial rhizopathy to coexist, such as arterial hypertension in 75% of patients or hemifacial spasm in 10% of patients [1, 2, 14].

Veins of the superior petrosal complex, particularly the transverse pontine vein, may also be the only cause of compression. The drainage points of the petrosal vein complex in the superior petrosal sinus, which are roughly near the trigeminal nerve, must be taken into consideration initially in this regard. Three drainage types can be distinguished in relation to this anatomical detail: type I, in which the petrosal vein empties into the superior petrosal sinus above and lateral to the internal acoustic meatus; type II, which is the most common, empties between the medial limit of the facial nerve in the internal acoustic meatus and the lateral limit of the trigeminal nerve in the Meckel's cave; and type III, which empties into the superior petrosal sinus above and medial to the Meckel's cave. Second, it is necessary to take into account the veins that join to form the superior petrosal complex and their relationship to the trigeminal nerve. Numerous arrangements of compression have been described in this regard, including compression by a small-caliber transverse pontine vein that crosses the nerve perpendicularly, anteriorly, or behind; compression by a small or large petrosal pontine vein that enters the Meckel's cave alongside the nerve; and, lastly, the relationship with the petrosal vein or the cerebellopontine fissure vein [1, 2, 11, 16].

Lastly, in 25% of cases, the compression may be mixed, meaning that venous and arterial structures may combine to generate the nerve compression.

18.3.1.2 Nerve Compression

Marc Sindou has conducted extensive research on the compression zone on the trigeminal nerve root and its connection to the somatotopy of pain distribution. Superolateral, inferior, and superomedial are the regions where nerve compression occurs. Only 10% of patients who have surgery have inferior compression; 90% of patients have superior compression, two-thirds have superomedial compression, and the remaining third have superolateral compression. In 75% of cases, superomedial compression is linked to solo or combined painful involvement of the V1 area, while inferior compression is considered uncommon. Superomedial compression is less likely to occur in patients with solitary or mixed painful involvement of the V3 area than in other patients. Lastly, the likelihood of compression is comparable for both directions in the event of single or mixed painful involvement of the V2 region. More often, compression of the anteroinferior cerebellar artery is associated with first-branch neuralgia, whereas compression of the superior cerebellar artery is associated with third- or second-branch neuralgia [14].

18.3.1.3 Pathophysiology

It is a well-known fact that, regardless of the compression modality, the trigeminal root exhibits structural changes such as distortion, discoloration, or atrophy in addition to the compression aspect. The pathophysiological basis for compression is focal demyelination of the thick Aβ nerve fibers, which permits ephaptic transmission—the transfer of stimuli from one axon to another—and hyperexcitability of the axons, resulting in the generation of ectopic impulses in response to mechanical stimuli with numerous subsequent high-frequency discharges. These anomalous stimuli reach the brainstem and are transmitted to higher levels, being interpreted by the patient as discharges of paroxysmal pain. The etiology of persistent concurrent pain would be associated with the degeneration of demyelinated C nerve fibers. In contrast to paroxysmal pain, this selective denervation would encourage the spontaneous activity of the neurons in the brainstem's sensory nucleus of the trigeminal nerve, producing ascending nociceptive impulses that produce pain with the characteristics of neuropathic pain due to deafferentation, which patients describe as tingling or burning [1, 2].

18.3.2 Secondary Trigeminal Neuralgia

In 15% of patients, TN is secondary to neurological diseases or tumors and structural lesions of the cerebellopontine angle. The neurological disease that most frequently causes NT is multiple sclerosis, although in some cases, microvascular compression may be associated. On the other hand, any tumor of the cerebellopontine angle can be associated with NT, which accounts for approximately 10% of the total (refer to *case 28 in* Chap. 21). In these cases, the nerve may be invaded by the tumor, compressed by the tumor, or by a vessel displaced by the tumor. The epidermoid cyst is the lesion of the cerebellopontine angle that is most frequently associated with NT (75%), while others are less frequently associated with NT, such as meningioma (35%) and vestibular schwannoma (10%). It is noteworthy that trigeminal schwannoma does not usually cause NT. In these cases, compression of the nerve by the lesion would produce focal demyelination, generating anomalous impulses in a similar way to what occurs with microvascular compression. Trauma to the branches of the trigeminal nerve and some systemic connective tissue diseases can also cause secondary NT.

18.3.3 Idiopathic Trigeminal Neuralgia

Diagnostic tests that verify the existence of any lesion or disease that could account for the NT are lacking in this type of NT, and microneurosurgical examination of the nerve root in the cerebellopontine angle does not reveal any compression. Five to ten percent of cases are in young individuals with a brief medical history, and pain can be unilateral or bilateral.

18.4 Clinical Considerations

TN is diagnosed based on clinical criteria defining a neuralgic or *paroxysmal pain* in the trigeminal territory. The *International Association of Headache Disorders* (ICHD), in 2018, describes the clinical criteria for TN as follows: "Disorder characterized by recurrent, brief, unilateral, electric shock-like pains of abrupt onset and termination, limited to the distribution of one or more divisions of the trigeminal nerve, and triggered by innocuous stimuli. The diagnostic criteria are as follows: (A) recurrent paroxysms of unilateral facial pain in the distributions of one or more divisions of the trigeminal nerve, without radiation beyond, and meeting criteria B and C; (B) the pain has all of the following characteristics: lasts from a fraction of a second to 2 minutes; is of severe intensity; and is electric shock-like, shooting, stabbing, or sharp in quality; (C) is precipitated by innocuous stimuli within the affected trigeminal distribution; (D) is not better explained by another diagnosis."

In 2018, the *International Association for the Study of Pain* (IASP) defined TN as follows: "Orofacial pain restricted to one or more divisions of the trigeminal nerve. With the exception of TN caused by multiple sclerosis, the pain affects one side of the face. It has a sudden onset and typically lasts only a few seconds (2 min at most). Patients may have spontaneous pain, but pain paroxysms can always be triggered by harmless mechanical stimuli or movements. The diagnostic criteria are: The patient has (1) orofacial pain that (2) is distributed in the trigeminal territory of the face or intraorally and (3) the pain is triggered by harmless maneuvers."

Both the ICHD and the IASP consider the possibility that a concomitant continuous pain associated with paroxysmal pain (*neuralgia with concomitant continuous pain*) may be associated in the same distribution, which occurs in a high percentage of cases (between 25% and 50% of patients, according to the series).

The description of the TN symptomatology that we have described is an idealized version of the clinical reality. All patients who come to the outpatient office of the neurosurgeon have a long history of the disease and have received or are receiving mono- or polytherapy medication therapy. Some have undergone more or less aggressive surgical treatments on the trigeminal nerve. Every patient experiences some level of reactive depression in response to the unsatisfactory course of their illness, along with anxiety stemming from it or from the hope of a final remedy.

Pain most frequently affects the V2 and V3 branches; V1 territory is affected in isolation in only 5% of patients and alone or in combination in one third; V2 territory is affected in isolation in 55% of patients and alone or in combination in 80%; V3 territory is affected in isolation in the remaining 40% of the patients and alone or in combination in more than half of patients. Pain is more frequent on the right side and can rarely be bilateral; it is more frequent in women than in men in a ratio of 2:3, and, finally, its frequency increases with age, with the typical age of onset being the fifth decade. The incidence is between 4 and 20 new cases per 100,000 inhabitants per year, being higher in developed countries due to the greater ease of diagnosis, with a prevalence of 0.1–0.3% of the population. It is associated with arterial hypertension and some neurological diseases, such as multiple sclerosis, Charcot-Marie-Tooth disease, and other cranial rhizopathies. Finally, there are frequent remission periods, lasting months or years. Remission can be spontaneous or as a response to pharmacological or surgical treatments.

Although a highly thorough or detailed examination may reveal extremely minor sensory abnormalities, the neurological evaluation is typically normal. Secondary TN should be suspected if the neurological examination reveals any positive deficiency findings. Paroxysmal pain can be produced during the examination with a harmless stimulus, such as rubbing the skin with a brush or piece of cloth or gentle percussion with the finger, applied to certain skin areas called *trigger zones*. During the interview, the patient may spontaneously present attacks of paroxysmal pain or may be asked to trigger them with specific maneuvers of daily life, such as talking, shaving, chewing, brushing teeth, drying the face, eating, drinking, or swallowing saliva. It is very interesting that some patients report and reproduce the attacks of paroxysmal pain with movements of the head, jaw, or trunk, yawning, or laughing. The crisis of paroxysmal pain is usually accompanied by blinking, grimacing, or a massive and coarse contraction of the homolateral facial muscles called *tic convulsive* or *tic doloreux*. In some cases, it is possible to observe subtle vasomotor changes or changes in the turgor and softness of the skin in the affected territories [1, 2, 14].

18.5 Diagnostic Considerations

All patients with TN should be studied with neuroimaging techniques, particularly magnetic resonance imaging (MRI), including T1-weighted TOF (*Time Of Flight angiography*) and T1-weighted sequences with gadolinium, as well as high-resolution T2-weighted sequences such as FIESTA (*Fast Imaging Employing Steady State Acquisition*). This study aims to rule out the existence of any tumor or neurological disease, to identify secondary neuralgia, and to demonstrate the microvascular compression to confirm the diagnosis of classic neuralgia (Fig. 18.2). The imaging of the different types of tumors and lesions of the cerebellopontine angle is described elsewhere in the chapters corresponding to each pathology.

The concept of classic TN contains a paradox, since the diagnosis can only be made when microvascular compression is demonstrated, and this can only be done precisely after microneurosurgical exploration of the trigeminal root, since imaging studies have a high percentage of false positives and false negatives. On the other hand, it is not necessary to demonstrate a vascular compression on MRI to presume that the compression actually exists. Thus, there is intraoperative confirmation of vascular compression in 80–100% of patients with TN regardless of the MRI findings. In imaging studies, vascular compression is detected in less than 60% of patients with TN, but also in more than 30% of people without TN and on the contralateral side in almost half of patients with TN. In autopsies, vascular compression of the trigeminal nerve has been demonstrated in 10–60% of people without neuralgia. Thus, it can be stated that the verification of vascular compression in MRI, by itself, should not be the only criterion on which to base decisions on the diagnosis of classic neuralgia, much less on the indication of a surgical exploration that demonstrates compression and allows for MVD. Another interesting finding is the demonstration of atrophy of the trigeminal nerve in half of the cases with neuralgia versus only in 10% of asymptomatic cases, and that can reach 20% of its volume. The study with DTI (*Diffusion Tensor Imaging*) MRI reveals the decrease in

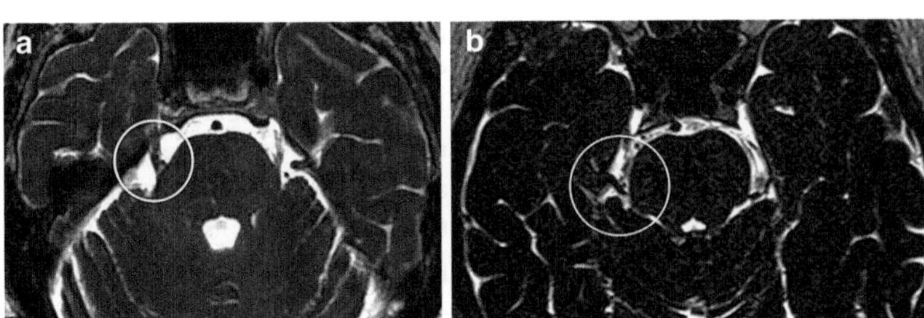

Fig. 18.2 Axial MRI sections in FIESTA sequence showing the relationship between a vascular structure and the right trigeminal nerve root at its exit from the pons in patients with classic trigeminal neuralgia. (**a**) Arterial vessel. (**b**) Vein

anisotropy due to demyelination. MRI can also show post-surgical and post-radiosurgery changes [5].

18.6 Surgical Types

When microneurosurgically exploring the cerebellopontine angle in patients with TN, there are essentially three scenarios [1, 2]. An anatomical cerebellopontine angle would be found in cases of idiopathic neuralgia and neuralgia resulting from neurological disorders (Fig. 18.1a). One or more vessels, either arteries or veins, compress the nerve in classic neuralgia (Fig. 18.1b). Lastly, a tumor or structural lesion compresses the nerve in neuralgia caused by cerebellopontine angle lesions (Fig. 18.1c).

18.7 Microneurosurgical Management

A retrosigmoid approach, which provides access to the trigeminal nerve root from its apparent exit from the pons to its entry into Meckel's cave, is currently the only approach used for microneurosurgical treatment of classic TN by MVD. This approach also enables the investigation of the vascular components that contribute to the development of classic TN [1, 3, 8]. Also, endoscopic approaches have been described [10]. In secondary TN, the retrosigmoid technique is also frequently utilized to treat various cerebellopontine angle lesions, whether they are tumors or something else that is causing the trigeminal nerve to become compressed.

18.7.1 Microvascular Decompression

The MVD strategy should follow the following steps: identification of the trigeminal nerve root and vascular elements of compression; vascular decompression; and, finally, maintenance of decompression.

18.7.2 Position and Craniotomy

There is no particularity in all that has been described in the chapter on the retrosigmoid approach regarding the position, anatomical references, incision, craniotomy, and dural opening. The retrosigmoid approach should ideally be high and framed by the angle formed by the confluence of the transverse sinus with the sigmoid sinus. The craniotomy does not need to be wide, since there is no intracranial space occupied by any lesion, and cisternal navigation is comfortable.

18.7.3 Cisternal Navigation and Superior Petrosal Vein Complex Dissection

A corridor created by the posterior aspect of the petrosal bone and the inferior surface of the tentorium can be accessed along the superior petrosal sinus if the craniotomy fits into the angle formed by the transverse and sigmoid sinuses. This corridor leads to the trigeminal root as it enters the Meckel's cave through the ostium and below the superior petrosal sinus, as well as to the superior petrosal vein complex as it drains into the superior petrosal sinus. The width of the cisterns can be predicted in imaging studies, and, in this sense, it is frequently observed that the cisterns of patients with TN are of a smaller volume than average. The spatula of the retractor must be placed on the most lateral part of the tentorial surface of the cerebellum to gain space. The next step is to section the arachnoid bands in the area with fine scissors, particularly those surrounding the veins of the upper petrosal complex, to isolate, mobilize, and maintain their anatomical integrity as far as possible (Fig. 18.3). The veins usually ascend towards the petrosal sinus, passing through an arachnoid hole, wider than the vein, which must be opened to facilitate the mobilization and preservation of the venous vessels. These arachnoid orifices are actually wider because under anesthetic conditions, the

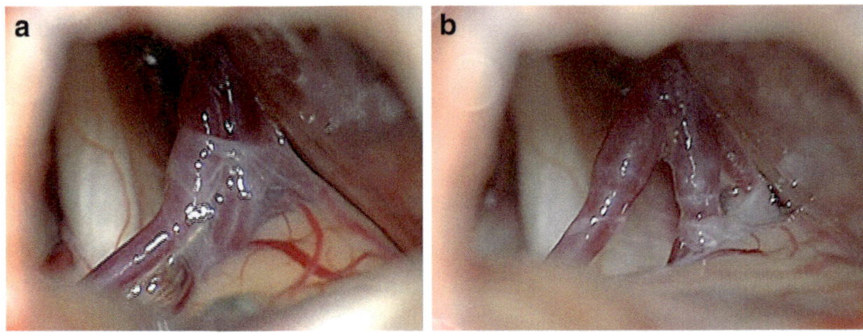

Fig. 18.3 Intraoperative pictures of the left cerebellopontine angle displaying different stages in the dissection of the superior petrosal venous complex from the arachnoid. The venous complex has an anatomical configuration. (**a**) Before dissection. (**b**) After releasing (left to right: trigeminal nerve; superior petrosal venous complex; tentorium)

veins are probably slimmed due to the facilitation of venous drainage by the posture and artificial ventilation. When the skull is closed, the veins are probably more enlarged, and physiological Valsalva maneuvers facilitate this expansion. Arachnoid stiffness and thickening, commonly referred to as focal arachnoiditis, can occasionally be discovered. This condition is not visible on imaging tests and appears to give patients a worse prognosis.

Since the trigeminal root is situated directly behind the veins in the retrosigmoid approach, routine identification, coagulation, and sectioning of the superior petrosal vein were advised in the early literature descriptions of the MVD procedure. This practice is currently not recommended, since the risk of developing symptomatic venous infarction is well known. Once the surgical level of the petrosal vein complex is reached, the trigeminal root must be effectively reached, so the position of the retractor and the angle of attack must be adjusted. The anatomical variations in the number, drainage point, and constitution of the superior petrosal vein make the described pattern highly variable.

18.7.4 Trigeminal Root Exploration

Once the trigeminal nerve has been identified, it must be cleared of the arachnoid to perform a systematic assessment of microvascular compression in the entry zone. The apparent exit point of the root from the pons is exposed, where it typically widens and some fascicles can be identified; later, the root trunk is exposed in its entire length, and, finally, the entry of the root into the Meckel's cave is explored. An attempt is made to identify areas of deformity, atrophy, or changes in brightness or color along the course of the nerve. On the other hand, the angle of the nerve at its entry into Meckel's cave when passing over the upper edge of the petrosal bone has also been considered in the pathophysiology of TN, although nowadays there is no microsurgical maneuver dedicated to its correction.

18.7.5 Microvascular Compression Assessment

Once the nerve is exposed, the vascular elements of compression are identified. Firstly, the unexpected finding of an undetected lesion in the imaging studies, whatever the type, is ruled out. The veins are then explored, usually more conspicuous and visible than the arteries, which, if they are related to the nerve, are freed from the arachnoid and mobilized. Finally, the arteries are explored.

The superior cerebellar artery can compress the root laterally or medially and is located on a level cranial to the nerve. The artery or its branches are positioned behind the root's entry zone and push the nerve in the direction of the surgeon in superomedial compression (Fig. 18.4); in superolateral compression, they are positioned in front of the root and force the nerve downward. The inferior compression of the root and its upward push are caused by the anterior inferior cerebellar artery.

Although the theoretical cause of TN is compression of the entry zone of the trigeminal nerve, it is not uncommon to find more distal compressions along the entire course of the root, so the exploration must be systematic throughout the entire course of the root and both in front of and behind the root. It is hypothesized that, in these cases of distal compression far away from the transitional zone, the vessels would exert traction on the root or that in this particular patient the transition zone would be more distal to the averaged.

18.7.6 Microvascular Root Decompression

Decompression should now be carried out, and depending on the situation, several options may be employed. The most common and traditional method involves placing a synthetic substance between the artery or arteries that are present and squeezing the root. Gelfoam was employed at first, but Teflon—an inert, non-adherent, nonabsorbable substance with little ability to function as a foreign body—is now favored. For every case, the author creates a little roll that is the right thickness and length, and it is carefully positioned between the artery vessels and the nerve. To maintain the position in the initial phases before the eventual arachnoid reaction fixes the structures, we apply a small amount of Tissucol, which is a human fibrin adhesive widely used as

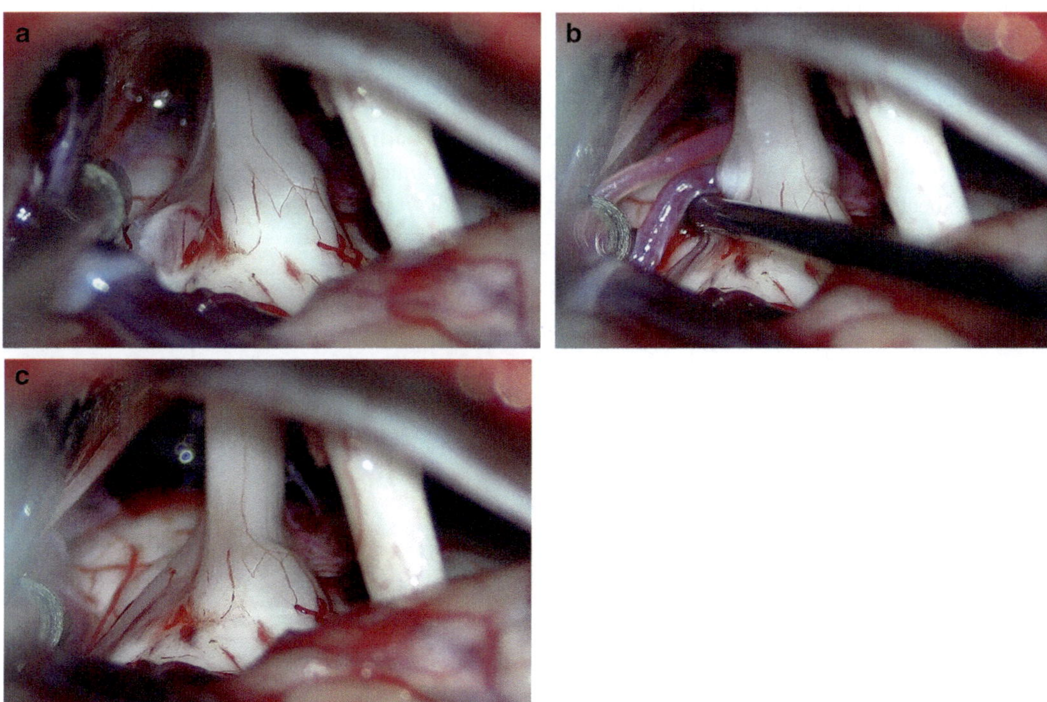

Fig. 18.4 MVD in a classic trigeminal neuralgia due to superomedial arterial compression by the right superior cerebellar artery. (**a**) Picture after arachnoid dissection, showing the superior cerebellar artery compressing the exit of the trigeminal nerve from the pons, surrounded by arachnoid. (**b**) Both branches of the superior cerebellar artery have been released and mobilized. (**c**) The entry zone of the trigeminal root shows an indentation due to chronic arterial compression

a sealant and hemostatic (*refer to case 30 in* Chap. 21).

To achieve decompression when dealing with larger caliber arterial vessels, more complex procedures have been described. Thus, large vessels, such as the basilar artery or vertebral artery, can be kept separated from the nerve by passing a loop of fascia or synthetic material that is attached to the dura mater with a stitch or vascular miniclip. The objective would be to maintain the separation without the interposition of any material that would remain in contact with the root and could exert a deleterious effect on it, thus improving the prognosis. However, for small arterial vessels, the pure transposition technique is difficult due to the lack of room, the size of the vessels, and the risk of injury or angulation leading to ischemia.

As far as veins are concerned, there are different options to achieve decompression. The problematic veins are released, but because of their brief free course, they are typically difficult to mobilize and must be coagulated and split. It is dangerous to perform venous decompression with interposed material since it will probably cause the vein to thrombose. Separation can be maintained by dragging the vein by pulling on its arachnoid sheaths and maintaining its position with adhesive material applied between the arachnoid and the dura mater. If the vein is clearly related to the root, coagulation and section of it is permissible, particularly if it is of small caliber or there are other free venous afferents to the superior petrosal sinus (Fig. 18.5). As indicated, coagulation and section of the superior petrosal venous trunk has a high risk of venous infarction on the superolateral side of the pons and superior cerebellar peduncle (*refer to case 29 in* Chap. 21).

In many cases, compression is mixed, and both arterial branches and venous channels may be involved. In this case, individual decompression of each component is performed, although arterial compression is usually given greater importance (Fig. 18.6).

18.7.7 Alternative Management When Microvascular Compression Is Not Found

In a percentage of cases, no element of trigeminal root compression is found to explain the patient's symptoms. In this case, there are other treatment options: partial sensory rhizotomy, internal neurolysis, and nontraumatic manipulation [7]. *Selective partial rhizotomy of the sensory root of*

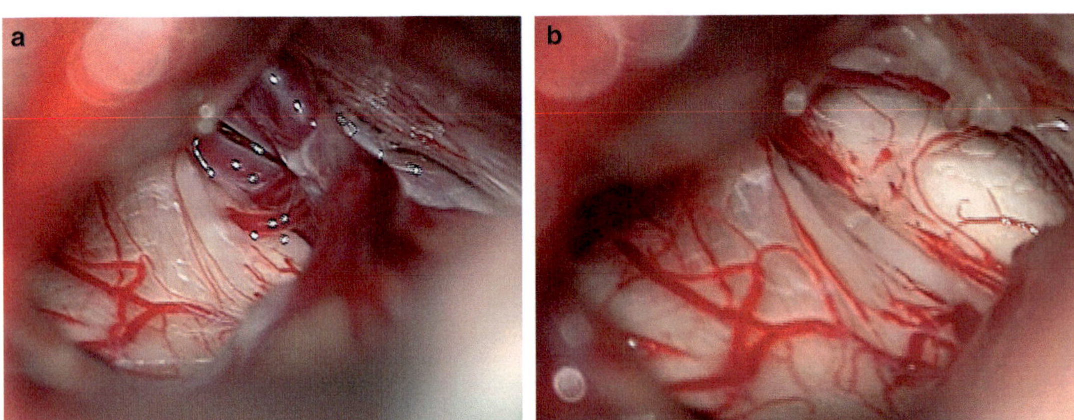

Fig. 18.5 MVD in a classic left trigeminal due to venous compression. (**a**) Picture after arachnoid dissection, where a venous plexus can be seen in relation to the trigeminal root (left to right: trigeminal root; veins; tentorium). (**b**) The nerve has been decompressed with the coagulation and section of all the venous channels, with the distal stump of the main drainage vein coagulated at its entry into the superior petrosal sinus being visible (left to right: trigeminal root; pons; tentorium)

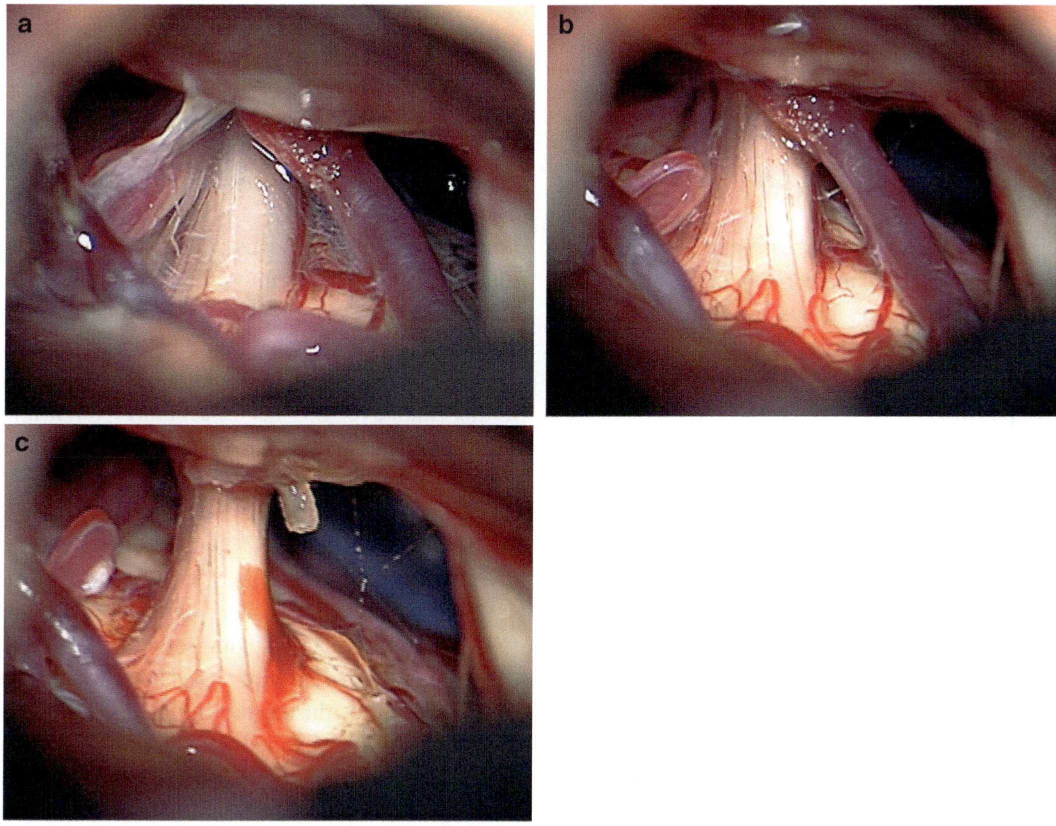

Fig. 18.6 MVD in a classic right trigeminal neuralgia due to arterial and venous compression. (**a**) Intraoperative picture displaying the right trigeminal root in relation cranially to the superior cerebellar artery and caudally to a venous channel coming from the pons and accessing the Meckel's cave. (**b**) Picture after arachnoid dissection. (**c**) The root has been decompressed with the mobilization of the superior cerebellar artery and coagulation and section of the venous channel, with the distal stump of the same coagulated being visible at its entry into the Meckel's cave (left to right: superior petrosal venous complex; superior cerebellar artery; trigeminal root; vein; facial-cochleo-vestibular complex)

the trigeminal nerve is the current version of that practiced by Dandy a century ago. The technique consists of sectioning half or two-thirds of the sensory root in its ventrolateral portion, near the pons, using fine-tipped microscissors. The technique is effective for paroxysmal pain, although with worse immediate and long-term results than with MVD, and is very frequently associated with facial hypoesthesia. Some authors propose associating rhizotomy with MVD in order to improve its effectiveness. *Internal neurolysis* consists of the longitudinal dissection of the trigeminal root with a straight dissector with a fine, blunt tip to separate the nerve fascicles in the most atraumatic way. The technique is effective for paroxysmal pain, with immediate disappearance of the pain, but with a high rate of relapses (more than 50% at 5 years) and is associated with intense facial paresthesia in the immediate postoperative period in many patients. Finally, some suggest performing a *nontraumatic manipulation of the trigeminal root* in the style proposed by Gardner. This is accomplished by applying jets of cold saline solution to the nerve (*barbotage*), gently alternating compression with the legs of a micro forceps, or mild percussion with the micro dissector.

18.7.8 Postoperative Care

Following surgery, the patient must continue taking medication to manage his pain for a few days before progressively lowering the amount in accordance with how the pain develops, with the ultimate goal of stopping all treatment entirely if at all possible.

18.8 Trigeminal Neuralgia that Requires Specific Treatment

18.8.1 Revision Surgery

Although MVD is the most effective technique for the treatment of classic TN when compared with the other available options, it is possible that it may be ineffective or that clinical relapses may occur after a period of painlessness [6, 15]. The initial failure rate is very low, probably less than 5%. Overall, the reported recurrence rate is around 10% of cases per year and increases to 20% after 10 years.

From a clinical point of view, there is consensus on reintroducing pharmacological treatment in an attempt to control the symptoms, but if the pharmacological treatment is not enough, a new neurosurgical treatment may be considered, either using percutaneous techniques or stereotactic radiosurgery. However, microneurosurgical revision of the MVD may be reconsidered, since reintervention yields clinical outcomes similar to those of the first intervention.

Many reasons have been offered to explain the recurrence, always demonstrated through the description and interpretation of the operative findings made by the neurosurgeon during the revision surgery (Fig. 18.7). The most common cause is probably inadequate decompression performed at the first surgery, particularly when there are poor initial results or early recurrence. One possibility is the development of a granuloma around the interposition material. Teflon is an inert material that should not produce a foreign body reaction, but this has been described, particularly when the Teflon is close to the dura mater. Other interposition materials may be less inert. Imaging investigations typically fail to detect this granuloma, and the presence of tiny cysts or a purported scar is neither pathognomonic nor conclusive as the cause of the clinical recurrence. Much more common seems to be the presence of a new compression of the nerve by an artery or vein, which is remarkable if decompression has already been done and, more importantly, if this maneuver has been successful for a long time. To explain this paradox, several justifications can be considered. It's possible that not all of the compressing vessels were identified, that the vessels were not sufficiently separated from the trigeminal root, and that the vessels that were sufficiently mobilized later regained a position that permitted a fresh compression. There are described cases of arterial vessels that were unrelated to the root during the initial operation that are seen to have changed their course and made unambiguous contact with the root during the revision procedure. This condition has been explained by the dissection and section of arachnoid bands carried out in the first decompression, often unnecessarily generous, which would allow the arteries to take a different course over time. Some authors have reported that these new compressing vessels are veins, and it has been postulated that new veins could develop, occluded veins could be recanalized, or the caliber of thin veins considered irrelevant in the first surgery could enlarge. Finally, a third explanation is that the development of adhesions and arachnoid scars produces distortion and displacement of the root and generates pain. Despite all these possible explanations, in almost a third of cases, no new compression is found to justify the recurrence.

However, the examination of the area allows the surgeon to attribute the causal relationship of the findings to the patient's symptoms and to propose a corrective action. In reality, the same decision tree is followed as in the first surgery. The most common actions are decompression with interposition of material if a vessel is involved; resection and release of arachnoid scar or cysts; and, in the case of granuloma, total or partial

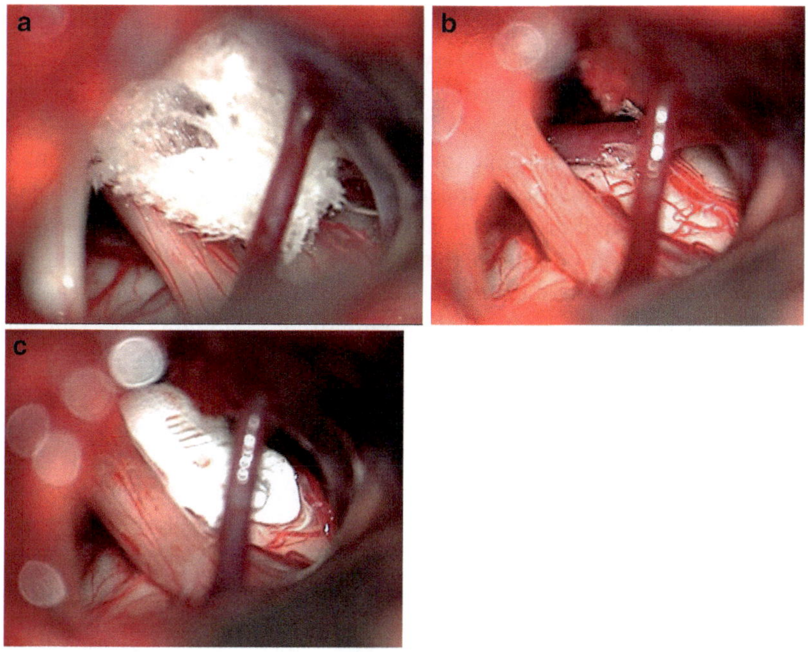

Fig. 18.7 Revision surgery for recurrent trigeminal neuralgia 3 years after MVD. (**a**) Intraoperative picture displaying the left trigeminal root with the interposition material placed (Gelfoam) in the prior intervention. No granuloma or arachnoid reaction is observed. (**b**) Picture after removal of the material. The nerve appears deformed, and the superior cerebellar artery can be seen behind it. (**c**) Final stage, after the placement of a new interposition material (Goretex) (left to right: facial-cochleo-vestibular complex; trigeminal root; interposed material; pons; venous complex superior petrosal)

resection, avoiding the root attrition and the placement of a new interposition material. If no new cause of compression is found, internal neurolysis or atraumatic manipulation of the nerve can be performed.

18.8.2 Secondary Trigeminal Neuralgia

In cases where TN is secondary to a structural pathology of the cerebellopontine angle, both the lesion and the compression must be solved. Regarding compression, the relationships between the lesion and the neurovascular elements have been classified into four different situations according to the pattern of the relationship between the tumor and the trigeminal nerve: the nerve is completely buried by the tumor, but without displacement; the nerve is compressed and distorted by the tumor; the nerve is displaced in a cranial or caudal direction by the tumor and is directly compressed by an artery on the opposite side of the nerve; and finally, the nerve is directly compressed by an artery displaced by the tumor located on the same side. In the first cases, the removal of the lesion ensures decompression of the nerve, while in the other two situations, the removal of the lesion must be accompanied by mobilization of the artery and, eventually, the placement of an interposed material to maintain the separation of the neurovascular elements (*refer to cases 17 and 28 in* Chap. 21).

18.9 Complications, Prevention, and Management

Complications related to the approach are those common to the retrosigmoid approach, as reviewed elsewhere. The selection of patients for less aggressive techniques in the case of systemic pathology or elderly patients, and the absence of pathology that allows for anatomical surgery allows for minimizing general and procedure-related complications. However, although MVD is not a damaging technique, it requires manipulation of the neurovascular structures of the upper group. Mandatory manipulation of the trigeminal nerve can produce hypoesthesia or neuropathic pain, while accidental manipulation of the neighboring nerves can produce hypoacusis, facial paresis, or diplopia. Vascular manipulation can produce arterial or venous rupture with intraoperative hemorrhage or ischemia due to spasm, angulation, or excessive compression of the arteries by the interposed material. These are conditions with very variable clinical expression, given the variability in the distribution of vascular territories between the superior cerebellar artery and the anteroinferior cerebellar artery. However, in the case of injury, it occurs in a very distal segment, where most of the perforating branches to the arteries to the brainstem have already given, so the clinical expression is not very relevant. Finally, venous infarction resulting from coagulation and section or thrombosis of the superior petrosal vein must be considered. In this case, a small percentage of patients may present changes in imaging studies and very varied clinical symptoms, generally minor and transient, which can be attributed to the individual variability of venous drainage through the petrosal vein. Symptoms include headache, ataxia, or facial paresis, which usually appear a few days after surgery and do not alter the prognosis for pain. A thorough understanding of the cerebellopontine angle's microsurgical anatomy and a masterful microneurosurgical technique are the foundations for preventing all of these issues.

18.10 Outcome, Prognosis, and Follow-Up

The clinical outcome of TN treatment is assessed using the *Barrow's Neurological Institute Pain Intensity Scale*, which has five grades: (1) meaning no pain and no medical treatment; (2) meaning occasional pain and no need for medical treatment; (3) meaning pain adequately controlled with medical treatment; (4) meaning pain not adequately controlled with medical treatment; and (5) meaning severe pain not controlled with medical treatment. Grades 1–3 are regarded as good results, whereas grades 4–5 are regarded as poor results. A parametric scale is also employed, combining the Pain Intensity Score for residual paroxysmal pain evaluation with the *Facial Numbness Score* for residual neuropathic pain evaluation. This scale has four grades: (1) meaning no facial numbness; (2) meaning mild facial numbness, not bothersome; (3) meaning facial numbness, somewhat bothersome; (4) meaning facial numbness, very bothersome. A result is rated as excellent if it receives a total score of 2 points, good if it receives 3 points, average if it receives 4 points, and poor if it is greater than five points. Some authors propose that the outcome of MVD should be assessed months after surgery, since the necessary manipulation required for decompression and interposition of the material could have a transitory effect on paroxysmal pain, as do percutaneous techniques or nontraumatic nerve manipulation.

Initial results of MVD show that more than 80% of patients have good short-term results in the immediate postoperative period, and at 10 years, more than 70% of patients maintain good results. The recurrence rate is <2% per year in the first 5 years and drops to <1% thereafter. Predictive factors for a good long-term prognosis after MVD have been identified, some of them imaging studies and others, more interesting, of a clinical nature (disappearance of pain immediately after the intervention; duration of neuralgia; compression by a single vessel; absence of venous compression; age under 70 years; male sex). Predictive factors for recurrence of pain after MVD have also been described (absence of vascular compression; previous percutaneous surgery or stereotactic radiosurgery; nature of the pain, with a worse prognosis for patients with sustained pain associated with paroxysmal pain;

pain affecting two or more branches; duration of neuralgia; female sex).

18.11 Management Modalities

18.11.1 Medical Treatment

Given that every treatment for TN is quite successful, the sequence in which the various treatments are administered is crucial. Every scientific society agrees that pharmaceutical treatment should be the first line of treatment for every patient. However, the time limits for treatment, the optimal number of drugs, and the pharmacological principles necessary to control pain before offering the patient the option of surgical treatment are not well defined. The general principles for guiding patients towards surgical treatment are: pain resistant to drugs (carbamazepine or oxycarbamazepine, combined with gabapentin, pregabalin, or lamotrigine); pain controlled with drugs, but at doses that produce serious or undesirable adverse effects for the patient; and, finally, the patient's desire to abandon medical treatment. There are no studies in which patients are offered neurosurgical treatment as a first option, and, naturally, there are also no comparative studies of surgical techniques with sham surgery control groups. When the patient comes to the neurosurgical office, he or she does so after months or years of pharmacological treatment and under the supervision of a neurologist who has ruled out a neurological disease. All patients have an imaging study, usually an MRI, which rules out a lesion in the cerebellopontine angle. Occasionally, patients have received minimally aggressive treatments, such as anesthetic blocks of peripheral branches of the trigeminal nerve. Fortunately, it is increasingly rare for patients to undergo surgical peripheral neurectomies, peripheral block of the branches of the trigeminal nerve with alcohol injections, radiofrequency, or cryolesions. Although the purpose of these procedures is symptomatic relief in exchange for producing an area of facial anesthesia, the result may be the development of neuropathic pain, like painful anesthesia.

18.11.2 Neurosurgical Treatment

Three surgical therapy options are available to the neurosurgeon: stereotactic radiosurgery, percutaneous methods, and MVD [1, 2, 8, 10, 12, 15, 16]. Therefore, choosing patients is crucial to prescribe the best course of treatment for their needs, which requires taking into account several factors. A thorough interview with the patient and their loved ones is essential in this regard. Below is a review of these elements.

18.11.2.1 Potential Damage to the Trigeminal Nerve

In theory, MVD is a technique that is neither damaging nor destructive, beyond the manipulation required during surgery to achieve decompression. By definition, any of the percutaneous techniques currently used is a technique that damages or destroys the nerve by applying thermal energy (radiofrequency thermocoagulation), mechanical energy (compression with an inflatable balloon), or chemical energy (glycerol injection). The nerve injury is partial, controlled, and reversible, especially affecting the thick myelinated fibers. Is the reversibility of the injury of the nerve fibers what explains the high rate of recurrences. Also, the repetition of the technique makes it necessary to injure more fibers to achieve the same initial effects, which triggers a higher rate of morbidity. Finally, stereotactic radiosurgery is also a damaging technique with the application of ionizing radiation of different types, either with a gamma knife or with a linear accelerator (LINAC).

18.11.2.2 General Risk Related to the Surgical Procedure

Stereotactic radiosurgery is a noninvasive and completely harmless technique, beyond the fixation of the stereotactic frame when it is considered necessary. Percutaneous techniques are minimally invasive and are performed in outpatient surgery settings or surgery without admission programs, but they are not harmless, and acute and relevant complications may occur. Finally, MVD is a major surgery since it requires a craniotomy and postoperative care in a neurological care unit for critical patients, with a potentially serious, specific acute or subacute morbidity. However, some studies report outpatient programs for MVD in selected patients.

18.11.2.3 General Condition and Age of the Patient

MVD is a major surgery, while any percutaneous technique is a minor surgery, of short duration and under local anesthesia and sedation, except for the need to deepen sedation for short periods of time with ultra-short-acting drugs. Therefore, percutaneous techniques should be recommended for older patients with high anesthetic risk, as well as for those who do not wish to undergo major or open surgery, while MVD is recommended for the rest of the cases, especially for younger patients. Stereotactic radiosurgery can be applied to any patient regardless of their general condition or age.

18.11.2.4 Acceptance of Paresthesia and Location of Pain

The purpose of percutaneous techniques is the controlled destruction of nerve fibers, so a necessary consequence of surgery is that parenthetic sensations and hypoesthesia will remain in the cutaneous area of the injured branch. In order to provide the patient, the opportunity to be aware of the feelings they might expect to experience in the postoperative period, some authors advise, prior to the intervention, performing an anesthetic blockade of the nerves that will be targeted. Only those patients who accept these sensations would be candidates for the percutaneous technique of choice. Classically, the involvement of the first branch of the trigeminal nerve has been rejected as an indication for these techniques since it is possible to produce corneal anesthesia with the consequent risk of corneal ulceration, infection, and loss of vision.

18.11.2.5 Patient Expectations

Both MVD and percutaneous techniques offer excellent results in the immediate postoperative period, while clinical improvement with stereotactic radiosurgery is only achieved over time. The probability of pain recurrence after MVD is much lower than after percutaneous techniques or stereotactic radiosurgery.

18.11.2.6 Availability and Surgical Practice

Percutaneous techniques require relatively simple equipment, can be carried out in a non-complex surgical environment such as an interventional radiology room, and are not very demanding for the neurosurgeon. In contrast, MVD requires expensive and complex equipment, must be carried out in a complex operating room with the support of an appropriate postoperative care unit, and requires a neurosurgical team with expertise in cerebellopontine angle surgery. Stereotactic radiosurgery requires the most expensive and scarce equipment, particularly if performed with the gamma knife, so access to these resources is much more difficult. Although any therapeutic technique must be carried out by specialized personnel with high technical training, it is clear that this level of experience is critical for MVD and stereotactic radiosurgery and of a lower level for percutaneous techniques.

18.11.2.7 Clinical Results

In terms of results, there is sufficient information obtained from clinical experience to offer a fairly precise view of the benefits and problems of each of the techniques. MVD is highly effective in controlling pain, and 60–90% of patients, according to published series, are pain-free at follow-up 3–11 years after surgery. Severe complications are rare (mortality 0.3%; edema, hemorrhage, or ischemia 0.6%; meningitis 0.4% and painful anesthesia 0.02%). Less serious complications, such as cranial nerve injury (4%), hearing loss (1.8%), and facial hypoesthesia (3%), are more frequent but transitory. With percutaneous techniques, the percentage of pain-free patients at 4–11 years is 30–80% for radiofrequency, 55–80% for balloon compression, and 20–60% for glycerol. The most frequent complications are facial hypoesthesia (19%), corneal hypoesthesia (5%), and trigeminal motor weakness (5%), with meningitis (0.7%) and painful anesthesia (0.5%) being the rarest and most serious complications. Finally, the literature review shows that stereotactic radiosurgery results in 50–55% of patients being pain-free without treatment. Patients reported hypoesthesia in 25% of cases, but other patients complained of dysesthesia, paraesthesia, dry eye, or keratitis.

Overall, it can be stated that MVD is the surgical technique of choice in classic TN, and should therefore be the first surgical procedure carried out in patients who have failed pharmacological treatment, provided that there is no formal contraindication or refusal by the patient. MVD performed after failure of percutaneous techniques or stereotactic radiosurgery is significantly less effective than if performed as a first procedure; fortunately, with the procedure-related morbidity being almost the same.

18.12 Key Messages

- *The most prevalent neurovascular compression in the cerebellopontine angle is classical TN.*
- *The recommended microneurosurgical technique for treating classic TN is the MVD of the trigeminal root in the cerebellopontine angle.*
- *The recommended microneurosurgical treatment for secondary TN brought on by tumors and other cerebellopontine angle lesions is to remove the lesion microsurgically, securing the decompression of the trigeminal root.*
- *For certain selected patients with TN, additional neurosurgical treatments such as stereotactic radiosurgery and percutaneous procedures are advised.*
- *Although all TN therapies are highly effective, each one has unique characteristics that require the neurosurgeon to choose carefully the right candidates.*

References

1. Bendtsen L, Zakrzewska JM, Heinskou TB, et al. Advances in diagnosis, classification, pathophysiology, and management of trigeminal neuralgia. Lancet Neurol. 2020;19:784–96. https://doi.org/10.1016/S1474-4422(20)30233-7.
2. Cruccu G, Di Stefano G, Truini A. Trigeminal neuralgia. N Engl J Med. 2020;383:754–62. https://doi.org/10.1056/NEJMra1914484.
3. González-Darder JM, Quilis-Quesada V, Capilla-Guasch P, de Oliveira E. Abordajes neuroquirúrgicos de la patología craneal y cerebral. 2nd ed. Barcelona: Elsevier España; 2020.
4. Kaufmann AM, Price AV. A history of the Jannetta procedure. J Neurosurg. 2019;132:639–46. https://doi.org/10.3171/2018.10.JNS181983. PMID: 30717044
5. Haller S, Etienne L, Kövari E, et al. Imaging of neurovascular compression syndromes: trigeminal neuralgia, hemifacial spasm, vestibular paroxysmia, and glossopharyngeal neuralgia. AJNR Am J Neuroradiol. 2016;37(8):1384–92. https://doi.org/10.3174/ajnr.A4683.
6. Hussain MA, Konteas A, Sunderland G, et al. Re-exploration of microvascular decompression in recurrent trigeminal neuralgia and intraoperative management options. World Neurosurg. 2018;117:e67–74. https://doi.org/10.1016/j.wneu.2018.05.147.
7. Liu Y, Yu Y, Wang Z, et al. Value of partial sensory rhizotomy in the microsurgical treatment of trigeminal neuralgia through retrosigmoid approach. J Pain Res. 2020;13:3207–15. https://doi.org/10.2147/JPR.S279674. PMID: 33299344
8. Park CK, Park BJ. Surgical treatment for trigeminal neuralgia. J Korean Neurosurg Soc. 2022;65:615–21. https://doi.org/10.3340/jkns.2021.0265.
9. Rhoton AL Jr. The posterior fossa: microsurgical anatomy & surgical approaches. Neurosurgery. 2000;47(Suppl 3):S1–S279. https://doi.org/10.1097/00006123-200009001-00013.
10. Tatagiba MS, Roser F, Hirt, et al. The retrosigmoid endoscopic approach for cerebellopontine-angle tumors and microvascular decompression. World Neurosurg. 2014;82:S171–6. https://doi.org/10.1016/j.wneu.2014.08.001.
11. Tsunoda S, Inoue T, Segawa M, et al. Vein-related trigeminal neuralgia: how to determine the treatment method of the causative vein: a technical note. Neurol Med Chir (Tokyo). 2022;62:105–9. https://doi.org/10.2176/nmc.tn.2021-0154.
12. Tuleasca C, Régis J, Sahgal A, et al. Stereotactic radiosurgery for trigeminal neuralgia: a systematic review. J Neurosurg. 2018;130:733–57. https://doi.org/10.3171/2017.9.JNS17545.
13. Patel SK, Markosian C, Choudhry OJ, et al. The historical evolution of microvascular decompression

for trigeminal neuralgia: from Dandy's discovery to Jannetta's legacy. Acta Neurochir. 2020;162:2773–82. https://doi.org/10.1007/s00701-020-04405-7.
14. Sindou M, Brinzeu A. Trigeminal neuralgias: a neurosurgical illustrated guide. Cham: Springer; 2023.
15. Theodros D, Rory Goodwin C, Bender MT, et al. Efficacy of primary microvascular decompression versus subsequent microvascular decompression for trigeminal neuralgia. J Neurosurg. 2017;126:1691–7. https://doi.org/10.3171/2016.5.JNS151692.
16. Wu M, Fu X, Ji Y, et al. Microvascular decompression for classical trigeminal neuralgia caused by venous compression: novel anatomic classifications and surgical strategy. World Neurosurg. 2018;113:e707–13. https://doi.org/10.1016/j.wneu.2018.02.130.

19 Other Neurovascular Compression Syndromes in the Cerebellopontine Angle

19.1 Introduction

Shortly after linking neurovascular compression of the trigeminal root with trigeminal neuralgia and proposing microvascular decompression (MVD) as a treatment, it was also Peter Jannetta (1932–2016) who expanded the list of neurological syndromes with the same pathophysiology and consequently with the same proposal for microneurosurgical treatment. This set of diseases was grouped under the name of *cranial rhizopathies*, which include trigeminal neuralgia, hemifacial spasm, glossopharyngeal neuralgia, vestibulocochlear dysfunction, masticatory hemispasm, and neurogenic arterial hypertension [1]. All of these are clinical syndromes secondary to neurovascular compression of the entry zone of the cranial nerve roots and are relieved by MVD of the responsible arterial or venous vessels [5]. With diagnostic techniques using magnetic resonance imaging (MRI) in highly T2-weighted sequences with very thin sections, it is possible to identify neurovascular compression in an increasing number of patients. These clinical syndromes were classified as primary, idiopathic, or essential when there was no neurological or structural disease to explain symptoms and as secondary when there was such a neurological or structural disease. The number of patients in the first category is declining as a result of imaging investigations that have made it possible to identify microvascular compression in many cases of essential or idiopathic cause. It also justifies surgical exploration of selected patients without neurological or structural pathology demonstrated in imaging studies, in search of neurovascular compression. After having reviewed trigeminal neuralgia in the previous chapter, in this chapter, we will review the different neurovascular compression syndromes that benefit from MVD.

19.2 Hemifacial Spasm

Hemifacial spasm is the second most prevalent syndrome brought on by neurovascular compression in the cerebellopontine angle. Hemifacial spasm was first accurately described by Babinski at the beginning of the last century. As with microvascular compression of the trigeminal root, it was also Walter Dandy (1886–1946), about a hundred years ago, who was the first neurosurgeon to observe the anatomical relationship between the facial nerve root and tumors or vascular loops and elongations in patients with hemifacial spasm, although again, as in the case of trigeminal neuralgia, he did not propose a causal relationship between the two events. In the sixties and seventies of the last century, it was James Gardner and Peter Jannetta who re-described this anatomical relationship and proposed MVD as a useful treatment [3]. The details and vicissitudes of these events have been

J. M. González-Darder, *Microneurosurgery of Cerebellopontine Angle*,
https://doi.org/10.1007/978-3-032-03091-7_19

detailed in the previous chapter devoted to trigeminal neuralgia.

19.2.1 Anatomical Considerations

The facial nerve root is part of the middle neurovascular complex described by Rhoton, which includes the abducens nerve, facial nerve, and vestibulocochlear nerve, together with the anterior inferior cerebellar artery (AICA). The facial and vestibulocochlear nerves originate laterally in the medullary-pontine sulcus, just above the supra-olivary fossa. Here, the origin of the facial nerve is slightly anterior and inferior to the exit of the vestibulocochlear nerve, and therefore, in the retrosigmoid approach, the facial nerve can be completely hidden by the vestibulocochlear nerve. The so-called intermediate nerve of Wrisberg is formed by a variable number of rootlets that originate and are located between both nerves, with adhesions to both. The facial-vestibulocochlear-intermediate complex runs superior-laterally to the internal auditory meatus (Fig. 19.1). The average length of the cisternal segment of the facial–vestibulocochlear nerve complex roots to the internal acoustic meatus is about 15 mm, with a similar length within the internal auditory canal. The total number of myelinated fibers of the facial nerve is between 10,000 and 15,000, and of the intermediate nerve, between 3000 and 5500, with less than 15% of unmyelinated fibers. The facial nerve carries motor, sensory, and parasympathetic fibers. The facial nerve has a relatively short number of nerve fibers in relation to the more than forty facial muscles that it must mobilize, apart from the fibers dedicated to conveying the parasympathetic function and the collection of sensitivity from a small cutaneous area of the ear and external auditory canal, and the taste sensation from the anterior two-thirds of the tongue. This explains the difficulty of the functional motor recovery of the facial nerve after it has been injured, since each muscle has a limited number of motor plates that must be activated again in a very precise and selective way in the process of Wallerian regeneration [17].

The anterior inferior cerebellar artery arises from the basilar artery (BA) trunk and divides into four parts: the anterior pontine segment, the lateral pontine segment, the flocculopeduncular segment, and finally, the cortical segment. The lateral pontine segment corresponds to the course of the anterior inferior cerebellar artery along the cerebellopontine angle, where the artery may be related to the facial and vestibulocochlear nerve roots and may contact, deform, or distort these nerves. The anatomical relationships and branches of the anterior inferior cerebellar artery in this segment are complex and variable. The trunk of the artery usually runs anterior and inferior to the nerves, and in two-thirds of cases, there is an arterial loop that runs to the internal

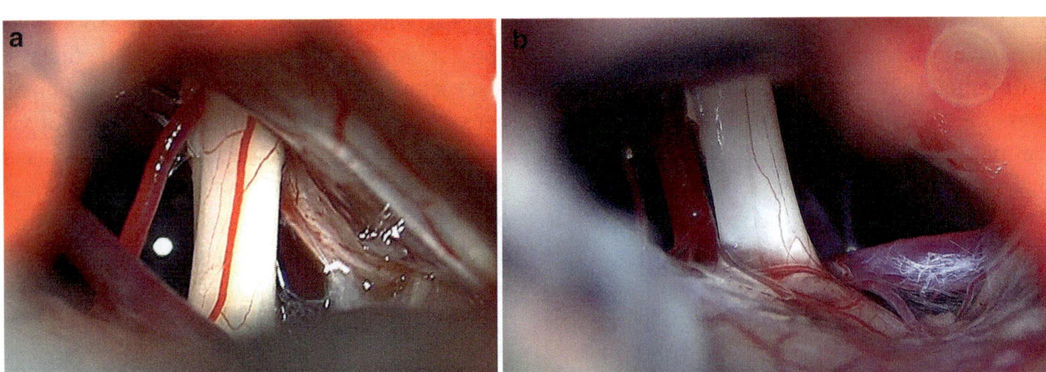

Fig. 19.1 Intraoperative pictures of the right facial–vestibulocochlear complex roots (left to right: facial–cochleovestibular nerves complex; petrosal bone). (**a**) Arterial loop of the anterior inferior cerebellar artery running between both nerves. (**b**) Vein running near nerves and a large anteroinferior cerebellar artery

auditory meatus. This meatal portion of the artery usually runs between the facial and vestibulocochlear nerves and may lie medial to the meatus, reach it, or enter the internal auditory canal. The meatal portion of the artery gives off the labyrinthine or internal auditory artery, which enters the internal auditory canal, giving off small branches to the bone, dura mater, and inner ear. After the meatal loop, the artery turns medially to supply the brainstem and cerebellum and to relate again to the facial and vestibulocochlear nerves. The facial nerve root is supplied with blood at the cerebellopontine angle by the confluence of proximal and distal root arteries. The proximal artery runs on the anterior surface of the nerve and is formed by the union of an arteriole arising from the premeatal segment of the anterior inferior cerebellar artery with a terminal branch of a short circumferential artery arising from the basilar artery, and sometimes with an arteriole arising from the anterior inferior cerebellar artery at its postmeatal segment. The distal artery has a double origin, with an arteriole arising from the anterior vestibular artery, a branch of the labyrinthine artery at the level of the horizontal crest of the fundus of the internal auditory canal, and/or from a branch arising from the loop of the anterior inferior cerebellar artery or its branches.

The venous drainage of this middle level of the cerebellopontine angle is mainly via the vein of the cerebellopontine fissure, formed by the confluence of several minor veins, and which runs cranially towards the superior petrosal venous complex. Another venous channel is the vein of the middle cerebellar peduncle, originating in the medullary-pontine sulcus and which also runs cranially towards the superior petrosal complex [11].

19.2.2 Pathology

As we have reported, Dandy was the first to observe the intimate anatomical relationships of the anterior inferior cerebellar artery with the root of the facial nerve in patients with hemifacial spasm. There are two etiopathogenic forms of hemifacial spasm: primary, which is associated with microvascular compression of the nerve root, and secondary, which is associated with any type of lesion that affects the nerve in its route from the motor nucleus in the brainstem to the stylomastoid foramen.

19.2.2.1 Primary Hemifacial Spasm

The pathophysiology of hemifacial spasm is considered to be the same as that of trigeminal neuralgia, that is, the formation of anomalous connections between nerve fibers in the so-called *entry zone* and *Obersteiner–Redlich transitional zone* that generate aberrant nerve impulses. In this area, the nerve fibers still have the glioneural sheath provided by oligodendroglia and the outermost support of astrocytes, before being protected by the myelin sheath provided by Schwann cells and the connective elements that form the endoneurium, such as fibroblasts and fibers of the extracellular matrix, such as collagen. The transitional zone between the central and peripheral myelin sheath does not occur at the same level in all fibers and adopts a conical morphology over a few microns throughout the root, that is, more distally in the center of the nerve. In the case of the facial nerve root, the average distance of the central myelin sheath is 3 mm, which represents less than 20% of the intracranial length of the root, which measures approximately 18 mm. This exit zone of the facial nerve is restricted to its course through the medullary-pontine sulcus [4].

The accepted underlying mechanism is that the pulsating mechanical energy of arterial compression produces focal demyelination of nerve fibers with the possibility of generating spontaneous anomalous nerve impulses (*ectopic excitation*) involving different axons connected by a kind of anomalous mechanical or chemical synapses (*ephaptic transmission*). These generated impulses could have a retrograde sense towards the motor nucleus of the facial nerve in the brainstem, causing neuronal hyperexcitability that in turn generates spontaneous motor impulses towards peripheral muscles. Alternatively, another possibility is that the impulses generated in the demyelination zone recruit neighboring fibers (*cross-talk mechanism*) that directly discharge towards peripheral muscles.

Microvascular compression is the cause of hemifacial spasm in approximately three-quarters of patients [4, 8, 9]. The vascular element responsible for the compression is usually an artery, the anterior inferior cerebellar artery, the posterior inferior cerebellar artery, or the vertebral artery. There are anatomical variations, with large elongations or loops. Asymmetry of the vertebral arteries before they join to form the basilar artery trunk is a risk factor. Compression may be caused by a single vessel or by several, but mixed compression of an artery and a vein is very rare. Only in a very small proportion of patients explored surgically is no vascular element found to be responsible. Although the distribution of the artery causing the compression varies according to the series, studies in the literature show that the posterior inferior cerebellar artery is the most frequent (50% of cases), followed by the anterior inferior cerebellar artery (45%), the vertebrobasilar complex in 17% of cases, perforating arteries in 10%, and veins in less than 10%. In diagnostic imaging series, there is an overrepresentation of facial nerve compressions by the vertebral arteries or the basilar artery, because they are more conspicuous in diagnostic studies. In these series, compression by these large dilated or elongated vessels reaches 20% of cases and is more frequent on the left side as it corresponds to the greater frequency of dominance of the left vertebral artery. A very characteristic type of compression is that produced by the loop of the anterior inferior cerebellar artery that enters the internal auditory canal. Different relationships between the arteries and the nerve root have been described: loop type, where the artery directly produces the compression; arachnoid type, where there are arachnoid trabeculae between the vessel and the brainstem that would transmit the tension; perforating type, where the perforating arteries of the compressing artery that go to the trunk of the nerve root; division type, where the nerve is trapped between the compressing artery and its branches; sandwich type, where the nerve is sandwiched between two different arteries; and, finally, tandem type, where one artery displaces another artery that in turn compresses the nerve. Thus, the location of the neurovascular compression of the facial nerve root can be observed in several areas: the exit point of the nerve root, the proximal segment of the root, the Obersteiner–Redlich transition zone between central and peripheral axonal myelination, the rest of the cisternal portion of the nerve, and, finally, in the intrameatal portion of the nerve. Surgical studies show a great variability in the point of compression, indicating that only in one quarter does the compression of the facial nerve occur in the proximal portion of the root, while in the other three quarters the compression is more distal.

19.2.2.2 Secondary Hemifacial Spasm

This includes neurological lesions of vascular, inflammatory, or demyelinating type located in the brainstem, as well as tumor and tumor-like lesions occupying the cerebellopontine angle. The most frequent tumors are vestibular schwannomas, epidermoid cysts, and meningiomas. In these cases, hemifacial spasm may be associated with other neurological problems with symptoms or signs of involvement of cranial nerves or the brainstem.

19.2.3 Clinical Considerations

Hemifacial spasm is clinically characterized by the involuntary contraction of the facial muscles on one side of the face [1, 7]. The spasms can vary greatly, from brief, more or less focused contractions of the facial muscles in the form of short-term crises to long-lasting mass contractions of all the muscles that produce an unpleasant grimace or disfigurement of the face that lasts over time. In most patients, the onset is insidious, with spasms of small muscle groups, involuntary and uncontrollable, and often synkinesis, in some cases associated with triggering or aggravating factors, such as anxiety, stress, fatigue, certain head positions, eating, or chewing. It usually begins with the muscles of the upper part of the face, so the eye closure predominates due to spasm of the orbicularis oculi. Over time, the affection of the muscles becomes more extensive. It can persist during sleep and, exceptionally, can be bilateral. During crises, the so-called *Babinski-2 sign* can occur, which consists of simultaneous elevation of the eyebrow and closure of the eye, which is almost pathognomonic of hemifacial spasm. This is because when the orbicularis oculi muscle contracts, closing the eye, the medial part of the frontal muscle contracts at the same time, raising the eyebrow. The female sex is predominant, and it affects mainly people in their fourth and fifth decades of life. A prevalence of 10 cases per 100,000 people has been calculated. The sustained spasm can produce a series of secondary symptoms, such as visual disorders due to the repeated and involuntary closure of the eye, dysarthria due to lack of motor coordination, or craniofacial pain due to muscle tension. Finally, the chronicity of the symptoms and their aesthetic impact can determine personality disorders, particularly of a depressive type.

As is currently the case with most neurosurgical disorders, the diagnosis is never made by the neurosurgeon, and patients are referred to the consultation by neurologists after diagnostic confirmation and lack of response to pharmacological treatment. The clinical differential diagnosis of hemifacial spasm includes a long list of neurological processes that have in common some type of paroxysmal motor disorder in the face. The most frequent clinical situations requiring differential diagnosis are psychogenic functional disorders, facial tics, and even facial paralysis. For example, Bell's palsy, especially in the recovery phase, may be accompanied by facial synkinesis that mimics hemifacial spasm and is restricted to the side of the face previously affected by the paralysis. The facial tic is a brief movement, sometimes alternating on the side, and the psychogenic spasms are anarchic in intensity, frequency, and distribution, although in both cases they predominate in the lower facial territory, and the Babinski-2 sign is absent. Other neurological problems to consider include, among others, facial myokines, post-encephalitis facial myoclonus, or facial dystonia such as blepharospasm, oromandibular dystonia, and Meige's syndrome.

19.2.4 Diagnostic Considerations

All patients with hemifacial spasm should be studied with neuroimaging techniques, particularly magnetic resonance imaging (MRI), including T1-weighted TOF (*Time Of Flight angiography*) and T1-weighted sequences with gadolinium, as well as high-resolution T2-weighted sequences such as FIESTA (*Fast Imaging Employing Steady State Acquisition*). The objective of this study is to rule out the existence of a tumor or neurological disease to identify secondary hemifacial spasm and try to demonstrate microvascular compression to confirm the diagnosis of primary hemifacial spasm (Fig. 19.2). The imaging of the different types of tumors and lesions of the cerebellopontine angle is described in the chapters corresponding to each pathology. On the other hand, it is not always possible to demonstrate vascular compression on MRI to presume that it exists, being easier when it is determined by large-caliber arteries, such as the vertebral or basilar arteries. However, the absence of vascular compression

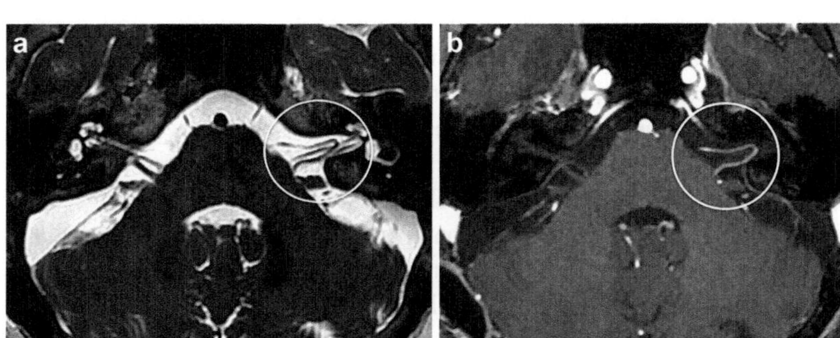

Fig. 19.2 Loop of the left anteroinferior cerebellar artery loop entering in to the internal acoustic canal. (**a**) Axial FIESTA slice. (**b**) Axial T1-weighted with gadolinium slice

does not exclude its finding in the microneurosurgical exploration of the nerve root, since this occurs and is found in practically all patients. The neurophysiological study is very useful to confirm the diagnosis. The activity of the needle electromyography (EMG) at rest shows spontaneous activity, and the activity in voluntary contraction is normal. Other nerve conduction tests demonstrate the existence of axonal short circuits. In the same way, the clinical diagnosis of hemifacial spasm is a task of the neurologist; it is the neurosurgeon's duty to get imaging studies that show with a high degree of probability the presence of microvascular compression of the facial nerve root before recommending a microneurosurgical exploration [5].

19.2.5 Surgical Types

Basically, there are two situations in the neurosurgical exploration of the cerebellopontine angle in patients with hemifacial spasm. In primary hemifacial spasm, the nerve root is compressed by one or more vessels, either arteries and/or veins [4]. In secondary hemifacial spasm, the nerve is compressed by a corresponding tumor or structural lesion of the cerebellopontine angle. Microneurosurgical exploration without findings of vascular or structural compression is exceptional.

19.2.6 Microneurosurgical Management

Currently, microneurosurgical treatment of hemifacial spasm is done exclusively through a retrosigmoid approach that allows access to the root of the facial nerve, from its apparent exit at the medullary–pontine junction in its cisternal course to its entry into the internal acoustic meatus and its exposure in the internal auditory canal, as well as the exploration of the vascular elements that are responsible for the compression [8, 9]. The retrosigmoid approach is also routinely used to solve the pathology of the cerebellopontine angle, whether tumoral or otherwise, responsible for the compression of the facial nerve in secondary hemifacial spasm.

19.2.6.1 Microvascular Decompression

The strategy for MVD should follow the following steps: identification of the nerve and the vascular elements of compression, vascular decompression, and, finally, maintenance of decompression. The retrosigmoid approach should be framed by the angle formed by the confluence of the transverse sinus with the sigmoid sinus. The craniotomy does not need to be extensive, since there are no intracranial space-occupying lesions, and cisternal navigation is comfortable. An alternative to the standard retrosigmoid approach with microsurgery is the endoscopic approach [15]. The width of the cisterns can be predicted in imaging studies, and, in this sense, it is frequently observed that the cisterns of patients with hemifacial spasm are of a smaller volume than average. The spatula of the retractor should be placed on the most lateral part of the petrosal surface of the cerebellum to gain space, centering it on the facial–vestibulocochlear complex.

The next step is to section the arachnoid adhesions in the area with fine scissors, in particular those that attach the nerve to the flocculus of the cerebellum, which allows more of the nerve complex to be exposed until the choroid plexuses that emerge at the cerebellopontine angle through the lateral recesses of the fourth ventricle and mark the level of the medullary-pontine sulcus, the anatomical level of emergence of the nerves, can be visualized. Access to this area can be facilitated by opening the petrosal fissure on the petrosal surface of the cerebellum, which allows space to be gained and also directs the path toward the flocculus and choroid plexus. Once the nerve complex has been identified, it must be cleared of arachnoid to perform a systematic evaluation of the nerve complex and microvascular compression. First, the facial nerve root is clearly identified with respect to the vestibulocochlear nerve due to its deeper anatomical location in the surgical field as it exits more medially. The facial nerve is whiter and brighter in appearance and also is helpful the neurophysiological response to direct electrical stimulation. At this point, the entire nerve root is visualized up to its entry into the internal auditory canal through the meatus. Once the facial nerve is exposed, the existence of any undetected lesion in the imaging studies is ruled out, and vascular elements are identified (Fig. 19.3a).

The veins are then explored, usually more conspicuous and visible than the arteries, which, if they are related to the nerve, are freed from the arachnoid and mobilized. The arteries are then explored. In the case of compression by the posterior inferior cerebellar artery or vertebral artery, compression occurs caudally, and arteries are mobilized in turn caudally and medially, releasing and dragging the perforating arteries that go to the brainstem. In the case of compression by the anterior inferior cerebellar artery, mobilization and decompression may be more difficult, since it is not unusual for the meatal loop to be located between the facial and vestibulocochlear nerve roots. Although the theoretical cause of hemifacial spasm is compression of the nerve entry area, it is not uncommon to find more distal compressions along the entire course of the nerve, so the examination must be systematic throughout the entire course of the nerve, both its anterior and posterior sides. In the particular case of a long loop that enters the internal auditory canal through the meatus, there is no other option than to carry out a transmeatal access, in the same way as described for intracanalicular vestibular schwannoma (Fig. 19.3b, c). However, in this case, the internal auditory artery that usually emerges from the end of the loop towards the inner ear must be identified and preserved, since otherwise there may be hearing loss due to ischemia. A highly complex situation is the decompression produced by large-caliber vessels that occurs in the most caudal portion of the nerve root. In this case, it has been proposed to access the nerve by taking a more caudal route, through

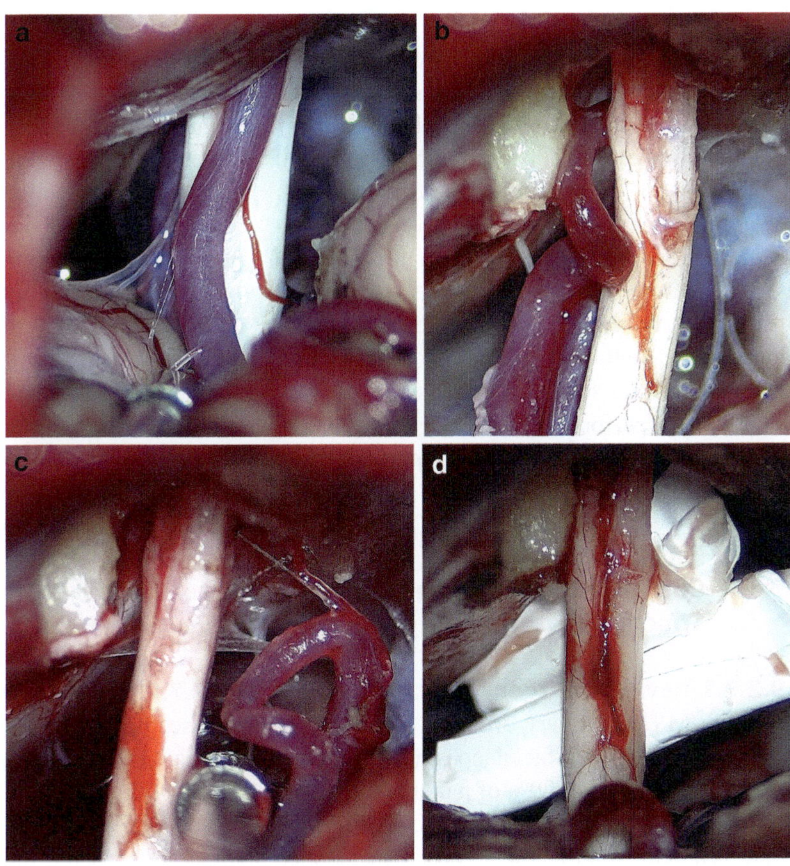

Fig. 19.3 MVD in a hemifacial spasm due to the intracanalicular compression of a loop of the left anteroinferior cerebellar artery. (**a**) Intraoperative picture after arachnoid dissection, displaying the proximal part of the arterial loop behind the nerves and the distal part in a direct view. (**b**) After drilling the auditory canal, the loop is fully exposed. (**c**) The arterial loop has been mobilized, and the internal auditory artery is seen arising from the convexity of the loop. (**d**) Picture displaying the interposed material (Goretex) and the normal appearance of the nerves and their microvessels running on the surface

the rootlets of the ninth and tenth cranial nerves, and to progressively mobilize the vertebral artery in a caudal, medial, and ventral direction while dragging the elongated vessels and loops of the anteroinferior cerebellar artery and posterior inferior cerebellar artery.

At this point, decompression should be performed, and for this purpose, different options can be used depending on the case. The most classic and frequent is the interposition of a synthetic material between the compressed artery or arteries and the nerve. Initially, Gelfoam was used, although Teflon is currently preferred, which is an inert, non-adherent, nonabsorbable material with little capacity to act as a foreign body. The author recommends making a small roll of appropriate length and thickness for each case, which we carefully place between the nerve and the vessels (Fig. 19.3d). To maintain the position in the initial time before the eventual arachnoid reaction fixes the structures, we apply a small amount of Tissucol, which is a human fibrin adhesive widely used as a sealant and hemostatic. Regarding the veins, there are different options to achieve decompression. The offending veins are released, but it is not usually easy to mobilize veins due to their short free path, so they must be coagulated and divided. Venous decompression with interposed material is unsafe, as it will most likely end up thrombosing the vein. In some exceptional cases, compression of the facial nerve root is mixed, and both arterial branches and venous channels may be involved. In this case, individual decompression of each component is performed, although arterial compression is usually given greater importance.

19.2.7 Facial Microvascular Compression That Requires Specific Treatment

19.2.7.1 Revision Surgery

Although MVD is a very effective technique in the treatment of hemifacial spasm, with long-term cure rates of over 90% of patients, there is a small percentage of patients where there is no initial clinical improvement or a recurrence occurs. The causes attributed to justify these poor results are various, although always demonstrated through the subjective interpretation of the operative findings by the surgeon. Probably the most frequent cause is inadequate decompression carried out in the first surgery, particularly in cases of poor initial results or recurrence shortly after. This is due to the fact that the exploration of the facial nerve has been incomplete and there are unexplored areas where there is unnoticed and unresolved compression, which is explained by the high frequency of compressions by multiple arteries or along the entire length of the nerve. The loop inside the internal auditory canal is an example of this problem, since to expose and mobilize this segment of the anterior inferior cerebellar artery, the auditory canal must have been drilled. Sometimes, the explanation would be the mobility of the vessels mobilized and separated from the nerve root, either because they are large and rigid vessels that return to their initial position or because of increased elongation. It is also possible that the displacement of the interposed material is placed. Finally, one possibility is the development of a granuloma around the interposition material, although Teflon is an inert material that should not produce a reaction to a foreign body, or that the arachnoid scar fixes or angles the arteries or the nerve, reproducing the compression.

The exploration of the area allows the surgeon to infer the causal relationship of the findings with the patient's symptoms and to propose a corrective action. In reality, the same decision tree is followed as in the first surgery. The most frequent actions are decompression with interposition of material if there is a vessel involved; resection and release of arachnoid scar; and, in the case of granuloma, total or partial resection without attrition of the nerve root and the placement of a new interposition material.

19.2.7.2 Secondary Hemifacial Spasm

In cases where hemifacial spasm is secondary to a structural pathology of the cerebellopontine angle, both the lesion and the compression must be solved. Regarding compression, the relationships between the tumor and the neurovascular elements have been classified into four different situations according to the pattern of the relationship of the tumor to the facial nerve: the nerve is completely buried by the tumor, but without displacement; the nerve is compressed and distorted by the tumor; the nerve is displaced in a cranial or caudal direction by the tumor and is directly compressed by an artery on the opposite side of the nerve; and finally, the nerve is directly compressed by an artery displaced by the tumor located on the same side. In the first two situations, removal of the lesion ensures decompression of the nerve, while in the others, removal of the lesion must be accompanied by mobilization of the artery and, eventually, placement of an interposed material to maintain the separation of the neurovascular elements.

19.2.8 Complications, Prevention, and Management

Complications related to the approach are those common to the retrosigmoid approach, as reviewed in another chapter. However, although MVD is not a damaging technique, it requires manipulation of the neurovascular structures of the middle group. The required manipulation of the vestibulocochlear nerve means that the most frequent neurological postoperative complication is hearing loss, present in less than 20% of patients and more frequent in elderly patients. Intraoperative neurophysiological monitoring with evoked auditory potentials of the brainstem (BAEP) and the preservation of the internal auditory artery, together with an exquisite microneurosurgical technique dissecting and sectioning all arachnoid adhesions, are the best ways to prevent this complication. An alarm criterion in preoperative BAEP is an increase in latency of 1 ms or a decrease in amplitude of 50% of wave V, since it is related to hearing loss in the postoperative period. Complete loss of wave V is not an alarm criterion, since it implies irreversible damage to the auditory pathway and is inevitably followed by cophosis. It is also necessary to rule out otological symptoms secondary to middle ear occupation by the retrosigmoid approach, which very frequently opens the mastoid cells, or by mechanical trauma to the cranial nerve during the approach or transmeatal access. Apart from auditory impairment, the most feared complication after MVD for hemifacial spasm is facial paresis or paralysis. Immediate facial paresis or paralysis is usually transient and secondary to nerve manipulation, heat from bipolar coagulation, or mechanical trauma from aspiration, irrigation, or interposed material. Late facial paresis or paralysis occurs several days after MVD, and its causal mechanism is not clear, having been suggested as viral infection from resident viruses in the nerve, although prognosis is equally good with spontaneous resolution in weeks or months.

19.2.9 Outcome, Prognosis, and Follow-Up

The prognosis of MVD in hemifacial spasm is very good, with an excellent long-term outcome rate of 90% [12]. There are different scales for assessing the outcome of MVD in hemifacial spasm, evaluating overall or by functional muscle groups, the improvement of motor symptoms, and, on the other hand, the degree of patient satisfaction. One of them, very simple and practical, is the one proposed by Marc Sindou, which establishes the following assessment by points: 0 or cure, with total disappearance of the spasm and the patient completely satisfied; 1 or subtotal non-disabling improvement, with occasional spasms in specific situations and the patient completely satisfied; 2 or partial disabling improvement of between 50–90% of the spasms and the patient dissatisfied with the result; and 3 or failure, with no substantial improvement in the spasm, still very disabling and with the patient dissatisfied and regretting having undergone the procedure. A score of 0–1 would be an effective surgery, and a score of 2–3 would be an ineffective surgery. Different studies of large series and systematic reviews or meta-analyses of the literature show very similar results. The good results of surgery reach 90% in most studies with an average follow-up of three years. Recurrence rates are less than 5%, and only a very low percentage of patients are reoperated on due to failure of the first surgery or recurrence. Good result rates are also very high in revision surgery, with results similar to those of the first surgery.

The clinical improvement is usually immediate after MVD, although in some patients, there is a latency period of days or a few weeks that is attributed to the remyelination processes of the injured nerve root fibers and the structural and functional reorganization of the neurons of the facial nucleus. This late healing can reach one third of patients and occur progressively days, weeks, or months after surgery, even exceptionally beyond the first year. This poses a problem when indicating an early surgical revision or delaying it while waiting for a late clinical improvement.

19.2.10 Management Modalities

Unlike with trigeminal neuralgia, there is no indication for the treatment of hemifacial spasm with stereotactic radiosurgery. Anecdotal cases of relief or cure of hemifacial spasm secondary to tumoral or vascular lesions of the cerebellopontine angle treated with stereotactic radiosurgery have been published, but the clinical improvement would be obtained by the resolution of the causal lesion. Therefore, the only alternative treatment to MVD is pharmacological treatment with botulinum toxin injection. This is a low-risk therapeutic option, available for about four decades, which allows transient symptomatic relief of the symptoms in almost 90% of patients. Indeed, the injection must be repeated every 3–6 months, but tolerance may develop; the diffusion of botulinum toxin can produce unpleasant side effects such as ptosis, diplopia, or blurred vision and, in the long term, muscle atrophy. Faced with this, MVD offers a pathophysiological and curative solution to the disease, theoretically without neurological involvement, although with the risk of morbidity and mortality related to cerebellopontine angle microneurosurgical exploration.

19.3 Vestibulocochlear Dysfunction

MVD has also been performed for the treatment of symptoms related to vestibulocochlear dysfunction caused by microvascular compression of the nerve root as it courses along the cerebellopontine angle [16].

19.3.1 Anatomical Considerations

The vestibulocochlear nerve is part of the middle neurovascular complex described by Rhoton and includes the abducens, facial, and vestibulocochlear nerves, along with the anterior inferior cerebellar artery. The facial and vestibulocochlear nerves originate more laterally, in the medullary-pontine sulcus, just above the supraolivary fossa. The facial–vestibulocochlear complex runs superior and laterally to the internal auditory meatus. The eighth cranial nerve consists of the cochlear and vestibular nerve roots, which have a total length of 17–20 mm between the brainstem and the internal acoustic meatus and extend another 10–15 mm into the internal auditory canal. In the cistern, the cochlear part occupies the most ventral and caudal portion of the nerve, while the vestibular part occupies the most posterior area of the nerve. In this cisternal portion, the nerve root is accompanied by the anterior inferior cerebellar artery and the internal auditory artery, and the facial nerve is placed more ventrally, while the vestibulocochlear is more dorsally, with the intermediate nerve between them. Within the auditory canal, the intermediate nerve joins the facial nerve before it enters the anterior superior quadrant of the bottom of the canal. The cochlear component will enter the fundus of the canal through the anterior inferior quadrant, and the two components of the vestibular nerve, the superior and the inferior, will do so through the superior and inferior posterior quadrants, respectively. In this intracanalicular path, the nerves are accompanied by the internal auditory artery and, only occasionally, by the meatal loop of the anterior inferior cerebellar artery. Above, when describing the microsurgical anatomy related to hemifacial spasm, we have reviewed the arterial and venous elements that are related to the facial and vestibulocochlear nerves, the most relevant being the anterior inferior cerebellar artery, particularly in its meatal loop from which the internal auditory or labyrinthine artery emerges [10].

19.3.2 Pathology

To explain vestibulocochlear dysfunction syndromes caused by neurovascular compression, the same theories have been used as in other cranial nerve rhizopathies. Therefore, it is accepted that the cause is the demyelination of the nerve fibers of the nerve root by the pulsating mechanical action of the offending artery. The entry zone of the vestibulocochlear nerve is very long, about 10 mm, and there have been described nerves where it extends to the bottom of the internal auditory canal, so the nerve root would be susceptible to demyelination in a long segment, both in its cisternal and meatal segments. Alternatively, it has been hypothesized that compression would produce ischemia of the nerve due to hypoperfusion, and others have suggested that the cause would be a narrow internal acoustic meatus, although none of these hypotheses have been proven.

19.3.3 Clinical and Diagnostic Considerations

Clinically, vestibulocochlear dysfunction syndrome includes hearing loss, tinnitus, and positional vertigo, either in isolation or in combination. Hearing loss and tinnitus are unilateral. The symptoms appear as paroxysmal attacks of tinnitus or vertigo lasting seconds or minutes, spontaneous or in certain head positions, which may be accompanied by facial spasm, hyperacusis, or otalgia. Hearing loss is progressive over time until cophosis occurs. It has been hypothesized that the variable anatomical relationships of the vestibular and cochlear nerve roots along their cisternal and meatal course could explain the different clinical presentation [1].

Imaging studies aim to demonstrate the relationship of the meatal loop of the anterior inferior cerebellar artery with the nerve root. For this purpose, MRI imaging studies with highly enhanced T2 sequences with a very thin section (FIESTA) are used. The results of the MRI study display different situations: no loop is observed in either the cistern or the auditory canal; a loop is observed in the cistern; and, finally, a loop is observed in the auditory canal [5]. The problem is that there is no clear relationship between these findings and the symptoms of the patients. The changes in the BAERs are also nonspecific.

19.3.4 Microvascular Decompression

The surgical technique regarding the approach, access to the nerve, exploration of its cisternal segment and in the auditory canal, and the mobilization and separation of the compressive vascular elements has no particularity in relation to that described for hemifacial spasm.

19.3.5 Outcome, Prognosis, and Follow-Up

The results of MVD are different depending on the symptoms. The best result is obtained for vertigo, which cures or improves in more than 75% of patients. The beneficial outcome is less likely for tinnitus, which improves in one-third of patients. The outcome depends on the duration of symptoms, and if tinnitus is present for more than 3–4 years, MVD would not be indicated if the goal is to cure tinnitus. Finally, the worst outcome is obtained for hearing loss, with improvement in less than 20% of patients and deterioration in some cases. In the selection of patients for surgery, if hearing loss in audiometry is greater than 60 dB, MVD would not be indicated if the goal is to improve hearing.

19.4 Glossopharyngeal Neuralgia

Glossopharyngeal neuralgia is a very rare type of craniofacial pain that reproduces many of the pathophysiological, clinical, and therapeutic features of trigeminal neuralgia.

19.4.1 Anatomical Considerations

The glossopharyngeal nerve, together with the vagal, spinal or accessory, and hypoglossal nerves, and the posterior inferior cerebellar artery, form the inferior neurovascular complex of the cerebellopontine angle described by Rhoton. The glossopharyngeal nerve is formed from one or, more rarely, two rootlets emerging from the lateral surface of the medulla oblongata in the posterolateral or retro-olivary sulcus, located between the lateral limit of the inferior olive and the cuneate fasciculus. After a short interval, several rootlets emerge caudally over a length of a few millimeters, forming the vagal nerve, and more caudally, the rootlets of the cranial portion of the accessory nerve. Glossopharyngeal and vagal nerve roots run laterally towards the jugular foramen, below the choroid plexus that protrudes from the fourth ventricle through the foramen of Luschka. The posterior inferior cerebellar artery has a very variable origin, course, and relationships. The posterior inferior cerebellar artery is divided into five parts: the anterior medullary segment, the lateral medullary segment, the tonsillar-medullary segment, the telovellotonsillar segment, and finally, the cortical segment. The anterior medullary segment is related to the roots of the hypoglossal nerve, and the lateral medullary segment is related in a variable way to the rootlets of the lower cranial nerves, always being inferior to the facial and vestibulocochlear nerves. The venous drainage of the inferior compartment of the cerebellopontine angle is through small veins that flow into the inferior petrosal sinus [10].

19.4.2 Pathology

Idiopathic glossopharyngeal neuralgia is distinguished from the secondary glossopharyngeal neuralgia associated with demyelinating neurological diseases, lesions of the cerebellopontine angle or skull base, and other much rarer vascular or inflammatory disorders. In most cases, idiopathic neuralgia is due to compression of the nerve entry zone by the posterior inferior cerebellar artery or the vertebral artery (Fig. 19.4). The length of the cisternal course of the glossopharyngeal nerve root is about 16 mm, but the entry zone is very short, only about 2 mm.

19.4.3 Clinical and Diagnostic Considerations

Clinically, glossopharyngeal neuralgia is characterized by paroxysmal pain in the form of intense,

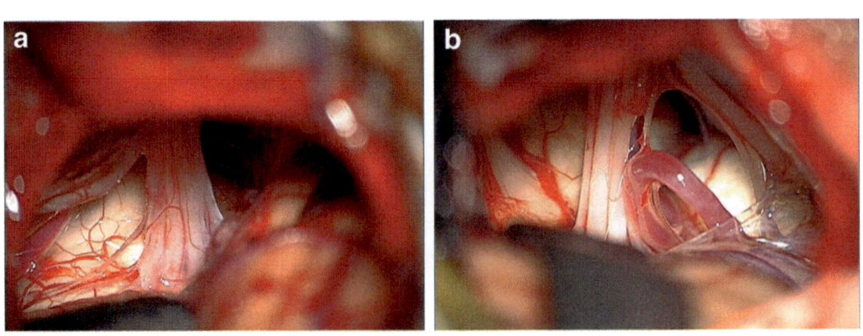

Fig. 19.4 Intraoperative pictures of the right glossopharyngeal and vagal rootlets. View through a right retrosigmoid approach (left to right: pons; glossopharyngeal and vagal rootlets; medulla oblongata). (**a**) Nerve roots have no vascular relationships. (**b**) Posteroinferior cerebellar artery loop

stabbing electrical discharges in the posterior pharynx, posterior third of the tongue, middle ear, angle of the jaw, and tonsillar fossa, lasting from a few seconds to minutes. Syncope may sometimes be associated. Pain crises may be spontaneous or triggered by speaking, swallowing, chewing, coughing, or yawning. It is a very rare disease, with an estimated incidence of 0.8 cases per 100,000 people per year [1]. To demonstrate neurovascular compression, MRI imaging studies with highly weighted T2 sequences with very thin sections (FIESTA) are used [5].

19.4.4 Microvascular Decompression

Glossopharyngeal neuralgia should initially be treated with anticonvulsant drugs, particularly carbamazepine. The treatment strategy is to increase the dose until the pain is controlled or undesirable side effects appear, in which case a second drug is used. Patients who are resistant to treatment, have side effects that prevent them from reaching therapeutic benefits, or who wish to stop drug treatment have different surgical treatment options. As with trigeminal neuralgia, there is the option of using invasive and non-lesive techniques on the nerve, such as MVD; invasive and lesive techniques on the nerve, such as rhizotomy; together with other minimally invasive but lesive techniques, such as percutaneous techniques; and finally, non-invasive but lesive techniques on the nerve, such as stereotactic radiosurgery.

When imaging studies show neurovascular compression, MVD is the technique of choice [16]. The microneurosurgical technique regarding the approach and access to the medullary-pontine sulcus has no particularities in relation to that described for hemifacial spasm. Now the approach can be a little more caudal, and access to the cerebellopontine angle is facilitated by the release of the arachnoid adhesions among the flocculus, facial–vestibulocochlear nerve complex, and the medullary-pontine sulcus, since the fascicles of the glossopharyngeal nerve exit the brainstem through the retro-olivary sulcus just below the medullary-pontine sulcus. Here, the artery that compresses the nerve root is identified, which in most cases is a loop or elongation of the posterior inferior cerebellar artery and, more rarely, the vertebral artery, which, once mobilized, is separated from the nerve with a Teflon fragment. Sometimes multiple compressions can be found, and the involvement of the veins is anecdotal.

When no relevant neurovascular compression is found, a glossopharyngeal rhizotomy can be performed instead. Some authors recommend associating it with MVD. Isolated rhizotomy may be considered when neurovascular compression has not been demonstrated in imaging studies and is not found in microneurosurgical exploration. If neuralgic pain is accompanied by syncope, rhizotomy of the upper fascicles of the vagal nerve may be associated, since it is considered that syncope would be a consequence of the involvement of the vagal nerve.

19.4.5 Outcome, Prognosis, and Follow-Up

The results of isolated MVD, combined with rhizotomy or stand-alone rhizotomy, are excellent, with immediate disappearance of pain in more than 90% of patients and maintenance of these good results for years, although with a slight decline over time. Some series show better outcomes combining MVD with rhizotomy, both in terms of cure and stability of the result over time, which would justify their combination. The most frequent complications are dysphagia, hoarseness, and cough, although these are transient and more frequent when an isolated rhizotomy is performed or associated with MVD, which would give arguments to avoid rhizotomy.

19.4.6 Management Modalities

Glossopharyngeal neural can be treated in selected patients with percutaneous techniques and stereotactic radiosurgery [2].

19.4.6.1 Percutaneous Controlled Thermocoagulation

Percutaneous techniques are based on controlled lesions to the glossopharyngeal nerve with thermocoagulation. Initially, the nerve was accessed through the jugular foramen, but more recently, a peripheral target has been used at an extracranial level, taking the tip of the styloid process as a reference. In both cases, the position of the electrode is confirmed with radioscopy or computed tomography imaging. It is mandatory to check the position of the electrode with electrical stimulation, thereby reproducing a pain similar to that the patient feels and in the same anatomical area that the patient suffers from. This distal approach to the nerve avoids complications related to the approach through the jugular foramen and minimizes the possibility of syncope and other intraoperative vasovagal reactions due to the lesion of the vagal nerve. The results of controlled thermocoagulation are good, with immediate disappearance of pain in more than 90% of patients, although there is a loss of effectiveness such that after five years only 50% of patients are pain-free. Complications related to the procedure are due to the transient affectation of the glossopharyngeal nerve, with dysphagia and paraesthesia in the posterior part of the tongue and pharynx.

19.4.6.2 Stereotactic Radiosurgery

Stereotactic radiosurgery should be reserved for patients who have one or more of the following circumstances: poor response to pharmacological treatment, absence of neurovascular compression in imaging studies, who do not wish for invasive treatment, or who are contraindicated for this invasive treatment due to associated systemic pathology. The target of stereotactic radiosurgery is placed in the glossopharyngeal fossa of the medulla oblongata or in the cisternal root segment of the glossopharyngeal nerve, with 75 Gy being the minimum radiation dose necessary for a satisfactory result. The results of stereotactic radiosurgery are poor; they need time to become evident and also decrease significantly over time, such that a year and a half after treatment, just over half of the patients maintain good results. However, stereotactic radiosurgery has no relevant side effects.

The selection of the ideal technique for a particular patient is made taking into consideration practically the same arguments as for trigeminal neuralgia, which have been discussed in the previous chapter, namely: potential damage to the glossopharyngeal nerve; general risk related to the surgical procedure; general condition and age of the patient; patient expectations; and, finally, availability and surgical practice. Overall, it can be stated that MVD is the surgical technique of choice in glossopharyngeal neuralgia and should therefore be the first surgical procedure carried out in patients who have failed pharmacological treatment, provided that there is no formal contraindication or refusal by the patient.

19.5 Masticatory Hemispasm

Masticatory hemispasm is a very rare disease that reproduces all the characteristics of hemifacial spasm but affects the masticatory muscles on one side of the face, particularly the temporal muscle and the masseter muscle, although the medial pterygoid muscle may also be involved. A small number of cases have been described, some secondary to irritation of the third branch of the trigeminal nerve in its peripheral course by tumors of the skull base and others secondary to neurovascular compression of the trigeminal root by the superior cerebellar artery. Pharmacological treatment is based in the use of local injections of botulinum toxin, but if compression is demonstrated with imaging studies, MVD of the trigeminal root is resolutive [14].

19.6 Neurogenic Arterial Hypertension

The relationship between arterial hypertension and neurovascular compression of the lateral aspect of the medulla oblongata was established by Peter Jannetta shortly after describing the relationship of trigeminal neuralgia with neurovascular compression of the trigeminal root. The first publication on this subject was in 1985 by Jannetta, reporting the results of 53 patients operated on since 1975, who associated arterial hypertension with any other type of neurovascular compression syndromes of the trigeminal, facial, or glossopharyngeal nerve roots, which founded the indication for microneurosurgical exploration of the cerebellopontine angle for MVD. In all these patients, after the MVD that justified the surgery, the exit from the brainstem and cisternal course of the rootlets of the glossopharyngeal and vagal nerves were explored, and any artery or vein related to them was searched for. In all patients with arterial hypertension except two, vascular compression by the posterior inferior cerebellar artery or vertebral artery was found, and an MVD with a Teflon fragment was performed in most of them [6]. This additional compression was constantly made up of an arterial loop of the offender artery that justified the indication of MVD. This additional compression in patients with arterial hypertension was located in the medulla oblongata ventrally itself, at the exit of the rootlets, on the retro-olivary sulcus of the medulla oblongata. Blood pressure improved significantly in almost all hypertensive patients in whom good decompression was achieved on the left side, while neither the hypertensive patients operated on in the right side nor the normotensive controls examined had microvascular compression or showed changes in their blood pressure. Despite these spectacular results, well described in the publication, the truth is that this indication for the treatment of arterial hypertension has not become popular.

19.6.1 Anatomical Considerations

The anatomical relationships of the rootlets of the glossopharyngeal and vagal nerves as they exit the medulla oblongata on their cisternal course running to the jugular foramen have been described above. The rostral-ventral-lateral (RVL) area of the medulla oblongata is an area where C1 adrenergic neurons accumulate, which control sympathetic nervous activity throughout the body. Peripheral sympathetic activity is increased in patients with arterial hypertension, congestive heart failure, diabetes, obesity, and chronic kidney disease, and its hyperactivity is a risk factor for cerebral and myocardial infarction. The hyperactivity of these C1 neurons is transmitted downward along the intermediolateral fasciculus of the spinal cord, which connects segmentally with sympathetic nerves to the heart (producing increased heart rate), arterioles (producing vasoconstriction), and kidneys (producing increased renin, angiotensin II, and Na^{++} reabsorption). All of these mediators are involved in essential or neurogenic hypertension. The location of these C1 neurons in the medulla oblongata is just below the retro-olivary sulcus, which anatomically corresponds to the apparent exit of the glossopharyngeal and vagal nerves from the brainstem, and where the offending vessels are found compressing the RVL area [10].

19.6.2 Pathology

The pathophysiological basis of the relationship between essential arterial hypertension and the benefit of MVD in patients with this condition is established in physiological studies and in the empirical relationship between MVD and the control of hypertension. Classic experimental studies demonstrate the fall in blood pressure with the section of the medulla oblongata caudally to the pontine junction and the rise in blood pressure when the RVL area of the medulla oblongata is electrically stimulated, an area in which nuclei clearly related to the control of cardiovascular function have been found. Experimental studies also demonstrated that pulsatile mechanical stimulation of this area on the left side induces an increase in blood pressure, while this does not occur on the right side. It is assumed that this difference would be related to the input from the heart to the left side. In patients with hypertension, this pulsatile compression would be produced by an artery, specifically the posterior inferior cerebellar artery (30% of cases), vertebral artery, or basilar artery (25%); vertebral artery or basilar artery together with the posterior inferior cerebellar artery (15%) and other multiple compressions.

19.6.3 Clinical and Diagnostic Considerations

Neurogenic hypertension is a type of hypertension characterized by increased sympathetic activity, and its etiology is not well understood [6, 11]. One imputed cause is microvascular compression of the RVL area of the medulla oblongata or the entry/exit zones of the glossopharyngeal or vagal cranial nerve roots. Neurogenic hypertension can be defined as that in which the sympathetic nervous system plays an important role in the genesis of hypertension. The clinical characteristics of this type of hypertension include atypical forms of hypertension, paroxysmal hypertension, labile hypertension, and resistance to combined treatment with ACE (*Angiotensin Converting Enzyme*) inhibitors and diuretics, severe and unexplained, resistant, with onset at an early age, associated with the ingestion of sympathomimetic agents or comorbidity such as stroke, alcohol abuse, chronic kidney disease, or sleep apnea. Many patients with hemifacial spasm or trigeminal neuralgia have neurogenic arterial hypertension, and, in clinical practice, most patients undergoing MVD associate both clinical situations. As in other neurovascular compression syndromes, the demonstration of neurovascular compression is made with MRI imaging studies with highly T2-weighted sequences and very thin sections (FIESTA) and T1-weighted TOF sequences (Fig. 19.5). Some studies have shown that microvascular compression of the RVL area of the medulla oblongata is significantly more frequent in hypertensive patients than in the non-hypertensive population.

19.6.4 Microvascular Decompression

The microneurosurgical technique regarding the approach and access to the medullary-pontine sulcus has no particularities in relation to that described for hemifacial spasm or glossopharyngeal neuralgia. The artery that compresses the RVL of the medulla oblongata is identified, which in most cases is a loop or elongation of the posterior inferior cerebellar artery and more rarely the vertebral artery, which, once mobilized, is separated from the nerve with a Teflon fragment. Sometimes multiple compressions can be found, and the involvement of the veins is anecdotal. In patients with associated neurovascular compression of the trigeminal or facial nerve, exploration and MVD of the affected nerve are performed.

19.6.5 Outcome, Prognosis, and Follow-Up

Following the seminal study by Jannetta, more recent studies have confirmed the beneficial effect of decompression of the RVL area and the glossopharyngeal or vagal rootlets in controlling arterial hypertension associated with patients undergoing MVD for another neurovascular compression syndrome. In these cases, blood

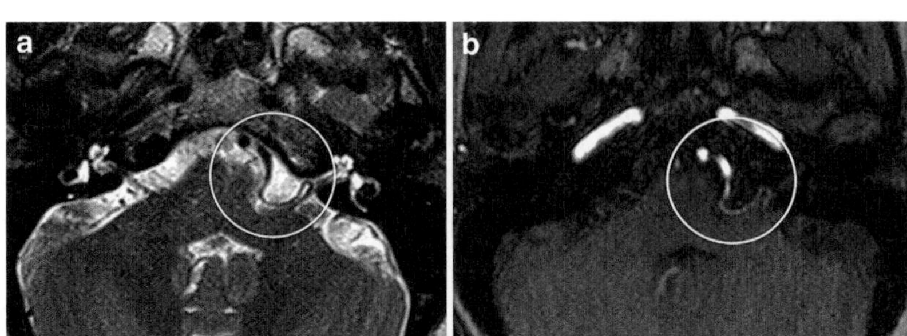

Fig. 19.5 Loop of the anteroinferior cerebellar artery compressing the left RVL area of the medulla oblongata. (**a**) Axial MRI-FIESTA slice. (**b**)MRI T1-weighted with gadolinium slice

pressure decreases in 70% of patients. However, there are only a few studies that have carried out decompression in patients with arterial hypertension without another associated neurovascular syndrome. These are patients with severe essential arterial hypertension resistant to treatment, in whom imaging studies show the presence of an isolated neurovascular compression of the RVL and/or the entry zone of the glossopharyngeal or vagal roots. In these patients, MVD controls blood pressure, although in some cases it would only do so temporarily. In this regard, the criteria for the indication of treatment of arterial hypertension with MVD have not been conclusively defined, but they should be at least the following: neurogenic arterial hypertension refractory to medical treatment, where the presence of compression of the RVL area and/or the exit zone of the glossopharyngeal and vagal roots is demonstrated, in which no comorbidity makes the intervention high risk. The complications observed are those related to the manipulated nerves, that is, dysphagia and hoarseness, most of the time transient [6, 11, 13].

In summary, the treatment of arterial hypertension with MVD cannot be advised in patients with isolated imaging studies that demonstrate microvascular compression. It seems mandatory, a safe diagnosis of neurogenic arterial hypertension refractory to treatment. In patients where hypertension is associated with trigeminal neuralgia or hemifacial spasm and there is neurovascular compression of the left RVL area in imaging studies, the patient should be offered decompression of both areas, while in those where there is no such compression, the patient should be offered exploration of this area to rule it out definitively.

19.7 Key Messages

- *Neurovascular compression syndromes, also referred to as cranial rhizopathies, are a family of neurological illnesses characterized by neurological dysfunction caused by offending vascular components compressing cranial nerve roots.*
- *The compressed structure is the root of a cranial nerve in its cisternal course, particularly in the so-called entry zone. Both arterial and venous compression are possible.*
- *Hemifacial spasm, glossopharyngeal neuralgia, vestibulocochlear dysfunction, masticatory hemispasm, and neurogenic arterial hypertension are among these syndromes, which are rather uncommon compared with trigeminal neuralgia.*
- *MVD of the vascular elements combined with the application of a soft separating material is the treatment of choice.*
- *The indication is predicated on the following: resistance to various noninvasive treatments, identification of neurovascular compression in imaging examinations, exclusion of other etiologies, and confirmation of the diagnosis.*
- *The clinical outcome of MVD is excellent and long-lasting. Complications are few, mild, and temporary.*

References

1. Baldauf J, Rosenstengel C, Schroeder HWS. Nerve compression syndromes in the posterior cranial fossa. Dtsch Arztebl Int. 2019;116:54–60. https://doi.org/10.3238/arztebl.2019.0054.
2. Berckemeyer MA, Suarez-Meade P, Carcelen MFV, et al. Current advances in the surgical treatment of glossopharyngeal neuralgia. Neurosurg Rev. 2013;46:47. https://doi.org/10.1007/s10143-023-01948-y.
3. Chaudhry N, Srivastava A, Joshi L. Hemifacial spasm: the past, present, and future. J Neurol Sci. 2015;356:27–31. https://doi.org/10.1016/j.jns.2015.06.032.
4. Dou NN, Zhong J, Zhou QM, et al. The mechanism of hemifacial spasm: a new understanding of the offending artery. Neurol Res. 2015;7:184–8. https://doi.org/10.1179/1743132814Y.0000000424.
5. Haller S, Etienne L, Kövari E, et al. Imaging of neurovascular compression syndromes: trigeminal neuralgia, hemifacial spasm, vestibular paroxysmia, and glossopharyngeal neuralgia. AJNR Am J Neuroradiol. 2016;37:1384–92. https://doi.org/10.3174/ajnr.A4683.
6. Jannetta PJ, Segal R, Wolfson SK Jr. Neurogenic hypertension: etiology and surgical treatment. I. Observations in 53 patients. Ann Surg. 1985;201:391–8. https://doi.org/10.1097/00000658-198503000-00023.

7. Lefaucheur JP, Ben Daamer N, Sangla S, et al. Diagnosis of primary hemifacial spasm. Neurochirurgie. 2018;64:82–6. https://doi.org/10.1016/j.neuchi.2017.12.003.
8. Mercier P, Bernard F. Surgical anatomy for hemifacial spasm. Neurochirurgie. 2018;64:124–32. https://doi.org/10.1016/j.neuchi.2018.04.008.
9. Mercier P, Sindou M. The conflicting vessels in hemifacial spasm: literature review and anatomical-surgical implications. Neurochirurgie. 2018;64:94–100. https://doi.org/10.1016/j.neuchi.2018.01.004.
10. Rhoton AL Jr. The posterior fossa: microsurgical anatomy & surgical approaches. Neurosurgery. 2000;47(Suppl 3):S1–S279. https://doi.org/10.1097/00006123-200009001-00013.
11. Sindou M, Mahmoudi M, Brînzeu A. Hypertension of neurogenic origin: effect of MVD of the CN IX-X root entry/exit zone and ventrolateral medulla on blood pressure in a prospective series of 48 patients with hemifacial spasm associated with essential hypertension. J Neurosurg. 2015;123:1405–13. https://doi.org/10.3171/2014.12.JNS141775.
12. Sindou M, Mercier P. Microvascular decompression for hemifacial spasm: outcome on spasm and complications. A review Neurochirurgie. 2018;64:106–16. https://doi.org/10.1016/j.neuchi.2018.01.001.
13. Song HD, Yang FJ, Liu RE. Efficacy of microvascular decompression on the vascular compression type of neurogenic hypertension: a meta-analysis. Rev Neurol (Paris). 2020;176:763–9. https://doi.org/10.1016/j.neurol.2020.02.002.
14. Sun H, Wei Z, Wang Y, et al. Microvascular decompression for hemimasticatory spasm: a case report and review of the literature. World Neurosurg. 2016;90:703.e5–703.e10. https://doi.org/10.1016/j.wneu.2016.02.088.
15. Tatagiba MS, Roser F, Hirt B, et al. The retrosigmoid endoscopic approach for cerebellopontine-angle tumors and microvascular decompression. World Neurosurg. 2014;82(6 Suppl):S171–6. https://doi.org/10.1016/j.wneu.2014.08.001.
16. Walijee H, Vaughan C, Munir N, et al. Microvascular compression of the vestibulocochlear nerve. Eur Arch Otorrinolaringol. 2021;278:3625–31. https://doi.org/10.1007/s00405-020-06586-4.
17. Yang SH, Park H, Yoo DS, et al. Microsurgical anatomy of the facial nerve. Clin Anat. 2021;34(1):90–102. https://doi.org/10.1002/ca.23652.

20 Facial Nerve Resuscitation: Hypoglossal-Facial Anastomosis

20.1 Introduction

Facial paralysis secondary to a complete and irreversible anatomic or functional lesion of the facial nerve causes severe functional and psychological disorders for the patient. Surgical repair techniques depend to a large extent on the anatomic location of the lesion, etiology, and time interval from the injury. Irreversible facial nerve injury is sometimes secondary to resection of cerebellopontine angle tumors, particularly vestibular schwannomas and brainstem, petrosal bone, middle fossa, or skull base tumors. Head trauma with skull base fracture is also a frequent cause of irreversible damage to the facial nerve. Different surgical attempts have been made by different surgical specialties to solve this troublesome problem. In the neurosurgical setting, facial nerve repair can be performed with direct neurotization techniques with facial nerve neurorrhaphy, with or without interposed nerve grafts, or via facial nerve reanimation techniques by transferring another donor motor nerve, such as the hypoglossal nerve, accessory nerve, or motor branches of the third branch of the trigeminal nerve, such as the masseter nerve, or using small distal branches of the contralateral facial nerve, also with or without interposed nerve grafts. Hypoglossal nerve transfer is one of the oldest techniques used for facial nerve reanimation by direct end-to-end suture with the facial nerve. The classic end-to-end hypoglossal-facial neurorrhaphy technique involved completely severing the hypoglossal nerve, with distressing sequelae for the patient due to the severe hemilingual atrophy and its consequences in swallowing, eating, and speaking. In 1991, May et al. proposed a side-to-end hypoglossal-facial neurorrhaphy technique, implanting the facial nerve in the dorsal aspect of the hypoglossal nerve. The hypoglossal nerve was cut to approximately one-third of its thickness, followed by microsurgical end-to-side epineural suture of the facial nerve on the hypoglossal nerve. To reach the hypoglossal nerve easily and to perform a tensionless suture, an interposition nerve graft was needed. Later, Atlas and Lowinger, in 1997 [2], and Asaoka et al. in 1999 [1], proposed an imaginative modification in the surgical technique that facilitated tension-free neurorrhaphy without interposition nerve graft by mobilizing the mastoid segment of the facial nerve. This is the modern side-to-end hypoglossal-to-facial neurorraphy (SEHFN) we use for facial nerve reanimation in patients with complete and irreversible facial nerve paralysis secondary to resection of brain stem or cerebellopontine angle lesions.

20.2 Anatomical Considerations

In this section, we will describe the anatomical tips of the facial nerve and hypoglossal nerve of interest for this particular microneurosurgical technique of SEHFN (Fig. 20.1) [3, 4].

J. M. González-Darder, *Microneurosurgery of Cerebellopontine Angle*,
https://doi.org/10.1007/978-3-032-03091-7_20

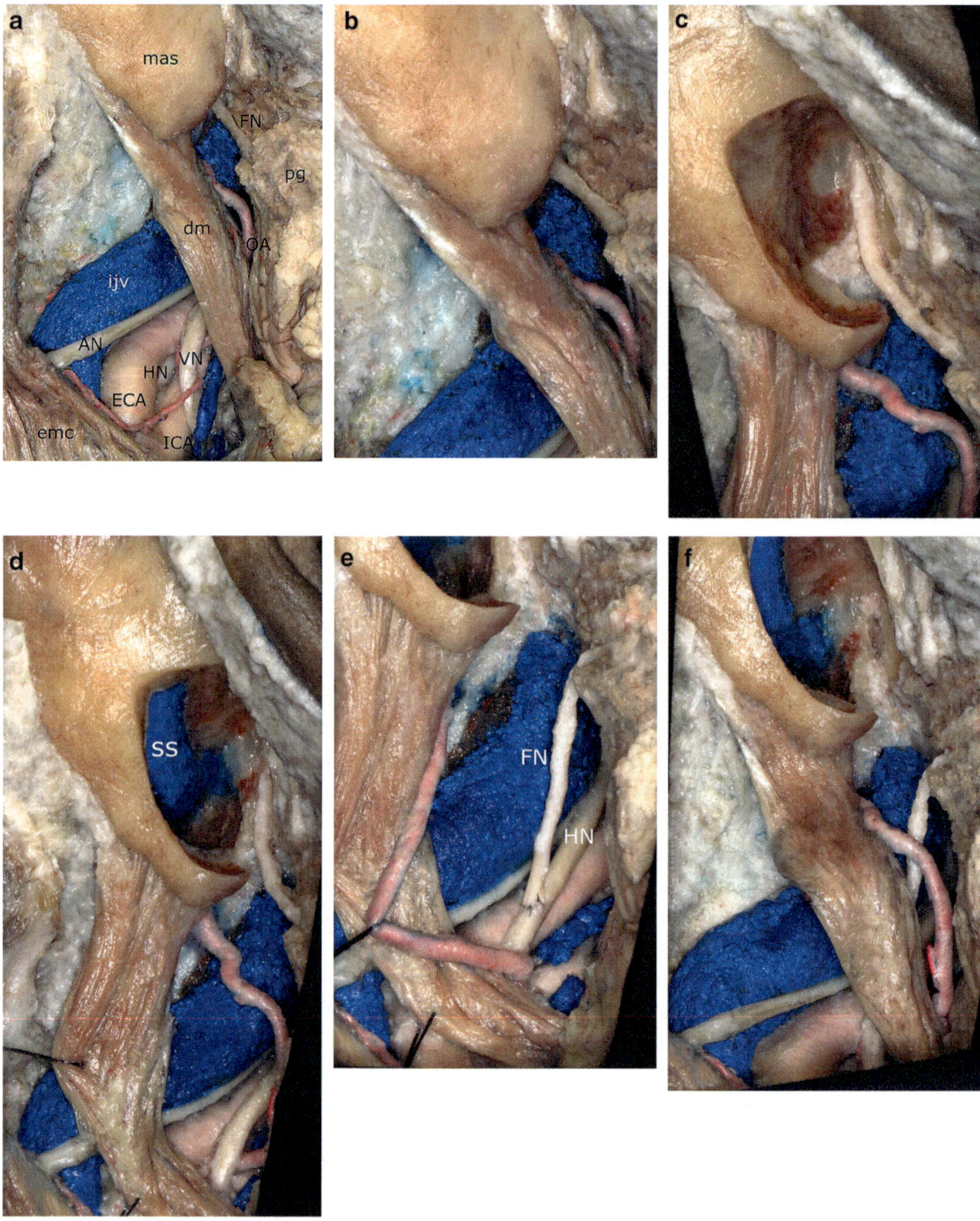

Fig. 20.1 Pictures of the anatomic study (right side). (**a**) Lateral view showing the mastoid and upper cervical region after release and posterior mobilization of the sternocleidomastoid muscle (emc). The digastric muscle (dm) is in the center, running from the digastric groove of the mastoid process (mas). The facial nerve (FN) is seen running to the parotid gland (pg). Other nerves are exposed: the accessory nerve (AN), vagal nerve (VN), and hypoglossal nerve (HN). Also, the most relevant vascular elements are dissected: internal carotid artery (ICA), external carotid artery (ECA), occipital artery (OA), and internal jugular vein (ijv). (**b**) Closer view of the extrapetrosal segment of the facial nerve. (**c**) The mastoid segment of the facial nerve has been fully exposed after mastoidectomy. (**d**) Overview of the anatomical area. The deep wall of the mastoid has been drilled to show the sigmoid sinus (ss), and the digastric muscle and occipital artery have been mobilized posteriorly to expose a segment of the hypoglossal nerve (HN). (**e**) The facial nerve (FN) has been cut and luxated inferiorly, approached to the hypoglossal nerve (HN), and end-to-side sutured. (**f**) Overview of the surgical field after repositioning the digastric muscle

20.2.1 Mastoid Segment of the Facial Nerve

The facial nerve has three parts in its course through the Fallopian aqueduct along the petrosal bone: the labyrinthine portion, between the cochlea and the labyrinth, until the geniculate ganglion; the tympanic portion, related to the middle ear; and, finally, the mastoid portion, until the stylomastoid foramen. The horizontal or tympanic segment directs the nerve to the stapes, and, after a change of direction of about 90°, the nerve enters the vertical or mastoid segment, of about 15 mm to the stylomastoid foramen. In the mastoid segment, the facial nerve releases two branches, the nerve of the stapedius muscle and, distally, about 3–4 mm from the foramen, a voluminous branch, the chorda tympani, which participates in salivary secretion and taste sensitivity of part of the tongue. Finally, at the exit of the facial nerve through the stylomastoid foramen is the extratemporal segment, of greater diameter (2–3 mm), which runs until penetrating the parotid gland, where it divides into two trunks in the *pes anserinus*.

The mastoid process has the shape of a quadrangular pyramid, with four walls, an upper base, and a truncated lower vertex: anterior wall, which in its upper half corresponds to the posterior wall of the external auditory canal; posterior wall that corresponds to the anterior face of the sigmoid sinus; medial wall, which is in contact with the presigmoid dura mater (Trautman's triangle) and with the semicircular canal above; lateral wall, which is the lateral surface of the skull, below the supramastoid crest; the upper base, which is a virtual plane that runs deep from the supramastoid crest to the basal temporal dura mater; and finally, the inferior apex or tip of the mastoid.

The mastoid contains numerous bullae or cavities covered with mucosa, filled with air, and connected to the middle ear. However, the most important element of the mastoid is the mastoid segment of the facial nerve. Mastoid cells vary considerably between people, but the trajectory of the mastoid segment of the facial nerve within the mastoid canal is quite constant. The mastoid portion of the facial nerve runs at a depth of about 15 mm from the lateral surface of the mastoid and is about 15 mm long. The stylomastoid foramen is at a depth of about 12 mm, slightly more superficial than the course of the nerve. In our anatomical studies, the distance in depth from the surface of cortical bone at the level of Henle's spine to the facial nerve in the mastoid canal is 13.45 mm (range, 12.3–13.7 mm).

To fully expose the mastoid process for the exposition of the mastoid segment of the facial nerve, it is mandatory to uncover anteriorly the posterior edge of the external auditory canal and locate Henle's spine; subsequently expose the mastoid surface until reaching a vertical line drawn caudally, approximately 1 cm anterior to the asterion; caudally expose the entire lateral aspect of the mastoid process after the sternocleidomastoid muscle dissection and mobilization; and finally, expose the mastoid surface cranially 4–5 cm from the tip of the mastoid process until reaching the level of Henle's spine. The mastoid is then drilled away to expose the mastoid segment of the facial nerve. The anteroinferior limit is the stylomastoid foramen, and the cranial limit is Henle's spine. Subsequently, an extension of 2–3 cm is needed for good exposure and to remove enough cortical bone covering the mastoid segment of the facial nerve. The cortical bone of the mastoid is drilled caudally and anteriorly between these lines to the tip of the mastoid. The mastoid cells are exposed, respecting the posterior wall of the external auditory canal. The internal structure of the mastoid is very variable. In the ideal case of a large pneumatization, the drilling must proceed to find the compact bone where the facial nerve canal runs. The canal has a hard, compact bone covering the facial nerve and is drilled along the mastoid facial nerve segment. The mastoid segment of the exposed facial nerve, from the spine of Henle level to the stylomastoid foramen, measures in our experience an average of 20.64 mm (range, 18.8–22.3 mm). Once the entire mastoid has been exposed, the extracranial segment of the facial nerve runs toward the parotid gland until its division into two main branches in the *pes anserinus*.

20.2.2 Cervical Course of the Hypoglossal Nerve

The hypoglossal nerve originates in the preolivary sulcus of the medulla oblongata. It passes through the hypoglossal canal at the level of the occipital condyle and exits to the extracranial space. It then runs down obliquely in an inferior-anterior direction and, at the end, follows a parallel direction to the digastric muscle until it reaches the intermediate tendon of the digastric muscle. In its extracranial way, the nerve is located anteromedial to the internal jugular vein and posterolateral to the internal carotid artery.

For identification of the hypoglossal nerve, the key point of reference is the digastric muscle. The sternocleidomastoid muscle is detached from the mastoid and reflected posteriorly, and the posterior belly digastric muscle is found in a deeper anatomical plane covering relevant neurovascular structures: the accessory nerve, going to the deep aspect of the sternocleidomastoid muscle; the hypoglossal nerve; the internal jugular vein and the internal carotid artery, with the vagal nerve in a deeper layer; the external carotid artery; and the occipital artery, running to the occipital region deeper to the digastric muscle (Fig. 20.1a). To show the exit of the hypoglossal nerve between the internal jugular vein and the internal carotid artery, the digastric muscle must be mobilized posteriorly. Here, the anatomic relationships between the hypoglossal nerve and the occipital artery are very variable, and the hypoglossal nerve must be isolated and mobilized by passing a rubber.

20.2.3 Ideal Location for the Anastomosis

In our anatomical studies, the average distance from the stylomastoid foramen to the easiest suture point of the hypoglossal nerve is 30.03 mm (range, 28.6–32.4 mm). The mobilized facial nerve portion, which includes both the mastoid segment and the predivision extrapetrossal segments, is referred to as the *anastomotic translocation portion* of the facial nerve. The average length of the anastomotic translocation portion of the facial nerve is 34.76 mm (range, 31.6–37.6 mm) in our anatomical studies. Therefore, the dislocation of the facial nerve allows enough length to be tensionless sutured on the hypoglossal nerve (Fig. 20.1e).

20.3 Pathology

The ESFHN is indicated in the event of a complete section of the facial nerve, that is, a *neurotmesis*. This lesion supposes the severing of all nerve fibers and connective elements supporting the nerve fibers and, consequently, the solution of continuity of the nerve trunk. In the peripheral nerve system, the nervous fibers degenerate and later regenerate following the rules of the Wallerian degeneration and regeneration, and in the proximal stump, regenerative sprouts, Schwann cell proliferation, and fibrous scar develop the so-called proximal neuroma. In the distal stump, a less conspicuous neuroma develops. However, in the cerebellopontine angle, there is no option for the development of a proximal or distal neuroma, because there are no Schwann cells or fibrous tissue in the nerve root. Nerve lesions in continuity have different degrees of intensity (nerve fiber section or *axonotmesis*, endoneural tube section, or fascicular section) and extension into the nerve (total or partial), but in any case, there is no solution of continuity of the nerve. In the peripheral nerve system, the final result is a neuroma in continuity, and there is a chance for a spontaneous partial or complete recovery of the function. Again, in the facial nerve root, it is not possible to develop a neuroma in continuity. Peripheral nerve and nerve root lesions in continuity open an undetermined outcome and selection of the most adequate management.

20.3.1 Internal Structure of the Facial and Hypoglossal Nerves

The facial nerve has a fascicular pattern in its extracranial portion. The diameter of the trunk is

1.2–1.4 mm in 70% of specimens, and the number of fascicles is one or two in 70% of the nerves. The facial nerve has a delicate vascular network, with intrinsic arteries placed superficially between the perineurium and epineurium. The total number of myelinated fibers of the facial nerve root in its cisternal segment is between 10,000 and 15,000, and of the intermediate nerve, between 3000 and 5500 [5]. The hypoglossal nerve has a monofascicular pattern along its most distal course, and the average number of myelinated axons for the hypoglossal nerve is around 9000–9500 fibers [6]. This means that there is a discordance between the number of fascicles between the facial nerve and the hypoglossal nerve, but the number of myelinated fibers is similar, accounting for the branches arising from the facial nerve along its petrosal way. This raises the question of how the facial nerve can be reinnervated by just a small portion of the hypoglossal nerve fibers. Experimental studies have shown in rats that both spontaneous collateral sprouting and regenerative sprouting of axons coexisted following ESFHN [7].

20.4 Clinical Considerations

SEHFN is indicated for patients with a complete anatomical lesion or neurotmesis of the facial nerve, where there is no possibility of spontaneous recovery of neurological function. Therefore, these are patients with House–Brackmann (HB) grade VI or complete paralysis. SEHFN could be indicated for patients without a complete anatomical lesion of the facial nerve but with a stable HB grade VI since the time of the nerve injury for at least 3 months, and where the electromyographic (EMG) study of the facial nerve does not show any degree of recovery. Caution should be taken with these EMG findings, since partial reinnervation of the injured nerve by the contralateral facial nerve is common. This reinnervation is usually not sufficient for functional recovery, but EMG findings can provide confusing data. Thus, the indications for SEHFN are based on the solution of continuity of the facial nerve and, in cases where this solution has not been demonstrated, on the evidence of an HB grade VI and absence of clinical improvement.

There are other elements to take into account. The time of evolution since the injury is an important factor. The hypoglossal fibers reinnervate the facial nerve following the endoneurial tubes. The structural damage to these endoneurial tubes as a guide for reinervation increases with time. However, the biggest problem with the passage of time is that the facial muscles, a very large group of muscles with a very small number of muscle fibers, will inevitably suffer a process of atrophy, fibrosis, and degeneration of the muscle fibers. On the other hand, a deformity of the face occurs due to the greater power of the healthy contralateral muscles, which must be overcome after the arrival of the axonal sprouts to the denervated muscle fibers. Thus, the more time passes, the lower the chances of functional recovery. The only way to favor the quality of the muscle fibers until the axonal sprouts arrive is to rehabilitate the facial muscles with massages, facial expressions, and gestures and botulinum toxin injections on the contralateral side. Six months is considered a waiting period that should not be exceeded before SEHFN, even if intensive rehabilitation of the facial muscles is maintained, although others extend this waiting time. Another element is the age of the patient, since with aging, the tone and elasticity of the facial muscles and soft tissues are reduced, and it is more difficult for the reinnervated muscles to perform their function. This makes the prognosis better in younger patients than in older patients, in whom it is advisable to have microneurosurgical treatment as soon as possible. Finally, the last element to consider is the nature of the process that has determined the injury to the facial nerve. In post-traumatic cases or secondary to a surgical injury in the treatment of benign tumors, the indication for treatment is clear, but in the case of malignancies, regional radiotherapy, short life expectancy of the patient, or severe associated pathology, SEHFN is not indicated, since the evident functional recovery of the facial nerve function can take a long time. Therefore, patients with HB grade VI are candidates for facial nerve resuscitation with SEHFN, but if the facial muscles show atrophy, there is severe deformity of the face on the affected side due to muscle paralysis, hypotonia, or atrophy of soft tissues or lack of elasticity, or due to hypertonia on the healthy side, the indication for resuscitation is very risky.

In summary, the indications for facial nerve resuscitation with the hypoglossal nerve are as follows. If there is evidence of anatomical loss of the facial nerve in surgery, early anastomosis is recommended before 6 months and, if possible, in the same surgical procedure. If there is anatomical preservation of the facial nerve, resuscitation is indicated after 6 months of absence of clinical recovery and with neurophysiological criteria of poor prognosis. Finally, if there is functional recovery, even if poor, resuscitation is not recommended, since it implies the loss of the recovered function, and the patient goes to an HB grade of VI; resuscitation does not ensure a better recovery, and, if this occurs, it takes months to achieve.

20.5 Diagnostic Considerations

The evidence of a complete anatomical severing of the facial nerve during surgery or neurotmesis is the most reliable method to assess the impossibility of spontaneous recovery of the function of the nerve. No diagnostic tests are necessary for this purpose in these patients. When the anatomic preservation has been assessed, but the functional status of the nerve shows an HB grade VI in the neurological examination 3 months after nerve injury, it is indicated that the sequential electromyographic study of the patient should be done every 3 months, looking for any electrical response. If neurophysiology does not improve, a neurological recovery must not be expected, and reanimation surgery must be proposed to the patient. If there is an electrical improvement but no neurological improvement, and HB grade VI continues, the electrical studies must be followed no more than a year before proposing SEHFN. If both electrical studies and neurological examination show improvement, the SEHFN is not indicated, because any functional recovery of the facial muscles achieved by the physiological regeneration will be lost with the sectioning of the facial nerve for reanimation. In patients submitted to a SEHFN, electrophysiology studies indicate that revitalization begins a mean of 4–5 months after neurorrhaphy, and clinical recovery begins a few weeks later.

20.6 Surgical Categories

SEHFN is only indicated for patients with a neurotmesis of the facial nerve. However, in real neurosurgery, selected patients with a severe axonotmesis, with HB grade HB and without EMG and clinical recovery over time, are also candidates for SEHFN. However, the microneurosurgical technique is exactly the same in both situations (Fig. 20.2), but the selection criteria are quite different.

20.7 Microneurosurgical Management

20.7.1 Position and Incision

The patient is placed in the supine position, with the head elevated and turned to the contralateral side. The previous standard retroauricular incision for the retrosigmoid approach is extended caudally below the angle of the jaw. The mastoid is localized, and the mastoid insertion of the sternocleidomastoid muscle is partially released and retracted backward. The posterior belly of the digastric muscle is identified, inserted in the digastric groove of the mastoid, taking care to preserve the small branch of the facial nerve that innervates this portion of the muscle. The posterior belly of the muscle is released to the tendon, and a rubber band is passed to mobilize the muscle anteriorly or posteriorly. The mastoid is now cleaned of any soft tissue anteriorly until the spine of Henle, taking care not to enter the external auditory canal, caudally exposing the entire tip of the mastoid, and posteriorly usually to the limit of the previous retrosigmoid craniotomy.

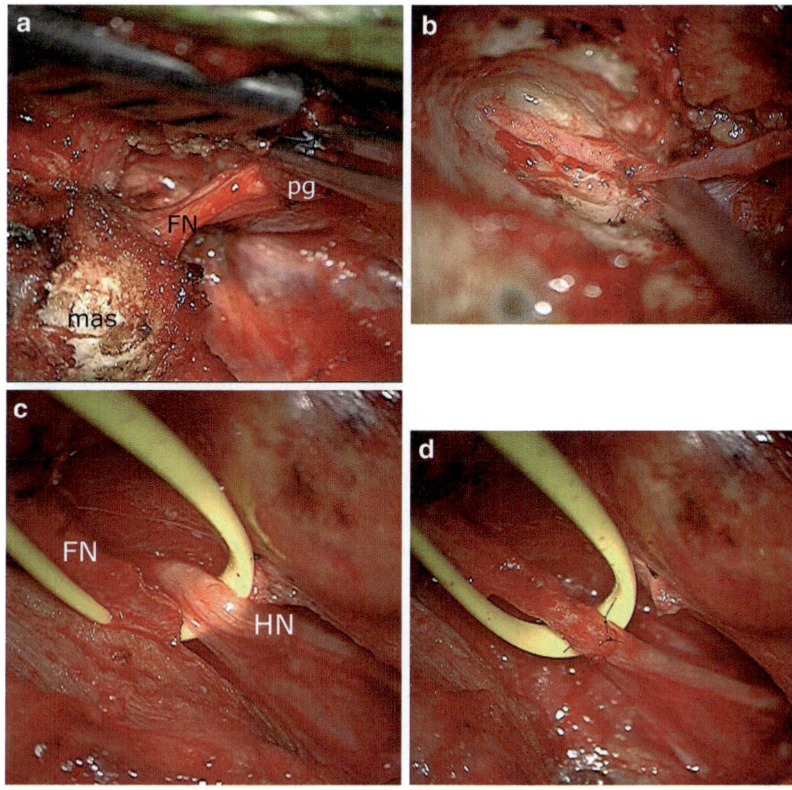

Fig. 20.2 Intraoperative pictures of the microneurosurgical approach (right side). (**a**) View of the extrapetrosal segment of the facial nerve (FN facial nerve, mas mastoid, pg parotid gland). (**b**) The mastoid segment of the facial nerve has been fully exposed after mastoidectomy. The tip of the sucker is in the stylomastoid foramen. (**c**) The facial nerve (FN) has been cut and luxated inferiorly, approaching the hypoglossal nerve (HN). (**d**) End-to-side suture completed

20.7.2 Exposure of the Facial Nerve

Usually, we proceed with the identification and isolation of the extrapetrosal portion of the facial nerve in its way from the stylomastoid foramen to the parotid gland, where it is followed until its main division or *pes anserinus* (Figs. 20.1b and 20.2a). The stylomastoid artery should be coagulated and sectioned. The mastoidectomy is carried out following the general principles described in the anatomical section. A horizontal line is marked with a pen on the mastoid surface from Henle's spine, and another vertical line from the tip of the mastoid that runs almost 1 cm posterior to the bony edge of the external auditory canal. Using a high-speed drill, the facial nerve is skeletonized in its entire mastoid segment and finally freed and mobilized. The nerve canal is opened in its posterior half. The facial nerve is covered by the periosteum of the facial canal and by its epineurium, so it has the characteristic of a regular peripheral nerve (Figs. 20.1c and 20.2b). The nerve is cut just at its more proximal point, where the mastoid nerve segment begins. All adhesions and branches are severed with delicate microscissors, grasping the epineurium of the stump of the facial nerve with jeweler-tipped forceps. The facial nerve is luxated in a caudal direction and carried near the hypoglossal nerve (Figs. 20.1d and 20.2c).

20.7.3 Exposure of the Hypoglossal Nerve

The hypoglossal nerve is located deeper and must be dissected proximally until its exit from the vascular aponeurotic sheath between the internal carotid artery medially and the internal jugular vein laterally, and distally until the nerve starts its curve going to the lingual muscles. This proximal and distal dissection of the hypoglossal nerve allows a free segment of the nerve of 2–3 cm, which can be maximized by mobilizing the digastric muscle and/or the occipital artery, even ligating and dividing the artery.

20.7.4 Nerve Anastomosis

We next pay attention again to the proximal section of the facial nerve, which is fully dislocated caudally to approximate the hypoglossal nerve. The epineural tissue of the facial nerve stump is removed with very thin scissors, and a section about one-quarter the thickness of the hypoglossal nerve is made at its concave dorsal aspect. We do not use any neurophysiological intraoperative tests because they have proven inefficient. The facial nerve is not functional at all, and the partial section of the hypoglossal nerve in its superior aspect has no functional or anatomical consequences for the patient. The end-to-lateral microsuture of the facial nerve to the hypoglossal nerve is done with 6–8 epineural 9/0 monofilament stitches (Figs. 20.1e and 20.2d).

20.7.5 Closure

The wound is closed by layers, taking care not to stretch the suture line. The mastoid cells are sealed, but it must be remembered that there is no risk of cerebrospinal fistula.

20.8 Complications, Prevention, and Management

Complications of ESHFN are few and of little relevance. There may be local pain, difficulty swallowing due to manipulation of the cervical region, or a hematoma from the wound. As it is an extracranial procedure, there is no risk of cerebrospinal fluid leak. Surgery without hospital admission may be considered.

20.9 Outcome, Prognosis, and Follow-Up

All facial nerve reanimation techniques are followed by months of waiting for functional recovery until regenerated axonal sprouts reach enough number of end plate neuromuscular targets. Therefore, facial nerve rehabilitation should be intensive and continuous from the first moment to preserve muscle and soft tissue elasticity and tone, avoid facial asymmetry, and prevent synkinesis. In addition, the eye must be actively protected by tarsorrhaphy or placement of a weight on the upper eyelid, if necessary.

The function of the facial nerve is evaluated with the HB grading, but a particular scale was developed by Pitty and Tator in 1992 for the evaluation of facial and hypoglossal nerve function after hypoglossal-facial anastomosis. A good outcome means good facial symmetry at rest, complete voluntary eye closure, mild to moderate mouth movement, minimal or absent synkinesis or mass movement, minimal or absent dysfunction in eating, swallowing, or speech, attributable to hypoglossal nerve section, and a feeling of major benefit from the procedure. Fair outcome means facial symmetry at rest; the patient is unable to obtain satisfactory closure of the eye, with marked synkinesis or mass movement, moderate dysfunction in eating, swallowing, or speech, attributable to hypoglossal nerve section, and a feeling of limited benefit from the procedure. Poor outcome should mean gross facial asymmetry at rest with total inability to close the eye and no mouth movement, marked synkinesis or mass movement, and a feeling of no benefit from the procedure. Finally, failure is no clinical evidence of reinnervation [8].

The SEFHN nerve must be followed by months of waiting for functional recovery until regenerated axonal sprouts reach enough number of end plate neuromuscular targets to begin any functional recovery. Electrophysiology studies indicate that revitalization begins a mean of 4–5 months after neurorrhaphy, but clinical recovery starts several weeks later. In our experience, almost all patients presented initial neurologic improvement 6 months after reanimation, moving the buccal angle. Twelve months after surgery, facial nerve function assessment with the HB scale showed that most of the patients with grade III. On the Pitty and Tator's scale, almost all patients achieved good recovery at 12 months. Later, recovery is very slow and unremarkable, and patients do not improve their HB or Pitty and Tator's scale grade. In clinical assessment and grading evaluation, it is necessary to consider that ocular closure function is improved by the ocular protection surgeries carried out in selected patients. However, no patients made a normal functional recovery in forehead mobility. No patients developed tongue atrophy, nor speech or swallowing disturbances [4].

Results of the SEHFN are usually analyzed in the literature, comparing this technique with the end-to-end hypoglossal-facial neurorrhaphy. Hamdi et al., in 2023, in a meta-analysis of the literature, summarize the results of both microneurosurgical techniques [9]. The proportion of good HB outcomes (HB I-III) did not differ by anastomosis type, end-to-side versus end-to-end anastomosis (73% vs. 59%). There was no difference in reported synkinesis rates between the anastomosis types. However, end-to-side anastomosis significantly developed less tongue atrophy than end-to-end anastomosis. Therefore, end-to-side anastomosis had significantly less speech and swallowing dysfunction than end-to-end anastomosis.

In the same way, some other factors have been considered in the prognosis of the nerve function recovery after end-to-side neurorrhaphy, particularly the age of the patient and the time between the nerve injury and reanimation. Some studies suggest that older people and a long delay in reanimation are risk factors for poor reinnervation, although results are not conclusive. In our opinion, patient age and time interval from facial nerve injury to reanimation might influence the quality of functional recovery through noncontrollable intermediate mechanisms, particularly muscular atrophy and fibrosis, soft tissue retraction, and elasticity loss. All these factors are more common in elderly patients and with a long interval from nerve lesion until reanimation. Also, the influence of rehabilitation, patient socioeconomic and health status, and the health center providing care may be relevant to the final clinical outcome [4, 8–10].

20.10 Management Modalities

The complete paralysis of the facial nerve muscles has been treated throughout history using different strategies.

20.10.1 Rehabilitation and Protection of Eye Complications

Rehabilitation of the facial nerve palsy is based on a daily routine based on massage maneuvers of the face and gesticulation in front of the mirror. Secondly, there is the periodic injection of low doses of botulinic toxin in the contralateral hypertonic muscles to avoid chronic deformity. Finally, patients with complete facial palsy can have disturbances in chewing, speaking, or swallowing, and they must be instructed to improve these functions. However, the most relevant question is the protection of the eye, because the lack of blinking and the dry eye favor recurrent conjunctival infections and corneal injuries, leading in some patients to severe complications with corneal opacity and loss of vision, unless a corneal transplantation is carried on. Eye protection is a question of applying adequate treatment at any stage of the disease, from artificial tears and protective creams, humid chambers, and artificial closure of the eyelid with tape, blepharoplasty if lagophthalmos, or gold eyelid weight procedures. These eye protection measures start just after the neurotmesis of the facial nerve, continue until the SEHFN, and are maintained indefinitely after, always tailored to the particular needs of each patient. Finally, the possible impact of the facial deformity suffered by the patient in their work, social, or family environment must be taken into account, evaluated, and adequately treated. This treatment can be purely psychological, involving coping strategies for acceptance of the deformity, or even pharmacological.

20.10.2 Facial Nerve Reanimation

Historically, different techniques of facial nerve resuscitation with neurorrhaphy to the hypoglossal nerve have been described. The oldest is the end-to-end epineurial neurorrhaphy (classic), with complete or incomplete section of the hypoglossal nerve and with or without the interposition of a nerve graft. End-to-side epineurial neurorrhaphy is currently used, with mobilization of the mastoid segment of the facial nerve and partial section of the hypoglossal nerve or without partial section of the hypoglossal nerve, suturing the facial nerve in an open window in the epineurium of the hypoglossal nerve. The advantages of end-to-side neurorrhaphy are that it has the same clinical results as end-to-end neurorrhaphy without the problems related to section of the hypoglossal nerve (hemilingual atrophy, dysphagia, dysarthria), it minimizes tongue atrophy and facial synkinesis, and it is especially interesting in cases of associated involvement of lower cranial nerves. In addition, the release of the mastoid segment makes it possible to avoid the use of an interposed graft and a double nerve suture.

20.11 Key Messages

- *The preferred microneurosurgical method for facial nerve resuscitation after neurotmesis is SEHFN.*
- *The patient's age, the amount of time after the neurotmesis, and the ongoing, rigorous rehabilitation program for the facial nerve injury are all factors that contribute to a positive functional outcome.*
- *Most patients achieve grade HB III clinical recovery 6 months following neurorrhaphy, and partial hypoglossal nerve section has no negative effects.*

References

1. Asaoka K, Sawamura Y, Nagashima M, et al. Surgical anatomy for direct hypoglossal-facial nerve side-to-end anastomosis. J Neurosurg. 1999;91:268–75. https://doi.org/10.3171/jns.1999.91.2.0268.
2. Atlas MD, Lowinger DS. A new technique for hypoglossal-facial nerve repair. Laryngoscope. 1997;107:984–91. https://doi.org/10.1097/00005537-199707000-00028.
3. Campero A, Socolovsky M. Facial reanimation by means of the hypoglossal nerve: anatomic comparison of different techniques. Neurosurgery. 2007;61(Suppl 3):41–9. https://doi.org/10.1227/01.neu.0000289710.95426.19.
4. González-Darder JM, Capilla-Guasch P, Escartín FP, et al. Side-to-end hypoglossal-facial neurorrhaphy for treatment of complete and irreversible facial paralysis after vestibular schwannoma removal by means of a retrosigmoid approach: a clinical and anatomic study. World Neurosurg. 2020;136:e262–9. https://doi.org/10.1016/j.wneu.2019.12.149.
5. Güerrissi JO, Gil Miranda MF. Intraneural topography of the extratemporal facial nerve: microsurgical nerve reconstruction. J Craniofac Surg. 2007;18:578–85. https://doi.org/10.1097/scs.0b013e318052feaa.
6. Mackinnon SE, Dellon AL. Fascicular patterns of the hypoglossal nerve. J Reconstr Microsurg. 1995;11:195–8. https://doi.org/10.1055/s-2007-1006531.
7. Liao C, Zhang W, Zhong W, et al. Facial-hypoglossal end-to-side neurorrhaphy: exploration of the source of axonal sprouting. J Reconstr Microsurg. 2016;32:599–607. https://doi.org/10.1055/s-0036-1584219.
8. Samii M, Alimohamadi M, Khouzani RK, et al. Comparison of direct side-to-end and end-to-end hypoglossal-facial anastomosis for facial nerve repair. World Neurosurg. 2015;84:368–75. https://doi.org/10.1016/j.wneu.2015.03.029.
9. Hamdi OA, Jones MK, Ziegler J, et al. Hypoglossal nerve transfer for facial nerve paralysis: a systematic review and meta-analysis. Facial Plast Surg Aesthet Med. 2024;26:219–27. https://doi.org/10.1089/fpsam.2023.0144.
10. Martins RS, Socolovsky M, Siqueira MG, et al. Hemihypoglossal-facial neurorrhaphy after mastoid dissection of the facial nerve: results in 24 patients and comparison with the classic technique. Neurosurgery. 2008;63:310–6. https://doi.org/10.1227/01.NEU.0000312387.52508.2C.

21 Atlas of Illustrative Cases

21.1 Case 1. Recurrent Vestibular Schwannoma with Multifocal Recurrence in the Cerebellopontine Angle Following Microneurosurgical Excision

A 62-year-old woman underwent surgery in 2008 for a Samii grade T3a left vestibular schwannoma (Fig. 21.1a), which involved a subtotal excision of the tumor to preserve the facial nerve. The extracanalicular segment of the tumor was entirely resected through a retro-sigmoid approach. The patient reported auditory impairment, tinnitus, and vertigo. After the surgery, she had cophosis, facial weakness rated as House–Brackman (HB) grade II in the early recovery stage, but she eventually improved. Sequential surveillance MRI imaging studies indicated a fast recurrence of the residual tumor (Fig. 21.1b). The patient underwent a second surgery two years later, involving the total excision of the extra and intracanalicular segments of the tumor, resulting in anatomical loss of the facial nerve a few millimeters beyond its emergence from the brainstem. This made it possible to directly resucitation of the facial nerve using Dott's tecnique. Specifically, it involved connecting the facial nerve from the brainstem to the facial nerve as it leaves the stylomastoid foramen, with help from a sural nerve graft placed in between. The proximal anastomosis between the facial nerve and the nerve graft was performed at the same surgical procedure as the removal of the vestibular schwannoma, whereas the distal anastomosis was conducted several weeks thereafter. The patient experienced total facial paralysis during the postoperative phase, ultimately recovering to an HB grade II. The MRI conducted six months post-surgery revealed a cup-shaped uptake at the fundus of the internal auditory canal and linear enhancement on the petrosal surface of the cerebellum, exhibiting scarring characteristics that have remained stable in subsequent examinations. During a routine imaging assessment, a novel punctate nodular enhancement was observed on the anterior surface of the pons (Fig. 21.1c). Subsequent examinations revealed an increase in size of this enhancement, along with the appearance of a new nodular lesion on the lateral surface of the medulla oblongata, related to the lower cranial nerves, which also exhibited rapid growth (Fig. 21.1d). Due to the growth of this new lesion, microneurosurgical excision was performed, revealing its relationship with the rootlets of the glossopharyngeal and vagal nerves. The histological examination revealed a typical schwannoma. The patient exhibited dysphagia throughout the postoperative phase, necessitating temporary gastrostomy feeding. The patient had no familial history or signs of neurofibromatosis, and the comprehensive genetic analysis revealed no mutations in the

J. M. González-Darder, *Microneurosurgery of Cerebellopontine Angle*,
https://doi.org/10.1007/978-3-032-03091-7_21

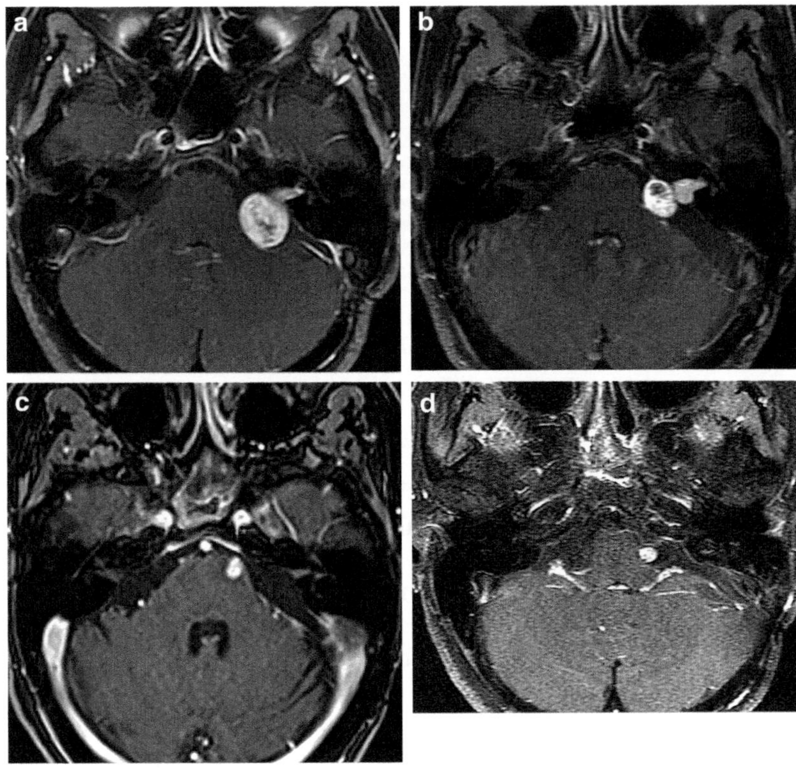

Fig. 21.1 Case 1. Recurrent vestibular schwannoma after microneurosurgical excision. (**a**) Axial image at the level of the internal auditory canal in a post-gadolinium MRI T1-weighted sequence showing a grade T3a vestibular schwannoma. (**b**) MRI imaging study showing the recurrence of the residual tumor. (**c**) MRI imaging study showing a new nodular enhancement on the anterior surface of the pons. (**d**) MRI imaging study showing a new nodular enhancement on the anterolateral surface of the medulla oblongata

NF2 gene. The pontine nodular lesion was subsequently treated using gamma knife stereotactic radiosurgery and remains stable five years post-treatment. The excised nodule has exhibited no recurrence, and no new nodules have emerged.

Comments This represents a case of unusual progression in vestibular schwannoma. Recurrence following subtotal resection is a potential outcome, but the recurrence rate of schwannomas excised with microneurosurgery is minimal; yet, it is elevated in instances of tumor remnants and increases with the size of the remnant. Recurrences occur with greater frequency and rapidity in neurofibromatosis type 2. The contamination of the surgical field during the resection of a schwannoma, accompanied by the emergence of additional lesions in the surrounding area, has not been documented. A scenario of mosaic neurofibromatosis type 2 may be postulated, wherein the mutation impacts just a subset of the patient's somatic cells, resulting in distinct topographic clinical manifestations.

21.2 Case 2. Microneurosurgical Excision of a Recurrent Vestibular Schwannoma Following Stereotactic Radiosurgery

A 58-year-old woman was diagnosed with a right vestibular schwannoma, rated as Samii grade T3a. She showed signs of hearing loss and trigeminal neuralgia, along with reduced sensation in the V2 and V3 branches' territories. Eight years ago, she had LINAC stereotactic radiosurgery for the schwannoma. However, her symptoms came back, along with slight facial weakness, HB grade II. The tumor size was diminished with stereotactic radiosurgery and exhibited rather steady intratumoral necrosis (Fig. 21.2a). The patient underwent surgery using a retrosigmoid approach, which showed a firm, fibrous, and hyaline tumor tightly attached to the cranial nerves (Fig. 21.2b). An initial opening of the internal auditory canal was executed to aid in resection. The tumor's origin was located in the

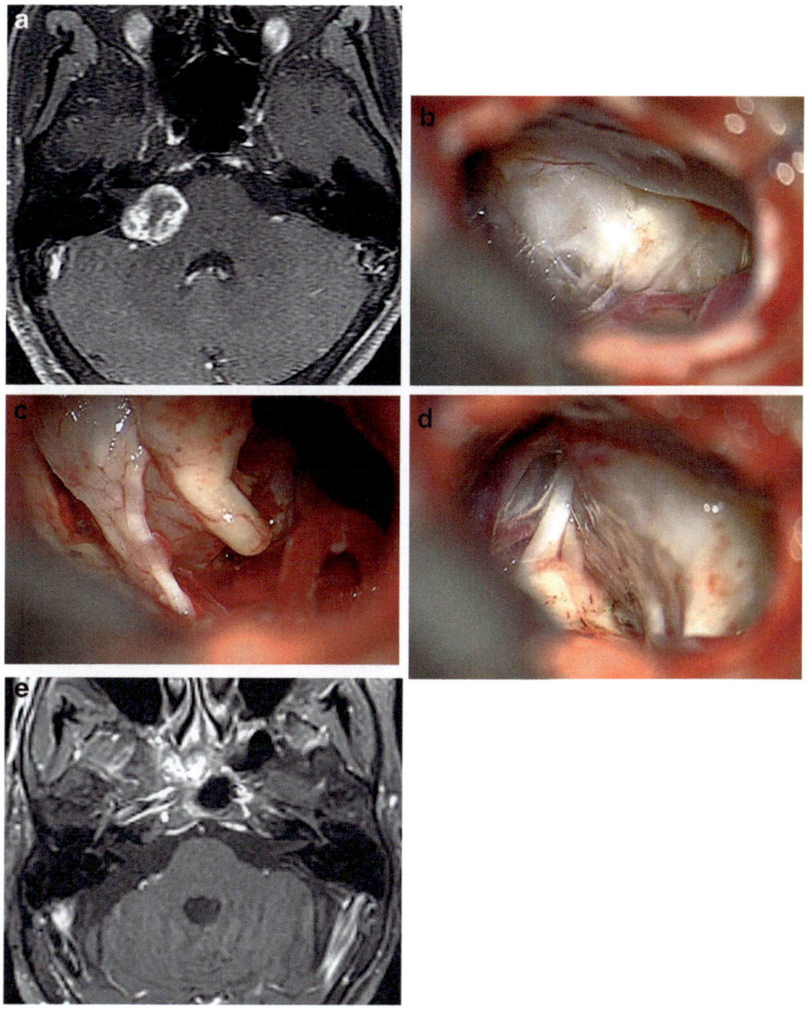

Fig. 21.2 Case 2. Recurrent vestibular schwannoma after stereotactic radiosurgical treatment. (**a**) Axial image at the level of the internal auditory canal in a post-gadolinium MRI T1-weighted sequence showing a grade T3a vestibular schwannoma after treatment with stereotactic radiosurgery, showing a central necrosis. (**b**) Intraoperative picture of the retrosigmoid transmeatal approach to the tumor. (**c**). Intraoperative picture showing over the tumor the trunk of the facial nerve (on the left), the transected vestibulocochlear nerve (in the center), and the anteroinferior cerebellar artery (on the right). (**d**) Intraoperative picture showing the final result of the excision and integrity of the trigeminal nerve and superior cerebellar artery. (**e**) Postoperative axial section at the level of the internal auditory canal in a post-gadolinium MRI T1-weighted sequence showing the total resection of the tumor

vestibulocochlear nerve, which was transected proximally near the brainstem (Fig. 21.2c). Nonetheless, the facial nerve could not be entirely separated from the tumor, resulting in a residual tumor that maintained the anatomical integrity and nerve conduction upon direct electrical stimulation of the facial nerve, albeit with a significant disparity in intensity between the proximal and distal segments, accompanied by the generation of substantial neurotonic discharges. The trigeminal nerve was shifted and twisted by the tumor, making contact with the superior cerebellar artery in its cranial segment (Fig. 21.2d). Postoperatively, total facial paralysis was noticed, exhibiting minimal improvement over time. Histopathological examination revealed the cellularity characteristic of a typical schwannoma. The patient had muscle transfers to enhance the functionality of the lower facial nerve-associated muscles and received a gold weight on the upper eyelid to facilitate eye closure. Trigeminal neuralgia resolved promptly post-surgery, and five years later, there are no findings of tumor recurrence (Fig. 21.2e).

Comments The stereotactic radiosurgical management of vestibular schwannoma controls the growth and clinical manifestations in a significant proportion of patients. In this case report, despite the patient's improvement from the trigeminal neuralgia endured for years, she experienced a relapse accompanied by sensory deficiency and subsequent facial paresis, prompting the proposal and acceptance of microneurosurgical excision. The tumor was confined to the vestibulocochlear nerve, which had to be severed. The tumor and fibrosis infiltrated and ensnared the facial nerve, hence exacerbating its functional impairment, while the anatomical and electrophysiological integrity was preserved post-resection. The trigeminal nerve was successfully decompressed, and there are no signs of recurrence eight years following the microneurosurgical excision.

21.3 Case 3. Postoperative Vestibular Schwannoma with Cerebrospinal Fluid Fistula

A 49-year-old lady with morbid obesity presents with a right vestibular schwannoma classified as Samii grade T3a (Fig. 21.3a), accompanied by complaints of hearing loss and tinnitus in the right ear. The bone CT scan shows widening of the meatus and internal auditory canal, clear air spaces in the petrosal bone, and air-filled cells in the back part of the internal auditory canal on both sides (Fig. 21.3b). Extensive openings were performed in the mastoid cells during the retrosigmoid approach. During the drilling of the meatus and the internal auditory canal, the cells of the posterior wall of the canal were also opened (Fig. 21.3c). All flaws were occluded with surgical wax, muscle pieces, dura mater grafting, and fibrin glue. An external lumbar drain is implanted and maintained for five days postoperatively, without rhinorrhea, until hospital release. Postoperatively, grade HB II facial paresis is noted and treated with steroids. The follow-up CT scan shows a large amount of fluid in the mastoid cells, drilling of the back part of the internal auditory canal, and fixing of the skull defect with titanium mesh (Fig. 21.3d). Two weeks later, the patient exhibits right rhinorrhea and mild swelling at the surgery site. The patient was hospitalized to commence therapy involving bed rest, the placement of an external lumbar drain, and the provision of prophylactic antibiotics, as the cerebrospinal fluid (CSF) culture test was negative. Seven days later, a sitting test was conducted, revealing continuing rhinorrhea; hence, a lumbo-peritoneal shunt was inserted, effectively managing the rhinorrhea, albeit resulting in a severe headache. Due to concerns over hyperdrainage syndrome, the valve's outflow pressure was adjusted, and the patient was released for home care. Three weeks post-discharge, the patient is readmitted, exhibiting signs of meningism, with *Streptococcus oralis* cultured from the cerebrospinal fluid. Consequently, antibiotic therapy was started per the antibiogram, the ventriculoperitoneal shunt was removed, and a new lumbar external drain was installed. A review of the surgical approach was conducted days afterward. The titanium mesh was taken out, and the condition of the dura mater was checked, which ruled out the chance of a fistula through the mastoid cells. The dura mater was opened, and the cerebellopontine angle was checked. This showed a bony defect on the back side of the petrosal bone that connects the cistern with the petrosal cells exposed during the tumor removal. The fibrinoid debris and scar tissue were excised, and a precise closure of the bone defect was executed with muscle and fibrin glue, and the external lumbar drainage was maintained for two weeks, and antibiotic therapy was extended for an additional three weeks until hospital discharge. The patient showed no new signs of CSF leak or infection and achieved the best possible recovery from facial nerve weakness (HB grade I) (Fig. 21.3e).

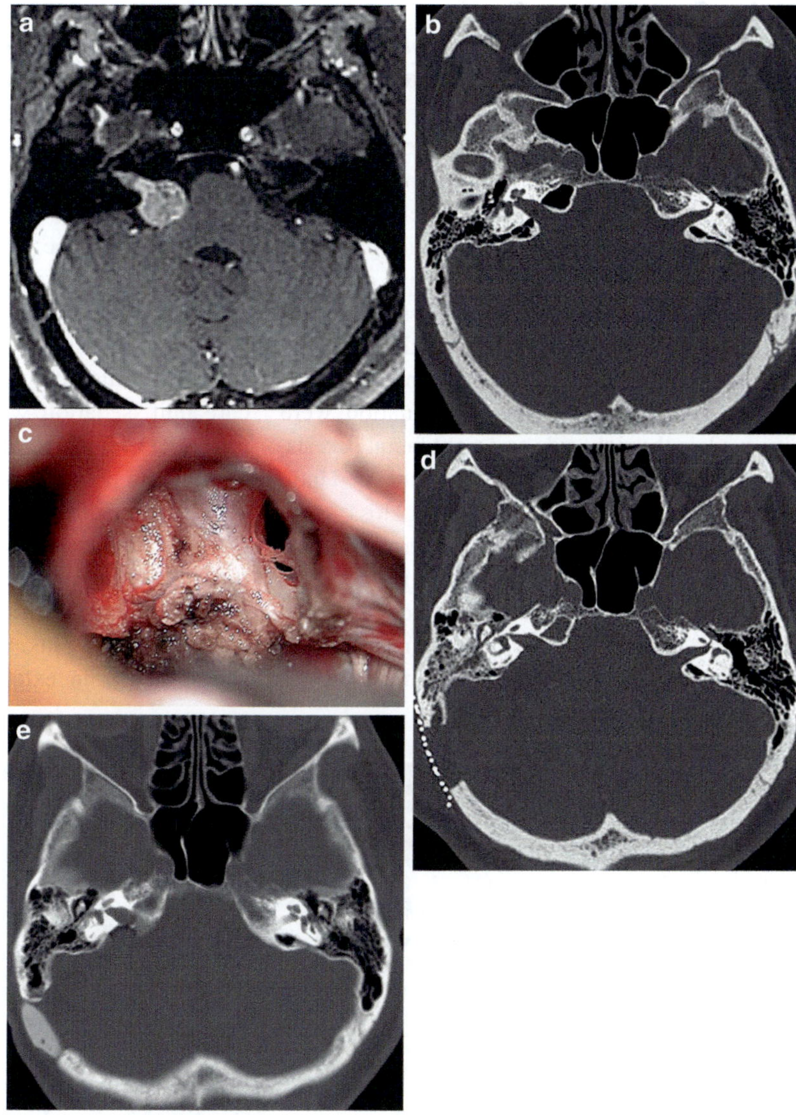

Fig. 21.3 Case 3. Postoperative cerebrospinal fluid fistula. (**a**) Axial image at the level of the internal auditory canal in a post-gadolinium MRI T1-weighted sequence showing a grade T3a vestibular schwannoma. (**b**) CT axial scan of the internal auditory canals, showing on the right side conspicuous pneumatized cells. (**c**) Intraoperative image of the retrosigmoid transmeatal approach, showing the intact tumoral intrameatal coverings and the opening of the air-filled cells (on the right). (**d**) A CT axial scan after surgery shows fluid in the mastoid cells, drilling of the back edge of the internal auditory meatus, and repair of the skull defect with titanium mesh. (**e**) Final CT axial scan after microsurgery to revise the CSF fistula, showing air in the mastoid cells and the skull defect closed with an acrylic cranioplasty

Comments Cerebrospinal fluid fistula is a prevalent complication associated with the retrosigmoid treatment for vestibular schwannomas. Cerebrospinal fluid leakage may arise at the surgical site due to inadequate watertight closure of the dura mater. It can also show as ipsilateral rhinorrhea, or the feeling of liquid swallowing when cerebrospinal fluid moves into the middle ear through open cells in the mastoid area from a craniotomy, which happens if the dura mater is not properly closed, or directly through the holes made when drilling the internal auditory canal. From the middle ear, the cerebrospinal fluid flows into the nasal cavity via the Eustachian tube. Corticosteroid usage and the patient's overweight may have contributed to the development or maintenance of the fistula. The case outlines a systematic approach to the adoption of preventive and treatment strategies for this prevalent complication.

21.4 Case 4. Large Cystic Schwannoma Accompanied by Surgical Hematoma

A 57-year-old patient was admitted following the detection of a large lesion in the right cerebellopontine angle. She presented a brief history of several months characterized by facial paresthesia and hypoesthesia, facial paresis, diplopia, dysphagia, and unilateral hearing loss, all affecting the right side. Recently, she had an uneven gait, necessitating assistance for ambulation. A modest tremor and motor incoordination were observed on the right side and right facial paresis, HB grade II, accompanied by synkinesis. Upon inquiry, she stated that the hearing loss commenced earlier, accompanied by intermittent tinnitus. The MRI showed a large right cystic vestibular schwannoma, rated as grade T5 based on Samii's classification, with no signs of hydrocephalus (Fig. 21.4a). The patient underwent a right retrosigmoid craniectomy, which exposed a polycystic lesion that was resected while preserving the anatomy and function of all cranial nerves except the vestibulocochlear nerve, achieving complete excision of both the extracanalicular and intracanalicular portions of the tumor through the opening of the internal auditory canal. Upon completion of the procedure, direct electrical stimulation of the facial nerve elicited an electromyographic response that mirrored the original one, utilizing similar stimulation parameters of intensity. Following transfer to the postoperative care unit, sedation was discontinued; however, the patient remained unconscious. Consequently, three hours post-intervention, an urgent CT scan was conducted, revealing hemorrhage in the surgical site that encompassed the entire volume of the excised tumor, accompanied by hydrocephalus without intraventricular bleeding (Fig. 21.4b). The patient was taken directly to the operating room, where an external ventricular drain was

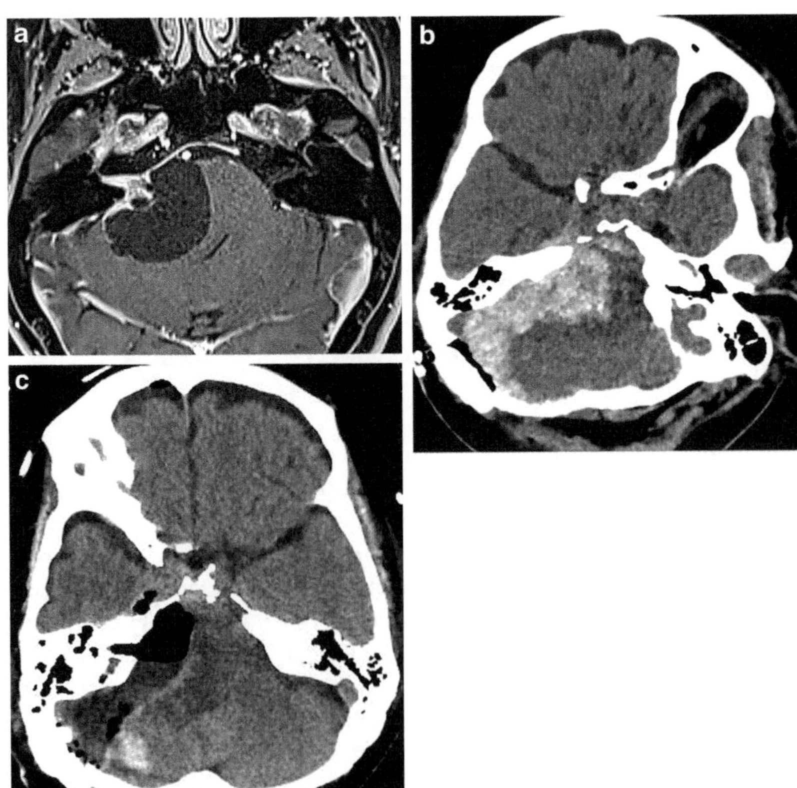

Fig. 21.4 Case 4. Postoperative hematoma. (**a**) Axial image at the level of the internal auditory canal in a post-gadolinium MRI T1-weighted sequence showing a T4 grade cystic vestibular schwannoma. (**b**) Postoperative CT scan showing a large cerebellopontine angle hemorrhage with compression of the brain stem. (**c**) Final CT scan after microsurgical removal of the hemorrhage

placed. The surgical area was reopened, and the hematoma was carefully removed using microneurosurgical techniques. This showed that the cranial nerves and the surface of the brainstem were unharmed. The hemorrhage was ascribed to a rupture of the superior petrosal vein at its junction with the superior petrosal sinus, which was subsequently sealed with hemostatic agents following hematoma evacuation. The following CT revealed total evacuation of the hematoma, with air present in the ear canal and improved decompression of the brain stem (Fig. 21.4c). The patient regained consciousness following the cessation of medication, and a few days later, her neurological status resembled that before surgery.

Comments Symptomatic postoperative hematoma is rare and precludes an emergent revision of the surgical approach. Blood in the surgical site is frequently seen in older patients with enlarged cisterns and does not need removal.

21.5 Case 5. Intracanalicular Meningioma Mimicking a Vestibular Schwannoma

A 60-year-old patient exhibited symptoms of left ear hearing loss and tinnitus for several months, thereafter developing a quickly progressing peripheral facial paresis graded HB III, unresponsive to steroid therapy. Audiometry revealed a decline in acute frequencies to 70 dB and bass frequencies to 30 dB. The CT examination revealed normal dimensions and morphology of both meatuses and internal auditory canals (Fig. 21.5a). The T2 and T1 MRI scans showed a tumor in the internal auditory canal that is 13 mm long and 5 mm wide. The tumor completely fills the canal but does not extend into the cistern of the cerebellopontine angle (Fig. 21.5b, c). The patient underwent surgery via a retrosigmoid transmeatal approach. A tumor reliant on the dura mater of the meatus was identified, and surgical biopsy verified it as a meningioma. The tumor

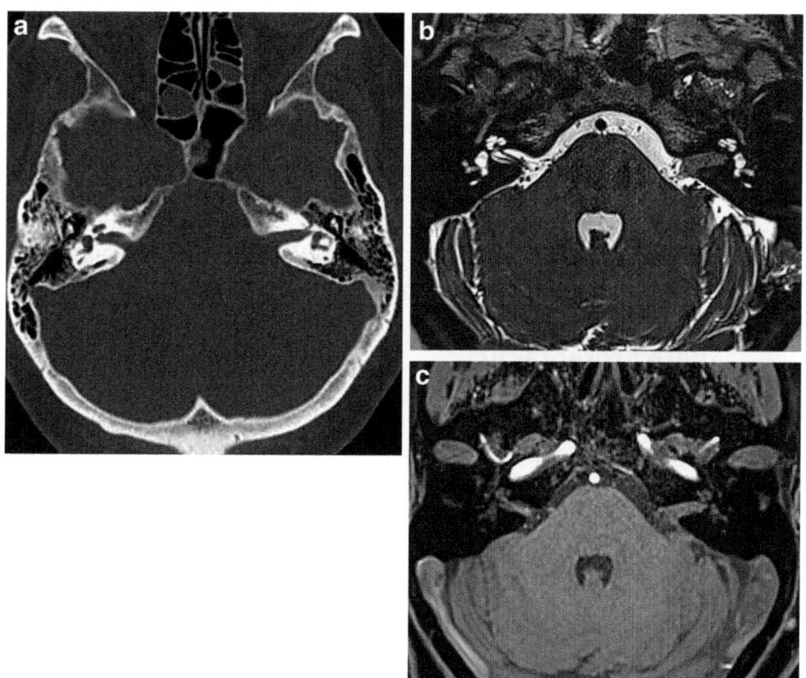

Fig. 21.5 Case 5. Intracanalicular meningioma. (**a**) CT axial scan section at the level of the internal auditory canals. (**b**, **c**) Axial images at the level of the internal auditory canal in an MRI T2- and T1-weighted sequence showing a tumor filling the internal auditory canal

was excised in fragments while preserving the anatomical integrity of the vestibulocochlear and facial nerves. Brainstem auditory evoked potentials (BAEP) exhibited reduced amplitude, with waves I to V absent and no modifications observed after the conclusion of the surgical procedure. The electromyographic recording showed regular neurotonic discharges in the muscles controlled by the facial nerve. It also showed a response to direct electrical stimulation of the facial nerve at 1.5 mA in the far side and at 4 mA in the near side after the resection of the tumor was finished. A definitive histological examination established that the lesion was a WHO grade I meningothelial meningioma. The patient's outcome was favorable, with restoration of facial nerve function to HB grade I, continued nonfunctional hearing loss, and no recurrence of the meningioma observed in imaging follow-up at 4 years.

Comments Intracanalicular meningioma is indistinguishable from intracanalicular schwannoma in imaging investigations and typically does not distort the meatus or the internal auditory canal. Clinically, it may exhibit more severe symptoms and progress more rapidly than a vestibular schwannoma.

21.6 Case 6. Progressive Intracanalicular Schwannoma and Treatment Problems Associated with Stereotactic Radiosurgery

A 60-year-old patient with considerable systemic diseases, including a lymphoproliferative disorder, was studied with MRI, revealing a few millimeter-sized right intracanalicular vestibular schwannoma in T1-weighted MRI with gadolinium enhancement. The patient reported bilateral hearing loss, more pronounced on the right side, accompanied by tinnitus (Fig. 21.6a). The lesion was monitored through imaging, showing growth in follow-up exams done at three years (Fig. 21.6b) and six years (Fig. 21.6c, d), with no signs of hydrocephalus or changes in clinical symptoms. Treatment was advised, and the lesion was treated using stereotactic radiosurgery with a gamma knife, delivering a maximum dose of 25 Gy. Several weeks later, the patient presented to the emergency department with complaints of headache, ataxia, disorientation, and diminished upper extremity function. The imaging investigation revealed ventricular enlargement with an Evans index of 0.38; however, the MRI flow scan did not yield definitive evidence of active hydrocephalus. Nonetheless, a comparison with prior imaging studies validated the evident dilation of the ventricular system (Fig. 21.6e). Symptomatic treatment commenced, resulting in partial and brief clinical improvement. After three weeks, a ventriculoperitoneal CSF shunt was placed, bringing the patient back to her normal condition. Imaging tests showed the ventricles had gotten smaller (Fig. 21.6f). The brain MRI done one year later shows that the lesion has increased in size and has a lot of necrotic tissue inside it. This condition was considered a pseudoprogression and is generally well tolerated (Fig. 21.6g).

Comments Small schwannomas may enlarge throughout the follow-up period, which should be monitored with imaging, as clinical complaints may not exhibit significant alterations. The etiology of hydrocephalus linked to schwannomas is inadequately comprehended. In this instance, where hydrocephalus occurs post-radiosurgery treatment, it may be associated with the production and discharge of proteins into the cerebrospinal fluid. Stereotactic radiosurgery causes significant intratumoral necrosis, resulting in tumor enlargement, typically asymptomatic, with the most probable diagnosis being pseudoprogression, which should be validated with follow-up imaging investigations.

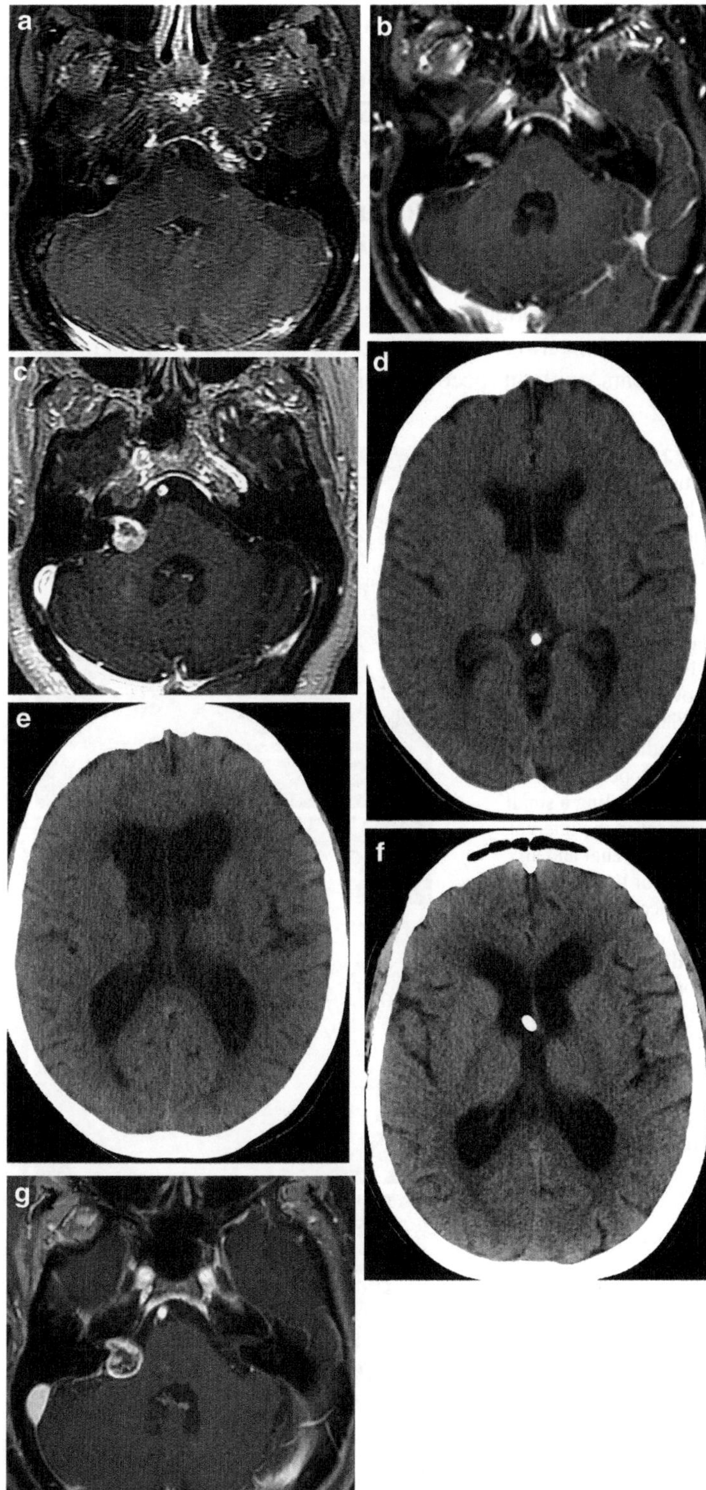

Fig. 21.6 Case 6. Growth of vestibular schwannoma. (**a**) Axial image at the level of the internal auditory canal in an MRI T1-weighted scan after gadolinium showing a tiny T1 grade vestibular schwannoma inside the canal at the time of diagnosis. (**b**) MRI study three years after diagnosis. (**c**) MRI study six years after diagnosis. (**d**) CT axial scan showing a normal-sized ventricular system. (**e**) CT scan showing an enlarged ventricular system following stereotactic radiosurgery treatment. (**f**) CT scan showing a reduction of ventricular size after shunting. (**g**) Axial image at the level of the internal auditory canal in an MRI T1-weighted scan after gadolinium showing a pseudoprogression of the tumor following stereotactic radiosurgery treatment

21.7 Case 7. Vestibular Schwannoma with Subtotal Resection and Residual Tumor Exhibiting Growth in the Postoperative Period, Managed with Stereotactic Radiosurgery, Resulting in Pseudoprogression

A 19-year-old patient presents with increasing right-sided hearing loss lasting approximately two years without accompanying tinnitus or vestibular complaints. Imaging examinations revealed a right vestibular schwannoma classified as Samii grade T4 (Fig. 21.7a). The patient possessed no functional hearing. The patient underwent microneurosurgical excision via a right retrosigmoid transmeatal approach. To safeguard the facial nerve, a small portion of the tumor was intentionally retained on the nerve. The intraoperative neurophysiological assessment showed strong neurotonic discharges, with the electromyographic response of the facial nerve muscles rising from 0.3 mA when the resection started to

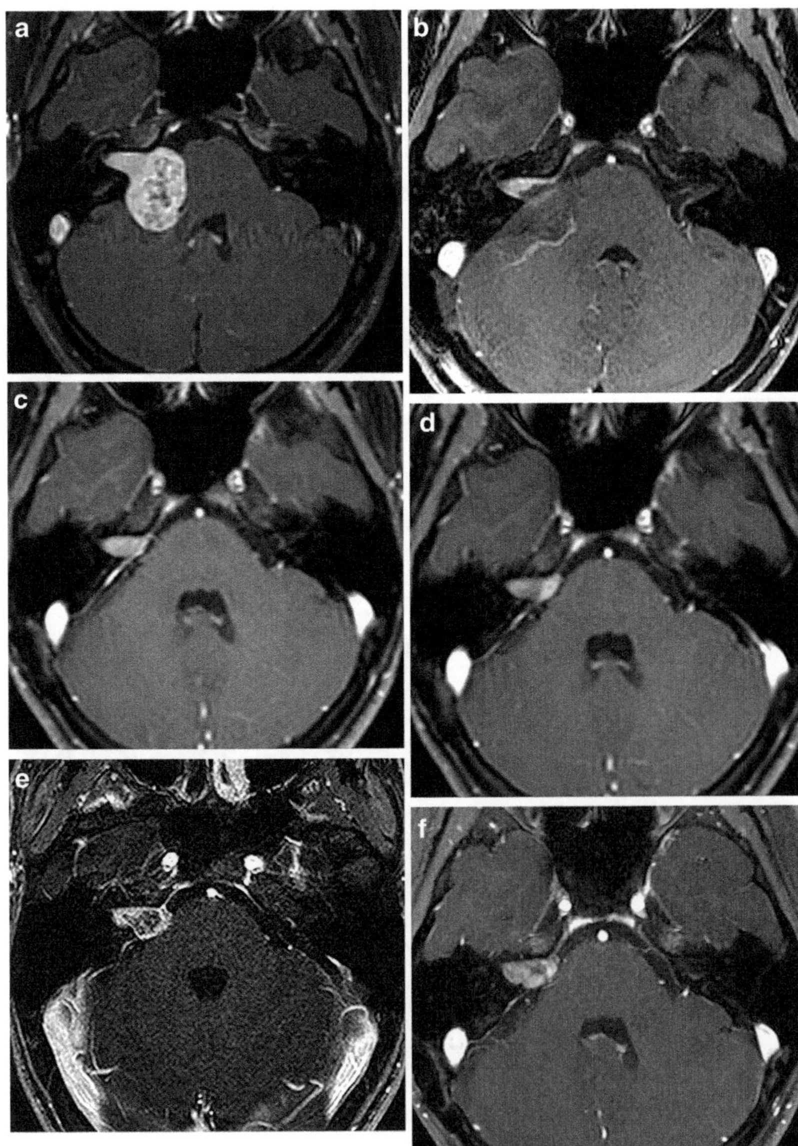

Fig. 21.7 Case 7. Growth of vestibular schwannoma after subtotal excision. (**a**) Axial image at the level of the internal auditory canal in a post-gadolinium MRI T1-weighted sequence showing a grade T4 vestibular schwannoma at the time of diagnosis. (**b**) Postoperative MRI study revealing a small remnant in the internal auditory canal and an extent of linear enhancement exhibiting inflammatory features. (**c, d**) MRI study six months and one year after subtotal excision. (**e**) MRI study six months after SRS treatment, showing a pseudoprogression. (**f**) MRI study five years after SRS treatment

0.9 mA when it ended. During the early postoperative period, trigeminal hypoesthesia, dysphagia, and dysphonia were apparent, resolving within a few weeks. Facial involvement was apparent with HB grade IV, although it progressed positively over a few weeks to HB grade I, with just the eye remaining dry. Cophosis manifested in the right ear. Several days after the surgery, an MRI was performed to assess the extent of the resection and the residual tumor volume. This revealed a small remnant in the internal auditory canal and a pronounced linear gadolinium enhancement along its walls, accompanied by a linear uptake in the cerebellar surface, both with distinctive inflammatory characteristics. (Fig. 21.7b). The remaining tumor had grown significantly during the follow-up done six months (Fig. 21.7c) and one year after surgery (Fig. 21.7d), leading to treatment with stereotactic radiosurgery using a gamma knife. The MRI conducted six months post-radiation revealed pseudoprogression characterized by intratumoral hyposignal, with no clinical worsening (Fig. 21.5e). Five years after radiosurgery, facial nerve function remains stable, and the remaining tumor has shown a slight increase in size compared to earlier evaluations (Fig. 21.5f).

Comments Near-total resection of schwannoma is a technique that intentionally leaves a small part of the tumor to help maintain hearing or the proper function of the facial nerve. The tumor remnant may be either treated using stereotactic radiosurgery or observed for growth.

21.8 Case 8. Vestibular Schwannoma with Incomplete Resection and Recurrence

A 20-year-old patient presents with gradual hearing loss and suboccipital pain. A grade 5 Samii left vestibular schwannoma was detected (Fig. 21.8a), and the patient had total excision without anatomical preservation of the vestibulocochlear nerve or the facial nerve. Three months after the surgery, a procedure was done to connect the hypoglossal nerve to the facial nerve to help the patient regain facial muscle movement, which led to a good recovery (HB grade II). Two years post-microneurosurgery, the MRI imaging examination revealed a recurrence in the internal auditory canal (Fig. 21.8b). Imaging has monitored this recurrence, revealing a gradual and

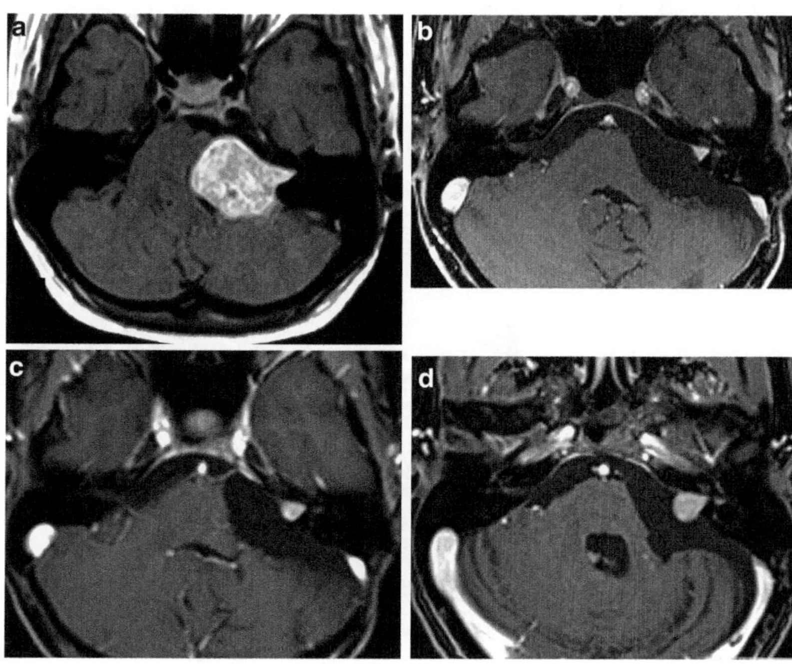

Fig. 21.8 Case 8. Growth of vestibular schwannoma after subtotal excision (**a**) Axial image at the level of the internal auditory canal in a post-gadolinium MRI T1-weighted sequence showing a grade T4 vestibular schwannoma at the time of diagnosis. (**b**) Postoperative MRI study revealing a small cup remnant in the internal auditory canal. (**c, d**) Sequential MRI studies showing the growth of the remnant

steady increase in size (Fig. 21.8c, d), with no clinical implications.

Comments Only imaging examinations can detect potential recurrence in individuals lacking vestibulocochlear or facial nerve function preservation. Checking for tumor growth in the cisterns is done using MRI, and if the tumor grows quickly, it shows changes suggesting it is becoming malignant or pressing on the brainstem it would require urgent microsurgical excision. This follow-up should be perpetual, and the recurrence should be excised. Styereotactic radiosurgery is not an advisable alternative, as there are no neurological or otological functions to maintain, except for contraindications to major microneurosurgery or the patient's preferences.

21.9 Case 9. Vestibular Schwannoma with Postoperative Cerebrospinal Fluid Fistula

A 50-year-old patient had surgical intervention for a grade T4 right cystic vestibular schwannoma (Fig. 21.9a). In the early postoperative period, the patient had cerebrospinal fluid accumulation in the surgical wound and right cerebrospinal fluid rhinorrhea, together with a sensation of middle ear fullness. The preoperative CT scan revealed significant pneumatization of both temporal bones, with cells extending to the posterior wall of the internal auditory canal and the apices of both petrosal bones (Fig. 21.9b). The tumor was removed from the internal audi-

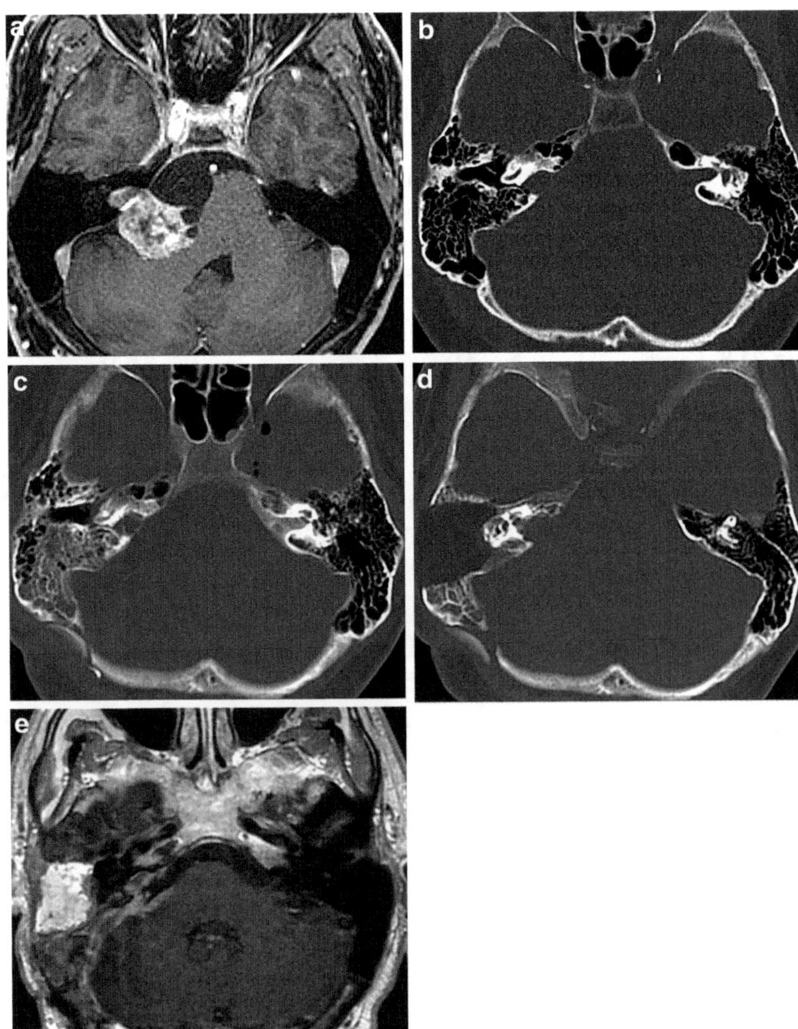

Fig. 21.9 Case 9. Postoperative cerebrospinal fluid fistula. (**a**) Axial image at the level of the internal auditory canal in a post-gadolinium MRI T1-weighted sequence showing a grade T4 cystic vestibular schwannoma. (**b**) CT axial scan of the internal auditory canals, showing conspicuous pneumatized cells extending to the posterior wall of the internal auditory canal. (**c**) Postoperative CT axial scan revealing fluid in the mastoid cells. (**d**, **e**) Final CT scan and MRI studies after radical microsurgical mastoidectomy, revision, and closure of the CSF fistula

tory canal, and no petrosal air cells were damaged. The postoperative CT scan revealed fluid accumulation in nearly all temporal cells (Fig. 21.9c). A sequential treatment was initiated due to the successive failure of all implemented procedures, including compression bandaging, bed rest, external lumbar drainage, and revision of the craniotomy to occlude the suspected open mastoid cells while exploring the intracranial region. There were no indications of cerebrospinal fluid infection; yet, the rhinorrhea showed no improvement. Since the problem was still not resolved and there was no proof of a connection related to the fistula, a radical mastoidectomy was performed. This involved sealing the cells and using an autologous fat graft, along with setting up a new temporary external lumbar drainage, which eventually led to the closure of the fistula (Fig. 21.9d, e).

Comments Cerebrospinal fluid fistula is a common complication following retrosigmoid surgical procedures for cerebellopontine angle tumors, particularly vestibular schwannomas, which necessitate drilling of the internal auditory canal. When less aggressive approaches fail, a strategy involving progressively complex and aggressive operations becomes necessary to address the fistula.

21.10 Case 10. Large Cystic Schwannoma Exhibiting Fast Growth and Increasing Clinical Manifestations

An 87-year-old patient was diagnosed with a Samii grade 3 left vestibular schwannoma (Fig. 21.10a), attributed to dizziness and gait instability. The patient had multiple systemic diseases yet remained autonomous in daily activities. He experienced bilateral hearing loss, absence of tinnitus or dizziness. Symptomatic management and imaging surveillance were advised. The lesion enlarged (Fig. 21.10b, c) six months later, and the patient's clinical condition deteriorated, particularly in terms of gait instability. An imaging exam done six months later showed that the tumor continued to grow, created several cysts, and was pressing on the brainstem and cerebellar peduncle. In the subsequent

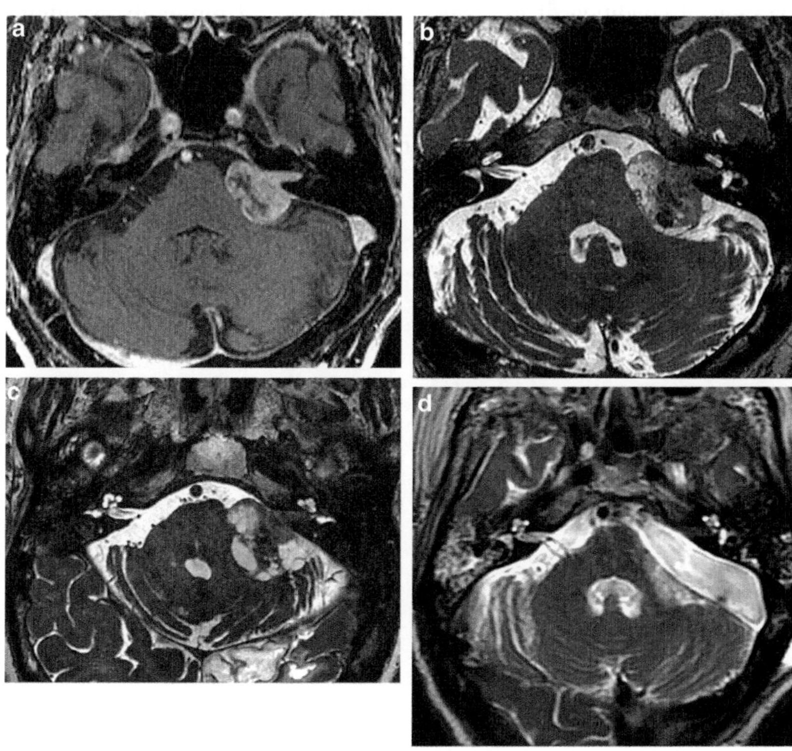

Fig. 21.10 Case 10. Growth of cystic vestibular schwannoma. (**a**) Axial image at the level of the internal auditory canal in a post-gadolinium MRI T1-weighted sequence showing a grade T3 vestibular schwannoma at diagnosis. (**b**, **c**) Axial images at the level of the internal auditory canal in an MRI T2-weighted sequence showing the enlargement of the vestibular schwannoma six months and one year later after diagnosis. (**d**) Postoperative MRI study after total excision

months, the patient's decline became increasingly evident, necessitating support for ambulation at home and a wheelchair for outdoor mobility. The patient experienced pain at the back of the head, hypoesthesia in parts of the face, and weakness in the facial muscles (HB grade III). The patient sought microneurosurgical intervention, which was performed via a left retrosigmoid approach. A cystic lesion was identified, pierced, and drained, resulting in internal decompression. The tumor walls exhibited a highly diverse look, with the contents displaying areas of necrosis and hemorrhage at various stages. The intracanalicular component was excised via transmeatal access. We achieved the anatomical and functional integrity of the facial nerve and all other cranial nerves, except the vestibulocochlear nerve. The procedure and recovery phase were unremarkable, with no deterioration in the function of the affected cranial nerves. Physiotherapy and rehabilitation commenced to facilitate ambulation recovery. Imaging investigations confirmed total excision of the tumor (Fig. 21.10d).

Comments The quick growth and worsening of the clinical condition of the patient with cystic schwannomas usually indicate a clear justification for microneurosurgery. The patient's age is a risk factor; nonetheless, it does not serve as an absolute contraindication for surgical intervention.

21.11 Case 11. Meningioma of the Foramen Magnum

A 48-year-old patient underwent cervical MRI for cervical syndrome, which identified a meningioma in the foramen magnum (Fig. 21.11a, b). The neurological assessment and somatosensory-evoked potentials were unremarkable. Microneurosurgical intervention was advised; however, the patient postponed the procedure for several years, during which no enlargement or exacerbation of neurological symptoms was observed. Ultimately, the tumor was entirely excised via an osteoplastic laminotomy of C1, accompanied by complete microneurosurgical resection of the tumor. The lesion was situated immediately under the dura mater (Fig. 21.11c). Following total excision, the dentate ligament is exposed, with the C2 posterior cervical rootlets intersecting, several rootlets of the accessory nerve ascending to the posterior fossa, and the hypoglossal nerve rootlets in a deeper plane (Fig. 21.11d). The surgical outcome and subsequent imaging assessments have been favorable (Fig. 21.11e).

Comments Meningiomas located behind the dentate ligament at the foramen magnum are easier to remove with microneurosurgery.

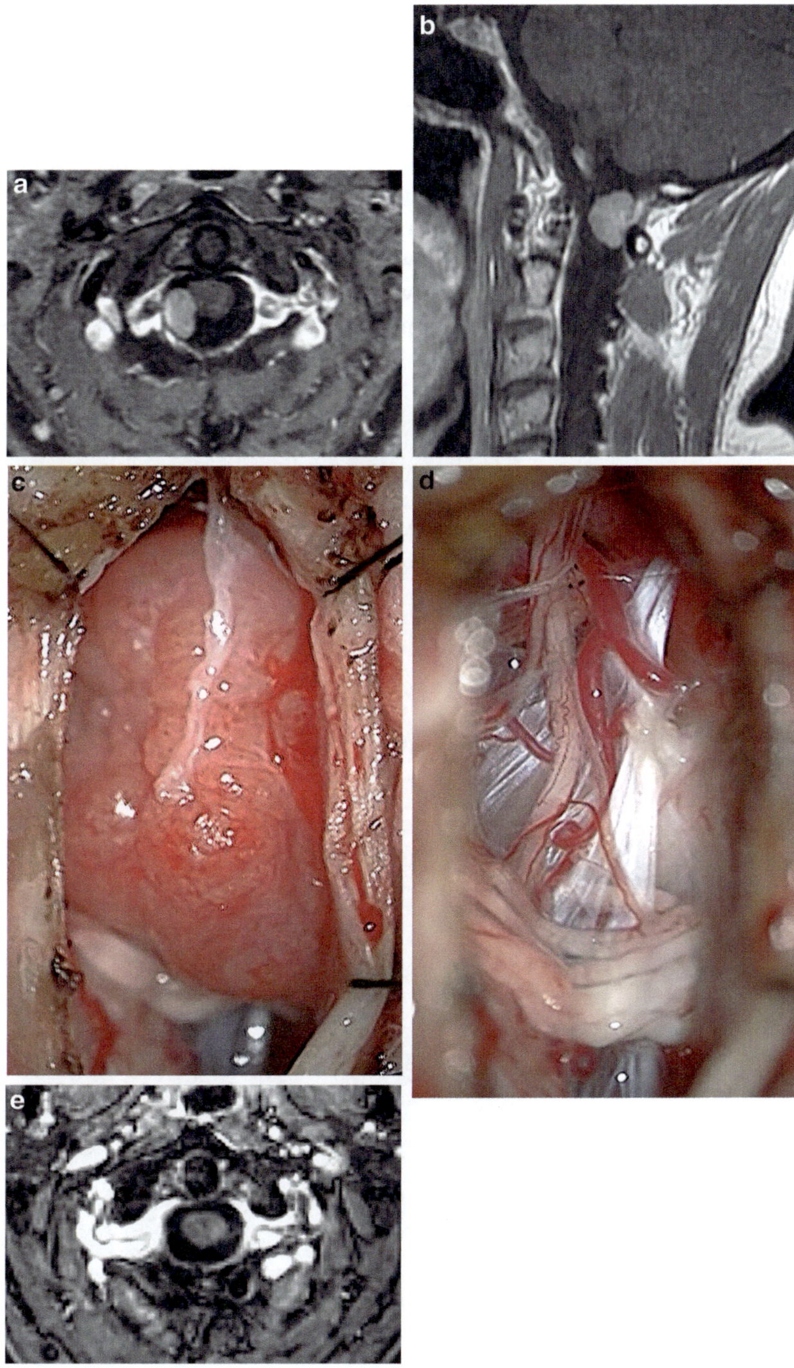

Fig. 21.11 Case 11. Foramen magnum meningioma. (**a**, **b**) Axial and sagittal images at the level of the foramen magnum in a post-gadolinium MRI T1-weighted sequence showing a small foramen magnum meningioma. (**c**) Intraoperative image of the C1 unilateral osteoplastic laminotomy, showing the tumor after opening the dura mater. (**d**) Intraoperative picture after radical excision of the tumor. (**e**) Postoperative MRI study after total excision

21.12 Case 12. Inframeatal Meningioma

A 45-year-old patient exhibits multiple acute and temporary neurological symptoms indicative of transient ischemic episodes, including dysphasia, visual abnormalities, and isolation from the surroundings. The imaging study showed a large tumor at the back of the clivus that was pushing on the brainstem and was likely a meningioma (Fig. 21.12a–c). The lesion was completely excised via a left retrosigmoid approach, revealing its origin in the left jugular tubercle, which had hyperostosis that required subsequent drilling. The tumor extended from the hypoglossal nerve to the trigeminal nerve and was situated between the two vertebral arteries. During the surgery, tests on the cranial nerves showed a strong response to electrical stimulation, but there was a significant decrease in somatosensory

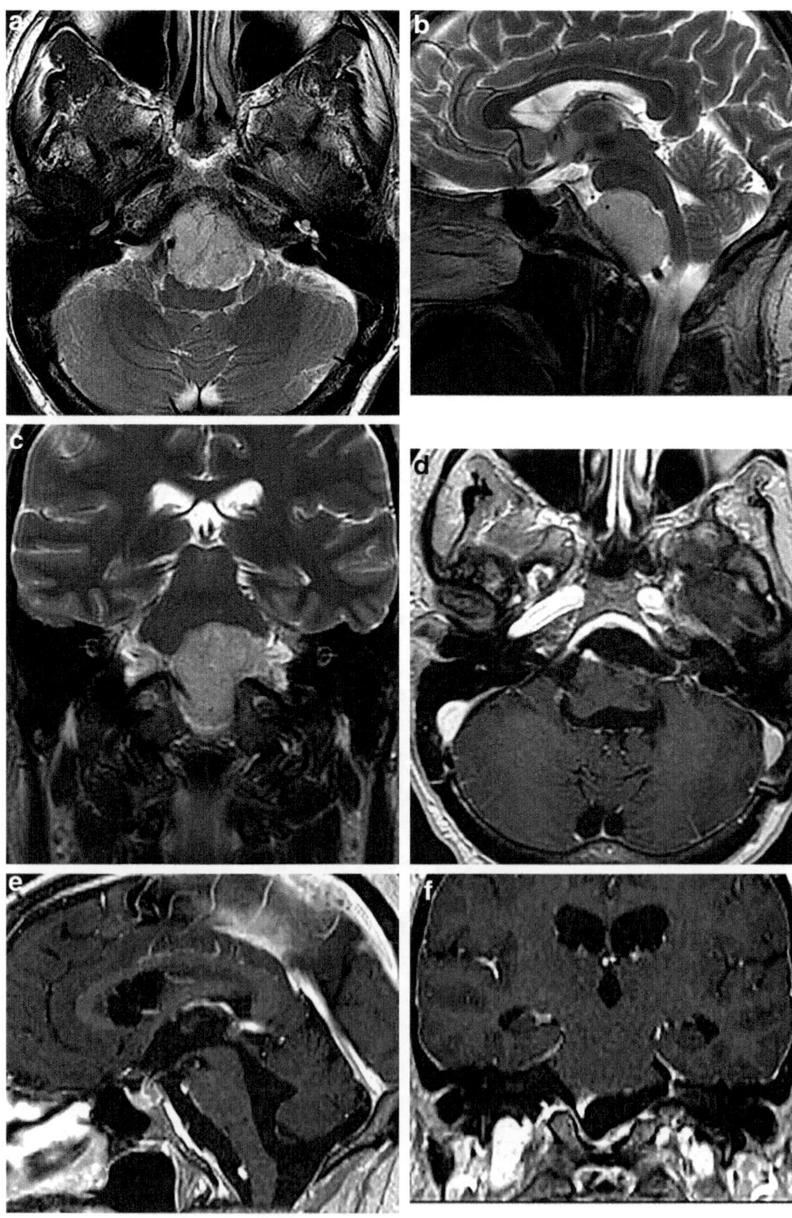

Fig. 21.12 Case 12. Inframeatal meningioma. (**a**–**c**) Axial, sagittal, and coronal images in an MRI T2-weighted sequence showing a large posterior fossa meningioma. (**d**–**f**) Postoperative axial, sagittal, and coronal in a post-gadolinium MRI T1-weighted sequence after complete resection

potentials on the left side. Post-surgery, the patient regained consciousness but experienced dysfunction of the sixth, seventh (HB grade III), eighth, ninth, and tenth cranial nerves, along with a global hemiparesis of 4/5 on the right side of the body. This necessitated a temporary external ventricular shunt, tarsorrhaphy, gastrostomy feeding, tracheostomy, and rehabilitation. The patient was admitted to a facility specializing in acquired brain damage for extensive rehabilitation. The patient's overall improvement was satisfactory, albeit with certain limits in daily tasks. Imaging controls indicated total excision of the tumor and an ischemic region in the left anterolateral segment of the medulla oblongata, implying involvement of the perforating branches of the anterior inferior cerebellar artery. The tumor has exhibited no indications of recurrence nine years post-surgery (Fig. 21.12d–f).

Comments Removing large cerebellopontine tumors requires handling cranial nerves, and even if the nerves are preserved, patients may experience varying degrees of clinical decline depending on how much damage was done. Ischemic lesions exhibit a poorer clinical and functional outcome.

21.13 Case 13. Petroclival Meningioma

A 50-year-old patient was identified with a left petroclival meningioma, attributed to trigeminal neuralgia and growing gait instability over several years (Fig. 21.13a–c). The patient underwent surgery via a left retrosigmoid approach, identifying the tumor's origin near the entrance of Meckel's cave and the inferior surface of the tentorium, requiring partial resection for excision. Electrophysiological monitoring of the cranial nerves revealed a robust electromyographic response to direct electrical stimulation in all nerves at the conclusion of the surgery; nonetheless, there were significant neurotonic discharges in the muscles innervated by the facial and tri-

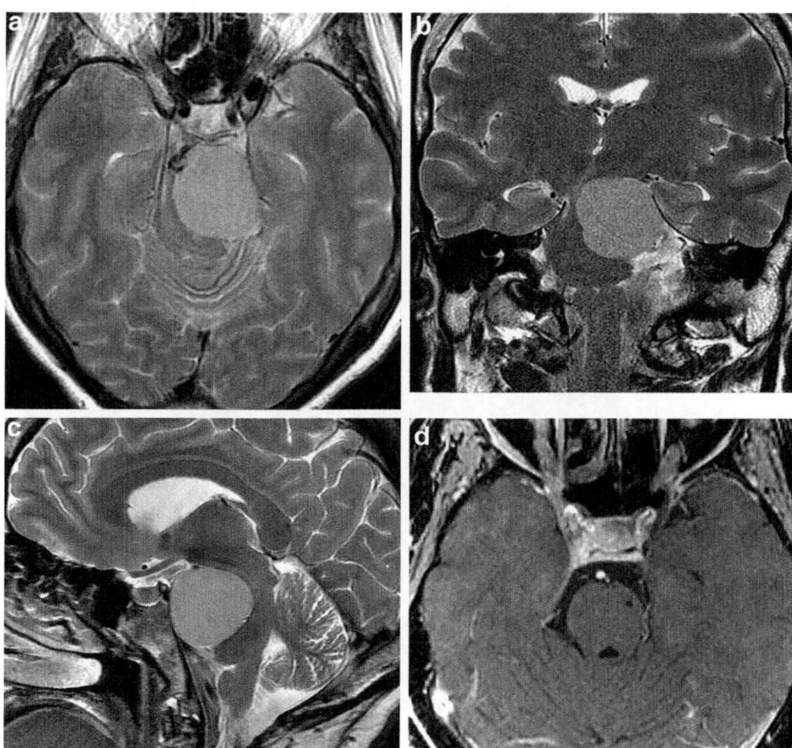

Fig. 21.13 Case 13. Petroclival meningioma. (**a**–**c**) Axial, sagittal, and coronal images in an MRI T2-weighted sequence showing a large petroclival meningioma. (**d**) Postoperative axial MRI T1-weighted study after total excision

geminal nerves. Post-surgery, there was a dysfunction of the fourth, seventh (HB grade II), eighth, and ninth cranial nerves, as well as a hemiparesis of 4/5 on the right side of the body. The patient was admitted to an acquired brain injury center for extensive neurorehabilitation. The patient's overall progress was satisfactory, albeit with some restrictions in everyday activities, accompanied solely by neuropathic pain in the facial region and the right side of the body. The imaging controls indicated whole tumor excision and a punctate ischemic region in the left anterolateral midbrain, implying involvement of the perforators of the superior cerebellar artery (Fig. 21.13d).

Comments The resection of large tumors in the cerebellopontine angle implies the manipulation of cranial nerves. Despite potential anatomical and electrophysiological preservation, it should be anticipated that a clinical deterioration of varying intensity and duration will occur, contingent upon the severity of the incurred nerve or vascular injury. Ischemic lesions exhibit a poorer clinical and functional outcome.

21.14 Case 14. Petroclival Meningioma Extending into Meckel's Cave

A 55-year-old patient exhibited symptoms of left trigeminal neuralgia accompanied by facial hypoesthesia and gait instability. Imaging examinations revealed a petroclival meningioma, causing compression of the brainstem and expansion into the Meckel's cave (Fig. 21.14a). A total resection was scheduled via the retrosigmoid approach. The tumor was located next to the superior petrosal vein complex, pressing down on

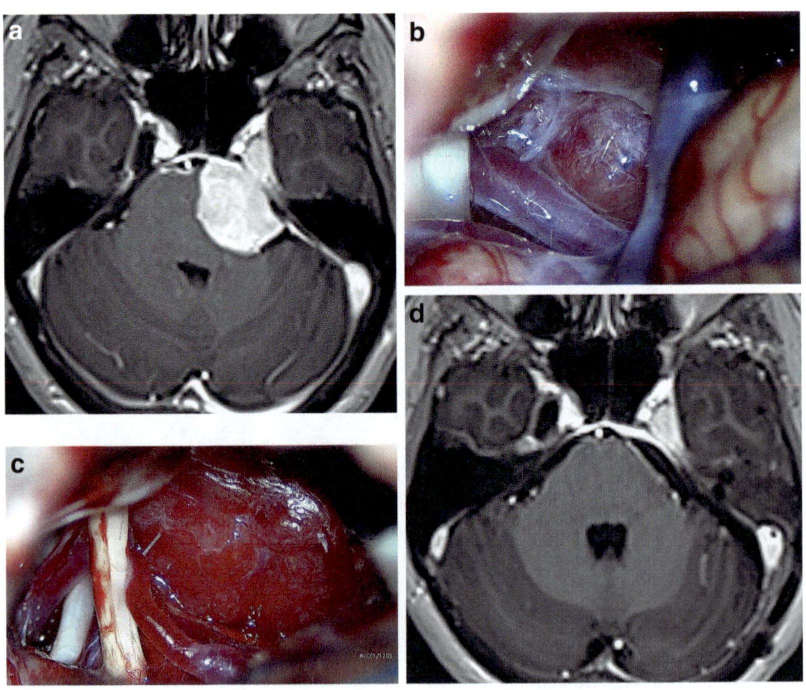

Fig. 21.14 Case 14. Petroclival and Meckel's cave meningioma. (**a**) Axial image at the level of the incisural foramen in a post-gadolinium MRI T1-weighted sequence showing a large petroclival meningioma extending into the Meckel's cave. (**b**) Intraoperative image of the retrosigmoid approach, showing the tumor covered by venous channels of the superior petrosal system. (**c**) Intraoperative image showing the tumor and the relationships between the tumor and the cranial nerves and vessels. (**d**) Postoperative axial MRI study after total excision of the cerebellopontine angle portion of the tumor, showing Meckel's cavum remnant

the facial and vestibulocochlear nerves. A substantial anterior inferior cerebellar artery traversed between the nerves and the tumor (Fig. 21.14b, c). We observed an enlargement of the tentorium and meatus of the Meckel's cave following internal decompression of the tumor. A tumor occupied the Meckel's cave, with no discernible separation from the trigeminal nerve fascicles. The trochlear nerve was unidentifiable, and the superior cerebellar artery was isolated. Moreover, during the surgical procedure, the electromyographic response of the trigeminal muscles to direct electrical stimulation was absent. Consequently, only the infratentorial excision of the tumor was performed. In the postoperative phase, the neuralgia resolves, leaving permanent facial hypoesthesia without functional motor impairment of the trigeminal muscles. The follow-up MRI at six months shows that the infratentorial tumor was completely removed, but there is still some tumor left in the Meckel's cave (Fig. 21.14d). After discussing various treatment options for the residual tumor, the patient decides to proceed with gamma knife stereotactic radiosurgery.

Comments Meningiomas of the cerebellopontine angle with multicompartmental extension may be excised in two or more surgical steps, ensuring complete resection of the targeted compartment in all instances. In our patient, resection was incomplete due to intraoperative findings, compelling an adaptive resection strategy.

21.15 Case 15. Meningeal Melanocytoma

A 46-year-old female presented with gait instability and diplopia. An axial T2-weighted MRI revealed a hyperintense lesion at the left cerebellopontine angle, displacing the midbrain (Fig. 21.15a), whereas a T1-weighted MRI with contrast demonstrated intense homogenous enhancement (Fig. 21.15b). The initial diagnosis suggested a left tentorial meningioma, so surgery through a retrosigmoid approach was advised. A brown lesion, mushy and tar-like in appearance, was found behind the petrosal vein complex during the surgical procedure (Fig. 21.15c). It appeared to originate from the dura mater and was entirely excised. The histological diagnosis identified meningeal melanocytoma. The postoperative recovery was satisfactory; however, diplopia lingered due to trochlear nerve paresis, which was alleviated using prism lenses. A control MRI conducted six months post-resection revealed a local recurrence, which was subsequently excised. Two years later, a T1-weighted MRI with gadolinium showed a return of the tumor in the area, marked by two spots that lit up with contrast: one on the surface of the cerebellar hemisphere and a smaller one deeper near the basilar artery (Fig. 21.15d). The patient underwent another microsurgical excision of both lesions. The superficial (Fig. 21.15e) and deep (Fig. 21.15f) lesions were excised. Notably, dark-hued pigmentation and microlesions were detected over the leptomeninges of the cerebellopontine angle, encompassing the cranial nerves, including the vestibulocochlear and facial nerves (Fig. 21.15g). The punctate lesions were recognized as deposits of melanocytoma in the histological examination. Treatment options, including beam radiation, stereotactic radiosurgery, chemotherapy, and immunotherapy, were examined but ultimately dismissed due to the ineffectiveness of any oncological intervention resulting from the absence of a *BRAF gene* mutation in the tumor cells. The patient had a steady decline in ambulation, necessitating the use of a wheelchair, while diplopia intensified and a severe homolateral cerebellar condition emerged. Several months later, an MRI follow-up showed new tumor growth with multiple nodules in the cerebellopontine angle (Fig. 21.15h, i), as well as various other implants of different sizes on the surface of the cervical spinal cord. A final microneurosurgical exploration was done, but the cerebellopontine area was filled with tumor nodules (Fig. 21.15j), so only a new biopsy was taken to gather material for molecular biology analysis of the tumor to check for any changes in tumor type. No more metastases were present at any point. The patient experienced a gradual decline in brainstem functions till her demise.

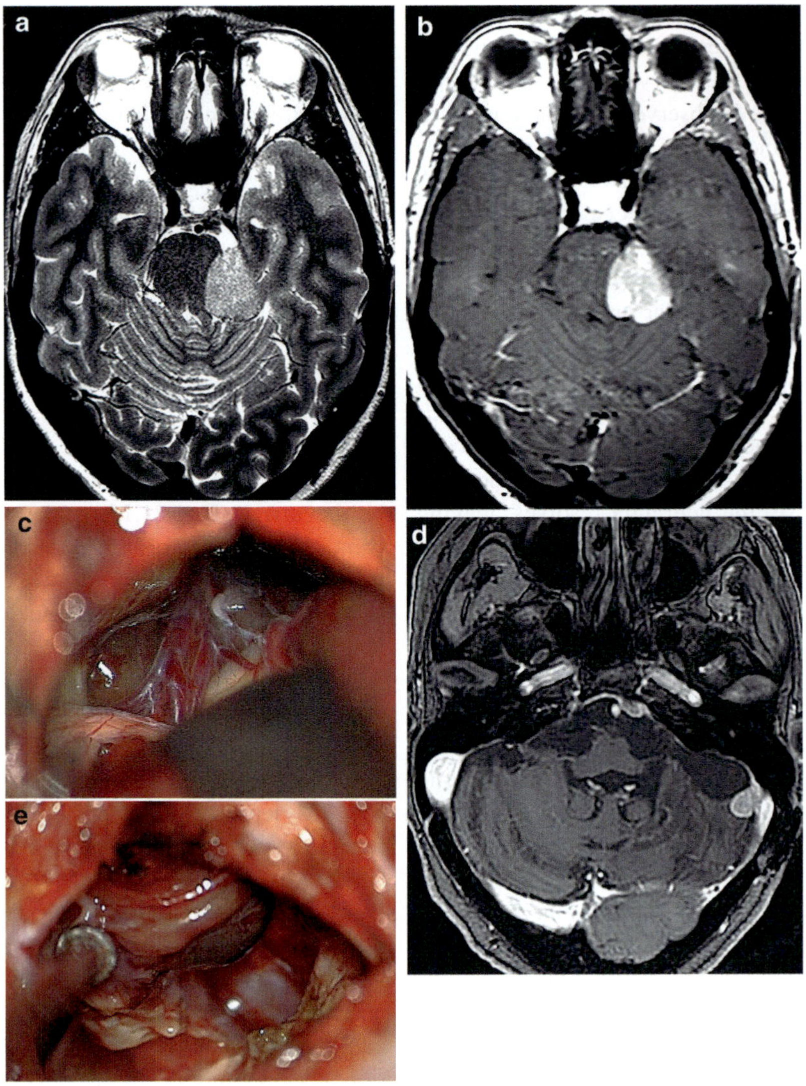

Fig. 21.15 Case 15. Meningeal melanocytoma. (**a**, **b**) Axial section at the level of the incisure foramen in an MRI T2- and T1-weighted sequence post-gadolinium showing a large lateral incisure tumor. (**c**) Intraoperative image of the retrosigmoid approach, showing a brown-stained tumor covered by venous channels of the superior petrosal system. (**d**) Postoperative axial image in a post-gadolinium MRI T1-weighted sequence showing a regional recurrence of the tumor with two noticeable lesions. (**e**, **f**) Intraoperative images of the revision retrosigmoid approach, showing both lesions. (**g**) Intraoperative image showing multiple punctate tumoral implants and spots. (**h**, **i**) Postoperative axial images in a post-gadolinium MRI T1-weighted sequence showing a massive multifocal posterior fossa recurrence. (**j**) Intraoperative images of the revision retrosigmoid approach, showing multiple tumoral implants

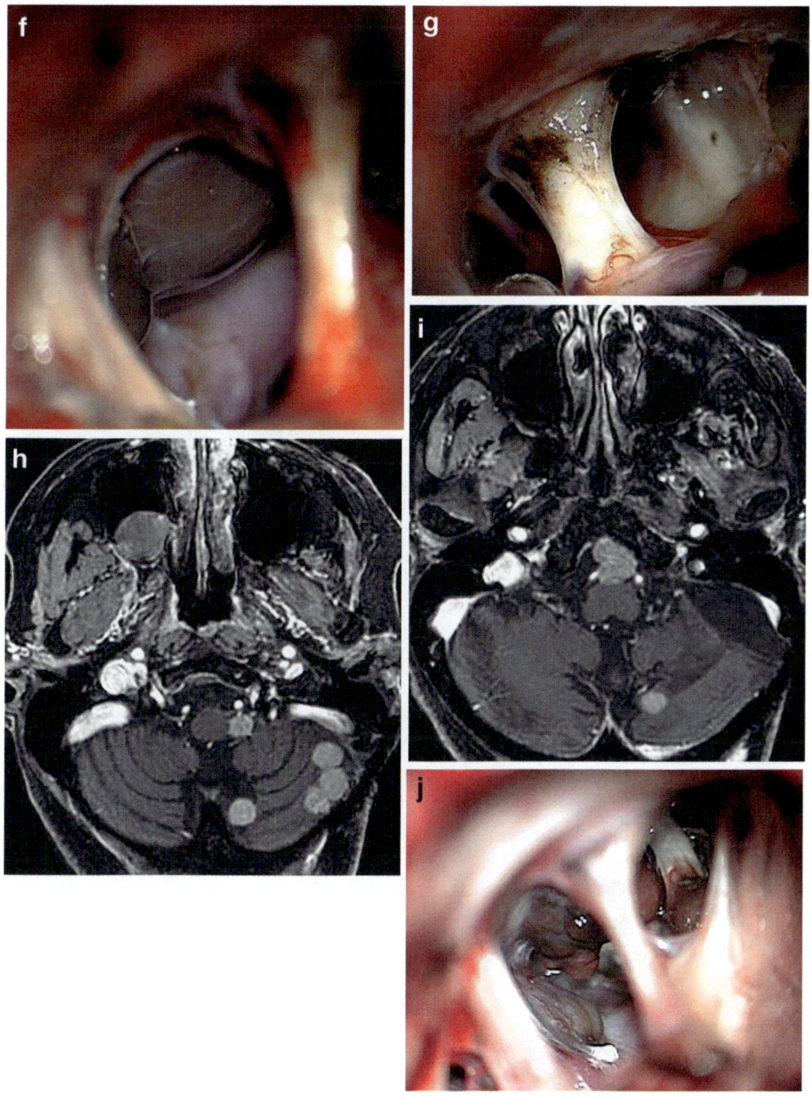

Fig. 21.15 (continued)

Comments Meningeal melanocytoma is a lesion that may mimic meningioma in imaging examinations. However, the microneurosurgical appearance is unequivocal. Resection is straightforward and thorough, as it originates from the leptomeningeal membranes without invading the dura mater or the bone. Nonetheless, there is a propensity for local and regional recurrence, which may ultimately prove fatal for the patient. Typically, the tumor exhibits no malignancy or dissemination beyond the nervous system, and repeated local resection constitutes the sole viable treatment.

21.16 Case 16. Epidermoid Cyst Located at the Cerebellopontine Angle

A 36-year-old woman has right trigeminal neuralgia involving the second branch, accompanied by hearing loss and facial muscle weakness. Neuralgia was effectively managed with medication. Imaging investigations indicated a lesion suggestive of an epidermoid cyst, as observed in the CT scan (Fig. 21.16a), T2-weighted MRI (Fig. 21.16b), and DWI MRI (Fig. 21.16c).

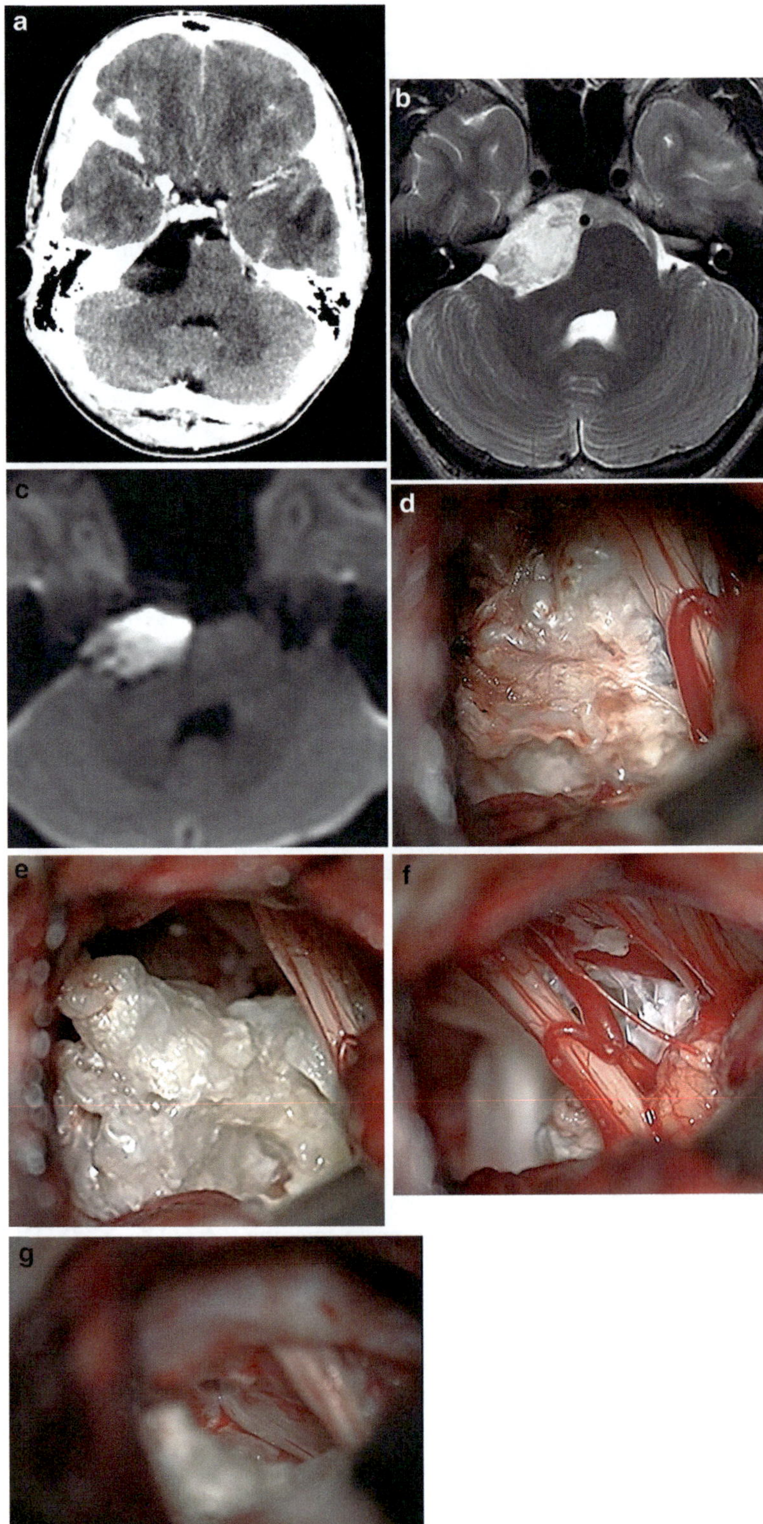

Fig. 21.16 Case 16. Cerebellopontine angle epidermoid cyst. (**a**) CT axial scan of the posterior fossa, showing a hypodense lesion in the cerebellopontine angle. (**b**, **c**) Axial sections in an MRI T2-weighted and DWI sequence. (**d**–**g**) Intraoperative images of the retrosigmoid approach, showing the sequential excision of the epidermoid cyst content and membranes, sparing cranial nerves and vessels

Surgical intervention was advised, resulting in the total excision of the lesion via a retrosigmoid approach. An epidermoid cyst was identified posterior and superior to the facial-cochleovestibular complex (Fig. 21.16d). The facial-cochleovestibular complex was decompressed (Fig. 21.16e), together with the glossopharyngeal and vagal rootlets and the posterior inferior cerebellar artery (Fig. 21.16f), and ultimately, the abducens nerve (Fig. 21.16f). The surgery and the initial postoperative period were unremarkable. Trigeminal pain has abated.

Comments Epidermoid cysts account for a significant proportion of secondary trigeminal neuralgia and other cranial nerve radiculopathies.

21.17 Case 17. Epidermoid Cyst Located at the Cerebellopontine Angle with Supratentorial Expansion

A 40-year-old lady exhibited headache, auditory impairment, right-sided tinnitus, and gait disturbance characterized by right ataxia. Notable was the neuralgic pain in the three branches of the right trigeminal nerve, which was unresponsive to pharmaceutical management and coupled with facial hypesthesia. An MRI scan showed a growth that looked like an epidermoid cyst in the right cerebellopontine angle, spreading into the area above the tentorium and filling the prepontine and ambiens cisterns (Fig. 21.17a, b). The patient underwent a retrosigmoid approach involving the exposure and excision of the tumor, alleviating compression of the trigeminal nerve (Fig. 21.17c). The removal of the tumor reached cranially the lower part of the third cranial nerve, and a Gore-Tex sheet was placed to mark the edge of the area that was removed. After the surgery, the patient temporarily had weakness in the facial and abducens nerves, but their hearing improved, and the pain from trigeminal neuralgia completely went away without any loss of sensibility. Six years later, the patient exhibited a complex partial temporal seizure, accompanied by gastrointestinal symptoms and dysgeusia, which was managed with anticonvulsant therapy. The follow-up imaging showed that the leftover tissue above the tentorium had slowly increased in size after the first surgery, which pushed on the inner part of the temporal lobe (Fig. 21.17d). No recurrence of the excised infratentorial part was observed. A new microneurosurgical procedure was performed using a pterional approach, which successfully removed the cyst completely and relieved pressure on the temporal lobe and lateral incisure area (Fig. 21.17e, f). During the postoperative phase, a temporary paresis of the trochlear nerve occurred. Months later, the anticonvulsant treatment was discontinued, and imaging assessments revealed no traces of the cyst, as demonstrated in the MRI DWI sequence (Fig. 21.17g, h), with no hypersignal indicative of diffusion restriction associated with cyst remains.

Comments Extra-compartmental expansion of the epidermoid cyst is prevalent. Generally, we should only conduct an aggressive excision of the compartment associated with neurological involvement that aligns with the patient's symptoms. Any residual in a separate compartment may be monitored using imaging, and excision via an alternative approach is warranted only if symptoms manifest or the growth becomes prominent.

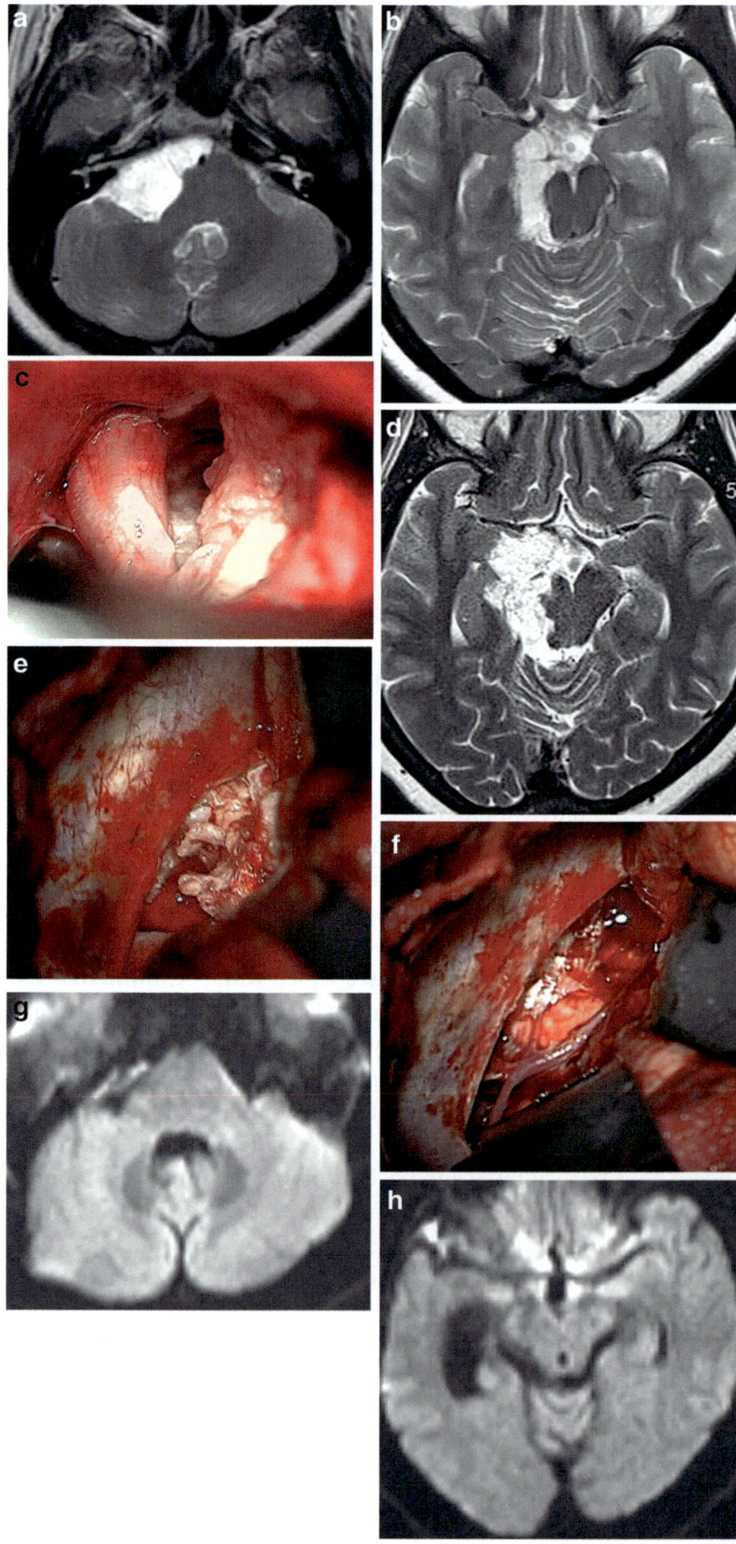

Fig. 21.17 Case 17. Cerebellopontine angle epidermoid cyst with supratentorial extension. (**a**, **b**) Axial sections in a T2-weighted sequence at the level of the internal auditory canal and midbrain. (**c**) Intraoperative image of the retrosigmoid approach, showing the excision of the infratentorial part of the epidermoid cyst, which released the trigeminal nerve. (**d**) Axial section in a T2-weighted sequence at the level of the midbrain, showing the growth of the cyst. (**e**, **f**) Intraoperative images of the pterional approach, showing the removal of the upper part of the epidermoid cyst, with the lateral incisure region clear of tumor. (**g**, **h**) Final axial MRI DWI sequence at the level of the internal auditory canal and midbrain without cyst remains

21.18 Case 18. Squamous Cell Carcinoma of the Cerebellopontine Angle

A 58-year-old man exhibited gait ataxia accompanied by hearing loss and left facial paresis for several months. MRI imaging revealed a lesion consistent with a small epidermoid cyst in the left cerebellopontine angle. An axial slice at the level of the internal acoustic meatus in T2-weighted FIESTA revealed a rounded hypointense lesion (Fig. 21.18a). The MRI DWI sequence exhibited a hyperintense signal indicative of restricted diffusion, consistent with an epidermoid cyst (Fig. 21.18b). The T1-weighted MRI with gadolinium demonstrated a non-enhancing lesion, accompanied by peripheral enhancement adjacent to the internal auditory canal (Fig. 21.18c). The patient received a retrosigmoid approach, resulting in the exposure and total excision of the cyst (Fig. 21.18d). The tumor's outer layer thickened at the internal acoustic meatus, affecting the facial and cochleovestibular nerves. Dissection of the facial nerve elicited significant neurotonic discharges in neurophysiological monitoring during excision. In the first few days after surgery, the patient still had trouble with balance, and there were also issues with the abducens, facial (HB grade III), and cochlear nerves. Several months later, there was a deterioration of neurological impairments, particularly ataxia on the left side. Due to the COVID-19 pandemic, a follow-up MRI was done about six months after the worsening of symptoms, showing a large mass that now filled the entire cerebellopontine angle and spread upwards, downwards, and towards the middle. This mass exerted significant pressure on the brainstem, accompanied by edema in both the brainstem and cerebellum (Fig. 21.18e). The mass exhibited an irregular shape without diffusion restriction in the DWI sequence (Fig. 21.18f) and demonstrated prominent contrast enhancement (Fig. 21.18g). The patient underwent reoperation, revealing an invasive, poorly defined, thick, hyaline tumor with extensive areas of necrosis (Fig. 21.18h). During the surgery, the tissue analysis confirmed the presence of squamous cell carcinoma, leading to the decision to perform a palliative internal decompression. The patient experienced a deteriorating neurological condition and subsequently acquired hydrocephalus, which was managed by a ventriculoperitoneal CSF shunt. We ruled out the possibility of a primitive carcinoma in any other area of the body. Three months later, he succumbed, having had no additional oncological treatment. The sample taken during the second surgery shows that he had a moderately developed adenocarcinoma with neuroendocrine differentiation. A thorough examination of all samples taken after the first procedure confirms that it was an epidermoid cyst.

Comments The transformation of an arachnoid cyst into squamous cell carcinoma is an uncommon, however conceivable, occurrence. The case demonstrates an exceptionally fast and lethal progression. One suggestion is that the early epidermoid cyst comprises regions of elevated cellularity. To support this idea, it's crucial to highlight how quickly symptoms developed before diagnosis, the presence of gadolinium enhancement in the preoperative MRI, and the poor clinical results shortly after surgery. The clinical and imaging findings from the MRI following the initial intervention are characteristic of carcinoma, as is the concerning postoperative progression. The absence of malignant tissue in the initial histological examination may indicate the alternative possibility of a rapid malignancy of the remains following the first operation.

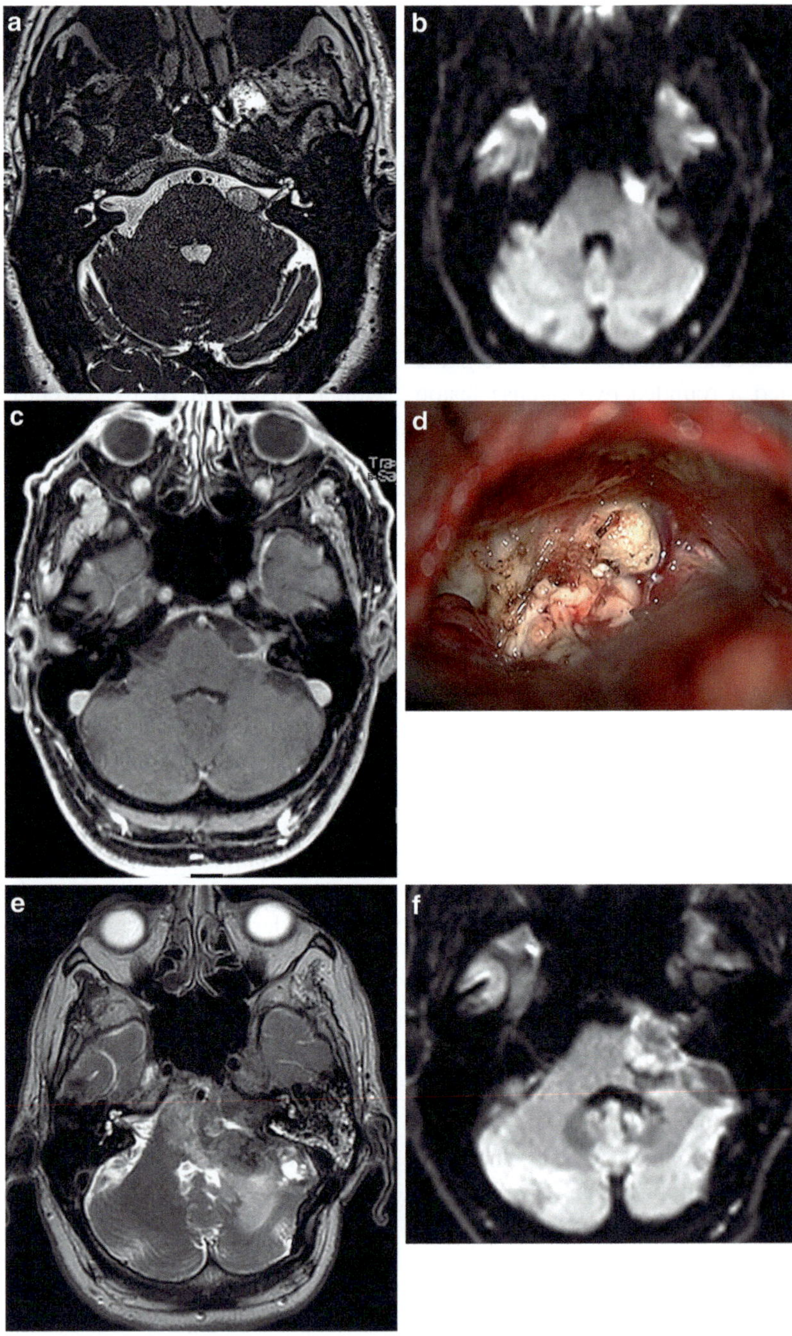

Fig. 21.18 Case 18. Cerebellopontine angle squamous cell carcinoma. (**a**) Axial section in a T2-weighted sequence at the level of the internal auditory canal. (**b**) Axial section in a DWI sequence. (**c**) Axial section in an MRI T1-weighted sequence post-gadolinium showing a peripheral enhancement adjacent to the internal auditory canal. (**d**) Intraoperative image of the retrosigmoid approach. (**e**) Evolutive axial MRI T2-weighted sequence. (**f**) Evolutive axial MRI DWI sequence. (**g**) Evolutive axial MRI T1-weighted sequence post-gadolinium. (**h**) Intraoperative image of the revision retrosigmoid approach

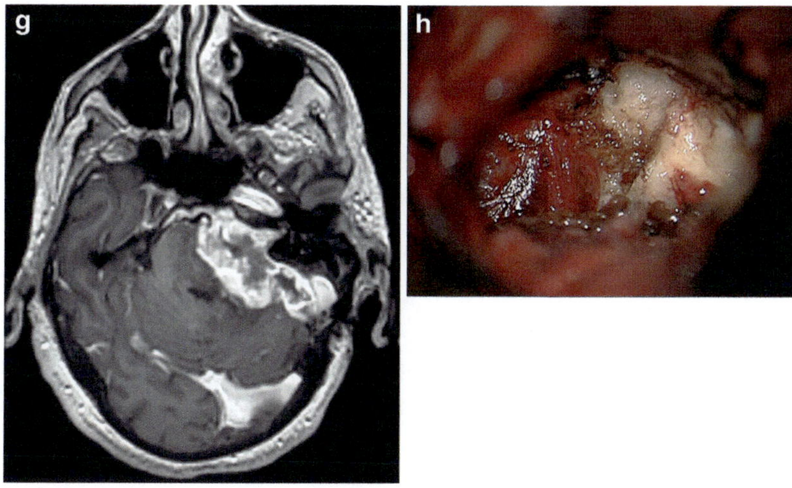

Fig. 21.18 (continued)

21.19 Case 19. Embryonal Epidermoid Cyst of the Middle Ear Extending into the Internal Ear Canal

A 40-year-old male underwent multiple otologic procedures for the excision of a recurring congenital epidermoid cyst in the left middle ear during a span exceeding ten years. The patient was sent for further evaluation after an imaging test showed an enlargement of the remnant and a new cyst in the internal auditory canal, as seen in the MRI scan that highlights a bright area where water movement is restricted (Fig. 21.19a). Currently, the patient exhibits chronic left cophosis and total facial paralysis, both of which are well tolerated. By widening the previous otologic surgery approach, we were able to reach the internal auditory canal through a labyrinthectomy, which helped to remove both the petrosal recurrence and the growth inside the internal auditory canal. The petrosal portion of the lesion was excised, and the osseous cavity was extensively curetted (Fig. 21.19b). The lesion resembles intracranial epidermoid cysts. We observed the intracranial portion of the cyst expanding along the facial–cochleovestibular nerves, which were transected for a radical en bloc resection (Fig. 21.19c, d). Post-surgery, there was a temporary otorrhea. Histopathology revealed a characteristic epidermoid cyst, devoid of indications of chronic infection or inflammation. The patient had no new neurological abnormalities, and the imaging conducted ten years later revealed no hypersignal in the DTI sequence of the MRI indicative of any remnants (Fig. 21.19e).

Comments Epidermoid cysts can develop in the middle ear of the petrosal bone. The epidermoid cyst of the middle ear differs from the cholesteatoma.

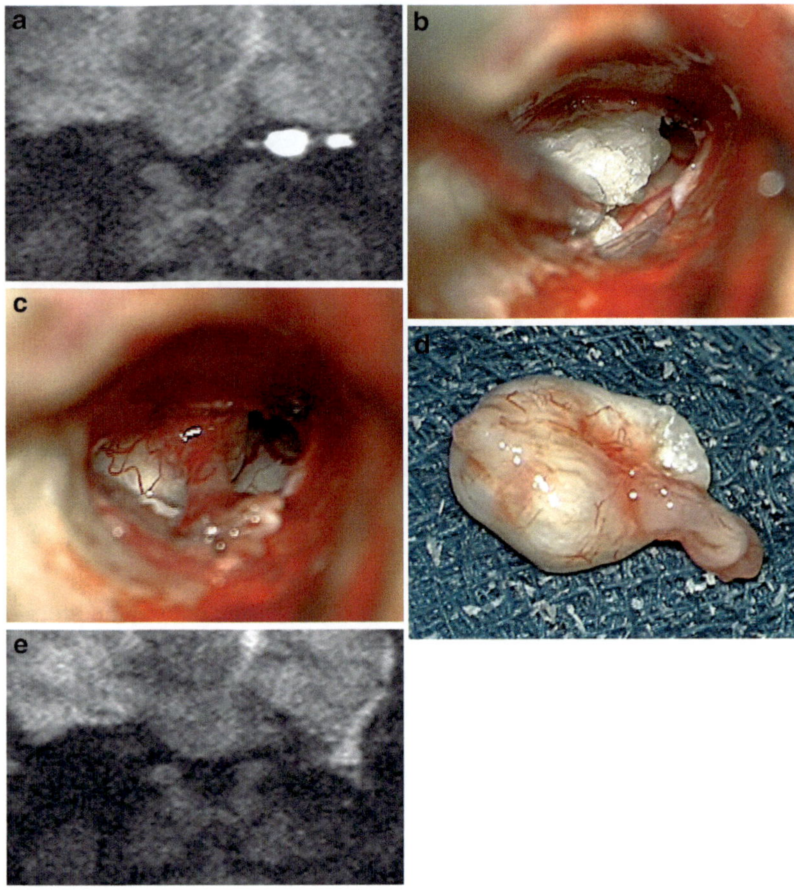

Fig. 21.19 Case 19. Petrosal embryonal epidermoid cyst. (**a**) Coronal section in a DWI-weighted sequence at the level of the internal auditory canals, showing two lesions: the external one, a middle ear recurrence, and the medial one, a cyst expansion into the internal auditory canal. (**b**) Intraoperative image of the translabyrinthine approach showing the middle ear cyst. (**c**) Intraoperative image of the translabyrinthine approach showing the internal auditory canal cyst attached to the facial-cochleovestibular nerves. (**d**) Excised internal auditory canal cyst and nerve stump. (**e**) Final MRI coronal section in a DWI-weighted sequence ten years after excision

21.20 Case 20. Ruptured Saccular Aneurysm at the Right Vertebrobasilar Junction: Endovascular Treatment

A 50-year-old patient presents with a WFNS (World Federation of Neurological Surgeons) grade IV subarachnoid hemorrhage and Fisher grade 3 on CT (Fig. 21.20a). Digital subtraction angiography (DSA) revealed a saccular aneurysm at the junction of the right vertebral and posterior cerebellar arteries, with the left vertebral artery being the dominant one (Fig. 21.20b). The aneurysm was successfully embolized using coils, resulting in total exclusion of the aneurysmal sac (Fig. 21.20c). The patient's condition improved, even though there were issues with vasospasm and hydrocephalus, which required placing a ventriculoperitoneal cerebrospinal fluid shunt. A year later, a control angiogram showed that the aneurysm had partially reopened (Fig. 21.20d). It was then retreated with embolization, which completely closed off the aneurysm (Fig. 21.20e).

Comments

Coil embolization with endovascular treatment is the optimal therapeutic approach for ruptured posterior fossa aneurysms, especially those situated deep within the brain and in patients exhibiting high-grade subarachnoid hemorrhage. Nonetheless, coiling is followed in a significant proportion of instances by recurrence and subsequent retreatment.

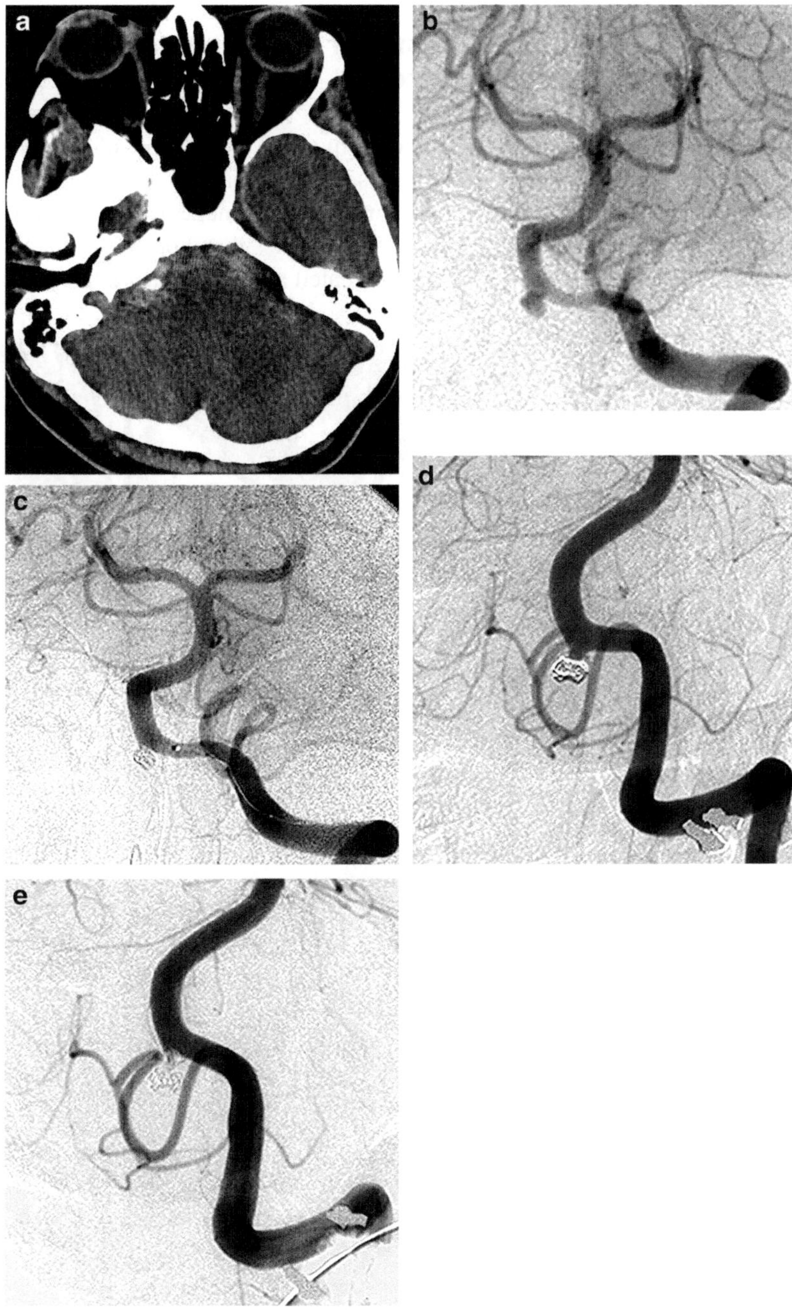

Fig. 21.20 Case 20. Saccular vertebral artery aneurysm. (**a**) CT axial scan of the posterior fossa, showing a diffuse subarachnoid hemorrhage. (**b**, **c**) Left vertebral DSA showing a saccular aneurysm before and after coiling. (**d**, **e**) Left vertebral DSA showing a partial recurrence of the saccular aneurysm before and after coiling

21.21 Case 21. Dissecting Aneurysms of the Posterior Inferior Cerebellar Artery

A 60-year-old patient with severe arterial hypertension and bipolar disorder was diagnosed with an unruptured aneurysm of the posterior inferior cerebellar artery in the lateral pontine-mesencephalic junction. The CT scan revealed a somewhat hyperdense rounded mass in the left cerebellopontine angle (Fig. 21.21a). The TOF (*Time Of Flight*) MRI showed a round growth linked to a blood vessel coming from either the upper part of the vertebral artery or the lower part of the basilar artery (Fig. 21.21b). The 3D image from the vascular CT showed a lesion that appeared linked to the posterior inferior cerebellar artery (Fig. 21.21c). At the same

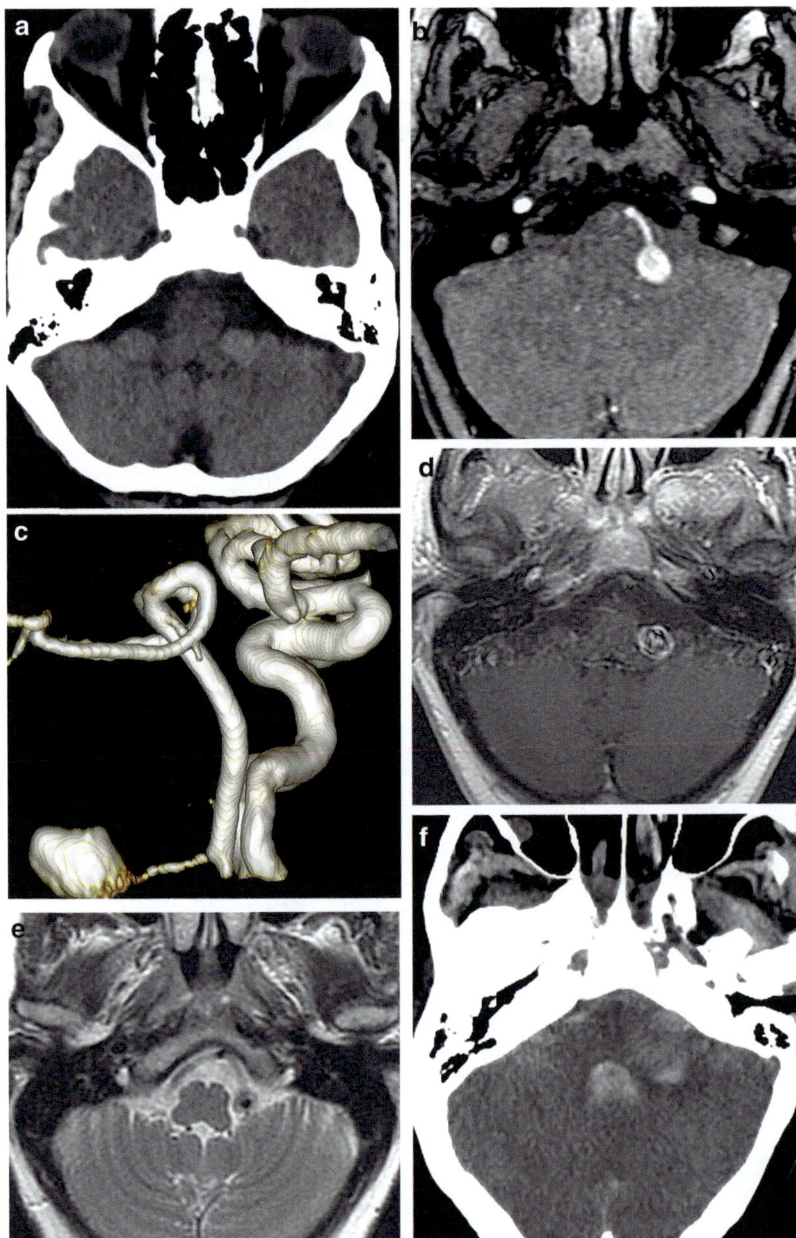

Fig. 21.21 Case 21. Dissecting vertebral artery aneurysm. (**a**) CT axial scan of the posterior fossa showing a round lesion in the cerebellopontine angle. (**b**) Axial section in a T1-weighted TOF study showing a round vascular lesion with an afferent vessel. (**c**) 3D angio-CT scan reconstruction. (**d**, **e**) 'Target sign' in axial sections in an MRI T1-weighted sequence following contrast injection and T2-weighted sequence. (**f**) CT axial scan of the posterior fossa showing bleeding in the cerebellopontine angle and fourth ventricle

time, the T2- and T1-weighted MRI after injection of gadolinium showed signs consistent with a dissecting aneurysm, known as the target sign (Fig. 21.21d, e). The patient declined treatment for the lesion and visited the emergency department multiple times for headaches and hypertensive crises. Approximately two years later, she experienced a WFNS grade IV subarachnoid hemorrhage and a Fisher grade 4 on CT imaging (Fig. 21.21f). The progression was swiftly disastrous despite the insertion of an external ventricular drain, and the woman succumbed a few hours after her admission to the critical care unit.

Comments Cerebral aneurysms that are allowed to progress exhibit a significant likelihood of hemorrhage, especially in the presence of vascular risk factors and those situated in the posterior circulation.

21.22 Case 22. Right Tonsillar Arteriovenous Malformation

A 46-year-old patient presents with hemorrhage in the posterior fossa, affecting the right cerebellar hemisphere and the fourth ventricle, accompanied by acute hydrocephalus (Fig. 21.22a). Upon admission, the Glasgow Coma Scale (GCS) score was 6, and an external ventricular drain was inserted. An arteriovenous malformation was seen in the DSA, located near the right tonsil, fed by branches of the posteroinferior cerebellar artery and with many small veins of drainage (Fig. 21.22b). Three-dimensional CT angiography reconstruction illustrates the morphology of the arteriovenous malformation nidus at the cerebellopontine angle and its association with skull base structures (Fig. 21.22c, d). Two weeks later, the patient underwent surgery via a right far lateral approach, revealing the tonsil harbouring the nidus of the arteriovenous malformation (Fig. 21.22e) and the segment V4 of the vertebral artery (Fig. 21.22f). The nidus of the arteriovenous malformation is resected along with the cerebellar hematoma (Fig. 21.22g). The patient's progress was uneventful, albeit gradual, requiring the placement of a ventriculoperitoneal shunt to control his hydrocephalus. The patient exhibits a respiratory infection and subsequently develops tetraparesis associated with a critical condition; despite early rehabilitation efforts, the patient was moved to a neurorehabilitation facility.

Comments This case presents significant neurological sequelae despite the effective management of the arteriovenous malformation and the evacuation of the cerebellar hematoma.

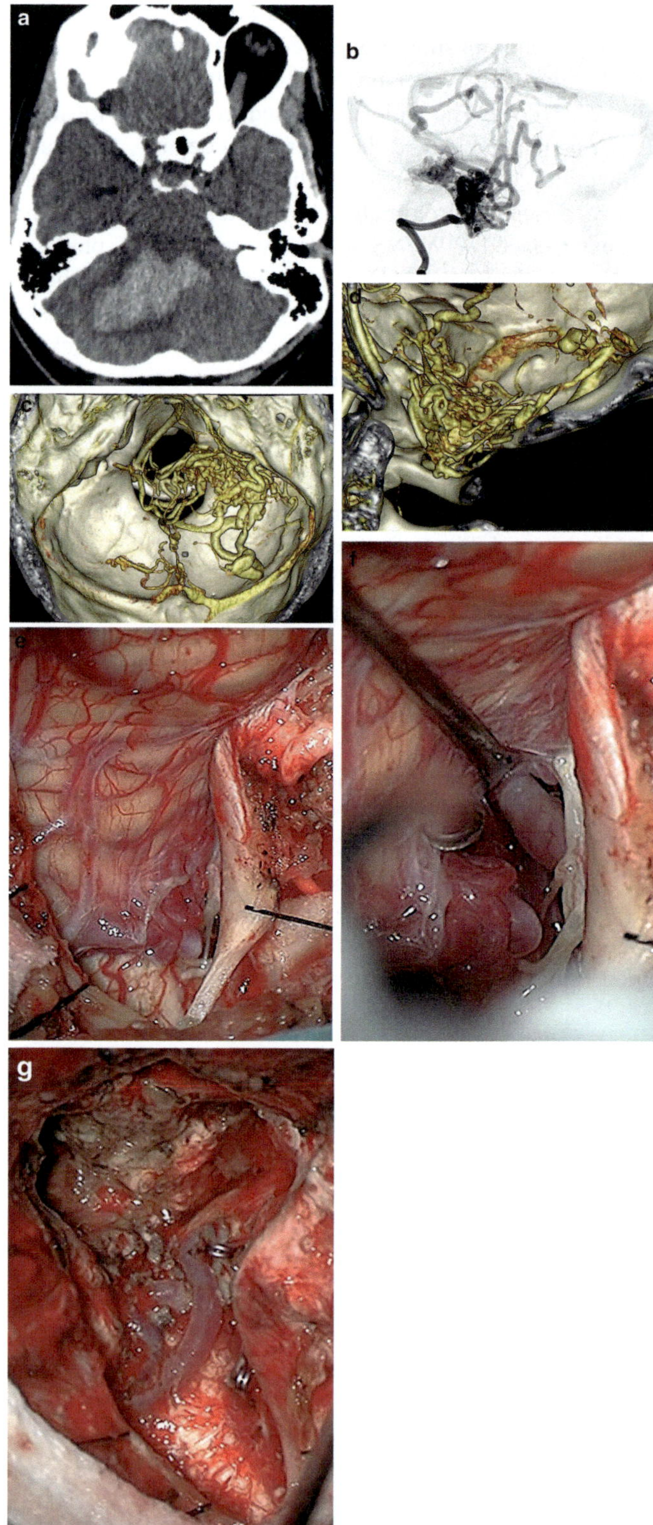

Fig. 21.22 Case 22. Tonsillar arteriovenous malformation. (**a**) CT axial scan showing a posterior fossa hemorrhage. (**b**) Right vertebral DSA showing an arteriovenous malformation in the tonsil. (**c, d**) 3D angio-CT scan reconstruction showing the arteriovenous malformation in a superior axial and a midline sagittal view. (**e, f**) Intraoperative images of the far lateral approach to the tonsil and vertebral arterial afferents. (**g**) Intraoperative image after complete excision of the lesion

21.23 Case 23. Left Lateral Medullary Arteriovenous Malformation

A 52-year-old woman had a hemorrhage in the posterior fossa, affecting the left cerebellopontine angle and the fourth ventricle, accompanied by acute hydrocephalus (Fig. 21.23a). The patient was admitted to another facility and diagnosed with a posterior fossa arteriovenous malformation that was ineffectively treated with embolization, resulting in a cerebellar infarction. Several months later, she sought consultation to complete the treatment. The patient had a normal level of consciousness, severe left cerebellar syndrome, total involvement of cranial nerves from seven through twelve on the left side, and a ventriculoperitoneal cerebrospinal fluid shunt. A DSA study showed a left arteriovenous malformation (Fig. 21.23b, c), fed by the anterior inferior cerebellar artery, with superficial venous drainage and enlarged veins. The left vertebral artery had nearly total occlusion. The patient underwent surgery via a left far lateral approach (Fig. 21.23d), allowing for the exposure of the partially thrombosed nidus, which was then mobilized along a gliotic plane (Fig. 21.23e, f). The nonfunctional cochleovestibular nerve's origin was situated within the nidus and scar, forcing sectioning to reveal the venous ectasia and facilitate its excision (Fig. 21.23g, h). The nidus of the arteriovenous malformation was entirely excised, preserving the anatomical integrity of the cranial nerves in the cerebellopontine angle, with the exception of the eighth nerve (Fig. 21.23i, j). The patient's outcome was favorable; the patient is independent in her everyday activities.

Comments This case involves failed embolization linked to cerebellar ischemia. The removal of the arteriovenous malformation was complete, helped by the pre-surgery embolization and the shrinkage of the cerebellum caused by the ischemia from the embolization. The vestibulocochlear complex sustained significant damage due to hemorrhage and was nonfunctional; therefore, it was excised to facilitate the excision of the nidus.

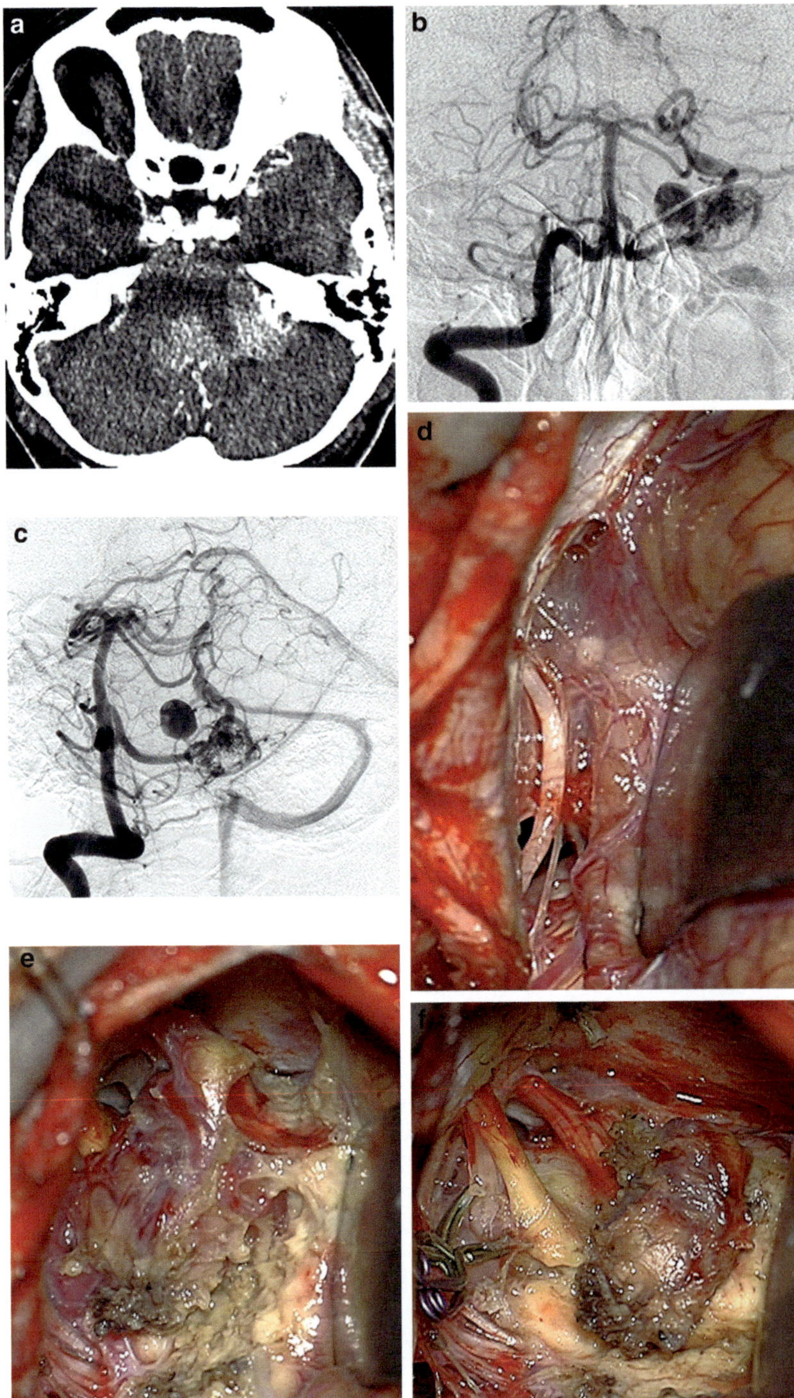

Fig. 21.23 Case 23. Medullary arteriovenous malformation. (**a**) CT axial scan showing a cerebellopontine angle and fourth ventricle hemorrhage and abnormal vessels. (**b**, **c**) Right vertebral DSA showing an arteriovenous malformation located in the lateral aspect of the medulla oblongata, accompanied by a conspicuous venous aneurysm, presented in both anteroposterior and oblique projections. (**d–g**) Sequential intraoperative images of the far lateral approach depicting the excision of the lesion. (**h**, **i**) Intraoperative images before and after excision of the venous aneurysm. (**j**) Final intraoperative image after the complete excision of the malformation

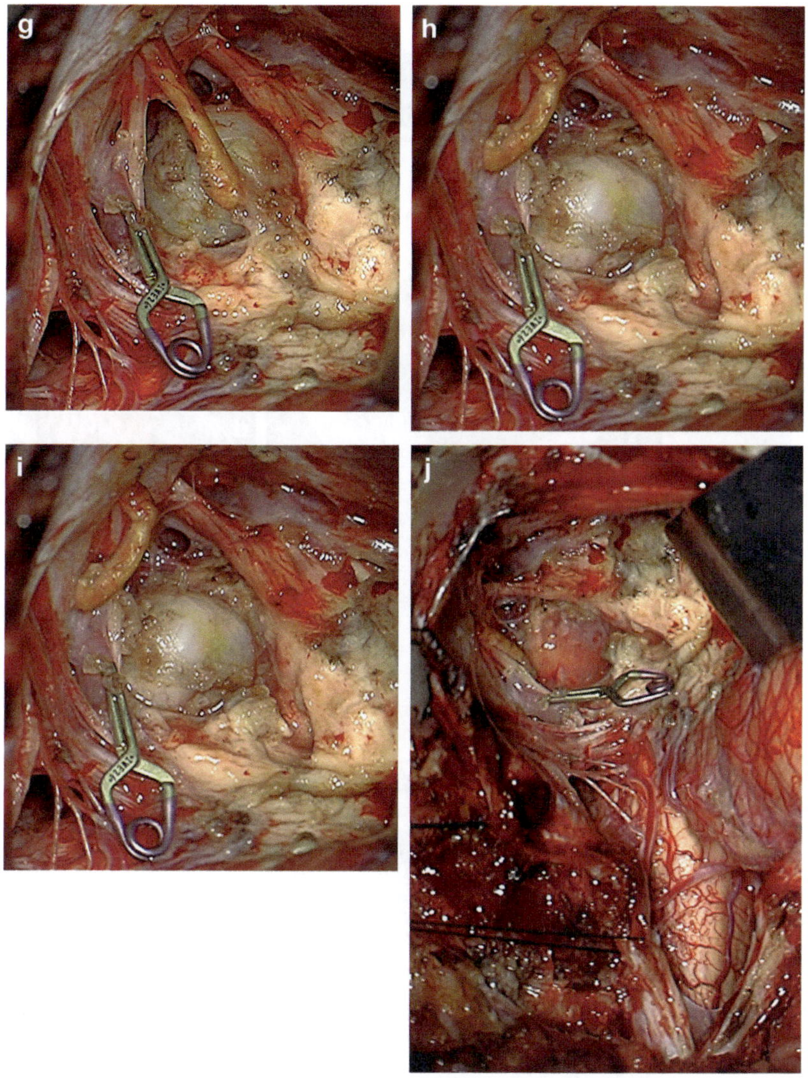

Fig. 21.23 (continued)

21.24 Case 24. Left Lateral Pontine Arteriovenous Malformation

A 64-year-old patient had a diffuse subarachnoid hemorrhage, classified as Fisher grade 3 and WFNS grade III (Fig. 21.24a), developing in hydrocephalus, which was managed with external ventricular shunting. The patient received a diagnosis of an arteriovenous malformation in the right cerebellopontine angle. The DSA revealed a right arteriovenous malformation supplied by the superior cerebellar artery and small branches of the anterior inferior cerebellar artery, with superficial drainage directed towards the vein of Galen (Fig. 21.24b, c). The patient's overall progression was favorable, exhibiting a normal level of consciousness; however, a severe right cerebellar syndrome appeared, characterized primarily by intentional tremor in the arm and gait instability, exacerbated by the patient's morbid obesity. He was released to a neurorehabilitation facility. Treatment for the arteriovenous malformation was advised; however, microsurgical intervention was deemed inappropriate due to MRI imaging confirming that the lesion penetrates far into the cerebellar peduncle

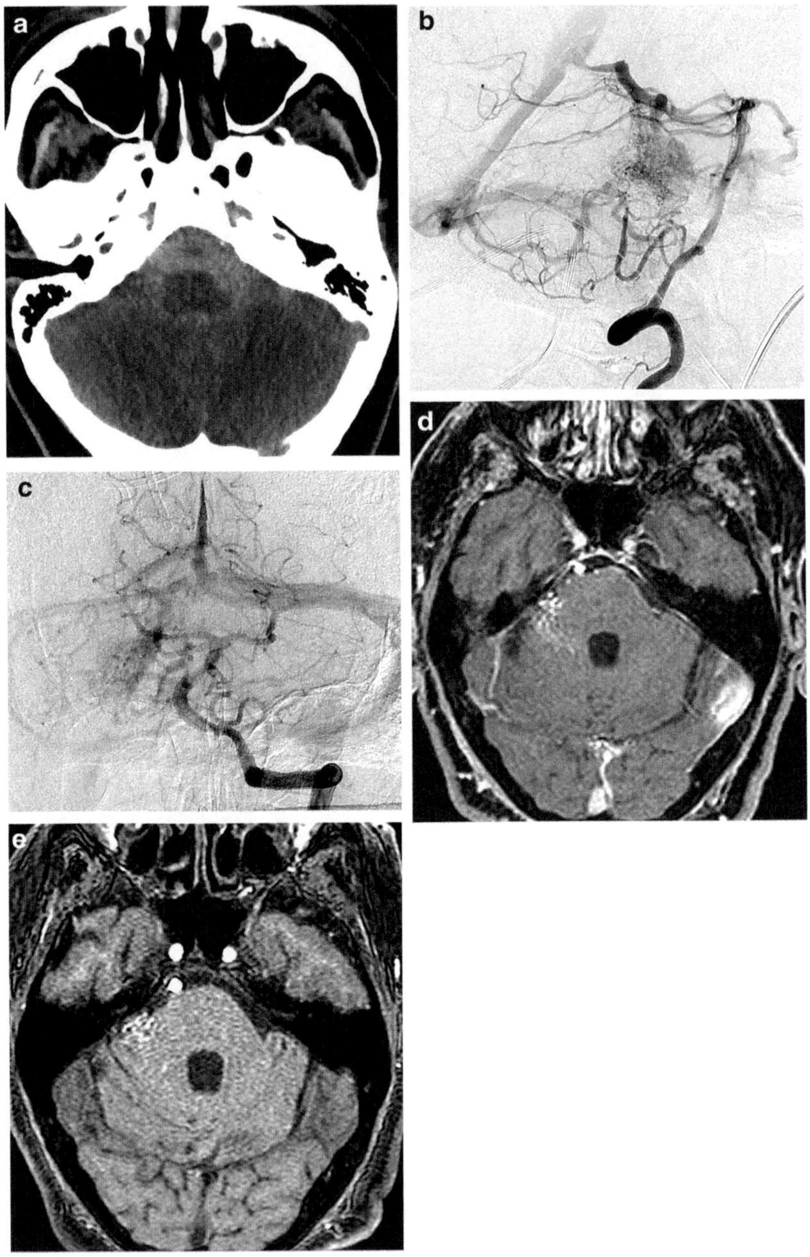

Fig. 21.24 Case 24. Pontine arteriovenous malformation. (**a**) CT axial scan showing a massive posterior fossa subarachnoid hemorrhage. (**b**, **c**) Left vertebral DSA showing a posterior circulation arteriovenous malformation in lateral and anteroposterior projections. (**d**, **e**) Axial images in a post-gadolinium MRI T1-weighted vascular sequence showing the lesion before and three years after SRS treatment

(Fig. 21.24d). Consequently, the patient underwent stereotactic radiosurgery utilizing a gamma knife. Three years post-treatment, the patient's clinical status is stable, and a decrease in the lesion's size is observable by the MRI examination (Fig. 21.24e).

Comments Stereotactic radiosurgery can effectively treat high-risk cerebellopontine angle arteriovenous malformations for microneurosurgical nidus excision, particularly in patients with elevated surgical risk.

21.25 Case 25. Recurrent Pontine Bleeding Resulting from Brainstem Cavernoma

The patient, aged 43, had a 25-year medical history of parathyroid carcinoma. She had undergone numerous surgical procedures to address local and regional recurrences, along with hormone replacement therapy. Nephrocalcinosis caused moderate renal insufficiency, but there was no arterial hypertension. The patient suddenly experienced a loss of feeling on the right side of the face in the V2 area, weakness on the left side of the face, weakness on the right side of the body with pyramidal signs, reduced sensation on the right side of the body, difficulty speaking, and uncontrolled eye movements (nystagmus). The imaging tests showed bleeding in the pons on the CT scan, about 28 × 20mm in size, which was pressing on the fourth ventricle but did not cause hydrocephalus. We identified two foci of bleeding, with one of them leveled (Fig. 21.25a). There was no visible contrast uptake. The MRI examination utilizing T2-weighted and gradient sequences corroborated the CT results (Fig. 21.25b, c). We conducted a DSA, which revealed no abnormal vascularization. The patient's neoplastic condition was reviewed, and local recurrence or systemic metastatic lesions were excluded. No further lesions were seen in the central nervous system. We diagnosed the patient with pontine hemorrhage due to a cavernoma, discharged him home, and scheduled microneurosurgical excision for two weeks later. However, surgery was postponed due to healthcare restrictions imposed by the COVID-19 epidemic. Four weeks after the first bleed, the patient had another major bleed, which led to them being taken to the emergency department with complete weakness on the left side, trouble swallowing with sialorrhea, and a lower level of alertness, along with the symptoms they already had. The CT scan revealed a substantial heterogeneous hematoma with peripheral hypointensity, measuring a maximum of 40 × 30 mm in the axial plane (Fig. 21.25d). In the T2-weighted MRI scan, blood at different stages was found in the right side of the pons, reaching up towards the area between the pons and midbrain and down towards the area between the medulla and pons, and it crossed the middle line, causing significant collapse and displacement of the fourth ventricle, but there was no hydrocephalus (Fig. 21.25e–g). An external ventricular shunt was inserted for safeguarding in anticipation of surgery. The patient underwent surgery using a right retrosigmoid approach, gaining access to the hematoma through the peritrigeminal safe entry zone. Following the evacuation of the hematoma, a more structured and nodular lesion was identified and excised en bloc. The somatosensory and motor-evoked potentials exhibited no alterations throughout the intervention. After 10 days, we released the patient to a neurological rehabilitation institution. The histological examination showed bleeding material at different stages of development, but there were no signs of blood vessel issues, tumors, or tumor spreading. The patient's neurological deficits improved, with a residual left hemisensory condition characterized by paresthesia, dysesthesias, and areas of hyperalgesia, indicative of neuropathic pain, with a residual right hemi-cerebellar syndrome as the end outcome. The imaging conducted two years post-surgery reveals postsurgical changes in the pons, exhibiting nearly complete restoration of normal structure (Fig. 21.25h).

Comments The brainstem cavernoma presents a significant risk of hemorrhage and recurrent hemorrhage. Nonetheless, early rebleeding is infrequent, and a prevalent treatment involves excising the cavernoma 4–6 weeks post-hemorrhage, allowing the partially liquefied hematoma to facilitate cavernoma resection.

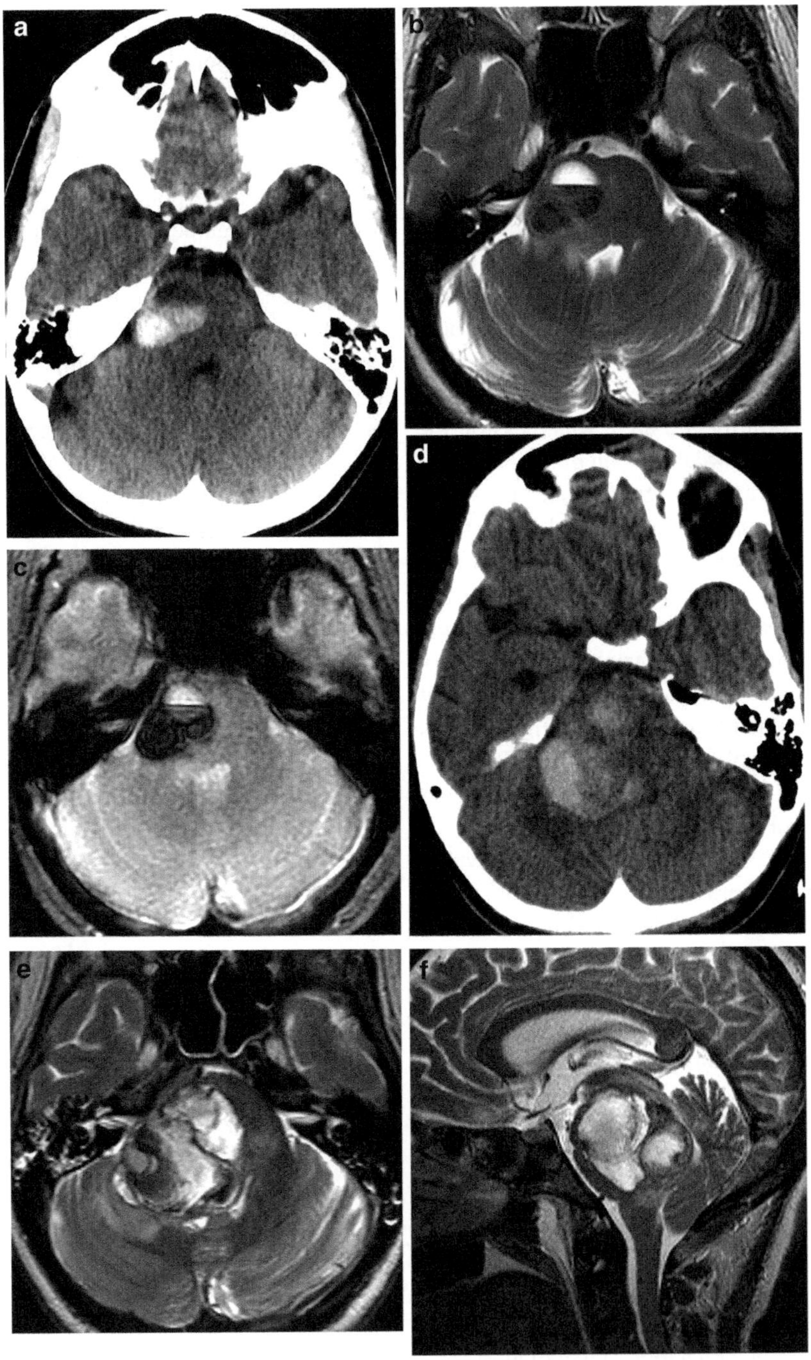

Fig. 21.25 Case 25. Brainstem cavernoma. (**a**) CT axial scan showing a pontine hemorrhage. (**b**, **c**) Axial images in an MRI T2-weighted and gradient sequence. (**d**) CT axial scan showing a massive pontine rebleeding. (**e–g**) Axial, sagittal, and coronal images in an MRI T2-weighted sequence. (**h**) Final postoperative axial image in an MRI T2-weighted after microsurgical treatment

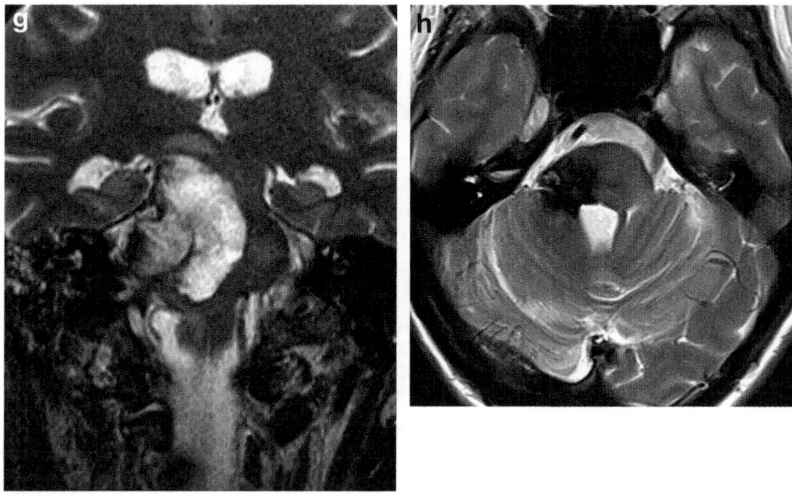

Fig. 21.25 (continued)

21.26 Case 26. Isolated Metastasis of Lung Cancer to the Pons

A 65-year-old patient was diagnosed with lung adenocarcinoma six years earlier, and his condition is currently under control. The patient presented with headache, clumsiness, and paresthesia on the right side of the body and had cerebral CT and MRI examinations. The CT scan showed a very calcified area in the pons that was slightly shifted to the left, along with some swelling around it (Fig. 21.26a). The MRI examination revealed a lesion approximately 2 cm in diameter on the T1-weighted sequence, which exhibited significant enhancement following gadolinium injection (Fig. 21.26b, c). In the T2-weighted sequence, the lesion manifested as a hypointense mass encircled by edema (Fig. 21.26d), while the T2-gradient-echo revealed a hyperintensity corresponding to the calcifications observed on the CT, although hemorrhage could not be ruled out (Fig. 21.26e). Systemic examinations revealed hilar pulmonary adenopathies, and systemic spread of the neoplastic disease was excluded. The patient received steroid treatment, resulting in a minor and temporary improvement of clinical symptoms. The calcification pattern, perilesional edema, and contrast enhancement, which suggested an isolated metastasis, warranted microneurosurgical intervention for the lesion. A left retrosigmoid craniotomy and a safe entry point near the trigeminal nerve in the pons provided access to the tumor (Fig. 21.26f). The tumor was entirely excised, and the histological analysis verified it as a metastasis of lung cancer (Fig. 21.26g). The patient exhibited a temporary exacerbation of long-tract symptoms and a disturbance in conjugate ocular movements accompanied by diplopia, with full recovery occurring after several weeks. The oncological treatment for his lung neoplasm was resumed. Two years later, the patient came back for a checkup because a lump had formed in the lower part of the retroauricular surgical scar, which was removed and found to be a skin metastasis of the adenocarcinoma, probably caused by contamination during surgery. Following 2.5 years, the control imaging analysis revealed no local recurrence and postoperative changes in the anterolateral region of the pons secondary to the surgical approach (Fig. 21.26h).

Comments Isolated metastases in the brainstem are an uncommon occurrence, and it is equally rare for the patient's clinical condition and progression to warrant surgical excision.

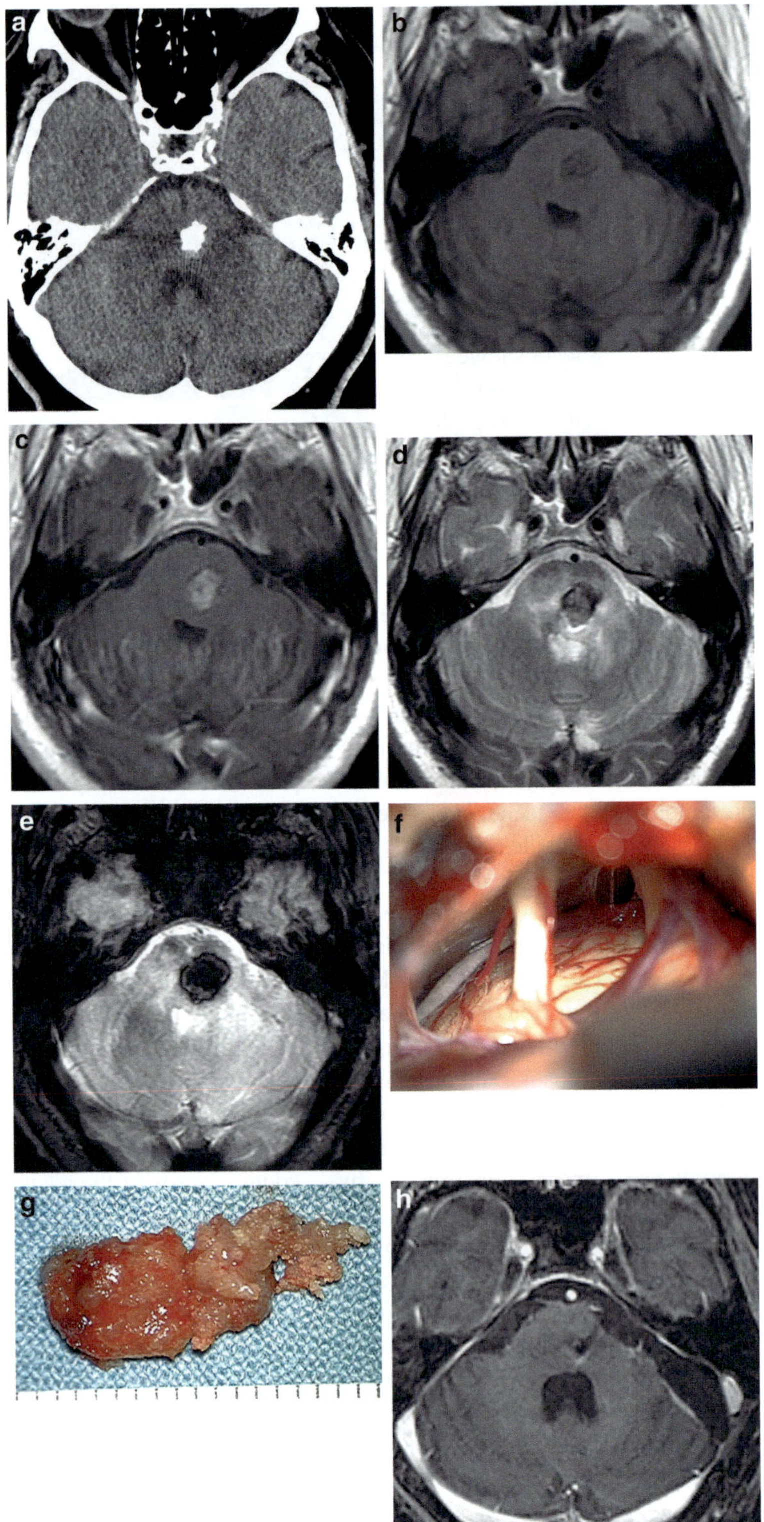

Fig. 21.26 Case 26. Pontine metastases. (**a**) CT axial scan showing a pontine calcified lesion. (**b**, **c**) Axial images of an MRI T1-weighted sequence before and after administration of gadolinium. (**d**) Axial image of an MRI T2-weighted sequence. (**e**) Axial MRI T2-gradient-echo weighted sequence. (**f**) Intraoperative image of the retrosigmoid approach showing the anterolateral surface of the pons. (**g**) Excised metastases. (**h**) Postoperative axial image of an MRI T1-weighted sequence after administration of gadolinium

21.27 Case 27. Trigeminal Neuralgia Secondary to a Microarteriovenous Malformation of the Trigeminal Root

A 67-year-old patient presented with a clinical manifestation of left trigeminal neuralgic pain affecting the first and second branches of the nerve, which had been progressing for several years. Imaging tests showed no problems in the cerebellopontine angle, but the persistent pain warranted surgery to check for possible trigeminal nerve compression from blood vessels. The patient underwent surgery via a left retrosigmoid approach, where a microarteriovenous malformation was located on the exit zone of the trigeminal nerve root (Fig. 21.27a). The nidus was excised, exposing a distorted trigeminal nerve root (Fig. 21.27b). Certain arterial branches reliant on the anterior inferior cerebellar artery were maintained apart by the interposition of Gore-Tex material (Fig. 21.27c). The pain subsided instantaneously in the postoperative phase, without the necessity for medication.

Comments This case exemplifies secondary trigeminal neuralgia, characterized by a normal preoperative MRI, which could only be recognized and addressed with microsurgical exploration of the trigeminal root.

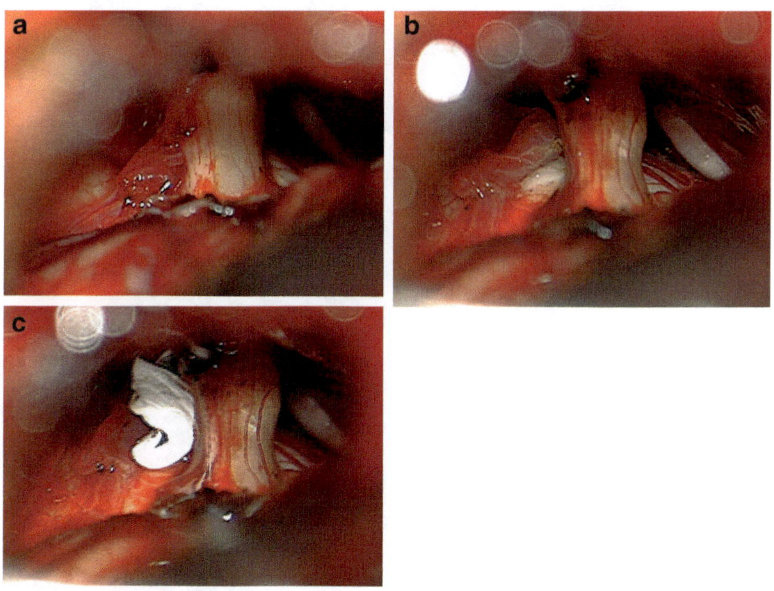

Fig. 21.27 Case 27. Trigeminal neuralgia secondary to arteriovenous malformation. (**a**) Intraoperative image of the retrosigmoid approach showing abnormal vessels around the trigeminal nerve root and pontine surface. (**b**). Intraoperative image after excision of abnormal vessels around the trigeminal root (center), with the superior cerebellar artery (on the left) and the facial-vestibulocochlear nerve complex (on the right). (**c**) Intraoperative image showing Gore-Tex material placed between the anteroinferior cerebellar artery and the trigeminal nerve root

21.28 Case 28. Trigeminal Neuralgia Secondary to a Cerebellopontine Angle Meningioma

A 57-year-old female presenting with paroxysmal left facial discomfort localized to the distribution of the second and third branches of the trigeminal nerve. There was a profound neuropathic pain, characterized by dysesthesia and accompanied by localized hypoesthesia. The patient responded favorably to the initial but temporary treatment with carbamazepine. The CT imaging study revealed a tiny meningioma in the cerebellopontine angle (Fig. 21.28a). The patient had surgery via a retrosigmoid approach, allowing for the exposure of the tumor situated behind the facial-vestibulocochlear complex (Fig. 21.28b). Post-excision of the meningioma, the trigeminal nerve appeared unimpeded, albeit flattened and twisted (Fig. 21.28c). Post-surgery, the patient experienced no facial discomfort and required no pharmacological treatment, with the facial hypoesthesia resolved.

Comments The present case exemplifies secondary trigeminal neuralgia, attributable to a small meningioma located on the petrosal bone, anterior to the internal auditory canal (premeatal).

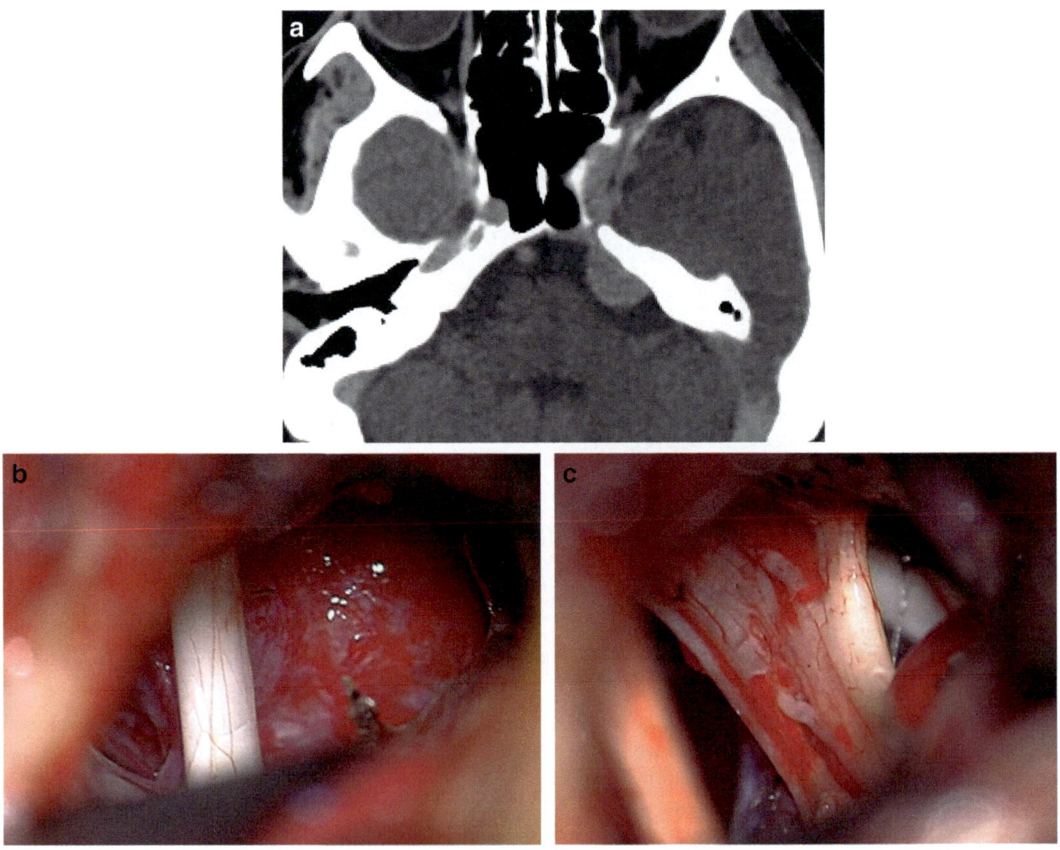

Fig. 21.28 Case 28. Trigeminal neuralgia secondary to meningioma. (**a**) CT axial scan showing a small cerebellopontine angle meningioma. (**b**) Intraoperative image of the retrosigmoid approach showing the tumor behind the facial-vestibulocochlear nerve complex. (**c**) Intraoperative image showing the trigeminal nerve after the meningioma excision

21.29 Case 29. Classical Trigeminal Neuralgia Resulting from Venous Compression

A 49-year-old female presented with paroxysmal right facial pain localized to the distribution of the second and third branches of the trigeminal nerve. The patient showed a favorable initial but temporary response to pharmaceutical treatment with carbamazepine and experienced a brief improvement following percutaneous thermocoagulation some years prior. The patient was referred by a neurologist to evaluate a new neurosurgical treatment, as her response to polytherapy was inadequate. Interestingly, the patient has never had an MRI examination, and she only agreed to undergo retrosigmoid surgery upon preoperative imaging verification of microvascular compression. A blood vessel was found running sideways near the right trigeminal root in MRI images taken after gadolinium administration (Fig. 21.29a, b). The vascular structure appears to traverse the nerve superiorly and encircles the pons, like a horizontal venous channel. The patient underwent surgery via a retrosigmoid approach, allowing for the exposure of the trigeminal nerve root, accompanied by a big vein. The superior cerebellar artery is anatomically positioned (Fig. 21.29c). The vein was separated from the arachnoid (Fig. 21.29d) and repositioned (Fig. 21.29e). An indocyanine green (ICG) fluorescence examination indicated that the vein was a substantial drainage channel, likely the transverse pontine vein, which was unsuitable for coagulation (Fig. 21.29f). The further dissection and mobilization of the venous channel revealed that it crossed between the pars minor and major of the trigeminal root (Fig. 21.29g). The vein was secured by inserting a roll of Teflon between the pars major and the vein (Fig. 21.29h). The microneurosurgical procedure and the outcome were unremarkable, resulting in immediate alleviation of pain without any sensory or motor deficits.

Comments This case exemplifies primary trigeminal pain resulting from venous compression, demonstrating a strong connection between MRI imaging and intraoperative observations.

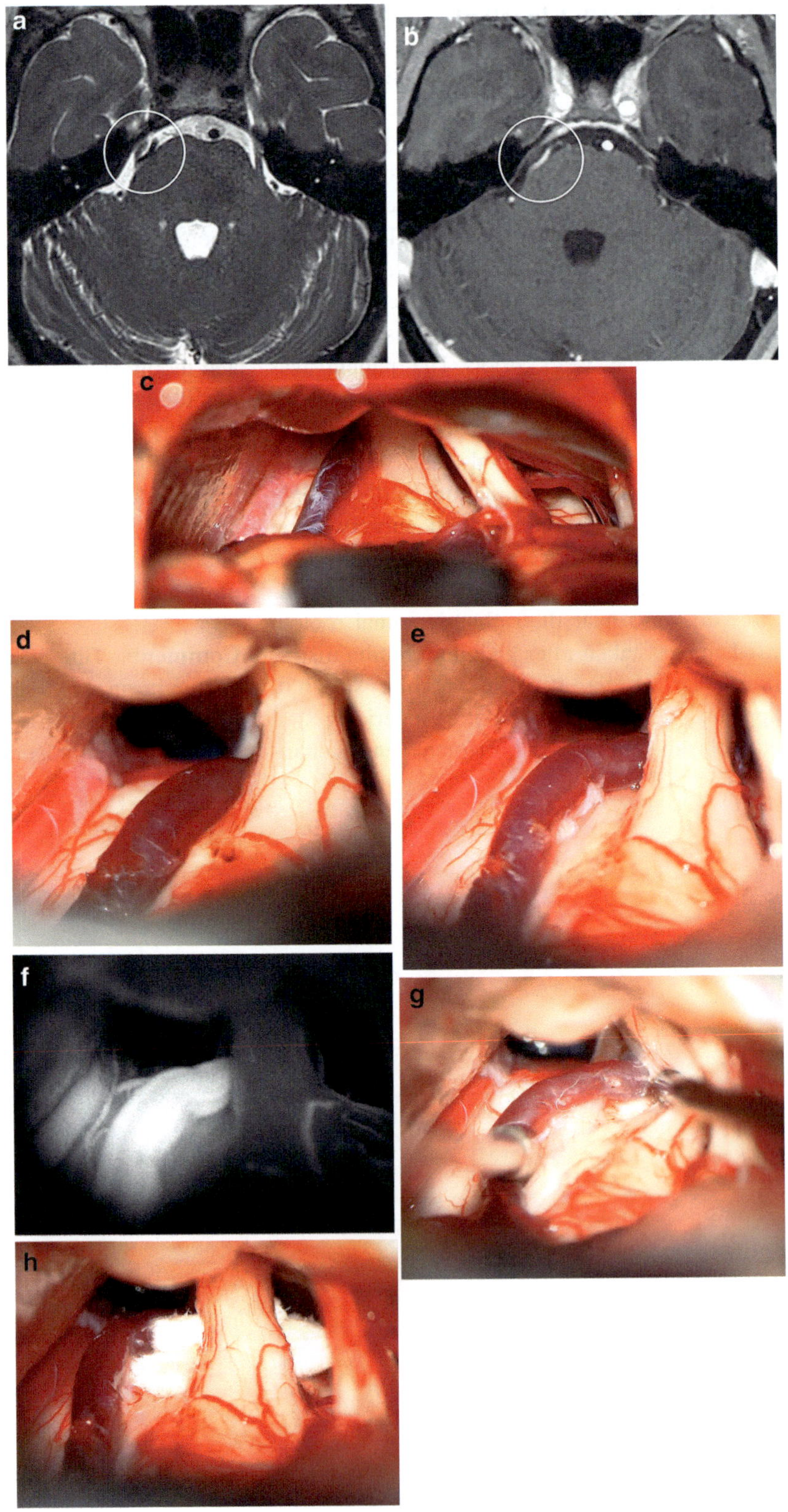

Fig. 21.29 Case 29. Classical trigeminal neuralgia due to venous compression. (**a**). Axial image of an MRI T2-weighted sequence showing a loop vessel in the prepontine cistern. (**b**) Axial image of an MRI T1-TOF-weighted sequence. (**c**) Intraoperative image of the retrosigmoid approach showing the superior cerebellar artery, the superior petrosal vein, the trigeminal nerve, and the facial-vestibulocochlear nerve complex (left to right). (**d**) Intraoperative image showing the superior cerebellar artery, venous channel, and trigeminal nerve relationships. (**e**) Intraoperative image showing the mobilized venous channel. (**f**) ICG (*Indocianyne Green*) fluorescence examination. (**g**, **h**) Intraoperative images showing the mobilization of the vein and insertion of a roll of Teflon between the trigeminal nerve and the vein

21.30 Case 30. Classical Trigeminal Neuralgia Resulting from Arterial Compression

A 69-year-old female presenting with paroxysmal left facial pain localized to the distribution of the third branch of the trigeminal nerve. The patient showed a favorable early but temporary response to carbamazepine treatment, prompting the neurologist to refer her for percutaneous surgery. However, a vascular structure was identified in proximity to the right trigeminal root in T2-weighted and T1-weighted axial MRI slices following gadolinium administration (Fig. 21.30a, b), leading to a proposed and accepted MVD by the patient. The patient underwent surgery via a retrosigmoid approach, allowing for the exposure of the trigeminal nerve root. The superior petrosal vein, connected to the superior petrosal sinus, was positioned away from the nerve root, whereas prominent arachnoid bundles were observed cranially to the root, encompassing the superior cerebellar artery (Fig. 21.30c). The arachnoid was excised, revealing the artery and its branches, along with evident compression of the trigeminal root by the inferior branch of the superior cerebellar artery (Fig. 21.30d). During the subsequent dissection and mobilization of the artery, a vein was revealed that traverses to Meckel's cave, which is situated between the nerve and the artery (Fig. 21.30e). The last vein was coagulated and severed, and several rolls of Teflon were used to sustain the arterial decompression (Fig. 21.30f). The microneurosurgical procedure and the outcome were unremarkable, resulting in immediate alleviation of pain without any sensory or motor deficits.

Comments This case exemplifies primary trigeminal neuralgia resulting from vascular compression, demonstrating a strong connection between MRI imaging and intraoperative observations.

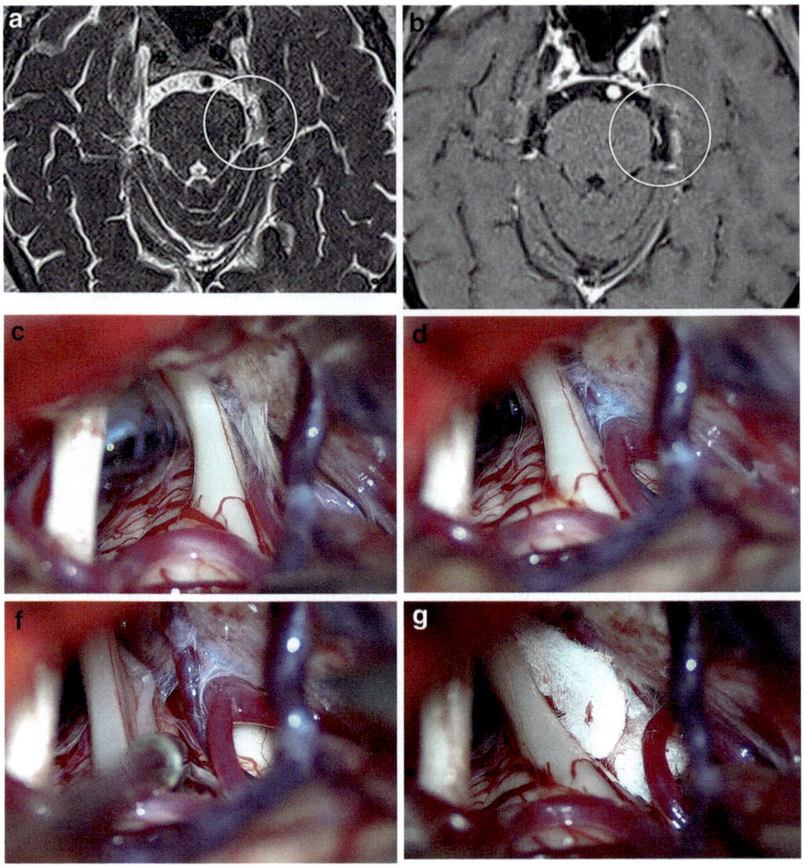

Fig. 21.30 Case 30. Classical trigeminal neuralgia due to arterial compression. (a) Axial image of an MRI T2-weighted sequence showing a loop vessel in the lateral pontine cistern. (**b**) Axial image of an MRI T1-TOF-weighted sequence. (**c**) Intraoperative image of retrosigmoid approach showing a general overview of the trigeminal nerve (center), with the facial-vestibulocochlear nerve complex (left) and arachnoid, tentorium, and petrosal vein complex (right). (**d**) Intraoperative image showing the superior petrosal vein, the superior cerebellar artery, and the trigeminal nerve (right to left). (**e**) Intraoperative image showing the dissection of the superior cerebellar artery. (**f**) Insertion of a roll of Teflon between the trigeminal nerve and the artery

GPSR Compliance

The European Union's (EU) General Product Safety Regulation (GPSR) is a set of rules that requires consumer products to be safe and our obligations to ensure this.

If you have any concerns about our products, you can contact us on ProductSafety@springernature.com

In case Publisher is established outside the EU, the EU authorized representative is:

Springer Nature Customer Service Center GmbH
Europaplatz 3
69115 Heidelberg, Germany

Batch number: 09091980

Printed by Printforce, the Netherlands